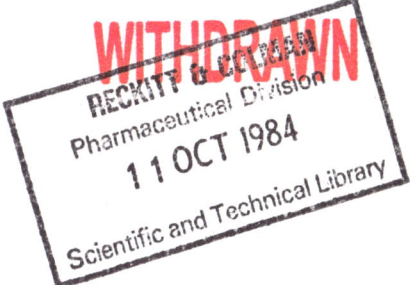

ADVANCES IN NEUROLOGY
Volume 33

Advances in Neurology

INTERNATIONAL ADVISORY BOARD

Advances in Neurology
Volume 33

Headache: Physiopathological and Clinical Concepts

Editors

Macdonald Critchley, M.D.,
F.R.C.P.

Private Consulting Room
The National Hospital
London, England

Arnold P. Friedman, M.D.,
F.A.C.P.

Neurological Associates of Tucson
Tucson, Arizona

Sergio Gorini, M.D.

Menarini International Foundation
Milan, Italy

Federigo Sicuteri, M.D.

Department of Clinical Pharmacology
Headache Center
University of Florence
Florence, Italy

Raven Press ▪ New York

Raven Press, 1140 Avenue of the Americas, New York, New York 10036

Made in the United States of America

Great care has been taken to maintain the accuracy of the information contained in this volume. However, Raven Press cannot be held responsible for errors or for any consequences arising from the use of the information contained herein.

Materials appearing in this book prepared by individuals as part of their official duties as U.S. Government employees are not covered by the above-mentioned copyright.

Library of Congress Cataloging in Publication Data
Main entry under title:

Headache, physiopathological and clinical concepts.

(Advances in neurology ; v. 33)
Papers of an international conference held in
Florence in 1980.
Includes bibliographical references and index.
1. Migraine—Congresses.   2. Headache—Psychosomatic
aspects—Congresses.   I. Critchley, Macdonald.
II. Series.   [DNLM: 1. Headache—Congresses.   2. Mi-
graine—Congresses.   W1 AD684H v.33 / WL 342 H432 1980]
RC321.A276 vol. 33   [RC392]   616.8s   80–5537
ISBN 0–89004–636–0   [616.8'49]

Advances in Neurology Series

Preface

As if in protest against the years of neglect, the subject of migraine has at long last attracted its share of attention. Today increasing numbers of physicians and clinics with an expressed interest in migraine and other varieties of headache are part of the medical community. The powerful cohorts of neurophysiology, biochemistry, pharmacology, and the pharmaceutical industry have stumbled upon considerable and lush pastures in which to graze. Their scrutiny has flipped from one promising clue to another, and no doubt the quest will go on, for the answer is obviously not yet in sight. It is a small wonder that the problem of head pain, one of the most common afflictions of mankind, should be the topic for one symposium after another throughout the world.

Italian physicians and scientists have been particularly prominent over the past 15 years among the advanced thinkers and workers in this field. They have always shown themselves to be stimulating colleagues and generous hosts.

One of the latest of these occasions, memorable in more ways than one, was the Internation Conference in Florence in 1980. Naturally there was an enthusiastic attendance from all parts of Italy, but delegates from the Americas, Australia, Great Britain, and other European countries eagerly participated. The publication of this symposium on headache contains 54 chapters by 113 contributors from 19 countries.

The communications all have contemporary interest and should stimulate further investigations and observations in the field of headache. Areas of overlap are inevitable, but it was thought desirable to permit various contributors to express their own viewpoints. It is hoped that this volume will provide the neuroscientists and clinicians with the current clinical initiatives and direction of research being pursued in the field of headache.

Macdonald Critchley, M.D., F.R.C.P.
Arnold P. Friedman, M.D., F.A.C.P.
Sergio Gorini, M.D.
Federigo Sicuteri, M.D.

Contents

Interrelationships Between Headache and Other Functions

Platelet Aggregation

Contributors

Charles S. Adler
Denver, Colorado 80220

W. H. Aellig
Experimental Therapeutics Department
Clinical Research Division
Sandoz Ltd.
Basle, Switzerland

A. Agnoli
Istituto di Neurologia
67100 L'Aquila, Italy

G. Amat
Centre de la Migraine
03200 Vichy, France

J. A. L. Amess
Department of Haematology
St. Bartholomew's Hospital
London, England

B. Anselmi
Clinical Pharmacology and Nuclear
*   Medicine Center*
50134 Florence, Italy

Michael Anthony
Division of Neurology
The Prince Henry Hospital
Sydney, Australia

E. Baldi
Department of Clinical Pharmacology
University of Florence
Florence, Italy

G. S. Barolin
Landes Nervenkrankenhaus Valduna
Neurologische Abteilung
6830 Rankweil, Austria

A. Bartolini
Istituto Interfacolta Di Farmacologia
50134 Florence, Italy

R. Bartolini
Department of Pharmacology
University of Florence
Florence, Italy

P. O. Behan
Institute of Neurological Sciences
Southern General Hospital
Glasgow, Scotland

Maria Boccuni
Department of Clinical Pharmacology
Headache Center
University of Florence
Florence, Italy

Francis Boismare
Department of Pharmacology
Hôtel-Dieu
Rouen, France

Mara Bonciani
Department of Clinical Pharmacology
University of Florence
Florence, Italy

G. Bono
Department of Neurology
Headache Center
University of Pavia
School of Medicine
Pavia, Italy

Jacques Boquet
Department of Pharmacology
Hôtel-Dieu
Rouen, France

R. Botolini
Department of Pharmacology
University of Florence
Florence, Italy

G. Broggi
Institute of Neurosurgery
University of Turin
Turin, Italy

G. W. Bruyn
Department of Neurology
Academic Hospital
State University
Leyden, The Netherlands

G. A. Buscaino
Clinica Malattie Nervose E Mentali
I Facota Di Medicina
80131 Naples, Italy

G. Cappelli
Department of Nuclear Medicine
University of Florence
50134 Florence, Italy

A. Carenzi
Laboratori Ricerche Zambon Farmaceutici
Milan, Italy

J. D. Carrol
Royal Surrey County Hospital
Guildford Surrey
GU2 5LX, England

F. Casacci
Zambon S.p.A. Research Laboratories
Bresso-Milan, Italy

E. Ceci
Department of Neurology
University of L'Aquila
L'Aquila, Italy

V. Centonze
Instituto de Semeiotica
Universita di Bari
Bari, Italy

T. C. Chen
National Institute of Neurological and Commu-
nicative Disorders and Stroke
National Institutes of Health
Bethesda, Maryland

Carlo Conti
Department of Clinical Pharmacology
Sexuality Section
University of Florence
Florence, Italy

A. Coppen
MRC Neuropsychiatry Laboratory
West Park Hospital
Epsom, Surrey, England

M. Criscuoli
Istituto Farmachimico Falorni
Florence, Italy

M. Da Prada
Pharmaceutical Research Department
F. Hoffmann-La Roche & Co.
CH 4002 Basel, Switzerland

Živan Deanović
Department of Experimental Biology and
Medicine
Institute Rudjer Bošković
Zagreb, Rebro, Yugoslavia

Pietro D'Egidio
Department of Clinical Pharmacology
Headache Center
University of Florence
Florence, Italy

Enrico Del Bene
Department of Clinical Pharmacology
Headache Center
University of Florence
Florence, Italy

P. L. Del Bianco
Headache Center
Department of Pharmacology
50134 Florence, Italy

D. Della Bella
Zambon S.p.A. Research Laboratories
Bresso-Milan, Italy

A. Denaro
Department of Neurology
University of L'Aquila
L'Aquila, Italy

Seymour Diamond
Diamond Headache Clinic
Chicago, Illinois 60625

Milivoj Dupelj
Department of Neurology
University Hospital
Zagreb, Rebro, Yugoslavia

Jens H. Eickhoff
Laboratory of Surgical Circulation Research
Department D
Rigshospitalet
Copenhagen, Denmark

P. Falaschi
V Medical Clinic
University of Rome
Rome, Italy

A. Fanchamps
Medical Counsel
Pharmaceutical Division
Sandoz Ltd.
Basel, Switzerland

Marcello Fanciullacci
Department of Clinical Pharmacology
Headache Center
University of Florence
Florence, Italy

V. A. Fasano
Institute of Neurosurgery
University of Turin
Turin, Italy

A. M. Forsythe
Department of Haematology
St. Bartholomew's Hospital
London, England

J. R. Fozard
Centre de Recherche
Merrell International
67074 Strasbourg, France

G. Franchi
Department of Clinical Pharmacology
University of Florence
Florence, Italy

Arnold P. Friedman
Neurological Associates of Tucson
Tuscon, Arizona 85712

M. J. Gawel
Department of Neurology
Charing Cross Hospital
London, England

G. L. Gessa
Istituto Di Farmacologia
Universita Degli Studi
09100 Cagliari, Italy

A. Giotti
Department of Pharmacology
University of Florence
Florence, Italy

M. Goldstein
Department of Health Education and Public
* Health*
National Institutes of Health
Bethesda, Maryland

S. Gori-Savellini
Department of Experimental Psychology
University of Florence
Florence, Italy

John R. Graham
The Headache Research Foundation
The Faulkner Hospital
Jamaica Plains, Massachusetts 02130

Henry J. Haigler
Department of Pharmacology
Emory University School of Medicine
Atlanta, Georgia 30322

Edda Hanington
Princess Margaret Migraine Clinic
Charing Cross Hospital
London, England

Albert Herz
Max Planck Institut für Psychiatrie
Department of Neuropharmacology
Munchen 40, West Germany

R. Horowski
Research Laboratories of Schering AG
Berlin (West) and Bergkamen
Federal Republic of Germany

Y. Hosobuchi
Neurological Surgery
University of California Hospital
San Francisco, California 94123

Brunon L. Imielinsky
Garyounis University
Benghazi, Libya

J. Jacob
Institut Pasteur
Paris, France

P. Jean Louis
Service de Cardiologie
Hôpital Croix Rousse
69317 Lyon, France

R. J. Jones
Department of Haematology
St. Bartholomew's Hospital
London, England

Lee Kudrow
California Medical Clinic for Headache
Encino, California 91436

James W. Lance
School of Medicine
University of New South Wales
Sydney, Australia

L. Lisci
Department of Clinical Pharmacology
* Headache Center*
University of Florence
Florence, Italy

C. Loisy
Centre de la Migraine
03200 Vichy, France

G. Lo Russo
Institute of Neurosurgery
University of Turin
Turin, Italy

P. Malmberg
Department of Pharmacology
University of Florence
Florence, Italy

L. Marianelli
Department of Pediatrics
University of Florence
Florence, Italy

M. Marini
Department of Clinical Pharmacology
Headache Center
University of Florence
Florence, Italy

E. Martignoni
Neurological Clinic
University of Pavia
Pavia, Italy

M. Martorana
Department of Experimental Psychology
University of Florence
Florence, Italy

P. Masturzo
Institute of Internal Medicine
University of Genoa
Genoa, Italy

Jose L. Medina
Diamond Headache Clinic
Chicago, Illinois

H. Merskey
University of Western Ontario
London Psychiatric Hospital
London, Ontario
N6A 4H1, Canada

S. Michelacci
Department of Clinical Pharmacology
University of Florence
Florence, Italy

Harvey Moldofsky
Department of Psychiatry
Toronto Western Hospital
Toronto, Canada

Nicholas Moore
Department of Pharmacology
Hôtel-Dieu
Rouen, France

Sheila Morrissey-Adler
Denver, Colorado 80220

Dorotea Mück-Šeler
Rudjer Boskovic Institute
Zagreb, Yugoslavia

E. Müller-Schweinitzer
Preclinical Research
Pharmaceutical Division
Sandoz Ltd.
Basel, Switzerland

G. Murialdo
Institute of Internal Medicine
University of Genoa
Genoa, Italy

G. Nappi
Istituto Di Neurologia
Centro Cefalee
Universita Degli Studi
27100 Pavia, Italy

Giovanni Nattero
Headache Center
Institute of Internal Medicine
10126 Torino, Italy

Jes Olesen
Department of Neurology
Department D
Rigshospitalet
Copenhagen, Denmark

S. Pelage
Centre de la Migraine
03200 Vichy, France

Agu Pert
Section on Biochemistry and Pharmacology
Biological Psychiatry Branch
National Institutes of Mental Health
Bethesda, Maryland 20205

Umberto Pietrini
Department of Clinical Pharmacology
Headache Center
University of Florence
Florence, Italy

Marco Poggioni
Department of Clinical Pharmacology
Headache Center
University of Florence
Florence, Italy

A. Polleri
Scientific Institute of Internal Medicine
University of Genoa
16100 Genoa, Italy

Edgard Raffaelli
Director Brazilian Headache Society
Sao Paulo, Brazil

N. H. Raskin
Department of Neurology
School of Medicine
San Francisco, California

F. Clifford Rose
Department of Neurology
Charing Cross Hospital
London, England

Robert E. Ryan, Jr.
St. Louis University School of Medicine
St. Louis, Missouri

Robert E. Ryan, Sr.
St. Louis University School of Medicine
St. Louis, Missouri

S. Salmon
Department of Clinical Pharmacology
Headache Center
University of Florence
Florence, Italy

F. Savoldi
Department of Neurology
Headache Center
University of Pavia
School of Medicine
Pavia, Italy

Pramod R. Saxena
Department of Pharmacology
Faculty of Medicine
Erasmus University
Rotterdam, The Netherlands

Rüdiger Schulz
Department of Neuropharmacology
Max Planck Instutut für Psychiatry
München, Federal Republic of Germany

Federigo Sicuteri
Department of Clinical Pharmacology
Headache Center
University of Florence
Florence, Italy

Bengt H. Sjolund
Department of Physiology and Neurosurgery
University of Lund
S-223 62 Lund, Sweden

Egilius L. H. Spierings
Department of Pharmacology
Faculty of Medicine
Erasmus University
Rotterdam, The Netherlands

C. C. Swade
MRC Neuropsychiatry Laboratory
West Park Hospital
Epsom, Surrey, England

Lars Terenius
Department of Pharmacology
University of Uppsala
751 23 Uppsala, Sweden

E. Testa
Institute of Internal Medicine
University of Genoa
Genoa, Italy

Peer Tfelt-Hansen
Department of Neurology and Laboratory of Surgical Circulation Research
Rigshospitalet
Copenhagen, Denmark

D. V. Thomas
Department of Pharmacology
Institute of Psychology
London, England

Julian E. Villareal
Instituto Miles De Terapeutica Experimental
Mexico D.F., Mexico

Barbara Wachowicz
Department of Biochemistry
Institute of Biochemistry and Biophysics
University of Lodz
Lodz, Poland

K. M. A. Welch
Department of Neurology
Baylor College of Medicine
Houston, Texas 77030

K. M. Wood
MRC Neuropsychiatry Laboratory
West Park Hospital
Epsom, Surrey, England

S. Zeme
Institute of Neurosurgery
University of Turin
Turin, Italy

Advances in Neurology, Vol. 33, edited by
M. Critchley et al. Raven Press, New York © 1982

Overview of Migraine

Arnold P. Friedman

Neurological Associates of Tucson, Tucson, Arizona 85712

Among all the symptoms for which the physician is consulted, head pain in one form or another is perhaps the most common. The clinical significance of headache is meaningful to the physician only if he understands the anatomical, physiological, and psychological factors that give rise to pain.

The most common and perhaps most baffling type of headache, migraine, acquired recognition as a symptom complex when described by Aretaeus of Capadocia toward the end of the first century A.D. (5). Even today, the definitions of migraine are far from uniform. For example, the term is used by many physicians to include only classic migraine, which comprises only about 10% of all migraine headaches. Others include tension headache and chronic vascular headaches as part of the migraine spectrum.

There is considerable evidence that heredity plays a part in the origin of migraine (17,23,37); apart from this factor, however, there is a lack of agreement as to the cause of migraine. The various theories proposed include pscyhological disturbances, allergy, endocrine disturbances, metabolic factors, endogenous or exogenous toxins, epilepsy, ocular dysfunction, and even disturbance of the cervical spine. These various hypotheses are supported by inconclusive evidence; none satisfactorily explains the fundamental cause of migraine.

Migraine may begin any time from early childhood to late in life, but the onset frequently occurs after puberty or in late adolescence. It is reported more frequently in females than in males. Motion sickness or attacks of cyclic vomiting may be precursors of migraine. In women, there is a frequent relationship between attacks of migraine and the menstrual period. The natural history of migraine is one of remissions and exacerbations for years, and migraine can recur after decades of quiescence in both sexes.

From a clinical standpoint, the classification of migraine provided by the Research Group on Headache and Migraine of the World Federation of Neurologists provides a practical outline for discussions of the subject (12). Migraine headache is defined as a familial disorder characterized by periodic recurrent headache widely variable in intensity, frequency, and duration. Attacks are commonly unilateral in onset, often associated with anorexia, nausea, and vomiting. They may be preceded by or associated with neurological and mood disturbances. The headache is modified by vasoconstrictors. These characteristics are not necessarily present in each attack or in each patient. Within the above definition are included the classic and common migraine and complicated migraine, or migraine accompagnée, which includes ophthalmoplegic, hemiplegic, vertebrobasilar, and dysphrenic migraine.

Varying therapeutic methods have been reported to be successful in the treatment of the migraine patient. This can be partially explained by the lack of uniformity in the definition of the term migraine, its natural history, and the importance of the physician-patient relationship. Not fully explained, however, are the reported successes with such diverse therapeutic measures as psychotherapy, both supportive and analytic, hypnotherapy, biofeedback, transcendental meditation, yoga, physical therapy, cervical traction, a variety of surgical procedures, pharmacological agents by the dozens, dietary restriction, and antiallergic therapy.

Over 35 years ago, my colleagues, the late Houston Merritt and Charles Brenner, and I suggested that a single causative agent or a constant disordered mechanism for migraine is unlikely (10). Furthermore, the large number of precipitating factors suggests a diversity of disordered functions and that migraine is more than a pain in the head but represents a total disturbance of bodily functions, both physiologic and biochemical. It was also emphasized that the supposition of having one specific drug or therapeutic technique for effective treatment of migraine is unlikely and oversimplifies this complicated problem. There is still no firm evidence that would change these suppositions.

PSYCHOLOGICAL ASPECTS OF MIGRAINE

Most studies on psychological factors in migraine have been on selected groups of patients who were attending a migraine clinic or who were deemed suitable by the family physician for psychiatric treatment. These patients may have a higher incidence of such personality traits as anxiety, obsession, overconscientiousness, and overconcern about health than do those who do not seek special aid for migraine (35,46,66); hence a bias exists in the skewed sample. There are no adequate published studies on migraine patients with control groups of similar age, sex, and social and economic backgrounds. Rees (54) has found the same traits common in patients with asthma, vasomotor rhinitis, thyrotoxicosis, and chronic urticaria. Furthermore, many patients with analogous emotional problems are not troubled with migraine.

In a study in 1949 of our migraine patients, we (9) reported that they had suppressed or unconscious strong feelings of resentment or anger, as well as a variety of other psychological patterns, including hysterical identification or conversion, interjection of hostility with subsequent depressions, or a process for identification with other members of the family. Later observations (21) substantiated our earlier findings and again pointed to the fact that no one personality type is characteristic of all migraine patients. The view that a special personality predisposes to migraine remains unproved. It was indicated that there must be an awareness of oversimplification and overgeneralization in categorizing the chronic headache patient. Furthermore, the same analytical, historical, and other material has been found in patients who do not have migraine or any psychophysiologic autonomic disorder. It is difficult to make a diagnosis of a psychosomatic disorder from a specific personality profile. We, as well as others, have observed migraine and ulcer symptoms concomitantly or attacks of asthma and neurodermatitis and migraine concomitantly.

There is no doubt that anxious and obsessive patients are often found with migraine, and most have not successfully learned to handle aggressive energy, either their own or that of others. During their earlier years, these patients were conditioned to value the approval of others more than their own. In addition, patients with migraine are generally exacting in requirements of themselves and of others and often become immersed in a morass of detail (6). Such behavior is bound to be frustrating because it cannot be maintained with consistency. Migraine patients have been conditioned to use their wits to the exclusion of feelings, with intellect assuming undue importance. The choice of the head as a focus of pain is perhaps a natural outcome. Many patients without migraine, however, demonstrate the same personality profile; all migraine patients do not fit into the same psychological mold.

Patients with migraine show transitory and prolonged depressions with withdrawn social behavior, irritability, and hostility. These occur not only during periods with headache but between attacks. In some patients, migraine and depression are an interchangeable pattern. Depression has some of the same dynamics as migraine and decreases the pain threshold; thus pain may be made more intense. Beneath depression may be many factors, including rage, recent loss, sense of failure, loss of respect or love, concealed secret, or a sexual problem with complications. Expressing emotions by means of a headache (a hurt, ache, or pain) may be a better solution than depression. The observation that patients with lifelong histories of migraine may suffer severe headaches late in life associated with a clinically identifiable depression indicates that if these patients are to be successfully treated, attention must be concentrated on the depression rather than on the headache.

The migraine patient has been depicted in the literature as having superior intelligence and being an overachiever, although Waters (65) showed in an epidemiologic study that there was no difference between migraine sufferers and the rest of the population. Our observations indicate that the migraine patient is usually intelligent but drives himself to achieve his goals.

A vivid description of the psychologic effect of a migraine headache on the sufferer and his family is provided by John Steinbeck in the person of Mrs. Pritchard in his novel *The Wayward Bus* (64). Her husband

> knew her headaches, and they were dreadful. They twisted her face and reduced her to a panting, sweating, grinning, quivering blob of pain. They filled a room and a house. They got into everyone around her. Mr. Pritchard could feel one of her headaches through walls. . . . The headaches usually came when she was nervous and when things, through no fault of her own, were not going well.

Steinbeck also touched on the extra cross that the migraine victim often bears, the accusation of malingering, here by Mrs. Pritchard's unfeeling daughter, who dismissed the pain as merely "psychosomatic." It was not so:

> They seemed to be selfish, these headaches, and yet they were not. The pain was real. No one could simulate such agonizing pain. Mr. Pritchard dreaded them more than anything in the world. A good one could make the whole house vibrate with horror.

PATHOGENESIS

The pain of migraine was long suspected to be of vascular origin. The temporal artery and its branches on the side of the headache were often seen to be conspicuously swollen and throbbing. However, it is only within contemporary experience that the experimental method was first used to give some understanding of the mechanisms of migraine headache. The prodromes of classic migraine, especially the visual and other sensory and motor phenomena, are indications of a central nervous system origin.

A possible sequence of events has been suggested by direct measurements of cerebral blood flow (49,52,62). First, there is a phase of vasoconstriction involving the intracranial arteries, with a reduction of blood flow of sufficient degree to produce the initial symptoms.

This is followed by the ischemic changes associated with the prodrome of the attack, and then a second phase of vasodilatation, primarily of the extracranial arteries, during which the headache occurs. The distribution of these vascular changes does not correlate well with the clinical features of the episode of migraine.

The two phases are not always sharply separated. For example, some cortical areas show vasodilatation at a stage when vessels in other areas are still constricted (20). This would account for those cases of migraine in which the usual temporal profile of an aura followed by a headache is disturbed, and symptoms of the aura continue into the headache phase. Furthermore, the reduction in cerebral blood flow may outlast the relatively brief aura time span. Similarly, the distribution of increased cerebral blood flow may not correlate well with the locale of the headache. Frequently, the intracranial vasodilatation may be hemispheric, while the headache is sharply localized to, for example, the frontal or temporal region. A recent study (57) of cerebral vasomotor responsiveness to 5% CO_2 in migraine patients indicated that during the headache phase of migraine, the cerebral hemisphere on the side of the headache showed significantly greater CO_2 response than the nonheadache hemisphere. During the prodrome of migraine, there was bilateral impairment of hemispheric CO_2 responsiveness.

Although observations make it clear that the scalp arteries dilate during a migraine headache, most patients turn pale and feel cold, despite their bounding temporal pulse. One explanation is that there is an imbalance between the caliber of large and small vessels. Heyck (42) presented evidence that transiently opening arteriovenous shunts occur with arterialization of the venous blood, and that the hemodynamic reductions in migraine are comparable to those encountered in an arteriovenous malformation. Permanent anatomically defined shunts exist in arteriovenous malformations, however; in migraine, there are no shunts during the attack-free interval. It must also be understood that vasodilatation itself is not usually uncomfortable; exertion, heat, and anoxia all produce vasodilatation.

This suggests that other factors, i.e., mediators of inflammation or vasoactive materials, are important to vascular permeability and are elaborated about the painful dilated arteries that characterize migraine. Studies carried out with patients suggest that the dilated migrainous arteries are hyperpermeable and are involved in a sterile local inflammatory reaction in which vasoactive substances and platelets participate (16). The vascular permeability may be influenced by the release of vasoactive substances from their reservoirs in the circulation or tissue sites. Present evidence implicates at least five and possibly more groups of vasoactive substances associated with arterial inflammation and increased permeability. Among the substances that have been suggested as being involved are the amines (serotonin, catecholamines, epinephrine or norepinephrine, histamine, tyramine, phenylethylamine) (3,4,40,44,58); the polypeptides (bradykinin and angiotensin) (61), and the free fatty acids, including prostaglandins (2,43). The question arises in all investigations as to whether we are studying the effects or the cause of migraine.

Platelets contain all the serotonin present in the blood and release it during aggregation. The observed changes in plasma serotonin levels in migraine (18) may be secondary to changes in platelet aggregation. It has been hypothesized that serotonin released from platelets in migraine first causes a vasoconstriction and is then adsorbed to the vessel wall, combining with histamine and kinins to increase the sensitivity to pain of the affected arteries (47). Second, the drop in plasma levels after adsorption and metabolism of the released serotonin diminishes the tonic constrictor effect that would normally tend to counteract that of any dilator substance, such as histamine, bradykinin, and

PGE_1 (2). The factor responsible for releasing serotonin is unknown, but free fatty acids, which have this potential, are known to be increased in the plasma during migraine. Levels of prostaglandins in the plasma of migraine patients show no changes, although intravenous infusion of PGE_1, a dilator, into normal subjects may produce a headache indistinguishable from migraine but without the aura.

The possible role of immune complexes must also be considered. Immunoglobulin gamma G, but not A, E, or M, can aggregate human platelets and cause a release of serotonin (41). A recent study by Moore et al. (51), however, showed no evidence of lowered complement levels, elevated immunoglobulin levels, or increased levels of immune complexes in patients with prodromal or nonprodromal migraine.

Irrespective of the role of metabolic, humoral, or immunological changes in the genesis of migraine, some explanation must be found for the asymmetry of the process. Headache and focal neurological symptoms usually implicate one side more than the other. The reason for selective involvement of parts of the vascular tree in migraine remains unknown.

CLINICAL FEATURES

The diagnosis of migraine is established by the patient's history. Migraine is characterized by its variability of symptoms and its periodicity. It may reappear after decades of quiescence in both females and males. The outstanding feature of the migraine syndrome is headache, but that is only a part of a widespread bodily disturbance.

The same individual may have classic migraine at one time and at other times may have a headache that may have some features of common migraine; or the headache may be difficult to classify. It is rare for a patient with migraine not to have muscle-contraction headaches at other periods in life.

Metabolic disturbances associated with migraine are electrolyte disturbances with retention of sodium and fluid before and during headache (63), sensitivity to insulin, with blood glucose levels significantly below those of control subjects during a 2-hr insulin hypoglycemic test (53), and an increase of free fatty acids in the blood of fasting patients with migraine greater than in those who do not (2). A high incidence of essential hypertension, increased incidence of toxemia of pregnancy (55), and abnormal blood clotting have been observed. How these events are directly related to the migraine process has not been established.

The issue remains clouded as to the exact role of foods in migraine headache. Some individuals are vulnerable to certain food substances and dietary modifications; for these, the elimination of certain food or drugs may prove beneficial. It is valuable to question all patients for possible links between headache and food or drug ingestion.

Migraine tends to be worsened in women at times of hormonal changes, such as menstruation, ovulation, menopause, and use of contraceptive drugs. It bears repetition that oral contraceptives and estrogen therapy worsen migraine in a large number of patients. Withdrawal of oral contraceptives may result in marked improvement of migraine in approximately 70% of the individuals taking them.

CLINICAL TYPES OF MIGRAINE

Migraine attacks can occur in a variety of patterns and profiles which can be classified into the following types (29).

Classic Migraine

Classic migraine occurs in approximately 10% of patients with migraine. The prodromes are sharply defined, contralateral, neurologic manifestations, usually of a visual nature; in some patients, the effects are sensory or motor, or a combination of these. The pain is unilateral and pulsatile, and anorexia, nausea, and vomiting are concomitant features.

Common Migraine

The prodromes of common migraine, the most common type encountered, are not sharply defined and may precede the attack by several hours or days. These include psychic disturbances, gastrointestinal manifestations, and changes in fluid balance. The actual headache is frequently longer than in the classic types; it may last from many hours to days and may be bilateral. Symptoms common to both types of migraine include local or generalized edema, irritability, pallor, dizziness, and sweating.

Cluster Headache

Cluster headache, known as migrainous neuralgia in Britain, may be defined as a unilateral head or facial pain of high intensity that rarely lasts longer than 2 hr and usually less. It is commonly associated with ipsilateral injection of the conjunctiva, lacrimation, and congestion of the nostril. It characteristically occurs in clusters of one or more daily bouts for a period of weeks or months separated by long intervals of complete freedom. An ipsilateral Horner syndrome occurs in about 20% of the affected patients. It has been reported that facial thermography revealed multiple spotted areas of dense coolness in one supraorbital region, always ipsilateral to the pain, in two-thirds of the patients studied (31). This thermographic finding was not found in other types of vascular headache.

Complicated Migraine

Although uncommon, the importance of complicated migraine is obvious because the neurological symptoms that distinguish it may be of any type or function (11). Such a disorder can be misdiagnosed as being caused by other intracranial pathology, and careful work-up of these patients is indicated. The recent introduction of computerized axial tomography should make the differential diagnosis less difficult (32,48). There is usually a family history of migraine in these patients and a history of migraine attacks earlier in life.

Ocular Complications

The hemianopic scintillating scotomata present in classic migraine may also occur without headache, in which case they can mimic the ischemic attacks caused by transient insufficiency of cerebral blood flow. Visual prodromes may be accompanied by electroencephalographic changes consisting of slowing of the rhythm in the affected occipital lobe. The usual attacks of transitory blindness due to ischemia (amaurosis fugax) are shorter in duration (seconds to 3 to 5 min) and, while usually monocular, are rarely hemianopic and are not accompanied by a hemianopic fortification spectrum (13).

The monocular visual loss in migraine may be total or partial. Occasionally, photopsias consisting of showers or stationary flecks of light that disappear quickly may occur, as may other types of scotomata. Patients with migraine may also have internal carotid artery disease with severe stenosis, and early recognition of the cause of these visual phenomena is important to avoid a possible catastrophe. Intraoptic disorders (visual phenomena or retinal disorders) and the episodic blindness of giant-cell arteritis are other considerations in the differential diagnosis.

Permanent field defects may result from damage to either the retina or the visual cortex in migraine patients exhibiting homonymous hemianoptic defects. The cause of the damage is not certain, but there is little doubt that infarction is the most likely end result. The absence of a cranial bruit and of epilepsy and subarachnoid hemorrhage makes an angioma extremely unlikely.

Ophthalmoplegic Migraine

The pain in ophthalmoplegic migraine, a rare type of migraine that may occur in the young adult, is moderate and on the same side as the ophthalmoplegia (33). It is accompanied by extraocular muscle palsies, usually involving the third cranial nerve (internal as well as external ophthalmoplegia). The other oculomotor nerves are rarely involved. There is pupillary dilatation and external strabismus with diplopia due to paralysis of the third cranial nerve. Often the paralysis occurs as the headache subsides, 3 to 5 days after the onset.

Repeated ophthalmoplegic attacks may cause permanent injury to the third cranial nerve, possibly from compression by swelling and edema of the posterior cerebral and superior arteries during the stage of vasodilatation. One should be alert for the presence in some of these patients of an intracranial aneurysm on the main trunk of the internal carotid or at the junction between the carotid and the posterior communicating artery or of a sphenoidal mucocele. Periarteritis of the carotid siphon (Tolosa and Hunt syndrome) also stimulates ophthalmoplegic migraine. It is characterized by a steady, gnawing, retrobulbar pain preceding or following paralysis of the oculomotor nerves. The course is variable; attacks may last for days or weeks, with or without visual deficit.

Hemiplegic Migraine

The syndrome of hemiplegic migraine includes both motor and sensory symptoms occurring in a unilateral distribution as part of a migraine attack (36,45). Transient hemiparesis or unilateral tingling and numbness may occur occasionally in the patient prone to frequent attacks of uncomplicated migraine. Usually, these focal symptoms are brief, lasting 10 to 60 min. Particularly characteristic of hemiplegic migraine is the complaint of pins and needles around both sides of the lip and tongue. The usually incomplete paralysis is succeeded by headache, nausea, and malaise, which testify to the migrainous nature of the attack. It is the brevity of the symptoms in a young person already known to suffer from uncomplicated migraine that permits the correct diagnosis to be made. In patients with recurrent attacks of hemiplegic migraine, the history may extend back for many years. About half of the patients with hemiplegic migraine have a family history of uncomplicated migraine and 20% of familial hemiplegic migraine.

The completeness of recovery after several days or weeks of spastic paralysis, a feature of migrainous hemiplegia, is most unusual in occlusive cerebrovascular disease due to atheromatous thromboembolism. Oral contraceptive agents have been reported to cause exacerbation of hemiplegic migraine in women (8).

Familial Hemiplegic Migraine

The symptomatology of familial hemiplegic migraine closely replicates that observed in hemiplegic migraine, but the weakness always recurs on the same side and outlasts the headache, lasting for hours and days. In some patients, it is accompanied by impairment of consciousness. Within the patient's family, the hemiplegic migraine also occurs on the same side. In contrast, the paralysis in ordinary hemiplegic migraine may be on either side, and relatives may have uncomplicated migraine or occasional hemiplegic episodes but not necessarily of the same variety.

Basilar-Artery Migraine

Bickerstaff (1) was the first to describe basilar-artery migraine as yet another variant of migraine types. The preheadache phase reflects circulatory disturbances of the basilar artery in the brainstem and thalamic, occipital, and cerebellar regions, all of which are fed by branches of the vertebrobasilar arterial system. The prodromal period may include visual loss and brainstem symptoms, ranging from paresthesias to vertigo, ataxia, and dysarthria. Ophthalmoplegic, sensory, autonomic, and bilateral visual disturbances can occur. Severe throbbing occipital pain and vomiting follow. Transitory loss of consciousness may occur with the attacks. This type of migraine occurs in young women, often associated with menstruation.

DIFFERENTIAL DIAGNOSIS

The diagnosis of migraine presents no problem if the clinical history fits the description of classic or common migraine. Difficulty arises if the patient presents with conditions that fall within the category of complicated migraine or with one of the various progressive neurologic syndromes that may be associated with head pain.

The neurologic part of the migraine syndrome may simulate the clinical picture of a vascular malformation, such as an angioma or an aneurysm, vascular disease, such as embolic or thrombotic stroke with cerebral ischemic attacks, tumor of the occipital lobe, and focal epilepsy. Other conditions that may have to be considered in the differential diagnosis of migraine include temporal arteritis, glaucoma, and pheochromocytoma.

There is no well-documented evidence that angioma or aneurysm is related to the presence or absence of migraine (28). It is coincidental if these two conditions are associated with migraine. The temporal profile of any given attack due to an angioma or an aneurysm usually reveals a very acute onset and, if bleeding occurs, a very intense headache. Aneurysm of the posterior communicating or internal carotid artery may cause a unilateral headache that occurs in the orbital or frontal region on the same side of the head as the aneurysm. Persistent defects in the visual field and sudden or increasing paralysis of the third or other extraocular cranial nerves suggest dilatation of an aneurysm.

The occurrence of head pain in patients with unruptured angioma is infrequent; they more commonly present with convulsive seizures. Neurologic disturbances, such as hemiplegia, hemianopia, or aphasia, may occur with or without headache. Auscultation of the skull may reveal a cranial bruit. Should hemorrhage occur, severe headache and stiff neck lasting many days associated with blood in the spinal fluid may be present.

Headache is a feature of large vessel involvement in cerebrovascular disease (50). Lucunar infarction of small vessels is not associated with headache. Basilar and carotid artery insufficiency may cause headache accompanied by sensory and motor disturbances. The pain frequently is throbbing and is probably secondary to dilatation of the extracranial arteries, the increased flow thus providing collateral circulation. Headache is present in approximately half of the patients with vertebrobasilar stenosis or occlusion and in about one-third of the patients with internal carotid artery and middle cerebral artery involvement. The headache is restricted to the occipital and nuchal areas or to the bifrontal area if the vertebrobasilar system is involved.

Although the neurologic part of the migraine syndrome may resemble focal seizures, the pacing and timing of the neurologic symptoms and attacks distinguish the condition from epilepsy. The aura of migraine is measured in minutes rather than seconds, and the migraine attack lasts hours rather than minutes and is rarely accompanied by loss of consciousness. A family history of migraine and a lack of the electroencephalographic changes usually seen in focal seizures are other features that differentiate the two diseases.

Headache associated with tumors of the occipital lobe can simulate migraine. If the patient has a history of periodic headache, vomiting, and homonymous visual hallucinations, careful examination of the visual fields is indicated and will usually reveal the presence of a persistent defect, which may increase in severity. Later, signs and symptoms of an intracranial space-occupying lesion will appear.

Temporal arteritis, often characterized by localized head pain, should be considered in the differential diagnosis of migraine. The headache may be unilateral or bitemporal. The intense pain is of a deep, aching quality, throbbing, persistent, with a burning sensation absent in most other vascular headaches. The throbbing usually diminishes or ceases after the early phase. Temporal arteritis usually begins after the age of 60 and affects both sexes equally. It has been suggested that cranial arteritis represents an example of immunologic vasculitis in which immune complexes are deposited within the walls of the blood vessels, producing localized vascular injury and inflammation (25).

During an acute attack, the superficial temporal arteries are tender to touch and cordlike (string sign felt by rolling the artery over a finger), and they may become thrombosed along part of their length. Pain on mastication, which may be the first symptom, is felt by many patients; often the presenting complaint is an ocular disturbance. Because partial or complete loss of vision threatens more than 50% of the patients, early diagnosis and treatment with steroids are essential. Systemic signs and symptoms (fever, malaise, anorexia, myalgia, weakness, anxiety, depression, and central nervous system disturbances) may be part of the syndrome.

The sedimentation rate is almost always elevated, and a mild leukocytosis and hypochromic anemia may occur. Examination by biopsy of the involved arterial segment establishes the diagnosis. A fairly long segment of the vessel should be obtained to avoid inadvertent biopsy of a normal area. Arteriography may demonstrate stenosis of the involved vessel.

Another condition that may have to be considered in the differential diagnosis of migraine in older patients is glaucoma, which may cause extremely severe orbital pain accompanied by nausea and vomiting. The presence of increased intraocular pressure is shown by tonometry.

MANAGEMENT

The present treatment of migraine presents an extreme diversification of therapeutic measures, each claiming some degree of success (52). Few conditions are as unpredictable in response to treatment as migraine; individualized therapy and close follow-up are necessary. An important aspect of the management of the migraine patient is the evaluation of factors that may precipitate an attack. These vary from patient to patient and include correction of psychologic or structural abnormalities and situational demands, reduction of emotional tension, regulation of social and occupational activities, the use of daily routine exercise, and elimination of foods or chemicals that trigger an attack, such as tyramine, nitrites, phenylethylalanine, and monosodium glutamate.

Pharmacotherapy

The array of pharmacologic approaches proposed for migraine is more remarkable for diversity than for therapeutic results. This diversity has been derived from a lack of insight into the disease disturbance, with subsequent reliance on various empirical treatments. The problem with a pragmatic approach lies mostly with the lack of adequate control data that would eliminate improvement due to the fluctuating course of the disease rather than to the treatment.

In prescribing drugs, the physician on occasion may find striking variations in therapeutic response to a given regimen, which can be satisfactory in one patient, ineffective in a second, and toxic in a third. These individual differences can be attributed to many factors, including variations in drug disposition (absorption, distribution, metabolism); an underlying disease process, such as low renal clearance, hepatic disease, and congestive failure; varying bioavailabilities of the drug formulations used; and interaction between drugs. Pharmacokinetic data, such as the relationship between drug dose and blood level and clinical effectiveness, and toxic potentialities have been monitored in only a small number of drugs (26).

The following discussion centers on established and proposed pharmacologic approaches to the treatment of migraine and touches only lightly on specific dosage information for these agents. More detailed information than that given in Tables 1 and 2 can be obtained from *AMA Drug Evaluation* (1). The principal pharmacologic agents that have been suggested for the treatment of migraine and their physiologic effects are summarized in Table 2.

Acute Attack

Treatment of an acute attack of migraine is directed toward preventing the painful dilatation of the cranial vessels that appears to be the source of the headache. Commonly used analgesics or small doses of codeine may be effective in mild attacks if administered early enough. Sedatives with salicylates are of special value in treating a migraine attack in children. Treatment of migraine headache in an emergency room setting is aimed at reducing pain, anxiety, and vomiting.

Of all the agents used and studied, ergotamine tartrate is still the most effective treatment for an acute migraine attack (26). Its beneficial effect is probably related to the restoration of the dilated scalp vessels to a nonpainful, normally constricted state and the pain threshold to normal. In addition to obliterative vascular reactions and gastrointestinal disturbances, prolonged use of ergotamine may lead to dependence with withdrawal symptoms if the drug is stopped. Although rare, the classic signs and symptoms of ergotism may develop if ergotamine is given in large doses, at frequent intervals, or when contraindicated (27).

Caffeine acts synergistically with ergotamine by potentiating the vasoconstrictor effect of the ergot alkaloid. Caffeine also causes faster, more complete intestinal absorption of ergotamine, thus reducing the total dosage required (24).

Sedatives and antiemetics may be used to control the nausea and vomiting that may occur during the migraine attack or be induced by the ergotamine itself. Meperidine combined with an antiemetic is occasionally necessary for treatment of an acute attack refractory to ergotamine.

If the migraine attacks are prolonged and not aborted by the usual antimigraine agents, steroids may terminate them. One method is prednisone in dosages of 25 to 60 mg administered orally, building up slowly from 10 mg daily, maintaining at maximum dosage for 3 to 4 days, then reducing slowly.

Interval Treatment

Most of the agents introduced for prophylaxis of migraine were first used to treat other disorders and then incorporated into the list of antimigraine agents (Table 2). It should be remembered that some studies have shown that placebos have reduced the frequency of migraine in more than 45% of patients.

Methysergide maleate (Sansert®), which acts as a competitive serotonin inhibitor, has proved to be an effective prophylactic agent in migraine (30,39). Because of its side effects, it should be used in only the limited number of situations in which attacks have not been controlled by any other method. Cyproheptadine (Periactin®), another agent that simulates the action of serotonin on receptor sites, has also been used in the prophylaxis of migraine (38). Both these drugs have antihistamine activity but block only the histamine H_1 receptors, whereas the extracranial circulation contains mainly H_2 receptors (60). Methysergide also potentiates the vasoconstrictor action of norepinephrine.

Propranolol hydrochloride (Inderal®), a beta-adrenergic blocker, has been reported effective in the prevention of common migraine (19,34). A caveat to keep in mind is the possibility that propranolol may precipitate or potentiate a heart failure or asthma. Angina pectoris has been reported following sudden withdrawal, particularly in patients with preexisting coronary disease (19).

Tricyclic antidepressants, such as imipramine hydrochloride (Tofranil®) and amitriptyline hydrochloride (Elavil®), are more effective than the anxiety-reducing drugs in the prophylactic treatment of patients with migraine who are also subject to depression (19,15). They act by inhibiting uptake of norepinephrine and serotonin. Other agents that have been used are those that prevent depletion of serotonin and possibly other vasoactive amines (catecholamines and histamines) by interfering with the action of their deactivating enzymes (monoamine oxidase inhibitors) (22).

Clonidine (Catapres®) directly stimulates arterial alpha receptors. Note that studies evaluating the effectiveness of clonidine have not generally shown a beneficial result surpassing that of placebos (56).

In certain patients, some headaches will recur even after the use of the chemical agents described above as well as those listed in Table 2.

TABLE 1. *Drugs for effective treatment of acute attack of migraine headache*[a]

Drug	Form	Dosage	Route	Action	Side effects	Contraindications
Gynergen (Sandoz) Ergotamine tartrate, 0.05 mg/cc	Ampul	1–2	Parenteral	Vasoconstrictive	Nausea, vomiting, weakness in legs, muscle pains in extremities, numbness and tingling in fingers and toes, angina-like precordial distress and pain, transient tachycardia or bradycardia, localized edema and itching	Septic infections, vascular diseases (e.g., marked arteriosclerosis, coronary artery disease, thrombophlebitis, Raynaud or Buerger syndrome, pregnancy)
Ergomar (Cooper) Ergotamine tartrate, 2 mg	Tablet	1–3	Sublingual	Same		
Medihaler-ergotamine (Riker) Ergotamine tartrate, 0.35 mg per dose	Aerosol	2–6	Oral inhalation	Same		
D.H.E. 45 (Sandoz) Dihydroergotamine Methanesulfonate, 1 mg/cc	Ampul	1–2	IM or IV	Same		
Cafergot P-B (Sandoz) Ergotamine tartrate, 1 mg Caffeine, 100 mg 1-Belladonna alkaloids (bellafoline), 0.125 mg Phenobarbital sodium, 30 mg	Tablet	2–6	Oral	Vasoconstrictive Antispasmodic Sedative	Nausea, vomiting, numbness and tingling of hands and feet, muscle pain in thighs and neck, abdominal pain, prostration, dryness of mucous membranes and skin, drowsiness	Septic infections, vascular diseases, coronary sclerosis, history of angina pectoris, pregnancy, hypertension, impaired renal or hepatic function, glaucoma
Ergotamine tartrate, 2 mg Caffeine, 100 mg 1-Belladonna alkaloids, 0.25 mg Pentobarbital, 60 mg	Suppository	1–2	Rectal			

Product	Dosage form	No.	Route	Action	Side effects	Contraindications
Wigraine (Organon) Ergotamine tartrate, 1 mg Caffeine, 100 mg 1-Belladonna alkaloids, 0.1 mg Phenacetin, 130 mg	Tablet or suppository	1–2	Oral or rectal	Vasoconstrictive	Same as for ergotamine tartrate + dryness of mucous membranes and skin	Same as for ergotamine tartrate + glaucoma
Migral (Burroughs Wellcome) Ergotamine tartrate, 1 mg Caffeine, 50 mg Cyclizine hydrochloride, 25 mg	Tablet	2–4	Oral	Vasoconstrictive Antiemetic	Same as for Wigraine	Same as for ergotamine tartrate
Midrin (Carnick) Isometheptene mucate, 65 mg Dichloralphenazone, 100 mg Acetaminophen, 325 mg	Capsule	2–5	Oral	Vasoconstrictive Analgesic Sedative	Drowsiness, dizziness, palpitations, weakness	Glaucoma, severe renal disease, hypertension, organic heart disease, hepatic disease, patients on MAO inhibitor therapy

[a] Adapted from ref. 22.

TABLE 2. *Drugs for prophylactic treatment of migraine headache*

Drug	Dosage
Those acting as competitive serotonin inhibitors by simulating action of serotonin on receptor sites	
Methysergide maleate (Sansert)	2 mg t.i.d.
Cyproheptadine (Periactin)	4–16 mg daily as tolerated
Those producing vasoconstriction, sedation; antispasmodic	
Ergotamine, phenobarbital, and belladonna	
Bellergal	1 tablet q.i.d.
Bellergal-S	1 tablet b.i.d.
Those preventing vasodilatation by blocking beta-adrenergic receptors on blood vessels	
Propranolol hydrochloride (Inderal)	40–120 mg daily in divided doses
Those inhibiting uptake of norepinephrine and serotonin, including tricyclic depressants	
Imipramine hydrochloride (Tofranil)	(50–150 mg in divided doses)
Amitriptyline hydrochloride (Elavil)	(or once daily at bedtime)
Those having a stimulating effect on arterial alpha receptors	
Clonidine (Catapres)	0.1 mg b.i.d. or t.i.d. (dosage may be increased gradually by increments of 0.1 mg)
Miscellaneous group	
Tranquilizers	
Sedatives	
Muscle relaxants	
Heparin	
Lithium carbonate	
Levodopa	
Bromocriptine	
Indomethacin	
Prednisone	
Estrogens	
Serotonin precursors	
Papaverine hydrochloride	
Anticonvulsants	

Adapted from ref. 22a.

Psychotherapy

Emotional factors frequently precipitate a migraine attack as well as muscle-contraction (tension) headaches. Treatment of psychologic aspects is paramount because the tensions developed in migraine patients over repeated frustrations, hostility, anxiety, and inability to meet personal standards of perfection often provide the setting in which the migraine attack occurs (15).

Environmental stress at home, at work, or in social situations may bring about more tension or anxiety than the patient can endure. One of the first steps in the treatment of migraine, greatly aided by the confidence engendered by the physician-patient relationship, is to remove as much adverse stress as possible from the patient's environment. This alone will likely decrease the number of headache attacks.

Autoregulatory Techniques

Various autoregulatory techniques have been introduced for treatment of migraine, e.g., biofeedback. Reports on the success of this technique have varied with different investigations (59). Types of meditation, such as zen, yoga, transcendentalism, and progressive relaxation, have also been used in the treatment of migraine. While some individuals who practice these secure temporary relief from their tension states and migraine, use of these techniques does not give the patient the needed insight into the causes of tension or provide methods for solving the underlying problems.

Other Procedures

Cook (14) has reported a 75% success in a 6-month follow-up of the use of cryosurgery, which involves freezing the occipital, superficial, temporal, and sphenopalatine arteries on the affected side. Insufficient data, including control studies, make it wise to withhold judgment as to the degree of temporary or permanent success of acupuncture with headache patients. Further research of the newly discovered endorphins and enkephalins by providing insight into the mechanisms of pain and its relief may explain some apparent successes of such methods as acupuncture.

SUMMARY

The most effective prescription for the treatment of migraine remains the physician who understands the mechanisms of the disorder, has made a correct diagnosis, has established a good relationship with the patient, and from knowledge has made appropriate use of the optimal treatment for the disease and relief of its symptoms.

REFERENCES

1. AMA Department of Drugs, in cooperation with American Society for Clinical Pharmacology and Therapeutics. *AMA Drug Evaluation,* 3rd edition. Littleton, Publishing Sciences Group, Massachusetts.
2. Anthony, M. (1977): The role of free fatty acids in migraine. Paper delivered at First International Migraine Symposium, London.
3. Anthony, M., and Lance, J. W. (1971): Histamine and serotonin in cluster headache. *Arch. Neurol.,* 25:225–231.
4. Anthony, M., Hinterberger, H., and Lance, J. W. (1967): Plasma serotonin in migraine and stress. *Arch. Neurol,* 16:544–552.
5. Aretaeus Cappadox (1923): Heter crania. In: *Corpus Medicorum Graecorum,* edited by C. Hude, vol. 3, p. 37, vol. 4, p. 149. Teubner, Leipzig.
6. Aring, C. D. (1962): Vascular headache. *Arch. Intern. Med.,* 109:18.
7. Bickerstaff, E. R. (1961): Basilar artery migraine. *Lancet,* 1:15–17.
8. Bradshaw, P., and Parsons, M. (1965): Hemiplegic migraine—a clinical study. *Q. J. Med.,* 34:65.
9. Brenner, C., Friedman, A. P., and Carter, S. (1949): Psychologic factors in the etiology and treatment of chronic headache. *Psychosom. Med.,* 11:53–56.
10. Brenner, C., Freidman, A. P., Merritt, H. H., and Denny-Brown, D. E. (1944): Posttraumatic headache. *J. Neurosurg.,* 1:370–391.
11. Bruyn, G. W. (1968): Complicated migraine. In: *Handbook of Clinical Neurology,* edited by P. J. Vinken and G. W. Bruyn, vol. 5, pp. 59–95. North-Holland, Amsterdam.
12. Cochrane, A. L. (ed.) (1970): The definition of migraine. *The Background of Migraine,* pp. 181–182. Heinemann, London.

13. Connor, R. C. R. (1962): Complicated migraine. A study of permanent neurological and visual field defects caused by migraine. *Lancet,* 2:1,072–1,075.
14. Cook, N. (1973): Cryosurgery of migraine. *Headache,* 12:143–150.
15. Couch, J. R., Ziegler, D. K., and Hassanein, R. (1976): Amitriptyline is the prophylaxis of migraine. *Neurology,* 26:121–127.
16. Dalessio, D. J. (1978): Mechanisms of headache. A symposium on headache and related pain syndromes. *Med. Clin. North Am.,* 62:429–442.
17. Dalsgaard-Nielsen, R. (1965): Migraine and heredity. *Acta Neurol. Scand.,* 41:287–300.
18. Deshmukh, S. V., and Meyer, J. S. (1977): Cyclic changes in platelet dynamics and the pathogenesis and prophylaxis of migraine. *Headache,* 17:101–108.
19. Diamond, S., and Medina, J. L. (1976): Double-blind study of propranolol for migraine prophylaxis. *Headache,* 16:24–27.
20. Edmeads, J. (1977): Cerebral blood flow in migraine. *Headache,* 17:148–152.
21. Friedman, A. P. (1956): The psychologic aspects of headache therapy. *NY State J. Med.,* 56:2,392–2,396.
22. Friedman, A. P. (1968): Drug treatment of migraine. In: *Handbook of Clinical Neurology,* edited by P. J. Vinken and G. W. Bruyn, vol. 5, pp. 96–102. North-Holland, Amsterdam.
22a. Friedman, A. P. (1980): Medicine for migraine. *Mod. Med.,* 48:36–49.
23. Friedman, A. P. (1972): Current concepts in the diagnosis and treatment of chronic recurring headache. *Med. Clin. North Am.,* 56(6):1,257–1,271.
24. Friedman, A. P. (1972): *JAMA,* 222:1,399–1,402.
25. Friedman, A. P. (1978): Migraine. A symposium on headache and related pain syndromes. *Med. Clin. North Am.,* 62:481–494.
26. Friedman, A. P. (1978): Pharmacological treatment of migraine and headache. *Drug Ther.,* 8:47–58.
27. Friedman, A. P. (1979): Ergotism. In: *Handbook of Clinical Neurology,* edited by P. J. Vinken and G. W. Bruyn, vol. 36, pp. 547–559. North-Holland, Amsterdam.
28. Friedman, A. P. (1979): Headache. In: *Clinical Neurology,* edited by A. B. Baker, vol. 2, Harper & Row, Hagerstown.
29. Friedman, A. P. (1979): Migraine. In: *Textbook of Neurology,* 6th edition, edited by H. H. Merritt, pp. 825–843. Lea & Febinger, Philadelphia.
30. Friedman, A. P., and Elkind, A. H. (1963): Appraisal in the treatment of vascular headache of the migraine type. *JAMA,* 184:125–128.
31. Friedman, A. P., and Wood, E. H. (1975): Thermography in vascular headache. In: *Medical Thermography, Theory and Applications,* pp. 80–85. Brentwood, Los Angeles.
32. Friedman, A. P., Buchsbaum, H. W., and Masland, W. S. (1978): Computerized axial tomography—Observation on its role in the examination of patients with headache. In: *Current Concepts in Migraine Research,* edited by R. Green, pp. 73–77. Raven Press, New York.
33. Friedman, A. P., Harter, D. H., and Merritt, H. H. (1962): Ophthalmoplegic migraine. *Arch. Neurol.,* 7:82–87.
34. Forssman, B., Henriksson, K-G., Johannsson, V. et al. (1976): Propranolol for migraine prophylaxis. *Headache,* 16:238–245.
35. Fromm-Reichmann, F. (1937): Contribution to the psychogenesis of migraine. *Psychoanal. Rev.,* 24:26–33.
36. Gilbert, G. J., Rappaport, A., and Trump, R. (1974): Retinal degeneration in hemiplegic migraine. *Headache,* 14:77–80.
37. Goodell, H., Lewontin, R., and Wolff, H. G. (1954): Familial occurrence of migraine headache. A study of heredity. *Arch. Neurol. Psychiatry,* 72:325–334.
38. Goodman, L. S., and Gilman, A. (1975): *Pharmacological Basis of Therapeutics,* 5th edition. Macmillan, New York.
39. Graham, J. R. (1964): Methysergide for prevention of headache. Experience in 500 patients over 3 years. *N. Engl. J. Med.,* 270:67–72.
40. Hannington, E., and Harper, A. M. (1963): The role of tyramine in the etiology of migraine and related studies on the cerebral and extracerebral circulation. *Headache,* 3:67.
41. Henson, P. M., and Spiegelberg, H. L. (1973): Release of serotonin from human platelets induced by aggregated immunoglobulins of different classes and subclasses. *J. Clin. Invest.,* 52:1,282–1,288.
42. Heyck, H. (1956): Neue Beitrage zur Pathogenese der Migraine. *Schweiz. Med. Wochenschr.,* 86:41.
43. Horrobin, D. F. (1977): Prostaglandins and migraine. *Headache,* 17:101–108.
44. Hsu, L. G. U., Crisp, A. H., Koval, J., Kalucy, R. S., Chen, C. N., Carruthers, M., and Zilkha, K. (1976): Electroencephalogram and plasma levels of catecholamines, tryptophan, glucose, insulin, free fatty acids, and prostaglandins during sleep preceding early morning migraine. In: *International Symposium, 16th–17th September, 1976,* pp. 11–12. The Migraine Trust, London.
45. Klee, A. (1968): *A Clinical Study of Migraine with Particular Reference to the Most Severe Cases.* Munksgaards, Copenhagen.
46. Kolb, L. C. (1963): Psychiatric aspects of the treatment of headache. *Neurology (Minneap.),* 13:34–37.

47. Lance, J. S. (1978): Migraine. In: *Recent Advances in Clinical Neurology, 2,* edited by W. B. Matthews and G. H. Glaser, pp. 145–161. Churchill Livingstone, Edinburgh.

48. Mathew, N. T., Meyer, J. S., Welch, K. M. A., and Neblet, C. R. (1977): Abnormal CT scans in migraine. *Headache,* 16:272–279.

49. Marshall, J. (1974): The regulation of cerebral blood flow—its relationship to migraine. *Arch. Neurobiol. (Madr.) [Suppl.],* 37:15–25.

50. Miller-Fisher, C. (1968): Cerebrovascular disease. In: *Handbook of Clinical Neurology,* edited by P. J. Vinken and G. W. Bruyn, vol. 5, pp. 124–156. North-Holland, Amsterdam.

51. Moore, T. L., Ryan, R. E., Jr., Pohl, D. A., Roodman, S. T., and Ryan, R. E., Sr. (1981): Comparison of immunoglobulin, complement, and immune complex levels in patients during a migraine headache and during a headache-free period. *Headache (in press).*

52. O'Brien, M. D. (1971): Cerebral blood flow changes in migraine. *Headache,* 10:139–143.

53. Rao, N. S., and Pearce, J. (1971): Hypothalamo-pituitary-adrenal axis studies in migraine with special reference to insulin sensitivity. *Brain,* 94:289–298.

54. Rees, W. L. (1971): Psychiatric and psychological factors. In: *Background to Migraine,* edited by J. N. Cumings, pp. 45–55. Heinemann, London.

55. Rotton, W. N. (1959): Migraine and eclampsia. *Obstet. Gynecol. Surv.,* 14:322–420.

56. Ryan, R. E., Sr., Diamond, S., and Ryan, R. E., Jr. (1975): Double-blind study of clonidine and placebo for prophylactic treatment of migraine. *Headache,* 15:202–206.

57. Sakai, F., and Meyer, J. (1981): Abnormal cerebrovascular reactivity in patients with migraine and cluster headache. *Headache, (in press).*

58. Sandler, M., Youdin, M. B. H., and Hannington, E. A. (1974): A phenylethylamine oxidizing defect in migraine. *Nature,* 250:335–337.

59. Sargent, J. D., Green, E. E., and Walters, E. D. (1973): Preliminary report on the use of autogenic feedback training in the treatment of migraine and tension headache. *Psychosom. Med.,* 35:129–135.

60. Saxena, P. R. (1975): Two types of histamine receptors in a vascular bed of relevance to migrainous headache. In: *Vasoactive Substances Relevant to Migraine,* edited by S. Diamond, D. J. Dalessio, J. R. Graham, and J. L. Medina, pp. 34–44. Charles C Thomas, Springfield, Illinois.

61. Sicuteri, F., Fanciullacci, M., and Anselmi, B. (1963): Bradykinin release and inactivation in man. *Int. Arch. Allergy Appl. Immunol.,* 22:77–84.

62. Skinhoj, E. (1973): Haemodynamic studies with the brain during migraine. *Arch. Neurol.,* 29:95–98.

63. Stanford, E., and Greene, R. (1970): A case of migraine cured by treatment of Conn's syndrome. In: *Background to Migraine,* edited by A. L. Cochrane, pp. 53–57. Heinemann, London.

64. Steinbeck, J. (1947): *The Wayward Bus.* Viking, New York.

65. Waters, W. E. (1975): Prevalence of migraine. *J. Neurol. Neurosurg. Psychiatry,* 38:613–616.

66. Wolff, H. G. (1937): Personality factors and reactions of subjects with migraine. *Arch. Neurol. Psychiatry,* 24:26–33.

Advances in Neurology, Vol. 33, edited by
M. Critchley et al. Raven Press, New York © 1982

Comments on A. P. Friedman's Report

Faustino Savoldi

Department of Neurology, Headache Center, University of Pavia School of Medicine, Pavia, Italy

The main feature of the psychosomatic approach is to stress the significance of the organic symptoms. Thus each symptom is found to have a significance different from that which it normally represents; that is, each symptom points to something different. In patients suffering from psychosomatic illness, organic symptoms are a symbolic realization of psychic disturbances, of conflicts, and especially of frustrations, which censorship renders unconscious. The basic mechanisms of this process are the conversion, somatization, and accompaniment. These mechanisms should permit what Freud (2), and later Deutsch (1), called "the mysterious leap from the mind to the body."

On the basis of this theory, many attempts have been proposed to define different types of "morbid personalities." Thus "ulcerous personalities" have been described as well as "tubercular," "rachialgic," and "migrainous."

A profound contradiction is hidden within the psychosomatic method—the constant search for a causality link and a significance link simultaneously. These two types of correlation are, in our judgment, incomparable. Psychosomatics cannot explain why or how a person becomes ill. They are aimed at refusing any dualistic perspective and at researching the "point of impact" (4), which can permit the attribution of an univocal value to the symptom, independently of its origin. In this case, however, a rigid and specific psychogenesis is emphasized, which again sanctions and maintains the subdivision between the body and the mind.

The hypothesis that pain may be purely psychogenic and therefore interpreted as the manifestation of a conversion mechanism is simplistic and unacceptable for most patients.

The psychosomatic approach, in our opinion, represents an intellectual method. Admitting that the symbolic function may underlie all our behavior and perception, it is evident that it cannot represent the ultimate term of the analysis. The search for the significance of a disease, when it is oriented toward a symbolic function, renders all illnesses equal, annuls any difference, reduces all to a false unity, and leaves no way to distinguish them from hysteria.

On the other hand, not even psychological testing may help us to resolve these problems. It can, however, help complete a patient's psychic picture. There is no test capable of establishing whether a patient's report of symptoms is of somatic or psychic origin. In fact, it is impossible to distinguish the effects of a chronic somatic pain state by conversion reaction. To this end, only careful reconstruction of the case history and observation of the way the symptoms are described, together with the sympathy of the physician, will furnish useful information. The contribution of psychological testing is limited only to the acquisition of cofactors and/or collateral aspects of the syndrome under study. Any attempt to distinguish psychic or functional from organic disturbances has proved insufficient. These tests, being psychological, can also indicate the existence of a thought or mood disturbance and quantify its severity, thus dictating psychopharmacological or psychotherapeutic cures.

Eventual organic disorders cannot be excluded. Regarding headache patients, in particular, it is known that both somatic and psychic factors can be involved and that the factors triggering the attacks can be numerous and often unidentified.

A distinction must be made between trigger events, among which are psychological stresses, and the constitution of the headache patient. This distinction has led several authors to attempt the description of the hypothetic migraine personality. A migraine subject would show a delayed affective development, sluggish intelligence, inadequate sexual development, a sense of personal insecurity, and perfectionist tendencies (5). Knopf's (3) description is similar: ambitious, reserved, authoritarian, depressed, lacking a sense of humor, and heterosexually maladjusted. Wolff's (6,7) classic description shows the migraine patient to be ambitious, perfectionist, rigid, and having an obsessive character. More recent research has indicated that migrainous and tension headache patients tend to be neurotic, sensitive, and less adaptable to stress. Unfortunately, such descriptions are applicable also to subjects with other diseases and with none at all.

The research of psychic disturbance in migraine calls to mind another problem: the relationship between migraine and epilepsy. In the past, because of the recurrent character of these patients, some authors have tried to include migraine and periodic headaches with epilepsy; but the clinical and electroencephalographic features have invalidated this hypothesis.

A psychoneurobiological approach may be able to help us to define, with reasonable accuracy, the fundamental characteristics of the migraine structure from both a biological and a psychic point of view.

REFERENCES

1. Deutsch, P. (1959): *On the Mysterious Leap from the Mind to the Body.* International University Press, New York.
2. Freud, S. (1952): *A General Introduction to Psychoanalysis.* Washington Square Press, New York.
3. Knopf, O. (1935): Preliminary report on personality studies in thirty migraine patients. *J. Nerv. Ment. Dis.,* 82:270–285.
4. Marty, P. (1951): Aspect psychodynamique de l'etude clinique de quelque cas de cephalalgies. *Rev. Franc. Psychoanal.,* 2:216–252.
5. Touraine, G. A., and Draper, G. (1934): The migrainous patient. A constitutional study. *J. Nerv. Ment. Dis.,* 80:1–23.
6. Wolff, H. G. (1935): Personality features and reactions of subjects with migraine. *Arch. Neurol. Psychiatry,* 37:895–921.
7. Wolff, H. G. (1963): *Headache and Other Head Pain.* Oxford University Press, New York.

Advances in Neurology, Vol. 33, edited by
M. Critchley et al. Raven Press, New York © 1982

What is Migraine?

James W. Lance

*Department of Neurology, School of Medicine, University of New South Wales; and Division of
Neurology, The Prince Henry and Prince of Wales Hospitals, Sydney, Australia*

Certain symptoms, such as mood changes (elation, irritability), increased appetite or thirst, a craving to eat sweets, and drowsiness may be noticed for as long as 24 hr before the onset of migraine headache. Nausea may precede headache by 30 to 60 min. These manifestations suggest that subtle changes are taking place in the hypothalamus or brainstem before the commonly recognized prodromal phase (aura) and vascular changes of migraine headache. The aura may occur without headache (migraine equivalent), or the headache may occur without a prodromal phase (common migraine). There are also those patients who do not fit easily into the present classification of migraine because they develop focal neurological symptoms or signs at the height of the headache without experiencing the conventional prodrome. If patients are subject to more than one of these varieties of migraine, are they suffering from more than one disorder or simply offering a glimpse of different segments of the migrainous spectrum? Should we speak of "the migraines" as we now speak of "the epilepsies" and therefore strive to separate entities that may conceal themselves within the general definition of migraine?

Lord and Duckworth (16) separated patients whose neurological symptoms precede the onset of headache (prodromal migraine) from those in whom such symptoms are present during the headache phase. Circulating immune complexes were detected in sera from nonprodromal migraineurs, and evidence was found of complement activation by the classical pathway. Serum complement levels did not change in patients with prodromal migraine, nor were immune complexes detected in this group. These findings suggest that an immune reaction may play a part in the pathogenesis of nonprodromal migraine, and that the definition of classical migraine should be restricted to attacks with prodromal symptoms, excluding those attacks in which focal neurological symptoms appear only during the headache phase.

MIGRAINE CLASSIFICATION

The above leads to a reconsideration of the classification of migraine in the following way, summarized in Table 1.

Premonitory Migraine

Premonitory migraine includes episodes in which mood changes, drowsiness, or alterations in appetite or thirst precede migraine headache by up to 24 hr. These symptoms may reflect central monoamine changes, particularly in the hypothalamus.

TABLE 1. *Proposed Classification of Migraine*

Group	Subgroup(s)
Premonitory migraine	
Prodromal migraine	
Classical	Retinal
Protracted prodromal	⎧ Vertebrobasilar ⎨ Migraine stupor ⎩ Hemiplegic
Migraine equivalent	Transient migrainous accompaniments
Nonprodromal migraine	
Common	Facial
Interposed	Ophthalmoplegic
Complicated migraine	

Prodromal Migraine

Classical Migraine

In classical migraine, visual disturbance or other focal neurological symptoms precede migraine headache by some 10 to 60 min. Retinal migraine appears to be a subgroup of classic migraine.

Protracted Prodromal Migraine

In protracted prodromal migraine, focal neurological symptoms persist into the headache phase. This group includes most cases of vertebrobasilar migraine (3), migraine stupor (15), confusional states of childhood, and hemiplegic migraine.

Migraine Equivalent

Gradual onset and subsidence of focal neurological symptoms in the manner of a migrainous prodrome without headache ensuing characterizes the migraine equivalent. An interesting subgroup in the middle-aged or older patient has been described by Fisher (7) as transient migrainous accompaniments (TMAs) to distinguish them from thromboembolic transient ischemic attacks (TIAs).

Nonprodromal Migraine

Common Migraine

Common migraine is an episodic headache, most commonly unilateral and associated with nausea, vomiting, and photophobia, without overt neurological symptoms or signs. Subgroups include most cases of premenstrual migraine, facial migraine (lower half headache), and those with features such as redness and watering of the eye and blockage of one or both nostrils, reminiscent of cluster headache.

Interposed Migraine

During interposed migraine, focal neurological symptoms or signs develop as the headache intensifies. Ophthalmoplegic migraine appears to be a subgroup of interposed migraine.

Complicated Migraine

Retinal or neurological deficit persisting after the usual duration of migraine headache or migraine equivalent is characteristic of complicated migraine, which may follow any form other than common migraine.

It is recognized that some syndromes overlap, and that one patient may suffer two or more forms of migraine at the same or different times of life. The above classification could be helpful in distinguishing groups with variations in pathophysiology and response to treatment. To use the analogy of epilepsy, it could be said that, in general, ethosuximide is not an effective anticonvulsant. Once the subgroup of petit mal absences with 3 Hz spike-wave paroxysms in the electroencephalogram is studied in isolation, it becomes apparent that ethosuximide is a highly effective anticonvulsant for this group selectively.

THE MIGRAINOUS PATIENT

Migrainous patients may complain of multiple symptoms, implicating many bodily systems, which may reflect their introspective nature or may be interpreted as dysfunction of the limbic system (21). There is good evidence that migrainous patients react more to stress than do controls (14). Migrainous children are more fearful, tense, sensitive, and vulnerable to frustration than their nonmigrainous peers (4). They are more tidy and perform various set tasks more slowly but with fewer errors than controls.

Each individual may have a "migraine threshold," a concept comparable with the "convulsive threshold" in epilepsy. It is not uncommon to find patients who have had only one, two, or three migrainous attacks in their lives; thus the frequency may range from one per lifetime to one almost every day. It is probable that any individual could have a migraine headache, just as anyone might have an epileptic seizure, given a suitable set of precipitating circumstances.

It would be of interest to have the "migraine threshold" quantified in a random sample of the population by graded stimuli, for example, hypoglycaemia, rapid changes in barometric pressure in a compression or decompression chamber, and the administration of vasodilator agents, such as alcohol, prostaglandin E_1, and reserpine. The migraine threshold appears to be a familial characteristic although not usually conforming to a standard mode of inheritance.

Thus, migraine may be regarded as a neurovascular reaction with a strong hereditary component, occurring more readily in individuals with certain personality characteristics, spontaneously or in response to certain trigger factors. The observation by Fanciullacci et al. (6) that migrainous subjects are more sensitive than controls to hallucinogenic agents, such as lysergic acid diethylamide (LSD) and psilocybin, may indicate that the migrainous patient differs in characteristics of blood-brain barrier or neurotransmitter pattern from his or her headache-free counterpart.

TRIGGER FACTORS

Probably the most common precipitant is emotional stress or excitement, the headache often appearing at the moment of letdown when the immediate crisis is past. Sustained physical exertion, the premenstrual fall in estradiol, and jarring of the head (footballer's migraine) are all well documented in provoking attacks. Sensitivity to food factors as a mechanism remains controversial. Tyramine in food may (13) or may not (17,18,23) trigger migraine; phenylethylamine in chocolate may (25) or may not (19) be a trigger factor. In many patients, no provocative factor can be found and they suffer migraine regularly without apparent cause.

PATHOPHYSIOLOGY

There is little doubt that the focal neurological symptoms of migraine, whether they occur before or during the headache phase, are the result of ischemia of the cerebral cortex (12,24). The cortex may become ischemic because of arteriolar and capillary constriction, the opening of arteriovenous anastomoses shunting blood away from the cortex, platelet aggregation, or a combination of these factors. It is unlikely that increased cerebral perfusion, which may or may not be caused solely by reactive hyperemia, is responsible for migraine headache. Headache has been reported in patients while cerebral blood flow remained normal, and has been abolished by ergotamine tartrate while cerebral blood flow was elevated (11). Moreover, the site of headache bears no constant relationship to the site of maximal cortical ischemia.

There is evidence for the release of serotonin and catecholamines and possibly histamine and a bradykinin-like substance as well during migraine. Adsorption of serotonin to the vessel wall combined with the effect of local bradykinin has been proposed as a mechanism for sensitizing the vessel so that pain is produced by modest distension of large cranial vessels.

The migrainous patient may have inherited a pattern of monoamine metabolism that renders him or her more vulnerable to stress; thus trigger factors cause changes in amine transmitters within the central nervous system as well as amine release peripherally, leading to the neural and vascular reaction described clinically as migraine. Small parenchymal brain vessels receive noradrenergic innervation from the locus ceruleus. A companion pathway has been described of serotonin-containing neurons which arise in the midbrain raphe nuclei of rats (22), providing a second system by which the brain could control its own microcirculation. A primary change in neurotransmitters in the hypothalamus and brainstem thus could initiate constriction of small vessels supplying the cerebral cortex as well as premonitory symptoms described above.

Norepinephrine synthesis in migraine patients even without headache (10), as measured by blood levels of the enzyme dopamine-β-hydroxylase (DBH), is almost double that in patients with tension headache and normal controls; it increases further during the migraine attack (1). The observation of Anthony et al. (2) that a serotonin-releasing factor is present in the blood during migraine headache has been amply confirmed (5, 20). The fall in blood serotonin level during migraine headache (2) is accompanied by a fall in plasma norepinephrine (8), the other potent naturally occurring vasoconstrictor in man, thereby removing normal humoral restraints on vasodilatation. The concept of platelet aggregation and serotonin release during migraine is strengthened by the finding of increased serum levels of beta-thromboglobulin, a protein formed during platelet release reactions, during migraine headache (9).

Whatever the amine changes within the nervous system, inside or outside the vessel wall, or in blood platelets, no satisfactory explanation has yet been proposed for the predominantly unilateral nature of focal neurological symptoms or of migraine headache. It is as though the normal, carefully controlled regulation of the cerebral and extracranial circulation has temporarily broken down and been replaced by chaotic, uncoordinated reactions, patchy and asymmetrical, involving both large and small vessels. It is a curious fact that the pattern is often remarkably consistent for a particular patient.

CONCLUSIONS AND SUMMARY

The migrainous patient appears to differ in reaction to stress or environmental changes from nonmigrainous subjects quantitatively rather than qualitatively. An inherited pattern of monoamine metabolism may render the patient more susceptible to such changes, which represent a threat, real or imagined, to the integrity of the brain. The migraine attack may thus be interpreted as a neurohumoral reaction aimed at protecting the brain from some noxious influence by shunting blood away from the cortex. The headache itself may be a by-product of such a reaction, serving, like any pain, to alert the organism to potential danger. The predominantly unilateral site of migraine remains unexplained.

A more comprehensive clinical classification of migraine is proposed in the hope that certain entities may prove to correlate with variations in pathophysiology and thus permit more selective therapy.

REFERENCES

1. Anthony, M. (1981): Biochemical indices of sympathetic activity in migraine. *Cephalalgia,* 1:83–89.
2. Anthony, M., Hinterberger, H., and Lance, J. W. (1968): The possible relation of serotonin to the migraine syndrome. *Res. Clin. Stud. Headache,* 2:29–59.
3. Bickerstaff, E. R. (1961): Basilar artery migraine. *Lancet,* 1:15–17.
4. Bille, B. (1962): Migraine in school children. *Acta Paediatr.* 51[*Suppl. 136*]:1–151.
5. Dvilansky, A., Rishpon, S., Nathan, I., Zoltow, Z., and Korczyn, A. D. (1976): Release of platelet 5-hydroxytryptamine by plasma taken from platelets during and between migraine attacks. *Pain,* 2:315–318.
6. Fanciullacci, M., Franchi, G., and Sicuteri, F. (1974): Hypersensitivity to lysergic acid diethylamide (LSD-25) and psilocybin in essential headache. *Experientia,* 30:1,441–1,443.
7. Fisher, C. M. (1979): Transient migrainous accompaniments (TMAs) of late onset. *Stroke,* 10:96–97.
8. Fog-Møller, F., Genefke, I. K., and Bryndum, B. (1978); Changes in concentration of catecholamines in blood during spontaneous migraine attacks and reserpine-induced attacks. In: *Current Concepts in Migraine Research,* edited by R. Greene, pp. 115–119. Raven Press, New York.
9. Gawal, M., Burkitt, M., and Rose, F. C. (1979): The platelet release reaction during migraine attacks. *Headache,* 19:323–327.
10. Gotoh, F., Kanda, T., Sakai, F., Yamamoto, M., and Takeoka, T. (1976): Serum dopamine-β-hydroxylase activity in migraine. *Arch. Neurol.,* 33:656–657.
11. Hachinski, V. C., Norris, J. W., Cooper, P. W., and Edmeads, J. G. (1978): Migraine and the cerebral circulation: In: *Current Concepts in Migraine Research,* edited by R. Greene, pp. 11–15. Raven Press, New York.
12. Hachinski, V. C., Olesen, J., Norris, J. W., Larsen, B., Enevoldsen, E., and Lassen, N. A. (1977): Cerebral hemodynamics in migraine. *Can. J. Neurol. Sci.,* 4:245–249.
13. Hanington, E., Horn, M., and Wilkinson, M. (1970): Further observations on the effects of tyramine. In: *Background to Migraine, Third Migraine Symposium,* edited by A. L. Cochrane, pp. 113–119. Heinemann, London.
14. Henryk-Gutt, R., and Rees, W. L. (1973): Psychological aspects of migraine. *J. Psychosom Res.,* 17:141–153.
15. Lee, C. H., and Lance, J. W. (1977): Migraine stupor. *Headache,* 17:32–38.
16. Lord, G. D. A., and Duckworth, J. W. (1978): Complement and immune complex studies in migraine. *Headache,* 18:255–260.

17. Medina, J. L., and Diamond, S. (1978): The role of diet in migraine. *Headache,* 18:31–34.
18. Moffett, A., Swash, M., and Scott, D. F. (1972): Effect of tyramine in migraine: A double-blind study. *J. Neurol. Neurosurg. Psychiatry,* 35:496–499.
19. Moffett, A. M., Swash, M., and Scott, D. F. (1974): Effect of chocolate in migraine: A double-blind study. *J. Neurol. Neurosurg. Psychiatry,* 37:445–448.
20. Mück-Šeler, D., Deanović, Ž., and Dupelj, M. (1979): Plasma serotonin (5-HT) and 5-HT releasing factor in plasma of migrainous patients. *Headache,* 19:14–17.
21. Raffaelli, E., Jr., and Menon, A. D. (1975): Migraine and the limbic system. *Headache,* 15:69–78.
22. Reinhard, J. F., Jr., Liebmann, J. E., Scholsberg, A. J., and Moskowitz, M. A. (1979): Serotonin neurons project to small blood vessels in the brain. *Science,* 206:85–87.
23. Ryan, R. E. (1974): A clinical study of tyramine as an etiological factor in migraine. *Headache,* 14:43–48.
24. Sakai, F., and Meyer, J. S. (1978): Regional cerebral hemodynamics during migraine and cluster headaches measured by the ^{133}Xe inhalation method. *Headache,* 18:122–132.
25. Sandler, M., Youdim, M. B. H., Southgate, J., and Hanington, E. (1970): The role of tyramine in migraine: Some possible biochemical mechanisms. In: *Background to Migraine, Third Migraine Symposium,* edited by A. L. Cochrane, pp. 103–112. Heinemann, London.

Advances in Neurology, Vol. 33, edited by
M. Critchley et al. Raven Press, New York © 1982

Migraine and the Mitral Valve Prolapse Syndrome

G. Amat, *P. Jean Louis, C. Loisy, †V. Centonze, and S. Pelage

*Centre de la Migraine, 03200 Vichy, France; * Service de Cardiologie, Hôpital Croix Rousse, 69317
Lyon, France; and † Instituto de Semeiotica, Universita di Bari, Bari, Italy*

Mitral valve prolapse (MVP), due to a myxomatous degeneration of the valve and chordae, corresponds to a faulty coaptation of the mitral leaflet, with hooding or prolapse of the posterior valve in the auricle and consequent intracardiac hemodynamic disturbances. Probably of a hereditary nature, this anomaly affects about 2 to 6% of the random population and is distinctly predominant in women. Suspected on hearing a midsystolic "click" with or without associated mid- to late-systolic murmur, MVP is confirmed by the "bowing" echocardiographic aspect and, secondarily, by angiocardiographic findings. The click is not permanent; it can appear only under certain conditions, and there can even be MVP silent on auscultation.

In the majority of cases, MVP is asymptomatic, but it can entail cardiothoracic symptoms (palpitations, dizziness, atypical chest pains), involving ventricular tachycardia, mitral regurgitation, rupture of the chordae, and endocarditis, as well as systemic or peripheric emboli whose exact origin is not known: *cul de sac* between the prolapsed valve and auricular wall, endothelium impairment producing platelet thrombi, or added atrial fibrillation (4,5).

Basing our study on the work of Litman and Friedman (7), which emphasizes an unusual frequency of migraine sufferers among patients with MVP (64 migraine sufferers of 230 patients, i.e., a prevalence of 27.8%, while the frequency of people suffering from migraines in the population is nearly 10%), we looked for MVP in a series of 195 headache sufferers examined during an 8-month period at the Centre de la Migraine in Vichy. Those 195 patients were distributed as shown in Table 1. In this series, we found 18 MVP verified by echocardiography, i.e., 9.23% of cases; all were found in the subgroup of vascular headaches, as shown in Table 1. The frequency of MVP found in vascular headaches, therefore, is 20.46%. In the general population, 6% have MVP, and 20% of women suffer migraine headaches. Thus these two ailments should not coincide in more than 1.2% of cases.

Migraine sufferers with MVP were predominantly women (17:1). Thoracic and associated symptoms (palpitations, dizziness, atypical chest pains, dyspnea) were noted in 10 of 18 patients. Symptoms evoking the possibility of an embolic (systemic or peripheric) accident were found in three of the 18 patients:

Case 141: Migraine with regressive right hemiparesia in 1972; negative arteriography.
Case 197: Migraines with several regressive episodes of hemiparesia of the left hand.
Case 240: Several episodes of leg failure before and during migraine attacks; Raynaud syndrome on the second and third fingers of the right hand.

TABLE 1. *Distribution of headaches in 195 patients*

	No. of patients	
Headache	Total	MVP[a]
Symptomatic and posttraumatic	5	—
Psychogenic and tensive	102	—
Vascular	(88)	(18)
Classic migraine	16	4
Common migraine	48	12
Cluster migraine	10	2
Cluster	14	0

[a] MVP was found in 18 of the 195 patients, or 9.46%, and in 20.46% of vascular headache patients.

Knowledge of this possible complication of MVP is important. In a recent case (not included in this study), we observed a patient with marked hereditary migraine antecedents in whom a migraine status was suddenly triggered at the age of 43 by a particularly severe right hemicranial attack, further complicated by a permanent blindness of the right eye. A thorough neurological study was performed (angiography, scanner) before our examination and showed only a right optical atrophy by acute ischemia of the head of the optical nerve. Despite the absence of "click," we carried out an echocardiography, which showed an MVP. We may therefore ask whether a certain number of ischemic strokes which have been described in migraine sufferers may be due to MVP; it should be sought systematically (1,7).

Basing our study on the work of Jean Louis (5), we looked for the following symptoms in our patients: (a) vertebrothoracic abnormalities (scoliosis and/or pectus excavatus and/or straight back) (17 of 18 cases), (b) obvious faciocorporal asymmetry (11 of 18 cases), (c) dermatological abnormalities (ichtyosis and/or lentiginosis and/or *café au lait* spots and/or lipomatosis) (12 of 18 cases), and (d) psychoneurotic troubles (patent or masked depression, anxiety neurosis, hypochondria, conversion hysteria) (17 of 18 cases). The link between MVP, vertebrothoracic, dermatological, and psychopathological abnormalities could be explained by a single neural crest and mesodermal embryonic tissue defect during the fourth to eighth week of embryonic development. From this point of view, MVP could be a manifestation of congenital neuroectomesodermal histodysplasia; the neurogenic factor (central and peripheral) would explain many symptoms and features associated with MVP.

Our 18 patients with MVP had been treated by DHE prior to our first examination. This treatment had little or no effect on 14, and four had noticeably improved. All these patients were treated by us with propanolol, as recommended by Litman and Friedmann (7). Sixteen patients were seen again after 4 to 6 months of treatment; 12 indicated excellent results from this beta-blocking agent, and four had little or no result (Table 2).

CONCLUSIONS

Our series is too small to allow final conclusions, but a number of hypotheses are possible. (a) MVP seems to be associated with vascular headaches with particular fre-

TABLE 2. *Results of 4 or 6 months treatment with DHE or propanolol*

Drug	Result	No. of patients
DHE[a]	Good	4
	Little or none	14
Propanolol[b]	Good	12
	Little or none	4

[a] $N = 18$.

[b] $N = 18$; but two patients were not seen again after the treatment period.

quency. (b) MVP should be systematically sought in all migraine sufferers, all the more so if they show embolic antecedents. In this research, echocardiography is of prime importance. (c) Because embolic risks are greater with patients with MVP, preventive treatment should be prescribed. (d) Migraineurs who show an MVP should be treated with propanolol. (e) Lastly, the frequency of the MVP-migraine association, if confirmed, could define a subgroup of migraine patients in whom the coexistence of a valvular myxomatous degeneration, vertebrothoracic abnormalities, faciocorporal asymmetry, dermatological abnormalities, and/or a psychopathological status might indicate a common congenital origin of these manifestations: neuroectomesodermal histodysplasia.

REFERENCES

1. Amat, G., and Loisy, C. (1980): Migraine et prolapsus valvulaire mitral. *Lyon Med.,* 243:265.
2. Barlow, J. B., and Pocock, W. A. (1979): Mitral valve prolapse. The specific billowing mitral leaflet syndrome or an insignificant non ejectional systolic click. *Am. Heart J.,* 97:277.
3. Barnett, H. J. M., Boughner, R. D., Taylor, D. W., Cooper, P. E., Roster W. J., Nichol, P. M. (1980): Further evidence relating mitral valve prolapse to cerebral ischemic events. *N. Engl. J. Med.,* 302:139–144.
4. Devereux, R. B. (1979): Mitral valve prolapse. *Am. J. Med.,* 67:729.
5. Jean Louis, P. (1980): Mitral valve prolapse: Possible manifestation of a congenital neuroectomesodermal histodysplasia. Communication to American College of Cardiology. March 9–13, 1980, Houston, Texas.
6. Jeresaty, R. M. (1979): Mitral Valve Prolapse. Raven Press, New York.
7. Litman, G. I., and Friedman, H. M. (1978): Migraine and the Mitral valve prolapse syndrome. *Am. Heart J.,* 96:610–613.

Advances in Neurology, Vol. 33, edited by
M. Critchley et al. Raven Press, New York © 1982

The Evolution of Thinking About the Role and Site of Action of Serotonin in Migraine

A. Fanchamps

Medical Counsel, Pharmaceutical Research, Sandoz Ltd., Basel, Switzerland

The hypothesis that serotonin (5-HT) might be involved in the mechanism of migraine was born in the late 1950s. While searching for humoral agents that might be responsible for rendering painful a normally painless extracranial dilatation, Wolff and his group (9,20) found that the local application of 5-HT lowers the pain threshold. Ostfeld (8), one of Wolff's co-workers, succeeded in provoking typical migraine attacks with intravenous 5-HT in four of 13 migraineurs; those four responded to a prophylactic treatment with the most potent 5-HT antagonist known, bromlysergic acid diethylamide (BOL 148). The conclusion was drawn that migraine is due, at least in part, to an excess of 5-HT. This was the starting point for the development of a series of antimigraine drugs with anti-5-HT properties. Since that time, the views regarding the role and site of action of 5-HT have been subject to astonishing changes (Table 1).

The finding by Sicuteri et al. (18) of an increased urinary excretion of 5-hydroxyindoleacetic acid, the main 5-HT metabolite, during the migraine attack confirmed the excess hypothesis. Sicuteri (13) proposed the theory that an increased local concentration of endogenous substances, which he termed "vasoneuroactive" (including not only 5-HT but also histamine, catecholamines, plasmakinins), could be responsible for the vascular and nervous disorders of migraine. The author was soon led to assume that the problem with 5-HT might be located in the brain as well as in the periphery (12). Surprisingly, when measuring the 5-HT blood level during migraine attacks, Lance and his group (5) did not find the expected increase, but a significant decrease. Migraine thus was linked not with an excess but with a deficiency of 5-HT.

A logical explanation emerged: experimental evidence demonstrated that at the beginning of a migraine attack, 5-HT is liberated from the blood platelets. Actually, it has been shown by various investigators that the platelets of migraineurs liberate 5-HT

TABLE 1. *Changing views on the role of 5-HT in migraine*

Investigators	Year	Hypothesis
Ostfeld et al.	1957	Excess of 5-HT in the periphery
Sicuteri	1963	Excess of 5-HT in the periphery and possibly in the brain
Lance et al.	1967	Lack of 5-HT in the periphery
Sicuteri et al.	1974	Lack of 5-HT in the brain

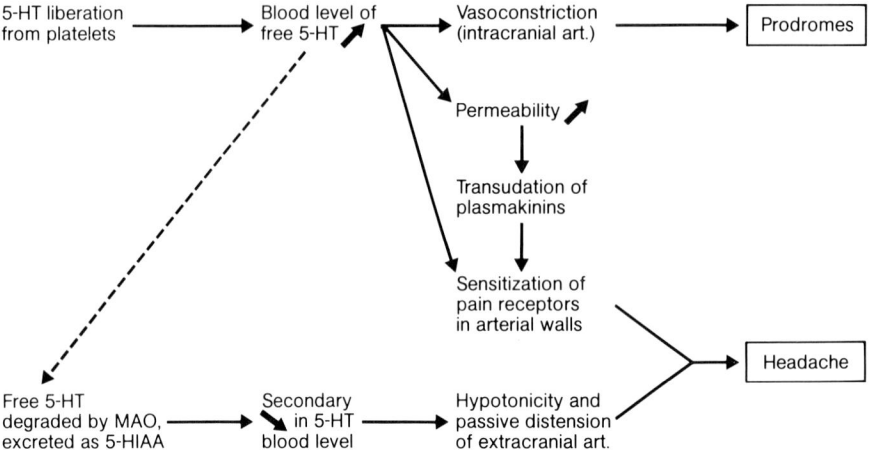

FIG. 1. Possible peripheral mechanism of the migraine attack. 5-HT, serotonin; MAO, mono-amine oxidase; 5-HIAA, 5-hydroxyindoleacetic acid; ↗, increase; ↘, decrease.

more readily than those of normal subjects (2), and that at the time of an attack, the plasma of migraine patients contains a 5-HT-liberating factor (1,6).

Free 5-HT constricts cranial arteries, especially of the internal carotid bed (7,11,19), which might account for some of the cortical prodromes. In addition, it increases perme-ability (10), thus favoring the transudation of plasmakinin into and around the vessel walls; also, it increases the sensitivity of the pain receptors (3,17). Secondarily, the degradation and increased excretion of 5-HT leads to the observed drop in 5-HT plasma level; this might favor the loss of tonus of extracranial arteries and the simultaneous capillary constriction that characterize the migraine attack (3,4). Migraine pain thus would result from the conjunction of the two factors already postulated by Wolff (20): hypotonicity and passive distension of an extracranial artery and, on the other hand, hypersensitivity of pain receptors in and around the wall of this same vessel (Fig. 1).

For the past several years, Sicuteri and his group (14–16) have been developing the hypothesis that migraine and other essential headaches result from a deficiency of brain 5-HT that would result in a lowering of the threshold for the central perception of pain. There is some evidence that 5-HT is acting in the brain as an inhibitor of nociceptive input. This theory is discussed elsewhere in this volume. In short, the peripheral and central theories are not incompatible; 5-HT disturbances can manifest themselves simulta-neously at a peripheral site—the cranial arteries—and in the brain centers.

REFERENCES

1. Anthony, M., Hinterberger, H., and Lance, J. W. (1969): The possible relationship of serotonin to the migraine syndrome. *Res. Clin. Stud. Headache,* 2:29–59.
2. Dalsgaard-Nielsen, T., and Genefke, I. K. (1974): Serotonin (5-hydroxytryptamine) release and uptake in platelets from healthy persons and migrainous patients in attack-free intervals. *Headache,* 14:26–32.
3. Fanchamps, A. (1974): The role of humoral mediators in migraine headache. *Can. J. Neurol. Sci.,* 1:189–195.
4. Lance, J. W. (1973): *The Mechanism and Management of Headache.* Butterworths, London.
5. Lance, J. W., Anthony, M., and Gonski, A. (1967): Serotonin, the carotid body, and cranial vessels in migraine. *Arch. Neurol.,* 16:553–558.

6. Mück-Šeler, D., Deanovic, Ž., and Dupelj, M. (1979): Platelet serotonin (5-HT) and 5-HT releasing factor in plasma of migrainous patients. *Headache,* 19:14–17.
7. Müller-Schweinitzer, E., and Weidmann, H. (1977): Regional differences in the responsiveness of isolated arteries from cattle, dog and man. *Agents Actions,* 7:383–389.
8. Ostfeld, A. M. (1959): Some aspects of cardiovascular regulation in man. *Angiology,* 10:34–42.
9. Ostfeld, A. M., Chapman, L. F., Goodell, H., and Wolff, H. G. (1957): Studies in headache. Summary of evidence concerning a noxious agent active locally during migraine headache. *Psychosom. Med.,* 19:199–208.
10. Rowley, D. A., and Benditt, E. P. (1956): 5-Hydroxytryptamine and histamine as mediators of the vascular injury produced by agents which damage mast cells in rats. *J. Exp. Med.,* 103:399–412.
11. Saxena, P. R., and De Vlaam-Schluter, G. M. (1974): Role of some biogenic substances in migraine and relevant mechanism in antimigraine action of ergotamine—Studies in an experimental model for migraine. *Headache,* 13:142–163.
12. Sicuteri, F. (1963): Prophylactic treatment of migraine by means of lysergic acid derivatives. *Triangle,* 6:116–125.
13. Sicuteri, F. (1966): Vasoneuroactive substances in migraine. *Headache,* 6:109 126.
14. Sicuteri, F. (1976): Hypothesis: Migraine, a central biochemical dysnociception. *Headache,* 16:145–159.
15. Sicuteri, F. (1979): The nature of pain in headache and central panalgesia. In: *Mechanisms of Pain and Analgesic Compounds,* edited by R. F. Beers, Jr. and E. G. Bassett, pp. 295–307. Raven Press, New York.
16. Sicuteri, F., Anselmi, B., and Fanciullacci, M. (1974): The serotonin (5-HT) theory of migraine. *Adv. Neurol.,* 4:383–394.
17. Sicuteri, F., Fanciullacci, M., Franchi, G., and Del Bianco, P. L. (1965): Serotonin-bradykinin potentiation on the pain receptors in man. *Life Sci.,* 4:309–316.
18. Sicuteri, F., Testi, A., and Anselmi, B. (1961): Biochemical investigations in headache: Increase in the hydroxyindoleacetic acid excretion during migraine attacks. *Int. Arch. Allergy Appl. Immunol.,* 19:55–58.
19. Spira, P. J., Mylecharane, E. J., and Lance, J. W. (1976): The effects of humoral agents and antimigraine drugs on the cranial circulation of the monkey. *Res. Clin. Stud. Headache,* 4:37–75.
20. Wolff, H. G. (1963): *Headache and Other Head Pain.* Oxford University Press, New York.

Advances in Neurology, Vol. 33, edited by
M. Critchley et al. Raven Press, New York © 1982

Impairment of Cerebral Serotonin and Energy Metabolism During Ischemia: Relevance to Migraine

K. M. A. Welch

Department of Neurology, Baylor College of Medicine, Neurosensory Center, Houston, Texas 77030

Decreased cerebral blood flow (CBF) has been reported during the prodrome of migraine (4). The cause of the flow decrease is popularly attributed to intracranial vasospasm, although a "steal" phenomenon between the extracranial and intracranial circulation has been proposed (13). The factor or factors that initiate the flow changes are unknown. This laboratory has reported cerebrospinal fluid (CSF) studies that indicated changes in central nervous system (CNS) energy and neurotransmitter metabolism during migraine and postulated that ischemia associated with the prodrome was responsible (15).

The purpose of the present study is to identify the metabolic changes in the brain during ischemia and reperfusion which could contribute to features of the migraine syndrome. To achieve this, the experimental model of transient cerebral ischemia in the gerbil has been studied. The findings are discussed particularly in relation to the role of serotonin and other neurotransmitters in the pathogenesis of migraine.

MATERIALS AND METHODS

Adult male and female Mongolian gerbils *(Meriones unguiculatus)* weighing 50 to 80 g were lightly anesthetized with ether A midline cervical incision was made, and the common carotid arteries (CCA) were exposed. Either the right or both CCA were occluded by the application of miniaturized Heifetz aneurysm clips. The animals were allowed to recover from anesthesia; those exhibiting the behavioral signs of ischemia, previously reported (14), were studied. The clips were removed after 10- to 30-min periods of occlusion. Reflow in the carotid artery was confirmed visually.

For the purpose of brain tissue studies, groups of animals were killed under liquid nitrogen immediately before removal of carotid occlusion and at intervals during reflow of up to 60 min. Samples of the cortices then were analyzed for energy metabolites, cyclic nucleotides, monoamines, and protein using established methodologies previously reported (9,14). Data were subjected to analysis of variance and Student's *t*-test. A *p* value of less than 0.05 was regarded as significant.

RESULTS

Decrease of ATP and phosphocreatine (PCr) and increase of AMP was observed during ischemia (Fig. 1). Both ATP and PCr rebounded rapidly after reflow to levels well above control. An initial although transient increase of ADP levels was probably related to recovery of AMP phosphorylation, since levels of the latter compound fell.

Brain glucose levels decreased during ischemia (Fig. 2); in the reflow period, however,

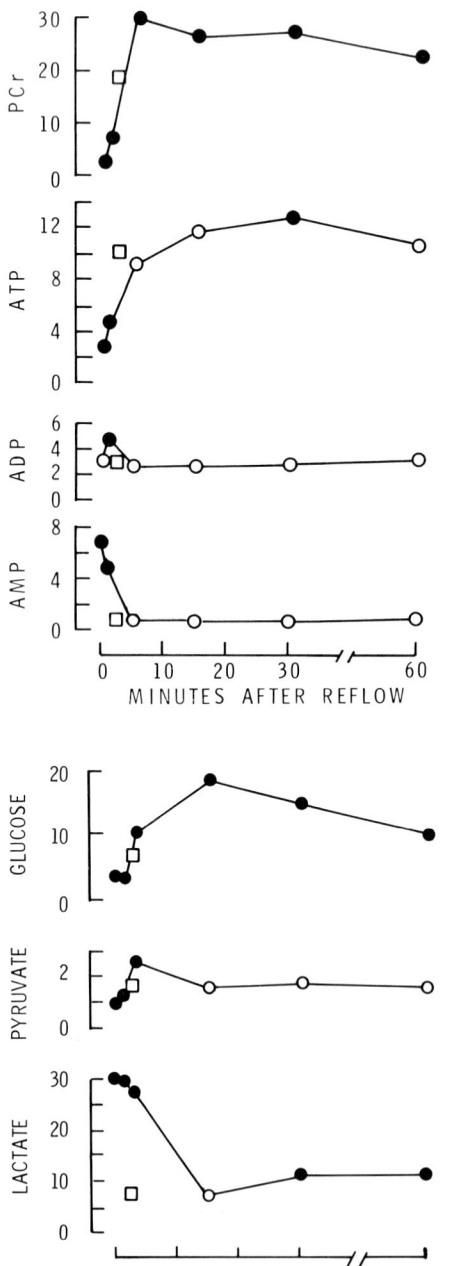

Fig. 1. Changes in cerebral cortex mean concentrations of PCr, ATP, ADP, and AMP during ischemia and reflow. Values are nmoles mg⁻¹ protein. *Filled circles,* changes significantly different from the mean *(open square)* of control sham-operated animals. Values at the zero time interval are at the end point of ischemia. *Open circles,* nonsignificant points.

Fig. 2. Changes in cerebral cortex mean concentrations of glucose, pyruvate, and lactate during ischemia and reflow. Values are nmoles mg⁻¹ protein. Symbols are as for Fig. 1.

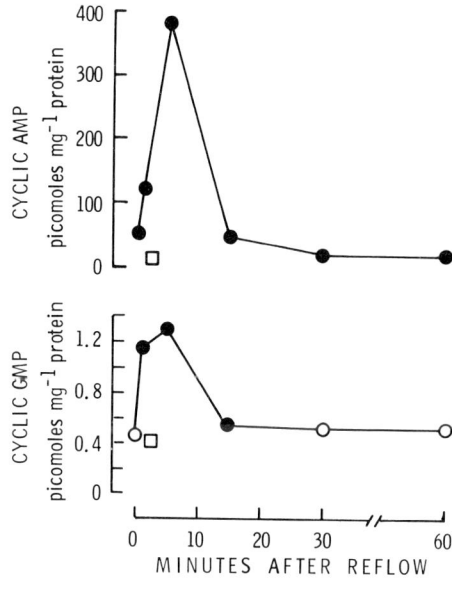

Fig. 3. Changes in cerebral cortex mean concentrations of cyclic AMP and cyclic GMP. Symbols are as for Fig. 1.

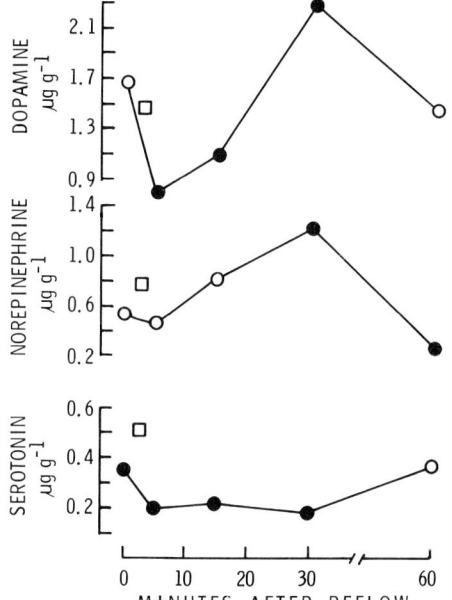

Fig. 4. Changes in cerebral cortex mean concentrations of monoamines during ischemia and reflow. Symbols are as for Fig. 1.

they increased to above control (see Fig. 2), coinciding with the high energy phosphate changes. Pyruvate levels were increased during ischemia but returned rapidly to control in the immediate reflow period (Fig. 2). Lactate levels, also high during ischemia, subsided during recovery but were still above control after 60 min of reflow.

Striking changes in cyclic nucleotide levels were recorded (Fig. 3). A three- to fivefold elevation in cyclic AMP levels during ischemia gave way to a 2,000-fold increase immediately upon reflow. Within 30 min, however, levels returned closer to control, although they remained elevated. Cyclic GMP levels were unaltered during ischemia but increased approximately fourfold in the first 15 min after reflow.

Depletion of 5-hydroxytryptamine (5-HT) occurred rapidly in ischemic brain and persisted throughout the reflow period (Fig. 4). Ischemia of up to 30 min duration produced no significant alteration in dopamine (DA) or norepinephrine levels. However, both catecholamines exhibited a marked rebound increase to above control levels after 30 min of reflow. That of DA followed an initial fall in level immediately upon removal of occlusion, which was presumably related to a washout of DA released during ischemia.

DISCUSSION

The factor or factors causing migraine are probably those that initiate the prodromal reduction of CBF. Some of the distressing clinical features of the syndrome, such as pain, nausea, and mental obtundation, could result from this flow decrease. The metabolic changes during ischemia and recovery must be known in order to support this concept. This discussion emphasizes not so much the mechanisms of the metabolic changes in ischemic brain as the possible relevance of these changes to clinical features of the migraine syndrome. Thus, the assumption is made that the metabolic changes in gerbil ischemic brain may resemble those in the human. The problems of making this assumption are accepted.

Ischemia

The induction of ischemia brought about changes in brain metabolism consistent with depletion of high energy phosphate reserves due to impaired oxidative phosphorylation plus a shift to anaerobic glycolysis causing tissue lactacidosis. Depletion of energy reserves leads to cellular changes manifested by neurological deficits and morphological abnormalities. Severe and prolonged ischemia leads to cerebral infarction. Although this is unusual in migraine, where ischemia is spontaneously reversible, cerebral infarction is recognized as a potential complication.

In this study, the neurotransmitter changes found during ischemia were limited to a rapid fall in 5-HT levels, probably due to release and synthesis inhibition. The relevance of this observation to migraine symptomatology is discussed below.

The reason for the spontaneous reversal of the ischemic phase of migraine is unknown. Large increases of two substances, lactate and cyclic AMP, however, take place in ischemic brain; both substances have vasodilator properties potentially capable of overcoming a vasoconstrictor influence (3,11).

Recovery

A puzzling aspect of reflow was the rebound increase in high energy phosphates. It is not clear whether this is due to a persisting neuronal depression with consequent decreased utilization of energy reserves or represents a form of reactive hypermetabolism. Brain glucose also reached greater than normal levels. Glucose uptake into brain is to an extent dependent on concentration gradients across the blood–brain barrier (BBB) (1); thus an increased blood glucose, perhaps as a result of stress, together with an impaired BBB caused by ischemia might be partly responsible for increased brain glucose.

The increased brain glucose may also be part of a metabolic adjustment related to enhanced anaerobic glycolysis; in the presence of above-normal high energy phosphate levels, this suggests a lack of glycolytic control. Tissue lactacidosis resulting from enhanced brain glucose utilization could be responsible for abnormally increased CBF and cerebral blood volume. The observation by Skinhøj (8) of lactate increase in CSF during migraine is relevant. Barbiturate treatment is somewhat protective against the effects of ischemia in experimental animals (10). Depression of neuronal function by this group of drugs decreases glucose utilization and tissue lactacidosis in ischemic tissue. These observations are interesting in view of the added benefit some patients gain from the addition of phenobarbital to ergot therapy for migraine headache.

A striking change in the immediate reflow period was the enormous further increase in cyclic AMP levels, coincidental with recovery of ATP. The amount of ATP available for synthesis of cyclic AMP was depleted during ischemia. Presumably, substances released during ischemia that stimulate adenyl cyclase (e.g., neurotransmitters, adenosine, and potassium) are still free to act when, in the reflow period, the availability of ATP increases. The later return to near normal levels of cyclic AMP probably indicates neuronal reuptake of these substances as brain energy status recovers. Similar mechanisms probably explain the less marked cyclic GMP changes, although substances that stimulate guanyl cyclase differ, e.g., acetylcholine and calcium. The cyclic AMP findings in this study add support to the postulate that the large increases of cyclic AMP found in the CSF of patients during a migraine headache might be related to the ischemic prodrome (15). The contribution of such changes to clinical features of the syndrome can be only speculative. The vasodilator influence of cyclic AMP has already been mentioned. Cyclic AMP, in increased amounts, can depress excitability of cortical neurons (9) and might be partly responsible for the mental obtundation, lethargy, and occasional electroencephalographic suppression during headache.

The Role of 5-HT

A profound depletion of 5-HT takes place in brain during ischemia and recovery. Pain supersensitivity related to depletion of 5-HT in the CNS is of importance in the migraine syndrome (6). In the rat, depletion of telencephalic 5-HT, either by ablative lesions of the medial forebrain bundle or by the inhibition of 5-HT synthesis with p-chlorophenylalanine (PCPA), results in increased pain sensitivity (2,12). Administration of PCPA to man also results in spontaneous pain syndromes (5). Depletion of brain 5-HT, secondary to the ischemic prodrome of migraine, could result in an enhancement of pain caused by dilatation and congestion of pain-sensitive vascular structures. Changes in central 5-HT also can be related to the disturbances of sleep, mood, temperature regulation, and appetite that may occur with the migraine syndrome.

Patients with migraine may have increased sensitivity of central DA receptors (7). This is based on an exaggerated propensity of migraineurs to develop headache and vomiting after being given either L-DOPA or the DA receptor agonist apomorphine. The rebound increase of brain DA during recovery from ischemia could also be considered to have a role in the production of similar symptoms during the migraine attack.

In conclusion, it should be borne in mind when searching for the cause of the multi-faceted syndrome of migraine that many aspects of the condition may be secondary to an ischemic prodrome. Thus it is reasonable to concentrate on the event that precipitates the ischemia.

ACKNOWLEDGMENTS

This work was supported in part by grant NS 09287 from the National Institute of Neurological and Communicative Disorders and Stroke, National Institutes of Health.

REFERENCES

1. Buschiazzo, P. M., Terrell, E. B., and Regen, D. M. (1970): Sugar transport across the blood-brain barrier. *Am. J. Physiol.,* 219:1503–1513.
2. Harvey, J. A., and Lints, C. E. (1965): Lesions in the medial forebrain bundle: Delayed effects on sensitivity to electric shock. *Science,* 148:250–252.
3. Meyer, J. S., and Welch, K. M. A. (1972): Relationship of cerebral blood flow and metabolism to neurological symptoms. In: *Progress in Brain Research, Vol. 35,* edited by J. S. Meyer and J. P. Schadé, pp. 285–347. Elsevier, Amsterdam.
4. O'Brien, M. D. (1971): Cerebral blood changes in migraine. *Headache,* 10:139–143.
5. Sicuteri, F. (1971): Pain syndrome in man following treatment with p-chlorophenylalanine. *Pharmacol. Res. Commun.,* 3:401–407.
6. Sicuteri, F. (1972): Headache as possible expression of deficiency of brain 5-hydroxytryptamine (central denervation supersensitivity). *Headache,* 12:69–71.
7. Sicuteri, F. (1977): Dopamine, the second putative protagonist in headache. *Headache,* 17:129–131.
8. Skinhøj, E. (1973): Hemodynamic studies within the brain during migraine. *Arch. Neurol.,* 29:95–98.
9. Skinner, J. E., Welch, K. M. A., Reed, J. C., and Nell, J. H. (1978): Psychological stress reduces cyclic 3′,5′-adenosine monophosphate levels in the cerebral cortex of conscious rats, as determined by a new cryogenic method of rapid tissue fixation. *J. Neurochem.,* 30:691–698.
10. Smith, A. L., Hoff, J. T., Nielsen, S. L., and Larson, C. P. (1974): Barbiturate protection in acute focal cerebral ischemia. *Stroke,* 5:1–7.
11. Tagashira, Y., Matsuda, M., Welch, K. M. A., Chabi, E., and Meyer, J. S. (1977): Effects of cyclic AMP and dibutyryl cyclic AMP on cerebral hemodynamics and metabolism in the baboon. *J. Neurosurg.,* 46:484–493.
12. Tenen, S. S. (1967): The effects of p-chlorophenylalanine, a serotonin depletor, on avoidance acquisition, pain sensitivity and related behavior in the rat. *Psychopharmacology (Berlin),* 10:204–219.
13. Welch, K. M. A., Spira, P. M., Knowles, L., and Lance, J. W. (1974): Effects of prostaglandins on the internal and external carotid blood flow in the monkey. *Neurology,* 24:705–710.
14. Welch, K. M. A., Chabi, E., Buckingham, J., Bergin, B., Achar, V. S., and Meyer, J. S. (1977): Catecholamine and 5-hydroxytryptamine levels in ischemic brain: Influence of p-chlorophenylalanine. *Stroke,* 8:341–346.
15. Welch, K. M. A., Chabi, E., Nell, J., Bartosh, K., Meyer, J. S., and Mathew, N. T. (1978): Similarities in biochemical effects of cerebral ischemia in patients with cerebrovascular disease and migraine. In: *Current Concepts in Migraine Research,* edited by R. Greene, pp. 1–8. Raven Press, New York.

Advances in Neurology, Vol. 33, edited by
M. Critchley et al. Raven Press, New York © 1982

Headaches and Transient Cerebral Ischemia: Comments on Welch's Report

Giuseppe Nappi and Giorgio Bono

Department of Neurology, Headache Center, University of Pavia School of Medicine, Pavia, Italy

Head pain, even when an obligatory phenomenon, represents one of the many clinical manifestations of primary headaches. Other functions, such as mood, sleep, appetite, and libido, may be involved. Sensory and motor function disturbances may precede or accompany headache attacks. These events in the CNS should not be ignored (14).

Headache studies initially were characterized by classifying descriptive aspects of the various symptoms. A more rational form of classification is proposed (15), in which, as a preliminary nosographic step, two subgroups of primary headache are identified: (a) those characterized by recurrent attacks, and (b) daily attacks (continuous or subcontinuous). In Fig. 1, the main clinical forms of headache are reported, regardless of their incidence.

Figure 2 reports the two spectrum diseases bordering on primary headaches: cerebro-

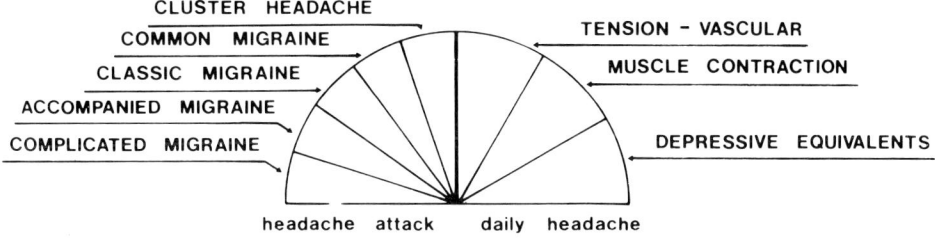

FIG. 1. Main clinical forms of headache, i.e., with recurrent or continuous attacks, are reported, independently from their incidence.

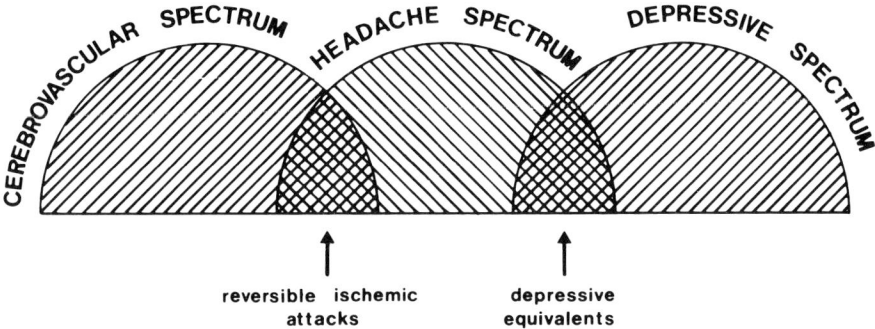

Fig. 2. Cerebrovascular and depressive diseases border with primary headache spectrum.

vascular disease (CVD) and affective disorders. Similarities and differences between migraine attacks and reversible ischemic attacks (RIAs) of CVD have been proposed (3,16).

According to Loeb (8), RIAs

> comprise two groups of cases: (a) transient ischemic attacks (TIAs), in which the focal symptoms last less than 24 hr, and (b) strokes with full recovery (SFR), in which full recovery takes place after more than 24 hr, often in a range of 3 weeks. The prerequisite for the definition of RIA still remains its complete reversibility.

RIAs are associated with a wide range of pathogenetic mechanisms, sometimes hemodynamic (i.e., recurring cardiac arrhythmias, orthostatic hypotension, carotid sinus hypersensitivity) and, more commonly, due to coagulation and platelet function disturbances. Atherothrombotic disease is the most frequent condition in which the platelet aggregation processes can play an etiologic role for cerebral ischemia (1).

Migraine can be defined as a familial disorder characterized by recurrent attacks of headache, commonly unilateral, and widely variable in intensity, frequency, and duration. In some cases, the attacks are preceded by, or associated with, neurological disturbances such as those observed in RIAs. Complicated migraine—a rare phenomenon—may lead to permanent ischemic damage (12).

An altered pain threshold due to a monoamine and neuropeptide genetic dysfunction at the level of specific areas of the central nervous system (CNS) has been proposed as a possible cause of primary headache. The experiments of Welch *(this volume)* and Mrsulja et al. (11) have demonstrated neurotransmitter depletion after experimental vascular occlusion and emphasize the similarities of rCBF and biochemical changes observed in migraine as well as in ischemic CVD (ICVD).

Cerebral ischemia can provoke disorders in neurotransmitter function, inducing an attack of migraine headache. The question then arises: are the ischemic attacks of CVD significantly preceded or accompanied by migraine-like headache? The results furnished by the various studies (4–7,9,10) are not in agreement (Table 1); however, some are prospective and others retrospective.

Our data concern 42 male subjects affected with RIAs. The cases were studied by means of a protocol of the Italian National Research Council (Finalized Program on Cerebral Atherosclerosis, directed by C. Fieschi, Rome). At the 18-month control point, headache as a symptom of ischemic events was found in 43% of the cases (Table 2), while of all patients, only 7 to 9% showed previous symptoms of family history of

TABLE 1. *Incidence of headache ICVD*

Reference	Tia (%)		Tia/infarct (%)		Infarct (%)	
	Carotid	VB	Carotid	VB	Carotid	VB
Mohr et al. (10)				9		
Fischer (6)			31	42		
Edmeads and Barnet (5)			35	51		
Grindal and Toole (7)		25				
Medina et al. (9)		64				
Edmeads (4)	26	17			25	27

TIA, transient ischemic attack; VB, vertebrobasilar system.

TABLE 2. *Headache and RIA: A prospective study*

System	Total population	RIA with headache	
		No.	%
Carotid	24	9	37
VB	18	9	50
Total	42	18	43

VB, Vertebrobasilar system.

headache. In the past, the main pathogenetic hypotheses formulated for headaches due to ischemia were: hypertension, ischemic edema, and collateral circulation development.

Table 3 shows that no correlation has been found between the occurrence of headache and hypertension, computed tomography (CT) findings of focal edema, and angiographic evidence of collateral circulation. Instead, considering the possible pathogenetic factors for ischemia, a lower incidence in RIAs without evidence of atherosclerotic (ATS) lesions can be found. This observation agrees with the opinion of Edmeads (4) concerning the relevant role of platelet aggregation and release reaction (platelet hypothesis) in these types of headache. The platelet disorder, in fact, is more important in atherothrombotic disease than in others. Only 20% of our patients showed an increased spontaneous aggregation rate (2), which was equally distributed in both RIA groups.

The phenomena examined are undoubtedly complex, as are the proposed pathogenetic mechanisms. Even for headaches due to ischemia, however, the central antinociception theory (15) may be accepted as a useful model for future studies.

The tendency to react to various trigger factors of headache represents a biological (or psychobiological) trait. This trait can be genetically determined (as in certain inherited migraine forms) or acquired during one's life (as with certain chronic posttraumatic headaches) (13). Considering the negative precedents for headache in these patients, another question arises: can atherothrombotic disease lead to a dysfunction of central

TABLE 3. *Correlation between RIA with or without headache and the main pathogenetic hypothesis of headache due to ischemia*

	RIA with headache ($N = 18$)		RIA without headache ($N = 24$)	
	No.	%	No.	%
Hypertension	10	56	6	25
CT focal edema	8	44	9	37
Angiographic findings				
Collateral circulation	2	11	2	8
ATS lesions[a]	11	61	5	21
No ATS lesions[b]	3	17	10	42
ATS and no ATS lesions	3	17	7	29
Normal	1	5	2	8
Platelet hyperaggregation[c]	4	22	5	21

[a] Occlusion, stenosis, atheromatic plaques or other signs.
[b] Arterial abnormalities in size, origin, distribution; mitral prolapse; osteoarthritis.
[c] From Breddin et al. (2).

pain threshold or determine the tendency to react with head pain to various trigger events, including RIAs?

Research is necessary. The postischemic changes in neurotransmitters demonstrated by Welch suggest that these changes can play a role in the pathogenesis of headaches symptomatic of ICVD. This experimental evidence stresses the role of RIAs as a clinical model for investigating the correlation between headache and cerebral ischemia.

REFERENCES

1. Barnet, H. J. M. (1979): Recent intervention studies on platelet suppressant drugs in cerebral ischemia—Clinical aspect. In: *Drug Treatment and Prevention in Cerebrovascular Disorders,* edited by G. Tognoni and G. Garattini, pp. 369–386. Elsevier, Amsterdam.
2. Breddin, K., Krzywanek, H. J., Zieman, J., Bayer, H., and Grün, H. (1977): Enhanced platelet aggregation as a risk factor for progress and complications of vascular disease. New findings with a platelet aggregation test and on the dependence of different aggregation tests on morphologic platelet changes. In: *Platelet Aggregation in the Pathogenesis of Cerebrovascular Disorders,* edited by A. Agnoli and C. Fazio, pp. 44–62. Springer-Verlag, Berlin.
3. Edmeads, J. (1979): Vascular headaches and the cranial circulation. Another look. *Headache,* 19:127–132.
4. Edmeads, J. (1979): The headaches of ischemic cerebrovascular disease. *Headache,* 19:345–349.
5. Edmeads, J., and Barnet, H. J. M. (1973): La cephalea en las affeciones cerebrovasculares occlusivas. In: *Cephaleas y Jacquecas,* edited by A. P. Friedman and G. F. Poch, pp. 89–100. Eudeba, Buenos Aires.
6. Fischer, C. M. (1968): Headache in cerebrovascular disease. In: *Handbook of Clinical Neurology,* edited by P. J. Vinken and G. W. Bruyn, pp. 124–156. North-Holland, Amsterdam.
7. Grindal, A., and Toole, J. (1974): Headache and transient ischemic attacks. *Stroke,* 5:603–606.
8. Loeb, C. (1979): Clinical evaluation of patients with transient ischemic attacks. In: *Cerebrovascular Disorders and Stroke,* edited by M. Goldstein, L. Bolis, C. Fieschi, S. Gorini, and C. H. Millikan, pp. 141–148. Raven Press, New York.
9. Medina, J., Diamond, S., and Rubino, S. (1975): Headaches in patients with transient ischemic attacks. *Headache,* 15:194–197.
10. Mohr, J. P., Caplan, L. R., Melski, J. W., Goldstein, R. J., Duncan, G. W., Kistler, J. P., Pessin, M. S., and Bleich, H. L. (1978): The Harvard cooperative stroke registry: A prospective registry. *Neurology (Minneap.),* 28:754–762.
11. Mrsulja, B. B., Mrsulja, B. J., Spatz, M., and Klatzo, I. (1976): Brain serotonin after experimental vascular occlusion. *Neurology (Minneap.),* 26:785–787.
12. Otis, S. M., Smith, R. A., Kroll, D. D., Krasny, S. E., Seltzer, K. A., and Dalessio, D. J. (1979): Vasospasm and vascular headaches: Selective vasoconstriction in the carotid vascular system measured by the Doppler ophthalmic method in migraineurs. *Headache,* 19:200–203.
13. Savoldi, F., and Nappi, G. (editors) (1979): *Headache Pavia 1979.* Tipo-litografica, Palladio, Vicenza.
14. Savoldi, F., and Nappi, G. (1979): Contributo all'identificazione di sottogruppi di cefalee primarie. In: *XXI Congr. Soc. Italiana Neurol.,* pp. 145–181, Catania, 8–10 Novembre (Atti).
15. Sicuteri, F. (editor) (1977): *Headache New Vistas.* Biomedical Press, Florence.
16. Welch, K. M. A., Chabi, E., Mell, J., Bartosh, K., and Meyer, L. S. (1976): Similarities in biochemical effects of cerebral ischemia in patients with cerebrovascular disease and migraine. In: *The Migraine Trust International Symposium,* p. 2. London, September 16–17, (Abstracts).

Advances in Neurology, Vol. 33, edited by
M. Critchley et al. Raven Press, New York © 1982

Serotonin and Cyclic Nucleotides in Migraine

Michael Anthony

Division of Neurology, The Prince Henry Hospital, Sydney, Australia

The migraine attack is known to be associated with dilatation of the cranial vessels, increased cerebral blood flow, and impaired autoregulation of the cerebral circulation (20). These changes have been attributed to the withdrawal of the vasotonic influence of serotonin on these vessels (3); there is general agreement that the migraine attack is associated with release of the amine from platelets (2,7,13,18). The mechanism of serotonin release remains unresolved, although it is likely caused by a plasma-releasing factor. Free fatty acids (FFA) have been suggested for this role; the migraine attack is accompanied by a significant rise of these acids in plasma, and some are known to release serotonin from platelets both *in vivo* and *in vitro* (1). The release of FFA during migraine is probably the result of catecholamine release due to sympathetic overactivity, since the most common precipitant of a migraine is stress, mental or physical; and plasma levels of these amines, as well as adenosine 3'5'-monophosphate (cAMP), rise significantly under such circumstances.

Monitoring functional cardiovascular parameters or plasma catecholamine levels as an index of sympathetic activity has generally been unrewarding, at least in migraine. On the other hand, monitoring several biochemical parameters, which are known to accompany catecholamine release, has been more satisfactory. As a result, the following three parameters were investigated.

Plasma cAMP

Catecholamines, particularly epinephrine, are known to stimulate the production of plasma cAMP, which may act as an index of catecholamine production (17).

Serum Dopamine Beta Hydroxylase Activity

Serum dopamine beta hydroxylase (DBH) catalyzes the conversion of dopamine to norepinephrine. The amount of DBH released via exocytosis from sympathetic nerve endings upon stimulation is known to parallel the amount of released norepinephrine (23). Furthermore, DBH appears to be present in some abundance in human cerebral vessels; there is proof that acute changes in its serum levels are an accurate index of sympathetic activity (24).

Total and Individual Plasma FFA

Catecholamines are probably the most potent releasers of FFA from storage sites. A rise in plasma levels of FFA probably reflects catecholamine action.

TABLE 1. *Changes in plasma cAMP, serum DBH, platelet serotonin, and plasma FFA during migraine headache*

Parameter investigated	No. of patients	Pre-HA[a]	HA	Post-HA	% Change
Plasma cAMP (pmoles/ml)	10	19.9	41.3	30.8	107.5
Serum DBH (% change from headache-free period)	20	112.0	147.7	138.1	31.9
Platelet serotonin (ng/10^9 platelets)	20	492	318	455	35.4
Plasma FFA (nmoles/ml)	10				
Total acids		340	485	322	42.6
Stearic		115.9	157.6	111.2	36.0
Palmitic		83.2	150.0	91.4	80.9
Oleic		143.0	278.8	156.3	95.0
Linoleic		41.3	98.1	72.6	135.8

[a] Pre-HA, preheadache period; HA, headache period; post-HA, postheadache period.

PATIENTS AND METHODS

Twenty patients suffering from frequent attacks of migraine were hospitalized for biochemical investigations. All forms of medication were suspended for 3 days before commencement of the study. Blood was collected three times daily before and after the migraine attack and every 4 hr throughout the period of the headache. Plasma cyclic AMP was estimated by the method of Frandsen and Krishna (11) using New England Nuclear cAMP (125) RIA, Kit. Total plasma FFA were estimated by alkali titration (22) and individual FFA by organic extraction and gas liquid chromatography (1). Serum DBH was assessed radiometrically (12) and platelet serotonin by a fluorometric technique (6).

Plasma cAMP and total and individual FFA were estimated in 10 patients. The above, together with serum DBH and platelet serotonin, were estimated in all 20 patients.

RESULTS

Statistically significant elevations during migraine were recorded in (a) plasma cAMP in nine of 10 patients, (b) total plasma FFA in eight of 10 patients, (c) individual plasma FFA, stearic, and palmitic acids in nine of 10 patients, and oleic and linoleic acids in all 10 patients, and (d) serum DBH in 19 of 20 patients. A statistically significant fall in platelet serotonin was noted in 18 of 20 patients. The results are summarized in Table 1.

DISCUSSION

It is generally accepted that β-adrenoreceptor stimulation leads to increased synthesis of cAMP. Thus intravenous infusion of norepinephrine causes much smaller changes in plasma cAMP than epinephrine in similar concentrations, and pure β-adrenergic stimulation increases plasma cAMP, whereas pure α-adrenergic stimulation increases plasma cGMP (15). Similarly, during surgery in humans, there was a significant and parallel increase in plasma concentration of both plasma epinephrine and cAMP, whereas little change was noted in plasma norepinephrine (17).

The mechanism of release of cAMP into plasma remains conjectural. Plasma concentrations of hormones or neurotransmitters may alter the intracellular concentration of the nucleotide or cell membrane permeability (16). One would expect that the intracellular concentration of cAMP would reflect more hormonal or neurotransmitter stimulation than would plasma levels. The action of these two groups of substances, however, occasionally develops with only minimal changes in tissue cAMP. In fact, increases so slight as to be barely detectable were recorded in the tissue content of cAMP when epinephrine, isoproterenol, or glucagon caused marked changes in carbohydrate metabolism in perfused liver and in isolated hepatic cells (9). It has been estimated that isoproterenol injections into rats in doses that failed to induce detectable increases in cAMP in the liver and muscles resulted in a fourfold increase in plasma cAMP (19). Therefore, the generation of "functioning" cAMP at an intracellular site might be reflected in an increase of plasma cAMP rather than its tissue content. Since endogenous catecholamines lead to a rise in plasma cAMP (15,17), estimation of plasma levels could serve as an index of adrenergic activity rather than estimation of catecholamine metabolites; (a) plasma cAMP estimation is simpler and more accurate; and (b) plasma levels of cAMP reflect β-adrenoreceptor-mediated action of catecholamines rather than their amounts in circulation. As a result, a closer correlation with cardiovascular and metabolic changes could be induced by catecholamines (21).

Another group of substances that affect the activity of adenyl cyclase are the prostaglandins of the E series (PGE). In low concentrations, PGE_1 stimulates the enzyme in a number of tissues, e.g., platelets, leading to a rise of cAMP; PGE_2 lowers cAMP (4). With respect to platelet function, inhibition of platelet aggregation by PGE_1 is mediated by cAMP; in the absence of this inhibitory agonist, the cAMP concentration in platelets is insufficient to exert any appreciable effect on platelet response.

The migraine attack is associated with reduced plasma levels of serotonin and the platelet release reaction (3,8). Furthermore, platelet aggregation is enhanced during the prodromal and the headache phases of the migrainous episode (8). At the same time, platelet aggregability to adenosine diphosphate (ADP) is increased during headache-free intervals, and there is a lower threshold for the platelet release reaction (5,8). It is not unreasonable to suggest that the high levels of plasma FFA are responsible for the changes observed in the platelets. FFA are capable of inducing the platelet reaction and also can be responsible for the accelerated synthesis of prostaglandins, particularly of the E series, which are potent vasodilating agents and which at the same time could be responsible for the reduced platelet aggregation observed during the latter part of the attack (8).

Plasma levels of both epinephrine and norepinephrine have been found to be increased 3 hr before nocturnal migraine attacks (14) and those of norepinephrine toward the later stages of the headache (10). Because DBH and catecholamines are released simultaneously from sympathetic nerve endings and the chromaffin cells of the adrenal medulla, it is not surprising that the majority of patients in this study showed a significant rise of serum DBH during the migraine attack.

CONCLUSIONS

The results reported in this study can be summarized as follows. Catecholamine release, as suggested by the raised levels of plasma cAMP and serum DBH, is induced by sympathetic stimulation as a result of emotional or physical stress. This leads to release of FFA; acting as releasers of platelet serotonin, they are responsible for the platelet release reaction. Simultaneously, by raising the levels of linoleic acid, FFA lead to accelerated formation of prostaglandins, the E series of which cause vascular dilatation. The combined effect of reduced vasotonic influence of serotonin and the vasodilating influence of prostaglandins leads to significant dilatation of the cranial arteries and the headache of the migraine attack.

REFERENCES

1. Anthony, M. (1978): The role of individual free fatty acids in migraine. *Res. Clin. Stud. Headache,* 6:110–116.
2. Anthony, M., Hinterberger, H., and Lance, J. W. (1969): The possible relationship of serotonin to the migraine syndrome. *Res. Clin. Stud. Headache,* 2:29–59.
3. Anthony, M., and Lance, J. W. (1975): The role of serotonin in migraine. In: *Modern Topics in Migraine,* edited by J. Pearce, pp. 107–123. Heinemann, London.
4. Bitensky, M. W., Keins, J. I., and Freeman, J. (1973): Cyclic adenine monophosphate and clinical medicine. Part 1. *Am. J. Med. Sci.,* 266:321–346.
5. Couch, J. R., and Hassanein, R. S. (1977): Platelet aggregability in migraine. Neurology, 27:843–848.
6. Crawford, H., and Rudd, B. T. (1962): A spectrofluorometric method for the determination of serotonin (5-hydroxytryptamine) in plasma. *Clin. Chim. Acta,* 7:114–121.
7. Curran, A. D., Hinterberger, H., and Lance, J. W. (1965): Total plasma serotonin, 5-hydroxyindoleacetic acid and p-hydroxy-m-methoxymandelic acid excretion in normal and migrainous subjects. *Brain,* 88:997–1010.
8. Deshmukh, S. V., and Meyer, J. S. (1977): Cyclic changes in platelet dynamics and the pathogenesis and prophylaxis of migraine. *Headache,* 17:101–108.
9. Exton, J. H., and Harper, S. C. (1975): Role of cyclic AMP in the actions of catecholamines on hepatic carbohydrate metabolism. *Adv. Cyclic Nucleotide Res.,* 5:519–528.
10. Fog-Moller, F., Genefke, I. K., and Bryndum, B. (1978): Changes in concentration of catecholamines in blood during spontaneous migraine attacks and reserpine-induced attacks. In: *Current Concepts in Migraine Research,* edited by R. Greene, pp. 115–119. Raven Press, New York.
11. Frandsen, E. K., and Krishna, G. J. (1976): A simple ultrasensitive method for the assay of cyclic AMP and cyclic GMP in tissues. *Life Sci.,* 18:529–541.
12. Henry, D. P., Johnson, D. G., Starman, B. J., and Williams, R. H. (1975): Kinetic characterization of rat serum dopamine-B-hydroxylase using a simplified radioenzyme assay. *Life Sci.,* 17:1,179–1,186.
13. Hilton, B. P., and Cumings, J. N. (1972): 5-Hydroxytryptamine levels and platelet aggregation responses in subjects with acute migraine headache. *J. Neurol. Neurosurg. Psychiatry,* 35:505–509.
14. Hsu, L. K. G., Crisp, A. H., Kalucy, R. S., Koval, J., Chen, C. M., Carruthers, M., and Zilkha, K. J. (1977): Early morning migraine, nocturnal plasma levels of catecholamines, tryptophan, glucose and free fatty acids and sleep encephalography. *Lancet,* 1:447–450.
15. Kunitada, S., Honna, M., and Ui, M. (1978): Increases in plasma cyclic AMP dependent on endogenous catecholamines. *Eur. J. Pharmacol.,* 48:159–169.
16. Mjos, O. D., Vik-Mo, H., Henden, T., and Wang, H. (1977): Increased plasma cyclic AMP concentrations in fasting man. *Scand. J. Clin. Lab. Invest.,* 37:439–442.
17. Nistrup Madsen, S., Fog-Moller, F., Christiansen, C., Vester-Adersen, T., and Enquist, A. (1978): Cyclic AMP, adrenaline and noradrenaline in plasma during surgery. *Br. J. Surg.,* 65:191–193.
18. Rydzcwski, W., and Wachowicz, B. (1978): Adenine nucleotides in platelets in and between migraine attacks. In: *Current Concepts in Migraine Research,* edited by R. Greene, pp. 153–158. Raven Press, New York.
19. Saitoh, Y., and Ui, M. (1976): Stimulation of glycogenolysis and gluconeogenesis by epinephrine independent of its B-stimulation in perfused liver. *Biochem. Pharmacol.,* 25:841–849.
20. Sakai, F., and Meyer, J. S. (1978): Regional cerebral haemodynamics during migraine and cluster headache by the 133 Xc inhalation method. *Headache,* 18:122–132.
21. Strange, R. C., Rowe, M. J., Mjos, O. D., and Oliver, M. F. (1976): The effect of antilipolytic agents on cyclic AMP, free fatty acids and total catecholamine concentration in plasma. *Acta Med. Scand.,* 199:421–424.

22. Trout, D. N., Estes, E. A., and Friedberg, S. J. (1960): Titration of free fatty acids of plasma: A study of current methods and a new modification. *J. Lipid Res.,* 1:199–202.
23. Weinshilboum, R. M., Thoa, N. B., Johnson, D. G., Kopin, I. J., and Axelrod, J. (1971): Proportional release of norepinephrine and dopamine-B-hydroxylase from sympathetic nerves. *Science,* 174:1,349–1,351.
24. Wooten, G. F., and Cardon, P. V. (1973): Plasma dopamine-B-hydroxylase activity. *Arch. Neurol.,* 28:103–106.

Advances in Neurology, Vol. 33, edited by
M. Critchley et al. Raven Press, New York © 1982

Rheumatic Pain Modulation Syndrome: The Interrelationships Between Sleep, Central Nervous System Serotonin, and Pain

Harvey Moldofsky

Department of Psychiatry, Toronto Western Hospital, Toronto, Ontario, Canada

Clinical experience and recent research suggest a relationship between sleep and pain. Most of us experience sleep to be refreshing, but sometimes we awaken in the morning feeling miserable, worse than on the previous evening. We might have slept in an uncomfortable position, perhaps disturbed by noise or worried about some personal matter. Fortunately, this "flu-like" miserable feeling—i.e., headache, generalized muscle aching, stiffness, loss of appetite, tiredness, lethargy, nervousness, and irritability—readily passes; but these noxious symptoms are common and particularly troublesome in certain clinical populations, specifically those who suffer acutely from migraine and chronically from fibrositis syndromes.

Approximately 30 years ago, Gans (5) drew attention to these symptoms in migraine patients. He observed, as did his predecessors, that migraine patients often complained of their neurasthenic symptoms upon awakening. He speculated that the symptoms were provoked by sleep disturbance. A similar situation is found in those who suffer from fibrositis syndrome, who complain chronically of widespread and variable musculoskeletal aching and stiffness, localized areas of tenderness (Fig. 1), easy fatigability,

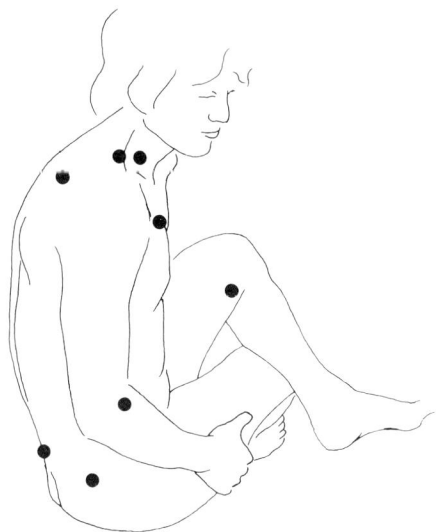

FIG. 1. Location of typical sites of deep tenderness in fibrositis. (Reproduced from ref. 27, with kind permission of H. A. Smythe and W. B. Saunders Company, Ltd.)

emotional distress (nervousness, irritability, and perhaps sadness), and light, restless sleep with intensification of their symptoms upon awakening in the morning. No biochemical, serologic, inflammatory, or structural pathology can be attributed to those symptoms (27,28). In both these disorders, recent studies suggest that sleep physiology and biogenic amine metabolism are important in influencing pain perception.

SLEEP AND MIGRAINE

Studies of sleep in patients predisposed to nocturnal headaches have shown that rapid eye movement (REM) sleep is temporally related to attacks of migraine, cluster headaches, or chronic paroxysmal hemicrania. Dexter and Weitzman (3), Hsu et al. (8) and Kayed et al. (10) found that their patients awoke with headache attacks out of REM sleep or within 10 min of a REM episode. Sleep shift studies by Dexter (4) support the concept that these nocturnal headache attacks are linked to sleep and not to other components of the 24-hr cycle. These studies suggest that specific physiologic mechanisms during sleep contribute to triggering acute attacks of nocturnal headaches.

SLEEP AND FIBROSITIS SYNDROME

Studies of sleep physiology in patients with fibrositis syndrome suggest the importance of sleep in modulating pain perception. Such patients often report that major stressful life situations had occurred at the onset of their sleep disturbance and musculoskeletal pain symptoms. In a recent study (14), most patients showed an overnight increase in measures of muscle tenderness and a coincident physiologic sleep disturbance, i.e., alpha non-REM sleep (Fig. 2). To determine whether a specific sleep disturbance is important, the sleep of healthy volunteers was disturbed by exogenous or noise stimuli (15). By interrupting EEG sleep stage 4 or delta sleep (0.5 to 2.5 Hz; > 75 μV) in these subjects, musculoskeletal aching and fatigue symptoms emerged that were similar to those symptoms found in patients with fibrositis syndrome. Moreover, a comparable alpha EEG sleep physiologic disturbance was artificially produced (see Fig. 2). The syndrome did not occur with noise interruption of REM sleep; therefore, specific features of sleep physiology appear to modulate pain perception.

To test this theory, alpha EEG frequency during sleep, a presumed feature of arousal during sleep, should be associated with an overnight increase in pain and mood symptoms. On the other hand, delta or slow wave EEG sleep should be related to amelioration of symptoms. Indeed, evidence consistent with those hypotheses was provided by a study in which sleep physiology was manipulated by 100 mg chlorpromazine or 5 g. L-tryptophan given orally at bedtime (19). While chlorpromazine influenced improvement in slow wave sleep, pain, and mood symptoms, L-tryptophan had no such effect but did shorten the time to sleep onset. Computerized quantification of the alpha frequency (the mean percent time per minute or mean percent power per minute) during sleep correlated with overnight increase in pain measures, hostility, and decrease in energy. On the other hand, delta frequency in sleep (mean percent time per minute) was related to overnight decrease in pain; delta power (mean percent power per minute) was related to overnight decreased anxiety, hostility, and increase in energy. Other EEG frequencies up to 30 Hz were not related to changes in these symptoms.

In another study of 18 patients with rheumatoid arthritis, a similar alpha EEG anomaly was found together with overnight increase in peripheral joint tenderness in both hands and in musculoskeletal tenderness (17). Grip strength, energy, anxiety, and hostility declined overnight. During the 2-week study period, one person experienced remission in joint and muscle symptoms while receiving acetylsalicylic acid. The EEG alpha frequency fell from a mean of 20% per minute during the initial 4 nights when he was acutely ill to 8% per minute on the last 2 nights 2 weeks later. Conversely, his delta frequency went from 30 to 41% per minute. The study suggests that intrusion of articular pain stimuli during sleep might induce physiologic arousal, as evidenced by the alpha EEG sleep anomaly and then subsequent morning nonarticular musculoskeletal aching, stiffness, and fatigue typical of the so-called fibrositis syndrome. Likely, there are other specific situations that evolve into this final common symptom pathway; for example, alcohol and opiate dependency withdrawal states and nocturnal myoclonus (which have been reported to be associated with the alpha sleep anomaly) may be associated with nonrestorative sleep and similar rheumatic pain symptoms.

These studies do not suggest that the alpha EEG sleep anomaly is necessarily or specifically involved in the emergence of chronic pain and fatigue. The sleep alpha frequency might serve simply as an indicator of a neurophysiologic arousal system within sleep. The studies do suggest that sleep physiology serves as a modulating influence on the noxious subjective experiences in patients with migraine and nonarticular and articular rheumatic disease. Furthermore, the constellation of nonrestorative sleep disturbance and overnight increase in musculoskeletal aching and stiffness, and subsequent daytime fatigue and emotional distress suggest a specific syndrome, the rheumatic pain modulation syndrome.

No explanation exists regarding how sleep physiology influences other features of the syndrome. However, studies of biogenic amine metabolism in migraine and fibrositis patients suggest that a metabolic transformation occurs within the nervous system that mediates the perception of pain. Evidence for the role of central nervous system (CNS) serotonin and pain perception in man comes from incidental observations by Van Woert and Sethy (33) and a series of studies on migraine or idiopathic headaches by Sicuteri and colleagues (24,25) and Hyyppa and Kangasniemi (9). Van Woert and Sethy (33) noted that a patient with postanoxic encephalopathy and myoclonus experienced spontaneous disappearance of generalized pain with L-5-hydroxytryptophan and a peripheral decarboxylase inhibitor. Sicuteri (24) observed a pain syndrome comparable to that found in fibrositis patients following the administration of ρ-chlorophenylalanine (PCPA). PCPA inhibits brain serotonin synthesis in animals. The drug was given for attempted prophylaxis against migraine. Sicuteri found that after PCPA was given, patients experienced pain in the muscles of the upper and lower limbs, trunk, scalp, and face. As in the fibrositis patients, the symptoms increased with physical effort and did not reflect active rheumatic disease. The symptoms disappeared when PCPA was stopped and recurred when the drug was administered again. Sicuteri suggested that this pain syndrome resulted from a deficiency of brain serotonin.

An inverse relationship between brain serotonergic activity and pain has been demonstrated in several animal studies. These studies have shown increased pain responsivity with neural lesion and pharmacologic and dietary depletion of brain serotonin (6,7,13,-22,31). On the other hand, decreased pain reactivity accompanies increased brain serotonin activity (1,7,13,20,23). The analgesic effect of narcotics is potentiated by serotonin precursors (2,12) and reduced by serotonin depletors (32). To translate these studies on brain serotonin metabolism and pain in man is not possible, but indirect approaches may be possible. Positive relationships have been demonstrated among plasma-free trypto-

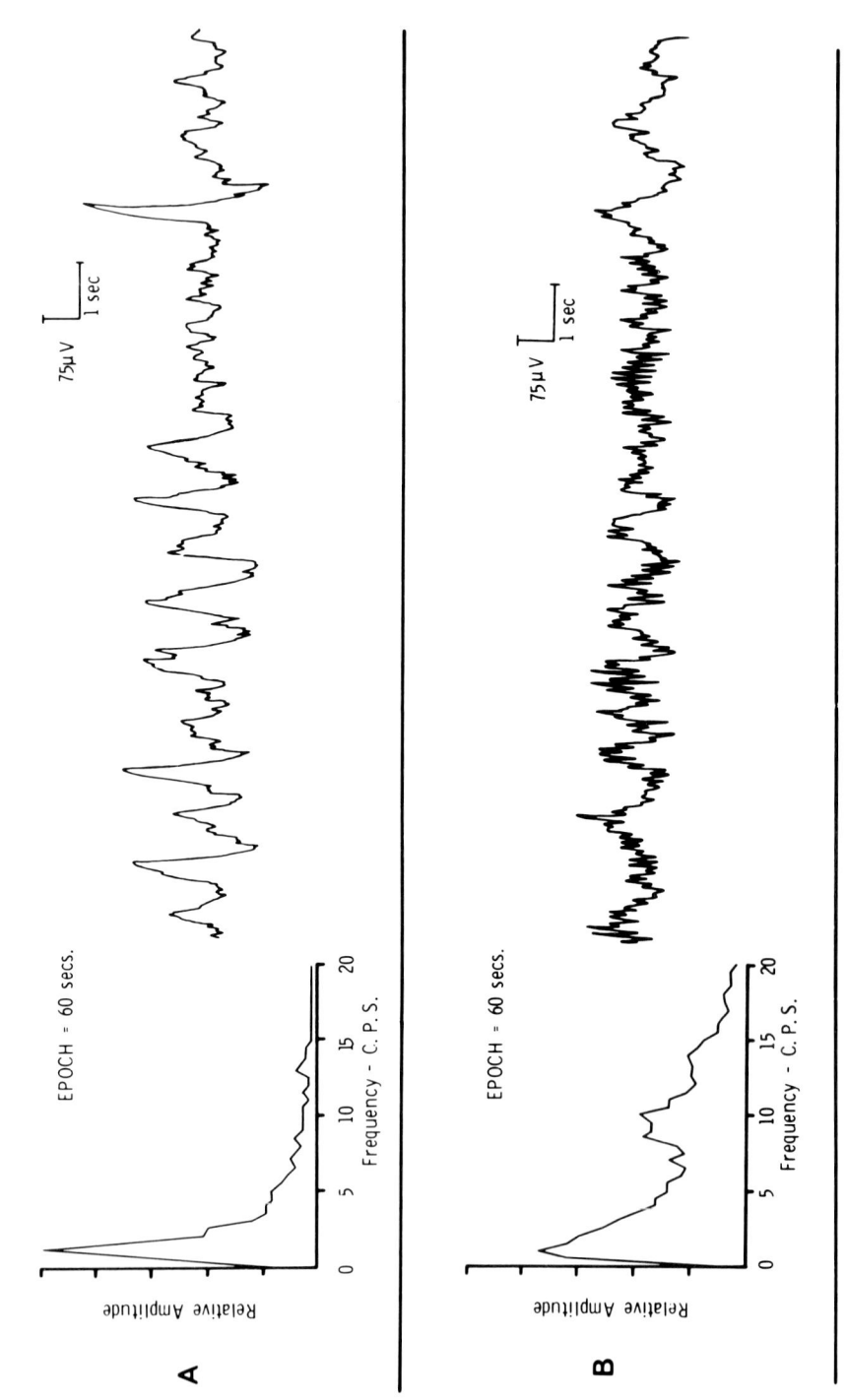

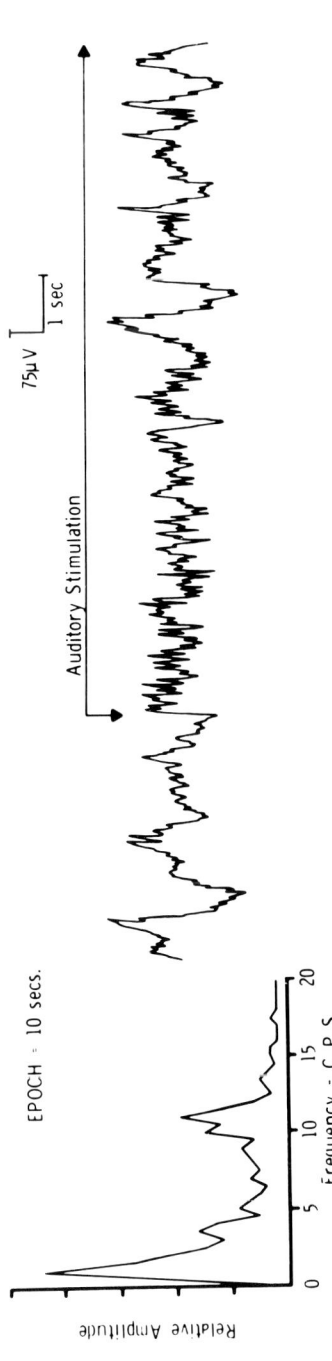

FIG. 2. Frequency spectra and raw EEG from **(A)** NREM (stage 4) sleep in a healthy 25-year-old subject. The spectrum shows that most amplitude is concentrated at 1 Hz (delta). **(B)** NREM sleep in a 42-year-old fibrositis patient. The spectrum shows amplitude at both 1 Hz (delta) and 8 to 10 Hz (alpha). **(C)** NREM sleep of a healthy 21-year-old subject during stage 4 sleep deprivation. There is a clear association between external arousal (auditory stimulation) and alpha onset in the EEG. Again, the frequency spectrum (obtained by 10-sec analysis from stimulus onset) shows amplitude concentrated in the delta and alpha bands. (Reproduced from ref. 15, with kind permission of The American Psychosomatic Society, Inc. and Elsevier North Holland, Inc.)

phan, brain tryptophan, and brain serotonin in studies in rats (11,29,30). Presuming that these relationships are applicable to man, then recent studies on plasma-free and bound tryptophan in migraine and fibrositis syndromes suggest a metabolic disorder of brain serotonin.

Moldofsky and Warsh (16) have shown that plasma-free tryptophan is inversely related to the subjective morning pain of fibrositis patients. Salmon et al. (21) found that the plasma-free tryptophan and the percent of plasma-free tryptophan/total plasma trypto-phan were significantly higher during migraine attacks. Hyyppa and Kangasniemi (9) found a similar but not significant increase in plasma-free tryptophan during the early headache stage. The total plasma tryptophan was lower in those with daily headache. These authors propose that with migraine, there is a lowering of brain serotonin which may displace tryptophan from its binding to plasma albumin through an unknown feed-back mechanism. Alteration in the central nervous metabolism of other biogenic amines may also be involved. Hsu et al. (8), in their nocturnal study of migraine, found that plasma total catecholamine and norepinephrine were increased in the 3-hr period before awakening with headache. No differences were found in plasma tryptophan, glucose, insulin, and free fatty acid levels.

Moldofsky and Warsh (18) found no significant relationship between urinary methy-droxyphenyl glycol (MHPG), an alleged derivative of brain norepinephrine, and pain measures in fibrositis patients. Furthermore, 5 g L-tryptophan at bedtime had no signifi-cant effect on pain symptoms in these patients (19). The observations on biogenic amine metabolism are not uniform because of population and methodologic differences. Never-theless, these data do suggest that such brain biogenic monoamines as serotonin and norepinephrine that have been found to be significant to sleep physiology are also impor-tant in influencing or modulating pain.

Sicuteri (26) recently suggested the term "central panalgesia" to be applied to those patients with such widespread pain symptoms as those found in idiopathic headache, migraine, and the fibrositis syndrome. Central panalgesia implies that CNS dysfunction is involved in evoking a generalized pain experience; but generalized pain is not a charac-teristic feature. The pain involves the musculoskeletal system and not typically viscera; the term panalgesia, therefore, is not quite accurate.

The research on the roles of sleep physiology and CNS biogenic amine metabolism influencing or modulating headache and nonarticular and articular pain is consistent with factors involving brain dysfunction. Moreover, a variety of external physical stimuli (e.g., weather change, heat, transcutaneous nerve stimulation, acupuncture) and psycho-logic factors (cognitive, affective, psychologic secondary gain, and social influences) also modulate pain perception. Rheumatic pain modulation syndrome is suggested to encom-pass the variety of factors, e.g., sleep and neurochemical, psychologic, and physical factors) that influence the perception of pain in these musculoskeletal disorders.

ACKNOWLEDGMENTS

We acknowledge the assistance of F. Lue, H. Smythe, and J. Warsh, and the support of the Ontario Mental Health Foundation, grant 753–78/80.

REFERENCES

1. Buchel, L., Levy, J., and Tanguy, O. (1958): Sur la potentialisation de l'action analgesique de la l-methadone par la 5-hydroxytryptamine (serotonine). *C.R. Acad. Sci. (Paris),* 246:2,947–2,949.
2. Dewey, W. L., Harris, L. S., Howes, J. F., and Nuite, J. A. (1970): The effect of various neurohumoral

modulators on the activity of morphine and the narcotic antagonist in the tailflick and phenylquinone test. *J. Pharmacol. Exp. Ther.,* 175:435–442.

3. Dexter, J. D., and Weitzman, E. D. (1970): The relationship of nocturnal headaches to sleep stage patterns. *Neurology,* 20:513–518.

4. Dexter, J. D. (1974): Studies in nocturnal migraine. *Arch. Neurobiol.* [*Suppl.*], 37:281–300.

5. Gans, M. (1951): Migraine as a form of neurasthenia. *J. Nerv. Ment. Dis.,* 113:315–331.

6. Harvey, J. A., and Lints, C. E. (1965): Lesions in the medial forebrain bundle: Delayed effects on sensitivity to electric shock. *Science,* 148:250–252.

7. Harvey, J. A., Schlosberg, A. J., and Yunger, L. M. (1975): Behavioral correlates of serotonin depletion. *Fed. Proc.,* 34:1,796–1,801.

8. Hsu, L. K. G., Crisp, A. M., Kalucy, R. S., Koval, J., Chen, C. N. et al. (1977): Early morning migraine. Nocturnal plasma levels of catecholamines, tryptophan, glucose, and free fatty acids, and sleep encephalographs. *Lancet,* 1:447–451.

9. Hyyppa, M. T., and Kangasniemi, P. (1977): Variation of plasma free tryptophan and CSF 5-HIAA during migraine. *Headache,* 17:25–27.

10. Kayed, K., Godtlibsen, O. B., and Sjaastad, O. (1978): Chronic paroxysmal hemicrania IV. "Rem Sleep Locked" nocturnal headache attacks. *Sleep,* 1:91–95.

11. Knott, P. J., and Curzon, G. (1972): Free tryptophan in plasma and brain tryptophan metabolism. *Nature,* 239:452–453.

12. Major, C. T., and Pleuvry, B. J. (1971): Effects of ρ-methyl-ρ-tyrosine, ρ-chlorophenylalanine, L-b-(3,4-dihydroxyphenyl) alanine, 5-hydroxytryptophan and diethyldithiocarbamate on the analgesic activity of morphine and methylamphetamine in the mouse. *Br. J. Pharmacol.,* 42:512–521.

13. Messing, R. B., Fisher, L. A., Phebus, L., and Lytle, L. D. (1976): Interaction of diet and drugs in the regulation of brain 5-hydroxyindoles and the response to painful electric shock. *Life Sci.,* 18:707–714.

14. Moldofsky, H., Scarisbrick, P., England, R., and Smythe, H. (1975): Musculoskeletal symptoms and non-REM sleep disturbance in patients with "fibrositis syndrome" and healthy subjects. *Psychosom. Med.,* 37:341–351.

15. Moldofsky, H., and Scarisbrick, P. (1976): Induction of neurasthenic musculoskeletal pain syndrome by selective sleep stage deprivation. *Psychosom. Med.,* 38:35–44.

16. Moldofsky, H., and Warsh, J. J. (1978): Plasma tryptophan and musculoskeletal pain in nonarticular rheumatism ("fibrositis syndrome"). *Pain,* 5:65–71.

17. Moldofsky, H., Lue, F., and Smythe, H. (1979): Alpha EEG sleep and pain in rheumatoid arthritis. *Sleep Res.* 8:236

18. Moldofsky, H., and Warsh, J. J. (1979): *Unpublished data.*

19. Moldofsky, H., and Lue, F. (1980): The relationship of alpha and delta EEG frequencies to pain and mood in "fibrositic" patients treated with chlorpromazine and L-tryptophan. *EEG Clin. Neurophysiol.* 50:71–80.

20. Riley, G. J., and Shaw, D. M. (1976): Total and non-bound tryptophan in unipolar illness. *Lancet,* 2:1,249.

21. Salmon, S., Fanciullaci, M., Bociani, I., and Sicuteri, F. (1978): Plasma tryptophan in migraine. *Headache,* 17:238–241.

22. Samanin, R., Gumulka, W., and Valzelli, L. (1970): Reduced effect of morphine in midbrain raphe-lesioned rats. *Eur. J. Pharmacol.,* 10:339–343.

23. Samanin, R., and Valzelli, L. (1972): Serotonergic neurotransmission and morphine activity. *Arch. Int. Pharmacodyn.,* 196:138–141.

24. Sicuteri, F. (1972): Headache as a possible expression of deficiency of brain 5-hydroxytryptamine (central denervation sensitivity). *Headache,* 12:69–72.

25. Sicuteri, F., Del Bianco, P. L., and Anselmi, B. (1979): Morphine abstinence and serotonin supersensitivity in man: Analogies with the mechanism of migraine. *Psychopharmacology,* 65:205–209.

26. Sicuteri, F. (1979): The nature of pain in headache and central panalgesia. In: *Mechanisms of Pain and Analgesic Compounds,* ed. R. F. Beers and E. G. Bassett. Raven Press, New York.

27. Smythe, H. A. (1979): "Fibrositis" as a disorder of pain modulation. *Clin. Rheum. Dis.,* 5(3):823–832.

28. Smythe, H. A., and Moldofsky, H. (1977): Two contributions to understanding of the "fibrositis" syndrome. *Bull. Rheum. Dis.,* 28:928–931.

29. Tagliamonte, A., Tagliamonte, P., Perez-Cruet, J., and Gessa, L. (1971): Increase of brain tryptophan caused by drugs which stimulate serotonin synthesis. *Nature* [*New Biol.*], 229:125–126.

30. Tagliamonte, A., Biggio, G., Vargiu, L., and Gessa, G. L. (1973): Increase of brain tryptophan and stimulation of serotonin synthesis by salicylate. *J. Neurochem.,* 20:909–912.

31. Tenen, S. S. (1967): The effects of ρ-chlorophenylalanine, a serotonin depletor, on avoidance acquisition, pain sensitivity, and related behaviour in the rat. *Psychopharmacologia (Berlin),* 10:204–219.

32. Tenen, S. S. (1968): Antagonism of the analgesic effect of morphine and other drugs by ρ-chlorophenylalanine, a serotonin depletor. *Psychopharmacologia (Berlin),* 12:278–285.

33. Van Woert, M. H., and Sethy, V. H. (1975): Therapy of intention myoclonus with L-5-hydroxytryptophan and a peripheral decarboxylase inhibitor, MK 486. *Neurology (Minneap.),* 25:135–140.

Advances in Neurology, Vol. 33, edited by
M. Critchley et al. Raven Press, New York © 1982

Endorphins and Modulation of Pain

Lars Terenius

Department of Pharmacology, University of Uppsala, Uppsala, Sweden

The endorphins, a family of structurally related peptides with affinity for opioid receptors, are formed in nerve and endocrine tissues. A brief outline of their distribution is given in Table 1. The active peptides are formed from larger precursor molecules. The precursor for β-endorphin, pro-opiocortin, has been defined chemically, and its processing to form active peptides has been characterized (7,19). The enkephalin precursor of the adrenal has been partially characterized. It is apparently a molecule with several enkephalin sequences and more methionine-enkephalin than leucine-enkephalin residues (15). The enkephalin sequences frequently are surrounded by pairs of basic amino acid residues which may be vulnerable to attack by trypsin-like enzymes, an arrangement found also among other peptide precursors. The enkephalin neurons may produce a number of peptides comprising the enkephalin sequence and extended at the C-terminus. Thus several such peptides have been identified (14,25). Another peptide containing the leucine-enkephalin sequence and not fully sequenced, dynorphin, may derive from yet another system (12). This brief summary of the presently known complexity both in terms of chemical structures and of organ distribution, serves to emphasize that there can be no simple relationship between any physiologic variable and "endorphinergic" activity. It is essential to define the activity in each individual system and establish its relationships to a particular physiologic function.

Also of concern is the complexity of opioid receptors. During the past 20 years, several lines of research have provided evidence of a family of opioid receptors. The

TABLE 1. *Outline of endorphin distribution*

Tissue	Endorphin
CNS	Enkephalins
	β-Endorphin
	Dynorphin
Pituitary	
Anterior	β-Endorphin
Posterior	Dynorphin
Adrenal	Enkephalins
Salivary gland	Enkephalins
Carotid body	
Gastrointestinal tract	
Nervous tissue	Enkephalins
Gland cells	Enkephalins

receptor most likely involved in the analgesic actions of powerful drugs, such as morphine, is the μ-receptor. This receptor is readily blocked by relatively low doses of naloxone (20). The endorphins have strong affinity for this receptor but also for another receptor, the δ-receptor, the function of which is not yet understood. At the receptor level, the enkephalins have lower affinity than β-endorphin (22). In test systems, such as the guinea pig ileum or mouse vas deferens, the longer peptides, β-endorphin and dynorphin, give more protracted effects and are far more potent than the enkephalins (27). The analgesic activity after intracerebral or intracerebroventricular administration is also much higher for the longer peptides than for the enkephalins. In fact, an analgesic effect of the enkephalins is hard to demonstrate unless high doses are given (2).

ASSESSMENT OF ENDORPHIN ACTIVITY IN MAN

Essentially two approaches have been taken to assess endorphinergic activity in humans. One is to administer the narcotic antagonist naloxone, the other to measure endorphins with biochemical techniques. Naloxone probes the μ-receptor, which is acceptable for evaluating endorphin action in relation to pain (see above). The chemical measurements of endorphin activity are complicated by their chemical variety. The approach we have taken is to use a receptor assay with a μ-receptor probe, dihydromorphine, as the competing radioactive ligand. Samples of cerebrospinal fluid (CSF) are subjected to a fractionation procedure. The resulting fractions are tested for affinity against a preparation of synaptic plasma membranes from rat brain (28). The assay monitors endorphin activity as a function of affinity and concentration. The procedure is detailed in Table 2.

The choice of CSF as the material for assays was dictated by the fact that endorphins are produced by tissues outside the central nervous system (CNS), such as endocrine glands (Table 1); the endorphin content of a plasma sample relates in a complex fashion to CNS activity. The CSF can also be considered an expansion of the extracellular fluid of brain, and its contents should reflect CNS activity. Our data suggest that endorphins are stable in CSF for fairly long periods of time. The choice of a receptor assay has the advantage that the functional activity is measured; it cannot yet be decided which endorphin is the most relevant in a particular clinical situation.

TABLE 2. *Protocol for CSF endorphin analysis* [a]

1. A 12.5-ml lumbar CSF sample is obtained with the patient in a supine position.
2. The sample is centrifuged for 5 min, and the clear fluid is frozen at $-20°C$ or lower until analysis.
3. The sample is filtered through a PM-10 ultrafilter (nominal exclusion limit; 10,000 MW), and 5 ml of the filtrate is run through a Sephadex G-10 column (2 × 50 cm).
4. The fraction I (15 ml; 1.3 V_o, V_o = void volume) is collected and lyophilized.
5. The lyophilized fraction is tested for competitive affinity against dihydromorphine-^{3}H in a receptor assay. A mixture of 0.2 mg synaptic plasma membrane protein from rat brain, test fraction, and label is incubated in 0.4 ml buffer, pH 7.4, in polypropylene centrifuge tubes. Following incubation, the tubes are cooled and centrifuged for 5 min in a Microfuge (Beckman). The tubes are inverted, and any remaining fluid is removed by centripetal forces induced by a rotary wheel. The tips of the tubes are cut and counted for radioactivity.

[a] From ref. 28.

Since many studies from our group have indicated a functional relevance of the fraction I endorphins (Table 2), we are currently trying to establish the chemical structures of the active components of this fraction. We have found (29) several components in the fraction, all fairly basic in nature and of a molecular weight around 1,500 to 2,000. One component also has affinity for antibodies directed against the sequence [1–13] of dynorphin. It also shows a chromatographic behavior similar to that of this dynorphin fragment. Since dynorphin and other basic peptides show much higher potency in a majority of bioassays (see above), the substances in fraction I may be functionally important. For instance, electrical stimulation causing pain relief in patients with chronic pain (8) increases the concentrations of the peptide related to dynorphin (23).

A MODULATORY ROLE FOR ENDORPHIN SYSTEMS IN CNS FUNCTION

Several lines of evidence suggest that the endorphin systems are dynamic, with respect to both biosynthesis and release and receptor function. Thus several investigators have observed a diurnal variation in pain sensitivity. In mice, this periodicity is quite marked; the animals are more sensitive to pain at the end of the activity period. The difference is largely abolished if the animals are pretreated with naloxone (9). In man, pain tolerance limits and pain thresholds are higher in the early morning than in the evening, i.e., in the early active period, in agreement with the observation in mice (11). Naloxone injections lower pain thresholds or change the amplitude of evoked potentials to sensory stimuli in the morning, while these effects are barely observable in the evening (4).

Opioid receptor mechanisms are particularly susceptible to desensitization (tolerance development). The mechanism for this phenomenon is not entirely clear. Events occurring after the actual opioid-receptor combination probably are responsible (21). For significant tolerance to occur, protracted exposure over days is necessary. Recently, other mechanisms for the development of opioid tolerance have been proposed; several groups have reported the existence of natural opioid antagonists. Our studies indicate that a compound with effects opposite to those of endorphins is present in increased amounts in CSF of narcotic addicts (30). This compound shows activity in the guinea pig ileum bioassay, where it produces an apparent reversal of the inhibition produced by opioids; however, it also potentiates the twitch in a morphine-naive preparation. Therefore, it may be a physiologic antagonist rather than a pharmacologic antagonist like naloxone. Other sites of action, such as on the smooth muscle, have been excluded.

The endorphin systems themselves have a number of autoregulatory sites involving biosynthesis, release, and receptor functions. In addition, generation of activity in systems that have an activity opposite to that of the endorphins themselves may occur. Evidence is lacking about how these systems are ultimately regulated or how the diurnal variation is maintained. Obviously, there are a number of possibilities, and measurement of only one variable has limitations.

ENDORPHINS IN ACUTE PAIN

There are comparatively few studies on the role of endorphins as modulators of acute pain. In one study, patients undergoing minor surgery for molar extraction were followed postoperatively and reported their pain level. Naloxone or placebo was given double-blind in a crossover design. There was a statistically significant although moderate effect of naloxone, which increased pain levels (17). This surgical procedure may not have been particularly traumatic. Using the same clinical setting, these authors reported that endorphin levels may increase by a placebo injection (16). This procedure was particularly effective in patients who reported high pain levels. Another factor contributing to differences in pain reactions is the interindividual variation. In a series of patients undergoing laparotomy, we were able to measure preoperative CSF endorphin levels. Postoperation, the patient was connected to a system that allows him to administer a narcotic analgesic on demand. This technique is attractive to the patient, who knows that he has the power to control the pain (6). The method also is useful in establishing the pain level in the patient objectively; if a short-acting analgesic is used, the patient will soon titrate his analgesic requirement to a steady state. Results from chemical analysis can be used to calculate a steady-state level of the analgesic in plasma and CSF. When related to the preoperative levels of CSF endorphins, an inverse relationship was found between the steady-state level of analgesic in CSF and the preoperative endorphin level. Thus a patient with high endorphin levels demands less analgesic than one with low levels (26). This finding reemphasizes the existence of interindividual differences in the activity of endorphinergic systems and also illustrates that endorphins serve a protective role as pain modulators.

ENDORPHINS AND NEUROPATHOLOGIC DISORDERS

Complaints of pain or headache are frequent in neuropathologic disorders. The opposite condition, indifference to pain, is much less common; however, it is anecdotally reported as a characteristic symptom in psychiatric disorders, such as schizophrenia. Schizophrenic patients seldom complain about venepuncture, lumbar puncture, or other painful diagnostic procedures. Not infrequently, they will self-mutilate (10). Recent studies have indicated that narcotic antagonists increase pain sensitivity in these patients (5), who often show increased fraction I endorphin levels in CSF (18). Increased endorphin activity also may occur in other clinical conditions. A single case with recurrent apnea and reduced pain sensitivity, responding to naloxone with improved ventilation, has recently been reported (3). This subject had strongly elevated fraction I levels. When he eventually died in respiratory arrest, radioimmunoassay analysis showed increased enkephalin levels in cortical and subcortical brain areas.

Clinical evidence suggests that chronic pain syndromes have a complex etiology. In some cases, the pain can be attributed to a well-defined lesion and has a definite somatotopic localization. In other cases, the patient's own description of the pain syndrome is vague and emotionally colored. The terms "organic" and "psychogenic" have been used to distinguish these subgroups of clinical pain syndromes. Although every chronic pain syndrome is likely to have both components, a clinical main type should be possible to identify and use for the selection of treatment modalities and prognostic purposes. A distinction between various pain syndromes can be made on the basis of endorphin measurements (Table 3).

The group of patients classified as having neurogenic pain is characterized by very low endorphin levels, indicating a low defense barrier for pain. In fact, these patients have lower pain thresholds and tolerance limits to experimental pain (31), react more strongly to visual stimuli (32), and belong to a vulnerable personality group (13). We suggest that such a patient is particularly prone to develop a pain syndrome, which may not be caused by excessive stimulation of a primary pain afferent but rather by a deficiency in the endorphinergic control mechanisms. In line with this hypothesis is

TABLE 3. *Distribution of cases with respect to CSF fraction I endorphin levels*[a]

Subjects	Fraction I endorphin (pmoles/ml CSF)[b]		
	< 0.6	0.6–1.2	> 1.2
Healthy volunteers	3	12	4
Pain syndromes			
Neurogenic	29	2	2
Other organic	2	3	3
Psychogenic	3	9	10

[a] Data compiled from refs. 1, 23, and 28.
[b] Calculated as methionine-enkephalin equivalents.

the observation that electroacupuncture produces naloxone-reversible pain relief (24). A biochemical correlate is increasing fraction I levels on stimulation (23). In clinical follow-up studies, it was found (8) that patients with neurogenic pain in particular experience relief by electrical stimulation; the pain relief outlasts the stimulation period. Patients in whom pain may be due to increased afferent activation, such as cancer or arthritis, do not benefit much from electrical stimulation therapy. The stimulus may be of insufficient strength to produce enough endorphin activation.

CONCLUSIONS

Our understanding of the role of endorphins in pain modulation is still incomplete. In the CNS, however, they probably can act as a "painstat," setting our pain modulatory capacity at a certain level. Differences in this setting could explain the well-known differences between individuals in tolerating clinical pain. In certain pathologic conditions, excessive production or deficiency may occur and give clinical consequences. In patients with chronic neurogenic pain, the endorphin systems are inadequate for pain modulation. Activation to a therapeutically significant extent can be achieved by strong electrical stimulation. In other painful conditions, such as cancer pain, electrical stimulation is not particularly powerful, indicating that the endorphin systems operate normally; in these conditions, pain is probably caused by excessive afferent input.

Future work should be directed to the identification of which endorphin system is particularly important for pain modulation and how activation is best achieved.

ACKNOWLEDGMENT

This work was supported by the Swedish Medical Research Council.

REFERENCES

1. Almay, B. G. L., Johansson, F., von Knorring, L., Terenius, L., and Wahlström, A. (1978): Endorphins in chronic pain. I. Differences in CSF endorphin levels between organic and psychogenic pain syndromes. *Pain,* 5:153–162.
2. Belluzzi, J. D., Grant, N., Garsky, V., Sarantakis, D., Wise, C. D., and Stein, L. (1976): Analgesia induced in vivo by central administration of enkephalin in rat. *Nature,* 260:625–626.

3. Brandt, N. J., Terenius, L., Brock Jacobsen, B., Klinken, L., Nordius, Å., Brandt, S., Blegvad, K., and Yssing, M. (1980): Hyper-endorphin syndrome in a child with necrotizing encephalomyelopathy. *N. Engl. J. Med.* 303:914–916.
4. Davis, G. C., Buchsbaum, M. S., and Bunney, W. E., Jr. (1978): Naloxone decreases diurnal variation in pain sensitivity and somatosensory evoked potentials. *Life Sci.,* 23:1449–1460.
5. Davis, G. C., Buchsbaum, M. S., van Kammen, D. P., and Bunney, W. E., Jr. (1979): Analgesia to pain stimuli in schizophrenics and its reversal by naltrexone. *Psychiatr. Res.,* 1:61–69.
6. Editorial (1980): Patient-controlled analgesia. *Lancet,* 1:289–290.
7. Eipper, B. A., and Mains, R. E. (1978): Analysis of the common precursor to corticotropin and endorphin. *J. Biol. Chem.,* 253:5,732–5,744.
8. Eriksson, M. B. E., Sjölund, B. H., and Nielzén, S. (1979): Long term results of peripheral conditioning stimulation as an analgesic measure in chronic pain. *Pain,* 6:335–347.
9. Fredrickson, R. C. A., Burgis, V., and Edwards, J. D. (1977): Hyperalgesia induced by naloxone follows diurnal rhythm in responsivity to painful stimuli. *Science,* 198:756–758.
10. Geschwind, N. (1975): Insensitivity to pain in psychotic patients. *N. Engl. J. Med.,* 296:1,480.
11. Glynn, C. J., Lloyd, J. W., and Folkard, S. (1976): The diurnal variation in perception of pain. *Proc. R. Soc. Med.,* 69:369–372.
12. Goldstein, A., Tachibana, S., Lowney, L. I., Hunkapiller, M., and Hood, L. (1979): Dynorphin-(1–13), an extraordinary potent opioid peptide. *Proc. Natl. Acad. Sci. USA,* 76:6,666–6,670.
13. Johansson, F., Almay, B. G. L., von Knorring, L., Terenius, L., and Åström, M. (1979): Personality traits in chronic pain patients related to endorphin levels in cerebrospinal fluid. *Psychiatr. Res.,* 1:231–239.
14. Kangawa, E., Matsuo, H., and Igarashi, M. (1979): α-Neo-endorphin: A "big" leu-enkephalin with potent opiate activity from porcine hypothalami. *Biochem. Biophys. Res. Commun.,* 86:153–160.
15. Kimura, S., Lewis, R. V., Stern, A. S., Rossier, J., Stein, S., and Udenfriend, S. (1980): Probable precursors of (Leu)enkephalin and (Met)enkephalin in adrenal medulla: Peptides of 3–5 kilodaltons. *Proc. Natl. Acad. Sci. USA,* 77:1,681–1,685.
16. Levine, J. D., Gordon, N. D., and Fields, H. L. (1978): The mechanism of placebo analgesia. *Lancet,* 2:654–657.
17. Levine, J. D., Gordon, N. C., Jones, R. T., and Fields, H. L. (1978): The narcotic antagonist naloxone enhances clinical pain. *Nature,* 272:826–827.
18. Lindström, L. H., Widerlöv, E., Gunne, L.-M., and Terenius L. (1978): Endorphins in human cerebrospinal fluid: Clinical correlations to some psychotic states. *Acta Psychiatr. Scand.,* 57:153–164.
19. Loh, P. Y. (1979): Immunological evidence for two common precursors to corticotropins, endorphins and melanotropin in the neurointermediate lobe of the toad pituitary. *Proc. Natl. Acad. Sci. USA,* 76:796–800.
20. Sawynok, L., Pinsky, C., and Labella, F. S. (1979): Minireview on the specificity of naloxone as an opiate antagonist. *Life Sci.,* 25:1,621–1,632.
21. Sharma, S. K., Nirenberg, M., and Klee, W. A. (1975): Morphine receptors as regulators of adenylate cyclase activity. *Proc. Natl. Acad. Sci. USA,* 72:590–594.
22. Simon, E. J., and Hiller, J. M. (1978): The opiate receptors. *Ann. Rev. Pharmacol. Toxicol.,* 18:371–394.
23. Sjölund, B., Terenius, L., and Eriksson, M. (1977): Increased cerebrospinal fluid levels of endorphins after electroacupuncture. *Acta Physiol. Scand.,* 100:382–384.
24. Sjölund, B. H., and Eriksson, M. B. E. (1979): The influence of naloxone on analgesia produced by peripheral conditioning stimulation. *Brain Res.,* 173:295–301.
25. Stern, A. S., Lewis, R. V., Kimura, S., Rossier, J., Gerber, L. D., Brink, L., Stein, S., and Udenfriend, S. (1979): Isolation of the opioid heptapeptide Met-enkephalin (Arg[6], Phe[7]) from bovine adrenal medullary granules and striatum. *Proc. Natl. Acad. Sci. USA,* 76:6,680–6,683.
26. Tamsen, A., Hartvig, P., Dahlström, B., Wahlström, A., and Terenius, L. (1980): Endorphins and on-demand pain relief. *Lancet,* 1:769–770.
27. Terenius, L. (1978): Endogenous peptides and analgesia. *Ann. Rev. Pharmacol. Toxicol.,* 18:189–204.
28. Terenius, L., and Wahlström, A. (1975): Morphine-like ligand for opiate receptors in human CSF. *Life Sci.,* 16:1,759–1,764.
29. Wahlström, A., and Terenius, L. (1980): Chemical characteristics of endorphins in human cerebrospinal fluid. *FEBS Lett.,* 118:241–244.
30. Wahlström, A., and Terenius, L. (1980): Factor in human cerebrospinal fluid with apparent morphine-antagonistic properties. *Acta Physiol. Scand.* 110:427–429.
31. von Knorring, L., Almay, B. G. L., Johansson, F., and Terenius, L. (1978): Pain perception and endorphin levels in cerebrospinal fluid. *Pain,* 5:359–365.
32. von Knorring, L., Almay, B. G. L., Johansson, F., and Terenius, L. (1979): Endorphins in CSF of chronic pain patients, in relation to augmenting-reducing response in visual averaged evoked response. *Neuropsychobiology,* 5:322–325.

Advances in Neurology, Vol. 33, edited by
M. Critchley et al. Raven Press, New York © 1982

Natural Opioids in Migraine

Federigo Sicuteri

Department of Clinical Pharmacology, Headache Center, University of Florence, Florence, Italy

Headache (Hd) and central panalgesia (CPA) (17) are clinical expressions of deficiencies in the endogenous opioid system (EOS). Because the EOS also controls the hedonia and the neurovegetative systems, anhedonia and dysautonomia present in Hd and CPA. The central nature of pain in Hd was suggested some years ago (18).

The reverent admiration for the pioneers in Hd studies should not be an obstacle, but rather a stimulus to improve knowledge in this difficult area. For instance, the vascular theory of Hd pain, so brilliant and convincing when first suggested (14), and when later applied to human pathology (27), cannot be maintained today. Vasoconstriction and vasodilatation do not provoke Hd in eunoceptors. Vasodilatation must be considered as an adjunctive, not obligatory, mechanism, able to increase pain, if manifest, to unmask it, if latent. In other words, vascular pain is a factor that emerges only when the pain threshold is locally lowered. When pain acquires a pulsating character, it does not mean that pain is vascular in nature. In normal subjects, somatoesthesia is regulated in such a way that the pulsations of the heart and arteries, as well as the congestion of veins, are not perceived; they are only perceived when the pain threshold is lowered. Therefore, the contraction of muscles of the scalp and neck become pain producing only when the pain threshold is depressed. Many anxious subjects exhibit scalp and neck muscle contraction, but not headache. The same is true of the exacerbation of pain from jolting or shaking the head: Shaking the head is not a pain producing factor in the eunoceptors, but it becomes so when the internal cranial walls have their pain threshold lowered. Insisting on considering the vascular, muscular factors as a primary mechanism of Hd is a conceptual misunderstanding today that hinders the progress of medical thought.

The investigator must constantly keep in mind the basic components of the disease (Fig. 1). The three basic components of Hd (we can consider as a prototype those of a migraine attack) are: (a) hypernociception ("spontaneous" ache exhibiting the well-known characteristics of central pain: poor localization, concomitant dysesthesias, ex-

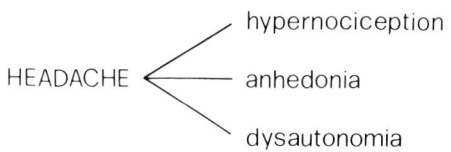

Fig. 1. Three functions are impaired in migraine attacks: nociception, well-being, and autonomia.

HYPOENDORPHIN SYNDROME

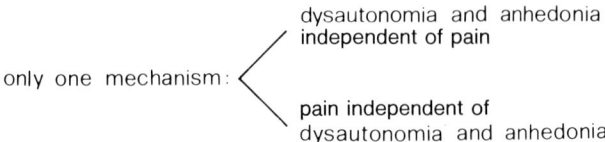

Fig. 2. In headache crisis (here intended as hypoendorphin syndrome), the chronological succession of the clinical phenomena (concerning the three impaired functions) is different according to individuals: this interindependence is compatible with a unique mechanism acting in various sequences in different discrete areas, rather than an interdependence, i.e., through a mechanism in cascade.

acerbation from sensorial stimuli, overreaction as intensity and duration); (b) anhedonia, i.e., loss of sense of well-being; and (c) dysautonomia: nausea, vomiting, impaired thermoregulation leading to fever, oliguria, poliuria, and sexual excitation in 10% of cases.

The components of the triadal syndrome (anhedonia, pain, dysautonomia) are interindependent. When the clinical phenomena of a disease emerge in different subjects in constant succession, this is indication that a primary noxious mechanism produces the first impairment that, in turn, provokes the other phenomena. The three groups of symptoms in a migraine attack do not present in a set order in all patients. The attack may start with any of the main components of Hd attacks. The variability in the succession of clinical components is compatible only with a unique mechanism that acts in various sequences in different discrete areas. (Fig. 2).

Dysautonomia, anhedonia, and hypernociception must be due to an acute recurrent impairment of a system able to subserve simultaneously the three groups of affected functions. I have been unable to find one different from the EOS. In fact, the EOS subserves: (a) the pain suppressor system, contributing to the modulation of pain; (b) hedonia, giving a feeling of well-being; and (c) the neurovegetative system, helping to maintain an excellent autonomic equilibrium (euautonomia). A deficiency of EOS is expected to provoke pain (apparently spontaneous, i.e., without peripheral causes), anhedonia, and dysautonomia. With reference to hypernociception, one may hypothesize that impairment concerns discrete anatomical areas of the suppressor pain system (Fig. 3). In this respect, it is particularly interesting to note the ability of enkephalinergic neurons to inhibit the release of P substance (a pain transmitter in the trigeminal nuclei) (1). As a matter of fact, pain in Hd—and particularly in migraine—concerns those regions subserved by trigeminal branches, the first one mainly.

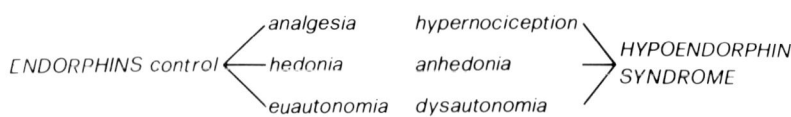

Fig. 3. Under impairment conditions of the endogenous opioids system, the main dependent functions are expected to be deficient or perverted.

CONDITIONS ANALOGOUS AND OPPOSITE TO HD

Morphine Abstinence

When one attempts to understand an enigma such as migraine, a fruitful way is to find a condition exhibiting analogous clinical phenomena. Morphine abstinence is the one such condition. (18,19). If one examines the effects of morphine abstinence, i.e., yawning, yen sleep, anxiety, restlessness, insomnia, sexual excitation, hot and cold flashes, gooseflesh, tremors, perspiration, increased temperature, oliguria, lacrimation, rhinorrhea, mydriasis, increased respiration, increased pulse rate, and aching bones and muscles (nausea and/or vomiting, so frequent in abstinence, are not listed in Fig. 4), one cannot but be surprised by the similarity of these phenomena to those of migraine attacks. Usually pain following heroin or morphine withdrawal is not complained of instantly, as pain appears late in abstinence. The addict self-administers opiates in order to interrupt the pain. When abstinence persists, pain becomes intense and spreads to the whole body, including the head. In rhesus monkeys, a protracted abstinence induces unbearable systemic pain, clearly expressed through high vocalization and grimaces (26). Pain is also a predominant phenomenon in animals that abstain. In rats, for instance, hyperalgesia is a method used to measure the extent of dependence (24). Sexual excitation during migraine or cluster headache attacks is present in 10% of patients; it appears that a positive correlation exists between the severity of an attack and the sexual arousal (7). Sexual arousal is also present in the same percentage during serious abstinence in man and in animals. The parallel between migraine and abstinence is even more suggestive when one considers the lowering or disappearance of morphinelike factors (MLF), or, more exactly, of metioenkephalin in cerebrospinal fluid (CSF) sampled during migraine and cluster headache (20). The enkephalin level is normal when CSF is taken during a period free from attacks; then its acute lowering during Hd pain

ITEMS ASSOCIATED WITH MORPHINE ABSTINENCE

yawning	hot cold flashes	lacrimation
"yen sleep"	gooseflesh	rhinorrhea
anxiety	tremors	mydriasis
restlessness	perspiration	increased respiration
insomnia	increased temperature	increased pulse rate
sexual excitation	oliguria	aching bones and muscles

Fig. 4. The type and succession of the clinical phenomena in a morphine abstinence crisis may be superimposed on those of a migraine attack. This list should also include nausea and vomiting, so frequent in abstinence as well as in migraine. (From Lancet 599–601, 1978, with permission.)

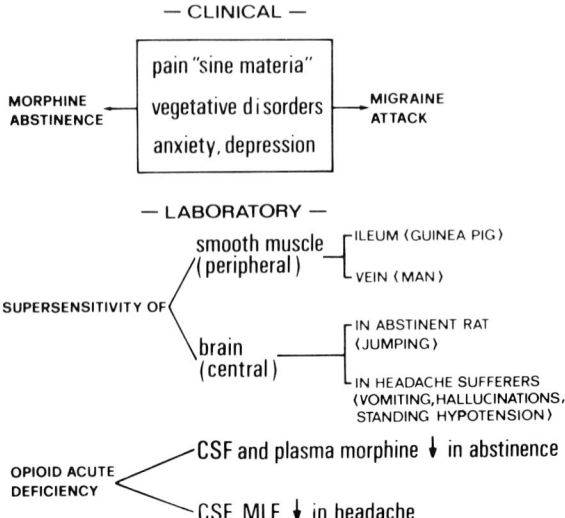

Fig. 5. The most convincing pattern of migraine attacks is the morphine abstinence crisis. Analogies concern not only the clinical phenomena but also some prominent chemical and pharmacological aspects. These items, concerning the supersensitivity of the α-adrenoceptors of the smooth muscle, must be supplemented with the one concerning the iris dilatator muscle (supersensitive to phenylephrine both in abstinent and migraine subjects).

is compatible with a failure of EOS in the area of the central nervous system (Fig. 5). The β-endorphin like immunoreactivity (β-ELI) serum is slightly increased during migraine, and is a credible indication of endorphin hypersecretion from pituitary gland as a consequence of the painful stress of the attack. Since endorphin acts strongly on the central nervous system in man when inoculated into CSF, and poorly when it is injected into the veins (13), one can infer that endorphin does not cross the brain–blood barrier. Its increase in serum, then, has little relevance in the mechanism of an attack. The difference in MLF levels (decreased in CSF and increased in serum) stresses further the hypothesis of EOS failure in the central nervous system during migraine.

Pregnancy

Effects experienced with pregnancy may be considered opposite those experienced with Hd. A happy pregnancy induces the well-known "state of grace" accompanied by: (a) a feeling of great well-being (hyperhedonia, euphoria); (b) excellent vegetative functions (euautonomia); and (c) conspicuous increase in threshold pain (hyponociception). This splendid enviable triadal condition emerges even more impressively when a woman is suffering from an opposite syndrome (anhedonia, dysautonomia, pain), i.e., from a serious Hd. Frequently, after delivery the Hd triadal syndrome emerges again. This prompted us to investigate the behavior of EOS in pregnancy (2). The increasing high levels of serum β-ELI can be an interpretation of the "state of grace" of pregnancy. After parturition the increased level of β-ELI returns to the normal state (2,3,5). If

β-endorphin is generated in the maternal brain, the disappearance of Hd could find an interpretation in a hyperactivity of EOS. Hypoalgesia of both the mother and fetus (the latter should be prone to terrible pains during the exit from uterus) could be explained in this way. As it is known, a fetus is insensitive to pain stimuli during the first hours of life.

Schizophrenia

The behavior of some schizophrenics recalls that of "nonlife problems," similar, even if perverted, to hyperhedonia. For a long time it has been known that a schizophrenic is rarely sensitive to noxious stimuli, owing to a high pain threshold. The analgesia of pain stimuli in schizophrenics is reversed by naltrexone, a long-acting, antimorphine drug (6). Most psychiatrists agree that only exceptional schizophrenics complain of headache. The hypothesis of a hypoendorphin condition in schizophrenia is supported by the increased level of endogenous opioids in CSF (8–12). Schizophrenics tolerate high doses of histamine without complaining of Hd: a dose that is lower by 20-fold is able to exacerbate or induce pain in Hd sufferers. These patients exhibit a very poor hypertensive arterial reaction (about 2–20-fold lower than normal) when treated with a venous bolus of norepinephrine *(unpublished observations),* which suggests hyporeactivity of the vascular smooth muscle, the opposite of the hyperreactivity of Hd sufferers and morphine abstainers.

"EMPTY NEURON" AND POSTRECEPTORAL SUPERSENSITIVITY

Postreceptoral supersensitivity (PRSS) is a condition of exaggerated reaction of cells, not due to an increase in quantity or sensitivity of pre- or postsynaptic receptors (this condition is known as receptoral supersensitivity) but to an increase in intrinsic potential, mainly correlated with the energy of a second messenger. Although receptoral supersensitivity (the prototype is that coming from denervation) concerns a neurotransmitter only, the PRSS appears with many transmitters, corresponding practically to the various receptors. A PRSS is found in nonorganic central pain (Hd and CPA), as well as in morphine abstinence, in animals (15,16) and in man (22). In painful conditions, the cells exhibiting PRSS apparently correspond to those that dispose of opiate receptors (morphine endorphin-dependent cells). These nerve and nonnerve cells are the same that spontaneously hyperreact when morphine concentrations in addicts decline and the pharmacological activity consequently ceases. Since the function of opiates is to modulate the neuroeffector junctions provided with opiate receptors, the PRSS represents a credible compensatory homeostatic mechanism to the overmodulation imposed by the excess of morphine. The PRSS is the basis for a positive conjunctival naloxone test (10). Those of the iris are one example of morphine-dependent adrenergic neurons in man. Morphine, acting on opiate receptors located in adrenergic neurons, causes the release of norepinephrine to slow down, thus resulting in cholinergic hypertonus and then miosis. Two examples of morphine sensitive adrenoneuroeffector junctions in animals are the nictitating membrane in the cat (25) and the vas deferens in the mouse (11). The other morphine-dependent neuroeffector junctions are cholinergic in nature.

If pain is due to a deficiency of autoanalgesia, one can postulate that PRSS is due to a mechanism quite different from that of morphine addiction. In fact, a deficiency in the EOS is expected to provoke a neuronal incontinence and then a chronic leakage

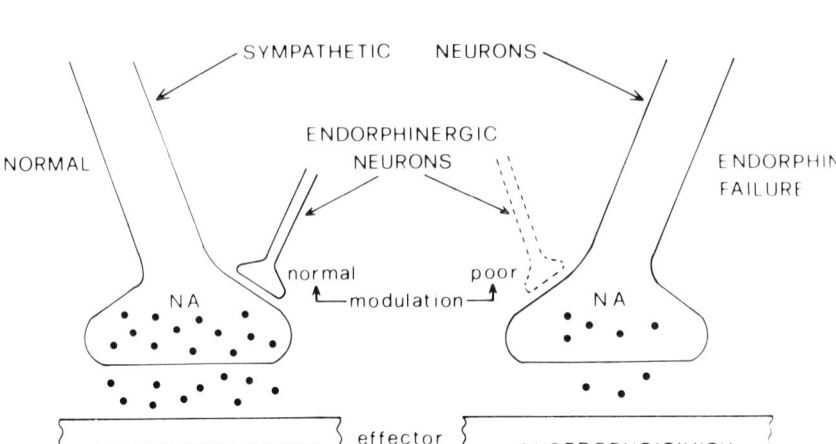

Fig. 6. A tentative interpretation of the postreceptoral supersensitivity of the effector cells due to the "empty neuron": neuronal hypomodulation and neurotransmitter exhaustion, ascribable to chronic leakage into the synaptic cleft, provoke an intracellular compensatory hyperactivity (postreceptoral supersensitivity).

of the neurotransmitter in the synaptic cleft of the endorphin-dependent neurons. The result will be an exhausted (and then "empty") neuron: the consequence will be an adaptive PRSS (Fig. 6). An example of "latent empty neuron" is the one recently detected in the iris of cluster headache sufferers. The homolateral pupil of the affected side does not dilate when the eye is tested with conjunctival instillation of tyramine (a norepinephrine releaser), while it dilates when tested with phenilephrine, an α-receptor agonist. Because this happens both in single crisis and in cluster headache, it may signify that the adrenergic neuron of the iris is chronically "empty" (9). The impressive PRSS in the muscle of the vein in men who abstain is similar in degree (200–1,000-fold higher than normal) and quality (to 5-HT, norepinephrine, DA, tyramine) to that detected in 50% of sufferers from CPA, a syndrome characterized by systemic generalized pains, central in nature (21).

IMPAIRMENT OF OPIATE RECEPTORS: FACT OR FICTION?

Opiate addiction in Hd sufferers is unusual; it occurs mainly because of the very poor (and promptly tachyphylactic) analgesia from morphine and heroin in Hd pain. This is apparently in contrast with the present Hd endorphin theory, since in migraine, intended as a "quasimorphine abstinence syndrome" (Fig. 7) (paraphrasing a well-known phrase in animal experiments (4)), the analgesizing effect of morphine must be enhanced, not reduced. The surprising lack of analgesia from morphine could depend on one or more mechanisms: (a) an increased inactivation or urinary excretion of morphine; (b) a deficiency of 5-HT in the brainstem that renders animals hyperalgesic and scarcely sensitive to morphine (23). Clinical investigations give indirect evidence that Hd sufferers have a poor 5-HT turnover in their antinociceptive system, and they easily display a

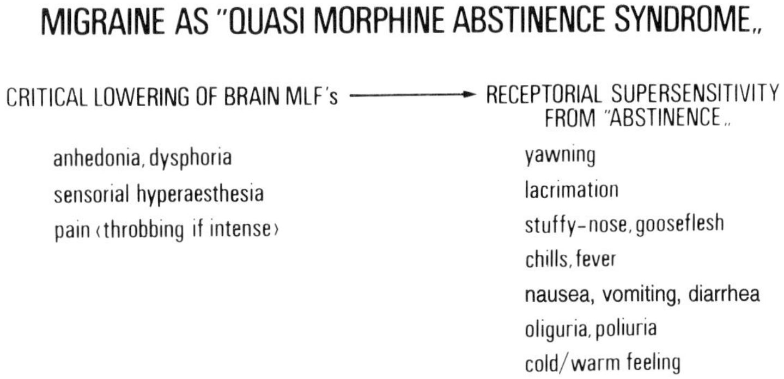

MIGRAINE AS "QUASI MORPHINE ABSTINENCE SYNDROME„

CRITICAL LOWERING OF BRAIN MLF's ⟶ RECEPTORIAL SUPERSENSITIVITY FROM "ABSTINENCE„

anhedonia, dysphoria

sensorial hyperaesthesia

pain (throbbing if intense)

yawning

lacrimation

stuffy-nose, gooseflesh

chills, fever

nausea, vomiting, diarrhea

oliguria, poliuria

cold/warm feeling

Fig. 7. By translating the concept from animal pharmacology (4) to human pathology, a migraine attack could be considered as a peculiar spontaneous crisis of "endorphin abstinence."

systemic reversible panalgesia when treated with clinical doses of p-chlorophenylalanine, an inhibitor of the 5-HT synthesis (17); (c) a poor response of opiate receptors (scarce affinity?, reduced number?) to morphine.

PSYCHOSOMATIC HEADACHE IN THE PERSPECTIVE OF ENDORPHIN THEORY

A history of serious Hd, following a long history of emotional stress (important school examination, promotional competition, conjugal and/or economical stress) occurs usually in the anamnesis of patients whose illness is labeled psychosomatic headache. The antinociceptive system is apparently stimulated only by emotions either pleasing (existential enjoyment, sexual excitation) or unpleasant (discomfort from pain, anxiety, interindivi-

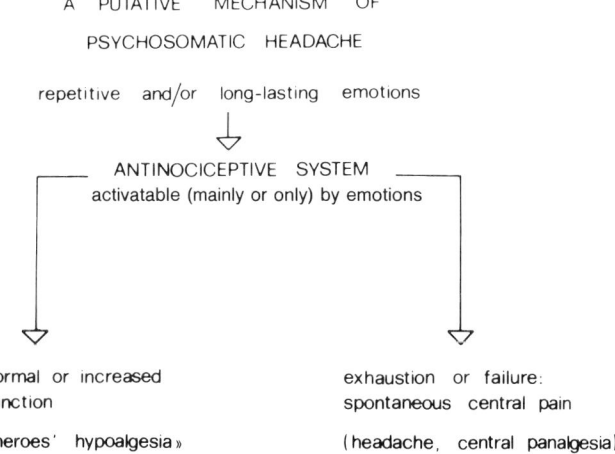

A PUTATIVE MECHANISM OF PSYCHOSOMATIC HEADACHE

repetitive and/or long-lasting emotions

ANTINOCICEPTIVE SYSTEM
activatable (mainly or only) by emotions

normal or increased function

«heroes' hypoalgesia»

exhaustion or failure:
spontaneous central pain

(headache, central panalgesia)

Fig. 8. Since the pain suppressor system is activated spontaneously by emotion only, it is overworked by long-lasting psychological tensions, regardless of any painful stimulus. If this system is solid and trainable, the result will be a reinforcement **(left)**; if fragile and exhaustible, a failure **(right)**.

dual conflicts, frustrations). All these emotions stimulate the pain suppressor mechanism (even if pain is absent) and the subserving EOS. If this system is efficient, stable, and adaptable, emotions leave it unimpaired or reinforce it. If the pain suppressor mechanism is phenotypically or genotypically fragile, repetitive emotional stress can provoke a weakening, a deterioration, and ultimately a failure of the analgesizing apparatus, resulting in hyperalgesia and spontaneous pain (Fig. 8). The failure of acupuncture in serious Hd (which is intended to stimulate the endorphin generation) is compatible with the unresponsiveness of a weak antinociceptive system. Finally, the "weekend Hd" can also be interpreted in the perspective of the endorphin theory. The daily emotions expressed in routine work maintain the antinociceptive system at a level of sufficient function. When this daily working EOS stimulation ceases (as during weekends), a deficiency of autoanalgesia emerges, thus resulting in Sunday Hd attacks.

CONCLUSION

Autoanalgesia depends on a delicate, complex multiintegrated system that is prone to dysfunction or disease, as any apparatus. The failure of the analgesic system presents clinically with spontaneous pain. The rostral section of the analgesic system, probably because of its close connection with the affective area, exhibits a higher fragility. This rostral section subserves the head, neck, and shoulders and this can explain the preferential localization of Hd pains in this area. Hd and other nonorganic central pains are the most common expression of the impairment of the analgesic system. The most important transmitters of antinociception are the endogenous opioids. Not only does the EOS modulate pain centrally, but it also modulates the well-being feeling and the neurovegetative equilibrium. Therefore, EOS deficiency is expected to provoke anhedonia (irritability and depression) as well as neurovegetative disorders, i.e., together with pain, the triadal syndrome of Hd. Obviously, in conditions of hypernociception, the vasodilatation as well as the contraction of the muscles of the scalp and the neck and the jolting of the head are able to exacerbate pain or unmask it, when latent. The triadal syndrome—spontaneous pain, anhedonia, and antonomic disturbances—is present only under two conditions: in Hd and in morphine abstinence. The opposite conditions (hypoalgesia, hyperhedonia, excellent vegetative balance) are found only in pregnancy and in some cases of schizophrenia. A deficiency and a hyperactivity of EOS are hypothesized, respectively, in the two opposite conditions. EOS modulates monoaminergic neurons; its chronic deficiency is expected to provoke a leakage of the transmitter, a neuron exhaustion, and emptying. Consequently, a compensatory hyperactivity of effector cells will arise.

These two conditions (poor release of transmitter and cell hyperactivity) appear to be the most salient phenomena of the hypoendorphin syndromes (Hd and CPA). The hyperreactivity of a cell, due to "empty neurons," is not receptoral but generic in nature, and it depends on a compensatory increased energy of the second messenger. Therefore it has been labeled as PRSS. This PRSS is a characteristic aspect in Hd as well as in morphine abstinence: it is detectable at the periphery (smooth muscle, intestine in animals, iris and veins in man) as well as at a central level (brain). The nerve and nonnerve cells showing PRSS correspond to those labeled as morphine dependent, in agreement with the map of opiate receptors and endorphinergic neurons (binding and histofluorescence methods). The map of the opiate-dependent cells of the body is also indicated more exactly when considering those functions impaired, in a stereotypic manner, when such cells are suddenly deprived of an excess of opiates, as happens during withdrawal in morphine-tolerant animals and humans.

In other words, the analysis of the clinical phenomena represents a valid tool to individualize the functions and the relevant structures provided by endogenous and exogenous opioid-dependent cells. There are two main differences between morphine abstinence and the putative endorphin failure: (a) the morphine action is invasive, i.e., it concerns all the opiate-dependent cells; in spontaneous pathological conditions, the failure of the endorphin-dependent cells is believed to involve some EOS structures; and (b) PRSS in morphine abstinence is due to excessive modulation on the neuronal release of transmitters, while in spontaneous condition the "empty neuron" is a sort of neuronal exhaustion caused by a chronic incontinence of a neurotransmitter, which, in turn, is due to a modulation defect. The poor endorphinergic modulation could depend on an impaired turnover of neuropeptides or on a receptoral disease or, finally, on both conditions.

The poor concentration of enkephalins in the CSF of Hd sufferers and the scarce analgesia from morphine and the deficient or absent inhibition from morphine of the 5-HT venospasm in few Hd and CPA patients, if confirmed, are all indirect evidence of a double (metabolic and receptoral) interdependent situation.

ACKNOWLEDGMENTS

This work was supported by a research grant from the National Research Council (CNR), Rome, Italy.

We acknowledge Comunicare S.n.c. Consulting Translators, Florence, Italy, for the language revision of the manuscript.

REFERENCES

1. Andersen, R. K., Lund, J. P., and Puil, E. (1978): Enkephalin and substance P effects related to trigeminal pain. *Can. J. Physiol. Pharmacol.,* 56:216–222.
2. Baldi, E., Branconi, F., Brocchi, A., Cappelli, G., Paladini, S., Salmon, S., and Sicuteri, F. (1979): Beta-endorphin-like-immunoreactivity (beta-ELI) in pregnancy. In: *Headache,* edited by F. Savoldi and G. Nappi, pp. 121–127. Fidia Research Laboratories, Padua, Italy.
3. Baldi, E., Branconi, F., Cappelli, G., Salmon, S., and Sicuteri, F. (1980): Hyperendorphinemia in pregnancy: Its relevance to migraine disappearance. *Neuroendocrinol. Lett.,* 2:164.
4. Collier, H. O. J., Francis, D. L., Henderson, G., and Schneider, C. (1974): Quasi morphine-abstinence syndrome. *Nature,* 249:471–473.
5. Csontos, K., Rust, M., Höllt, V., Mahr, W. W., Kromer, W., and Teschemacher, H. J. (1979): Elevated beta-endorphin levels in pregnant women and their neonates. *Life Sci.,* 25:835–844.
6. Davis, G. C., Buchsbaum, M. S., Van Kammen, D. P., and Bunney, W. E. (1979): Analgesia to pain stimuli in schizophrenics and its reversal by naltrexone. *Psychiatr. Res.,* 1:61–69.
7. Del Bene, E., and Sicuteri, F., (1979): Headache and sexual behavior. In: *Headache,* edited by F. Savoldi and G. Nappi, pp. 168–172. Fidia Research Laboratories, Padua, Italy.
8. Domschke, W., Dickschas, A., and Mitznegg, P. (1979): CSF beta-endorphin in schizophrenia. *Lancet,* 1:1024.
9. Fanciullacci, M., Del Bianco, P. L., and Sicuteri, F. (1978): Iris and vein adrenoreceptors in migraine and central panalgesia. In: *Recent Advances in the Pharmacology of Adrenoreceptors,* edited by E. Szabadi, C. M. Bradshaw, and P. Berton, pp. 295–303. Elsevier, Amsterdam.
10. Fanciullacci, M., Boccuni, M., Pietrini, U., and Sicuteri, F. (1980): The naloxone conjunctival test in morphine addiction. *Eur. J. Pharmacol.,* 61:319–320.
11. Henderson, G., Hughes, J., and Kosterlitz, H. W. (1972): A new example of a morphine-sensitive neuro-effector junction: Adrenergic transmission in the mouse vas deferens. *Br. J. Pharmacol.,* 46:764–766.
12. Lindstrom, L. H., Widerlöv, E., Gunne, L. M., Walström, A., and Terenius, L. (1978): Endorphins in

human cerebrospinal fluid. Clinical correlations to some psychiatric states. *Acta Psychiatr. Scand.,* 57:153–164.

13. Oyama, T., Iin, T., Yamaya, R., Ling, N., and Guillemin, R. (1980): Profound analgesic effects of beta-endorphin in man. *Lancet,* 1:122–124.

14. Pickering, G. W. (1939): Experimental observations on headache. *Br. Med. J.,* 1:907–912.

15. Schulz, R., and Herz, A. (1976): Aspects of opiate dependence in the myenteric plexus of the guinea pig. *Life Sci.,* 19:117–128.

16. Schulz, R., and Herz, A. (1977): Naxolone precipitated withdrawal reveals sensitization to neurotransmitters in morphine tolerant/dependent rats. *Nauynyn Schmiedebergs Arch. Pharmacol.,* 299:95–99.

17. Sicuteri, F. (1971): Pain syndrome in man following treatment with p-chlorophenylalanine. *Pharmacol. Res. Commun.,* 3:401–407.

18. Sicuteri, F. (1979): Headache as the most common disease of the antinociceptive system: Analogies with morphine abstinence. In: *Advances in Pain Research and Therapy, Vol. 3,* edited by J. J. Bonica, J. C. Liebeskind, and D. G. Albe-Fessard, pp. 359–365. Raven Press, New York.

19. Sicuteri, F. (1980): Vascular supersensitivity to serotonin and other monoamines in migraine and in morphine abstinence: A related mechanism? In: *Vascular Neuroeffector Mechanism,* edited by J. A. Bevan, T. Godfrain, R. A. Maxwell, and P. M. Vauhotte, pp. 357–359. Raven Press, New York.

20. Sicuteri, F., Anselmi, B., Curradi, C., Michelacci, S., and Sassi, A. (1978): Morphine-like-factors in CSF of headache patients. In: *Advances in Biochemical Psychopharmacology, Vol. 18,* edited by E. Costa and M. Trabucchi, pp. 363–366. Raven Press, New York.

21. Sicuteri, F., Anselmi, B., and Del Bianco, P. L. (1978): Systemic nonorganic central pain: A new syndrome with decentralization supersensitivity. *Headache,* 18:133–136.

22. Sicuteri, F., Del Bianco, P. L., and Anselmi, B. (1979): Morphine abstinence and serotonin supersensitivity in man: Analogies with the mechanism of migraine? *Psychopharmacology,* 65:205–209.

23. Tenen, S. S. (1976): The effect of p-chlorophenylalanine, a serotonin depletor, on avoidance, acquisition, pain sensitivity and related behavior in rats. *Psychopharmacology,* 10:204–219.

24. Tilson, H. A., Rech, R. H., and Stolman, S. (1973): Hyperalgesia during withdrawal as a means of measuring the degree of dependence in morphine dependent rats. *Psychopharmacology,* 28:287–300.

25. Trendelburgh, V. (1957): The action of morphine on the superior cervical ganglion and on the nictitating membrane. *Br. J. Pharmacol. Chemother.,* 12:79–85.

26. Villareal, J. E. (1973): The effects of morphine agonists and antagonists on morphine dependent rhesus monkeys. In: *Agonist and Antagonist Action of Narcotic Analgesic Drugs,* edited by H. W. Kosterlitz, H. O. G. Collier, and J. E. Villareal, pp. 73–93. Macmillan, New York.

27. Wolff, H. G. (1963): *Headache and Other Head Pain.* Oxford University Press, New York.

Advances in Neurology, Vol. 33, edited by
M. Critchley et al. Raven Press, New York © 1982

Endorphins in the Pathogenesis of Headache

D. Della Bella, A. Carenzi, F. Casacci, *B. Anselmi, *E. Baldi,
and *S. Salmon

*Zambon S.p.A. Research Laboratories, Bresso-Milan, Italy; and *Department of Clinical
Pharmacology, University of Florence, Florence, Italy*

The presence in several mammalian tissues of different peptides with morphine-like properties has been demonstrated. Methionine-enkephalin (met-enk) and leucine-enkephalin (leu-enk) were isolated from pig brain (17) and identified as two similar pentapeptides differing only in the last amino acid (18). Endorphins were isolated from hypothalamus (15) and pituitary (14) and consist of 30 amino acids. The morphinomimetic activity of beta-endorphin in different experimental preparations is more potent than that of morphine, while enkephalins and alpha-endorphin are weaker agonists (9). Evidence now indicates that the enkephalins are neurotransmitters of specific neuronal systems in the brain that mediate the sensory information dealing with pain and emotional behavior. Morphine-like factors (MLF) are also present in human cerebrospinal fluid (CSF); Terenius et al. (24) have shown that a significant variation of MLF content occurs in the CSF of psychotic patients. Since MLF have been involved in the modulation of pain, hedonia, and neurovegetative system (4,22), we investigated the possible relationship between the contents of CSF MLF and serum endorphins and a disease, such as headache, characterized by the presence of pain, neurovegetative disorders, and dysphoria.

MLF CONTENT IN CSF OF HEADACHE SUFFERERS: CLINICAL OBSERVATIONS

CSF samples were collected from patients hospitalized in the Department of Clinical Pharmacology, University of Florence, Italy, who underwent a diagnostic spinal puncture. Great care was taken to exclude all cases of psychogenic pain. CSF samples were collected, ultrafiltered, frozen, and purified in a Sephadex G 10 column according to Terenius and Wahlström (23); two different fractions were obtained. As previously reported (2,7), the elution patterns of the first and second fraction are similar to that of beta-endorphin or leu-enk, respectively. Because a similar chromatographic profile does not differentiate the peptides into the two fractions, the substances thus obtained and endowed with morphine-like properties were named morphine-like-factors (MLF). The samples related to the two fractions were pooled separately and lyophilized, then resuspended in a small volume of buffer and tested for their potency of displacing ^{3}H-dihydromorphine (^{3}H-DHM) from the opiate receptors (20).

We have published in detail most of the cases we studied (2,7,21); Table 1 summarizes the results. The displacing potency of CSF fractions on ^{3}H-DHM binding is expressed as if due to met-enk. In our experiment, the first fraction did not show any displacing property, which, on the other hand, is easily detectable in the second fraction of almost all the samples tested. Unfortunately, no CSF samples from healthy volunteers were available. Therefore, a comparison was made between the MLF content in the CSF of headache patients collected both during periods of pain and in the absence of pain. As reported in Table 1, the MLF concentration in the CSF collected during the attacks is clearly lower than that in pain-free periods. Moreover, high levels of MLF are present in the CSF of patients affected by different neurological (not painful) diseases (epilepsy, cerebral atrophy, Guillain-Barré syndrome, polyencephalomyelitis). Despite the small number of CSF samples collected in the absence of pain, the difference in MLF content of the two groups suggests a correlation between the presence of pain and the low levels of MLF in CSF. Similar results have been obtained by Von Knorring et al. (25), who studied the endorphin content in CSF of patients with chronic pain of organic or neurogenic origin.

Since the content of MLF in CSF may reflect central processes involved in pain syndromes, we focused our attention on the possibility of affecting the enkephalinergic system as a means of relieving pain or increasing the pain threshold. Evidence indicates that enkephalins are rapidly metabolized by exopeptidases. Aminopeptidase, peptidyl dipeptidase, and carboxypeptidase A have been suggested as possible catabolizing enzymes of enkephalins (16,17,19). It has been shown in animals that the inhibition of exopeptidases increases the analgesic effect of exogenously applied met-enk or endogenously released MLF (6,12). Since d-phenylalanine, a well-known inhibitor of carboxypeptidase A (11), has been used safely in humans (13), we attempted to relieve headache by treating three different patients with 250 mg d-phenylalanine orally 4 times/day. Unfortunately, no improvement was seen in pain intensity or attack frequency after 1 week of treatment. The failure of these preliminary observations can be ascribed to the following: (a) the dosage of d-phenylalanine was not high enough to inhibit *in vivo* carboxypeptidase; (b) the treatment period was too short; (c) in man, the inhibition of carboxypeptidase without affecting aminopeptidase and peptidyl dipeptidase is not relevant to the production of significant variation of enkephalin availability at the synaptic level. At present, we are measuring the levels of enkephalins in CSF and tissues of animals treated with different doses of d-phenylalanine and other peptidase inhibitors. In fact, exopeptidase inhibitors of theoretical clinical importance should potentiate the effects of enkephalins by increasing the turnover of these neuropeptides.

TABLE 1. *MLF content in CSF of headache sufferers and of patients with different neurological diseases*

No. of patients	Mean age (years)	Pathology	CSF collected during	MLF content (pmoles met-enk)
19	39.56 ± 2.86	Idiopathic headache	Attack period	2.27 ± 0.30
5	36.35 ± 4.61	Idiopathic headache	Free period	13.34 ± 5.11[a]
4	41.80 ± 1.15	Different neurological diseases	Free period	25.62 ± 10.86[a]

[a] $p < 0.01$.

TABLE 2. *Serum beta-ELI in controls and in headache sufferers*

No. of subjects	Mean age (years)	Sample collected in	Beta-ELI (pg/ml)
21	38.56 ± 2.12	Healthy volunteers	369.95 ± 35.08
33	37.60 ± 2.00	Headache sufferers (free period)	334.66 ± 33.97
13	42.77 ± 3.02	Headache sufferers (attack period)	315.00 ± 43.33
7	37.93 ± 2.97	Headache sufferers (at end of attack)	1152.57 ± 319.06[a]

[a] $p < 0.01$.

BETA-ENDORPHIN-LIKE IMMUNOREACTIVITY IN SERUM OF HEALTHY VOLUNTEERS AND HEADACHE SUFFERERS

Serum beta-endorphin-like immunoreactivity (beta-ELI) was determined by a radioimmunoassay technique (KIT Inc., Minnesota) partially modified as described elsewhere (3). The antiserum for beta-endorphin cross-reacts with beta-lipotropin, therefore, a direct assay in serum samples does not allow the valuation of beta-endorphin alone; thus the term beta-ELI is used.

Samples were collected from healthy volunteers and from headache sufferers in pain-free periods or at different stages of the attack. As shown in Table 2, no difference was found in the serum beta-ELI content of control subjects and headache patients when samples were obtained during a pain-free period or during the attack, whereas it was significantly higher at the end of the attack. Since it has been reported that stress induces a release of beta-endorphin and related peptides from pituitary (1), our findings suggest that the high levels of endorphins found at the end of the attack may be associated with the degree of stress provoked by headache pain. However, as has been previously pointed out in the explanation of the acupuncture-induced analgesia mechanism (8), the increased endorphin release may play an important role in attenuating the crisis and restoring the state of well-being (2). Recently, high levels of serum beta-ELI, with the maximum peak in the last trimester, have been found in pregnant women (3,5,10). This finding is pertinent to the observation that during pregnancy the autonomic system is well balanced, mood is clearly euphoric, and preexistent headache frequently disappears.

CONCLUSIONS

The role of endorphins in a number of diseases and metabolic disorders remains to be clarified. However, several studies suggest the involvement of these peptides in neuronal functions related to the pain-modulating system and certain psychic and behavioral conditions. A simultaneous impairment of these functions is present in idiopathic headache sufferers, suggesting that the unbalanced endorphin system might be involved in the pathogenesis of this disease. Assuming that the MLF content in CSF may be an index of neuronal activity in the brain, the low MLF levels found during the attack might confirm this hypothesis. Moreover, morphine, the potent central analgesic, is ineffective in relieving headache. This apparent discrepancy requires further considerations concerning the functional significance of endorphin content in CSF and plasma. Indeed, low endorphin levels might not necessarily reflect an impaired function of the peptidergic system in the brain, since the reliable biochemical index of neurotransmitter dynamics is the turn-over rate measurement. On the other hand, the presence of various opiate receptors with different affinities for morphine and enkephalins (7a) suggests that endogenous opiates may have effects different from those of narcotic alkaloids.

Despite the failure to define this discrepancy, it is likely that the high levels of endor-phins detected in the serum of patients at the end of the crisis may reflect an increased release of opioid peptides from the pituitary; i.e., the peptides participate in restoring the state of well-being, as a consequence of the stress produced by pain.

ACKNOWLEDGMENT

We acknowledge the National Research Council for financial support.

REFERENCES

1. Akil, H., Madden, J., Patrick, R. L., and Barchas, J. D. (1976): Stress-induced increase in endogenous opiate peptides: Concurrent analgesia and its partial reversal by naloxone. In: *Opiates and Endogenous Opioid Peptides,* edited by H. W. Kosterlitz, pp. 63–70. Elsevier, Amsterdam.
2. Anselmi, B., Baldi, E., Casacci, F., and Salmon, S. (1980): Endogenous opioids in cerebrospinal fluid and blood in idiopathic headache sufferers. *Headache,* 20:294–299.
3. Baldi, E., Branconi, F., Brocchi, A., Cappelli, G., Paladini, S., Salmon, S., and Sicuteri, F. (1979): Beta-endorphin-like-immunoreactivity (beta-ELI) in pregnancy. In: *Headache,* edited by F. Savoldi and G. Nappi, pp. 121–127. Fidia Research Laboratories, Padova, Italy.
4. Byck, R. (1976): Peptides transmitters: An unifying hypothesis for euphoria, respiration, sleep, and the action of lithium. *Lancet,* 10:72–73.
5. Cappelli, G., Brocchi, A., Milani, S., Paladini, S., Branconi, F., Baldi, E., Salmon, S., and Sicuteri, F. (1980): Beta-endorphin-like-immunoreactivity (beta-ELI) in pregnancy: Its relation to other hormones *(this volume).*
6. Carenzi, A., Biasini, I., Frigeni, V., and Della Bella, D. (1980): On the enzymatic degradation of enkepha-lins: Pharmacological implications. In: *Advances in Biochemical Psychopharmacology, Vol. 22,* edited by E. Costa and M. Trabucchi, pp. 237–246. Raven Press, New York.
7. Carenzi, A., Casacci, F., Sicuteri, F., and Della Bella, D. (1979): Livelli di morphine-like factors nel liquido cefalorachidiano di soggetti affetti da cefalea o da sindromi neurologiche diverse. *Riv. Farmacol. Ter.,* X:109–115.
7a. Chang, K. J., and Cuatrecasas, P. (1979): Multiple opiate receptors, enkephalins and morphine bind to receptors of different specificity. *J. Biol. Chem.,* 254:2610–2618.
8. Clement-Jones, V., McLoughlin, L., Lowry, P. J., Besser, G. M., Rees, L. H., and Wen, H. L. (1979): Acupuncture in heroin addicts: Changes in met-enkephalin and beta-endorphin in blood and cerebrospinal fluid. *Lancet,* 25:380–382.
9. Cox, B. M., Goldstein, A., and Li, C. H. (1976): Opioid activity of a peptide, beta-lipotropin- (61–91), derived from beta-lipotropin. *Proc. Natl. Acad. Sci. USA,* 73:1,821–1,823.
10. Csontos, K., Rust, M., Hollt, V., Mahar, W., Kromer, W., and Teschemacher, H. J. (1979): Elevated plasma beta-endorphin levels in pregnant women and their neonates. *Life Sci.,* 25:835–844.
11. Delange, R. J., and Smith, E. L. (1971): Leucine aminopeptidase and other N-terminal exopeptidase. In: *The Enzymes, Vol. 3,* edited by F. D. Boyer, pp. 81–119. Academic Press, New York.
12. Della Bella, D., Carenzi, A., Frigeni, V., and Santini, V. (1979): Effect of carboxypeptidase inhibition on the in vivo and in vitro pharmacological properties of morphine and enkephalins. *Neuropharmacology,* 18:719–721.
13. Ehrenpreis, S., Balagot, R. C., Comaty, J. E., and Myles, S. B. (1979): Naloxone reversible analgesia in mice produced by D-phenylalanine and hydrocinnamic acid, inhibitors of carboxypeptidase A. In: *Advances in Pain Research and Therapy,* edited by J. J. Bonica, pp. 479–488. Raven Press, New York.
14. Goldstein, A. (1976): Opioid peptides (endorphins) in pituitary and brain. *Science,* 193:1,081–1,086.
15. Guillemin, R., Ling, N., and Burgus, R. (1976): Endorphines, peptides d'origine hypothalamique et neurohypophysaire à activité morphinomimétique. Isolement et structure moléculaire de l'alpha-endor-phine. *C.R. Acad. Sci. Paris,* 282:783–785.
16. Hambrook, J. M., Morgan, B. A., Rance, M. J., and Smith, C. F. C. (1976): Mode of deactivation of the enkephalins by rat and human plasma and rat brain homogenates. *Nature,* 262:782–783.

17. Hughes, J. (1975): Isolation of an endogenous compound from the brain with pharmacological properties similar to morphine. *Brain Res.,* 88:295–308.
18. Hughes, J., Smith, T. W., Kosterlitz, H. W., Fothergill, L. A., Morgan, B. A., and Morris, H. R. (1975): Identification of two related pentapeptides from the brain with potent opiate agonist activity. *Nature,* 258:577–579.
19. Meek, J. L., Yang, H. Y. T., and Costa, E. (1977): Enkephalin catabolism in vitro and in vivo. *Neuropharmacology,* 16:151–154.
20. Pert, C. B., and Snyder, S. H. (1973): Opiate receptors: Demonstration in nervous tissues. *Science,* 179:1,011–1,014.
21. Sicuteri, F., Anselmi, B., Curradi, C., Michelacci, S., and Sassi, A. (1978): Morphine-like factors in CSF of headache patients. In: *Advances in Biochemical Psychopharmacology, Vol. 18,* edited by E. Costa and M. Trabucchi, pp. 363–366. Raven Press, New York.
22. Terenius, L. (1979): Endorphins in chronic pain. In: *Advances in Pain Research and Therapy, Vol. 3,* edited by J. J. Bonica, J. C. Liebeskind, and D. G. Albe-Fessard, pp. 459–471. Raven Press, New York.
23. Terenius, L., and Wahlström, A. (1975). Morphine-like ligand for opiate receptors in human CSF. *Life Sci.,* 16:1,759–1,764.
24. Terenius, L., Wahlström, A., Lindström, L., and Widerlöv, E. (1976): Increased CSF levels of endorphins in chronic psychosis. *Neurosci. Lett.,* 3:157–162.
25. Von Knorring, L., Almay, B. G. L., Johansson, F., and Terenius, L. (1978): Pain perception and endorphin levels in cerebrospinal fluid. *Pain,* 5:359–365.

Advances in Neurology, Vol. 33, edited by
M. Critchley et al. Raven Press, New York © 1982

Neuronal Sensitivity and Opiate Tolerance/Dependence

Albert Herz and Rüdiger Schulz

*Department of Neuropharmacology, Max Planck Institute for Psychiatry,
Munich, Federal Republic of Germany*

The phenomenon of drug addiction, constituted by a tolerance to and physical dependence on a particular drug class, reflects an adaptation of neurons to continuous exposure to the drug in question. These adaptive compensatory changes establish a new equilibrium, the disturbance of which by withdrawal of the addictive drug produces pathophysiological changes manifested as withdrawal signs.

Among the several theories advanced to explain the compensatory mechanisms leading to tolerance and dependence (see ref. 13), those of Collier (3) and Jaffe and Sharpless (15) emphasize the importance of changes in neuronal sensitivity; other theories also implicate the significance of such events. Collier postulated that postsynaptically located neurotransmitter receptors become supersensitive upon prolonged opiate-induced presynaptic inhibition of the release of the excitatory neurotransmitter, resembling the phenomenon of denervation or disuse supersensitivity (15). Other theories postulate adaptive changes, such as an altered sensitivity of the opiate-responsive neurons themselves (4). All these theories imply that the ability to induce changes in neuronal sensitivity is not specific to opiates (or other addictive drugs), since such changes are an expression of the general regulatory capacity of cells to adapt to the requirements of an altered functional state. In this chapter, some recent results concerning changes in neuronal sensitivity which occur during the cycle of opiate dependence are reviewed. The data obtained in intact animals, in isolated preparations, and upon recording from single neurons are mutually complementary and offer a basis for a discussion of the mechanisms involved in the development of tolerance and dependence (12).

EXPERIMENTS IN INTACT ANIMALS

A generalized increase in neuronal excitability during opiate abstinence is suggested by the lowered seizure threshold observed in withdrawn animals (1,10). More definitive information is obtained from behavioral studies, which show an increased sensitivity of the central nervous system (CNS) to certain specific effects of individual neurotransmitters or receptor agonists during opiate withdrawal. Thus several reports point to an increase in the effectiveness of catecholaminergic agents in inducing or enhancing aggression (18), stereotypes (6), increased motor activity (25), circling (11), or dyskinesias (5) in the withdrawn animal. Other reports indicate an increased responsiveness to cholinergic agents during abstinence from morphine (28).

In accord with the data obtained from these studies in abruptly withdrawn rats, recent observations show remarkable alterations in the responsiveness to intracerebroventricularly administered neurotransmitters or neurotransmitter receptor agonists after precipitation of withdrawal by naloxone (22,23). In these experiments, the test substances were injected after withdrawal jumping evoked by naloxone had ceased (Fig. 1). Neurotransmitters, such as dopamine, norepinephrine, or serotonin, as well as the dopamine receptor agonist apomorphine and the adrenoceptor agonist clonidine, were able to reiniti-

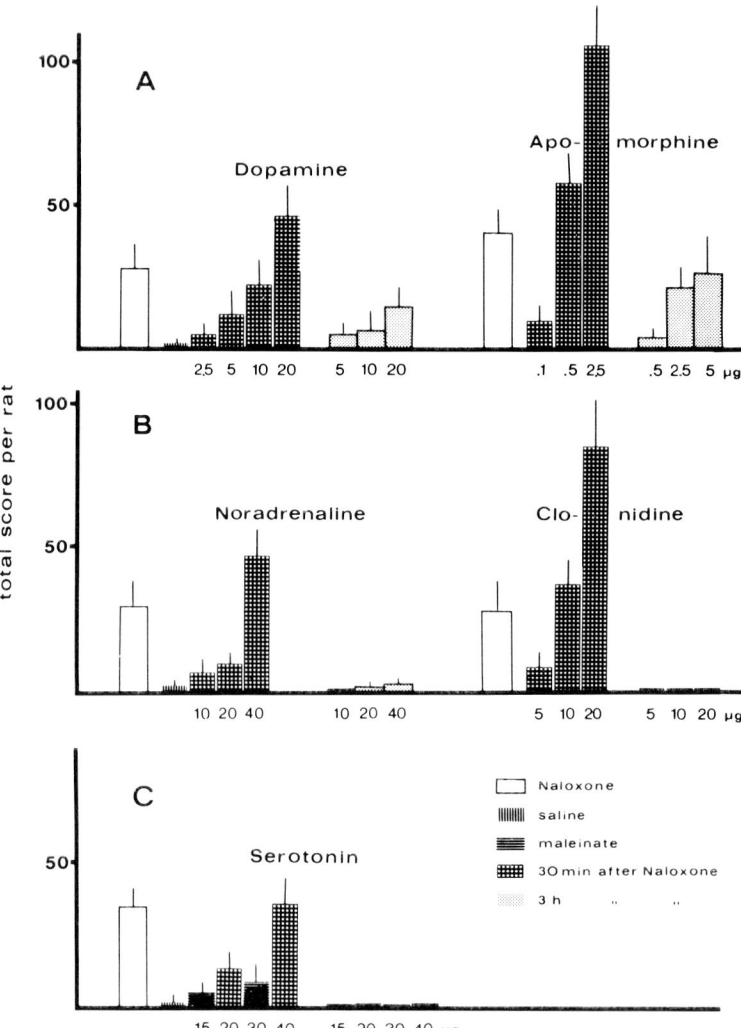

FIG. 1. Response of morphine-tolerant dependent rats, either not withdrawn or after naloxone (10 mg/kg, i.p.)-induced withdrawal, to intracerebroventricular (i.c.v.) administration of neurotransmitters or their receptor agonists. Naloxone-caused jumping *(open columns)* ceased after 20 to 40 min. Five minutes after cessation of jumping, the first i.c.v. injection was performed *(hatched columns)*. The second i.c.v. injection was conducted 3 hr after naloxone treatment *(stippled columns)*. Each column represents the mean total score of jumping. Rats not withdrawn *(bars)* failed to respond to i.c.v. drug administration. Abscissa: doses (μg base) given i.c.v. (For details, see ref. 22.)

ate jumping in a dose-dependent manner. Of all the transmitter receptor agonists tested, dopamine and apomorphine proved to be most effective in reinitiating jumping. These compounds were effective even after 3 hr of continuous exposure of the animals to naloxone. After this time, norepinephrine, clonidine, and serotonin no longer exerted any effect. In contrast, acetylcholine and prostaglandin E_1 (PGE_1) completely failed to reinitiate jumping.

Since even at high dosages these substances failed to induce jumping when applied intracerebroventricularly to naive rats or to tolerant/dependent rats prior to precipitation of withdrawal, one may speak of "neuronal sensitization" to the test drugs but not of "supersensitivity," which implies a shift of the dose-response curve; this does not in fact occur.

THE ISOLATED GUINEA PIG ILEUM AS A MODEL FOR TESTING ADAPTIVE MECHANISMS IN RESPONSE TO OPIATES

Isolated preparations with nervous structures less complicated than the CNS offer the possibility for a more mechanistic study of changes in sensitivity. The longitudinal muscle-myenteric plexus preparation of the guinea pig ileum represents a useful tool for the testing of opiates. In this preparation, opiates cause inhibition of electrically evoked contractions. Neurotransmitters/neuromodulators interfere with the activity of the preparation; e.g., 5-hydroxytryptamine (5-HT) and PGE_1 exert excitatory, epinephrine and dopamine inhibitory, actions. In preparations from guinea pigs rendered tolerant/dependent by morphine pellet implantation, changes in sensitivity to these compounds can be demonstrated (9,20,21) (Fig. 2). (In these experiments, the preparations were set up in the presence of 200 nM normorphine to prevent spontaneous withdrawal.)

As shown above, the effective concentration (EC_{50}) of normorphine in inhibiting electrically evoked contraction increases from about 100 nM in the naive preparation to about 2,000 nM in the tolerant preparation. As long as normorphine is present at the receptor, sensitivity to PGE_1 and 5-HT is not changed in comparison to naive preparations. Upon withdrawal by naloxone, however, the sensitivity to both excitatory agents dramatically increases. At the same time, the inhibitory action of epinephrine and dopamine is reduced, whereas the sensitivity to acetylcholine, the neurotransmitter acting mainly at the neuromuscular junction, is unchanged (9). The increased sensitivity for 5-HT and PGE_1 is obviously masked in the presence of the opiate but becomes visible after its removal from the receptors.

Dose-response curves for 5-HT and PGE_1 show a parallel shift to the left (indicating supersensitivity in the strict sense), with a maximum apparent immediately after withdrawal precipitation. At the same time, a withdrawal sign (that is, a contracture of smooth muscle) is precipitated by naloxone. Repeated washing results in a continuous reduction of the degree of tolerance and of supersensitivity, although even after 3 hr of washing, a normal sensitivity to morphine, 5-HT, and PGE_1 is not reached. The possibility to precipitate a further withdrawal contracture disappears, although supersensitivity still exists. This emphasizes the importance of a differentiation between manifestation of dependence (that is, the withdrawal sign) and tolerance/dependence (that is, supersensitivity). Thus a withdrawal sign may not be inducible although supersensitivity still exists. This altered sensitivity is suggested to be associated with tolerance and dependence.

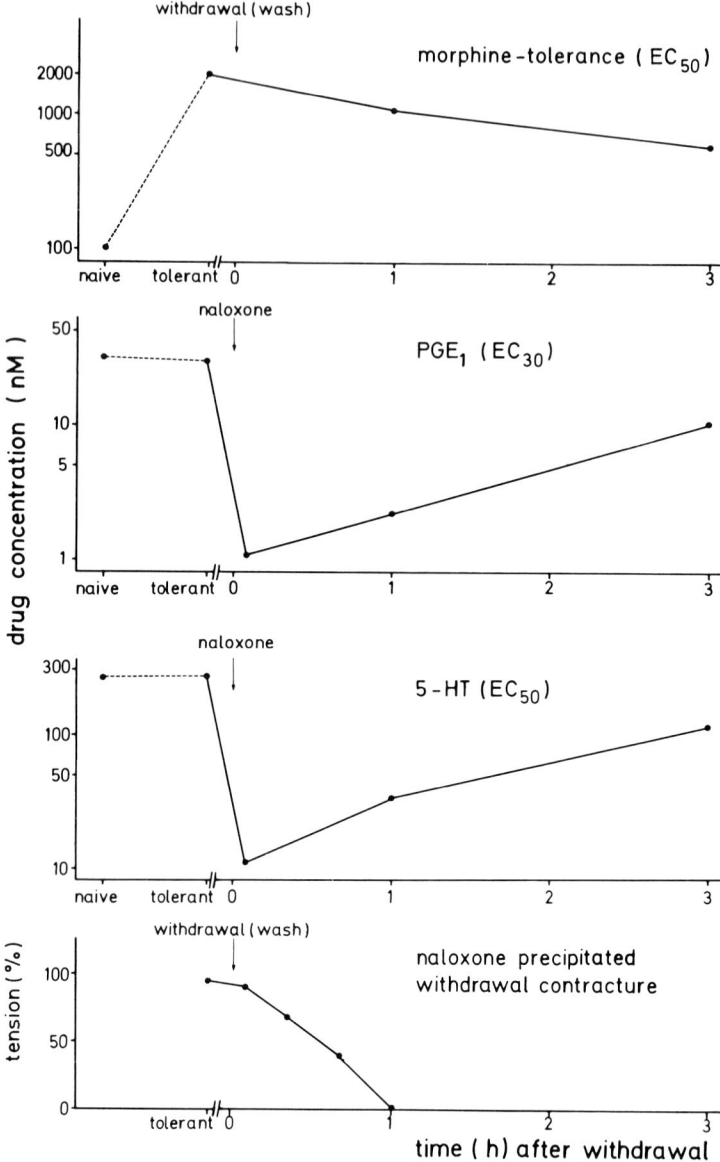

FIG. 2. Demonstration of morphine tolerance, change in neuronal sensitivity, and withdrawal contracture of the isolated longitudinal muscle-myenteric plexus preparation from chronically morphinized guinea pigs. The preparations were set up *in vitro* in the presence of 200 nM normorphine. Tests were conducted either before or after induction of withdrawal by naloxone *(arrow)*. The median effective concentrations (EC_{50} and EC_{30}) are plotted against time and a logarithmic scale. The intensity of withdrawal contracture precipitated by naloxone (50 nM) is expressed as percent of the twitch tension evoked by electrical stimulation. (Adapted from ref. 21.)

SENSITIVITY CHANGES AT THE SINGLE NEURON LEVEL

In studies with single neurons, it is possible to detect changes in the sensitivity of the response to neuroactive compounds directly from the tolerant/dependent neuron. Only a few studies based on this principle have been undertaken; but they have clearly shown changes in sensitivity, generally consistent with the indication derived from other approaches (19,29). In rats made highly tolerant to morphine, a significant increase in the sensitivity of cortical neurons was observed upon testing their excitatory response to glutamic acid or to acetylcholine applied microiontophoretically. These animals did not receive naloxone prior to testing. That such an increased sensitivity was detected under these conditions may be due to the partial spontaneous withdrawal of the tolerant/dependent rats. In more recent experiments (8), the sensitivity of striatal neurons to microiontophoretically applied glutamic acid and acetylcholine was tested in tolerant/dependent rats both before and during local (iontophoretic) application of naloxone. (+)-Naloxone, the pharmacologically inactive isomer of naloxone, was ineffective in changing the response to the excitatory compounds. Induction of local withdrawal by (−)-naloxone, however, induced not only spontaneous discharge activity but also an increased response to *l*-glutamate and acetylcholine.

POSSIBLE MECHANISMS UNDERLYING CHANGES IN NEURONAL SENSITIVITY

An increase in the responsiveness to a neurotransmitter may be caused either by a quantitative change in transmitter binding sites or by changes in the mechanisms through which ligand/receptor binding is translated into a given effect.

Changes at the Receptor Level

Thus far, little evidence suggests that the development of opiate tolerance/dependence is associated with an alteration of the receptor binding of neurotransmitters or with an increase in the number of these receptors, at least with respect to dopamine. Thus, displacement of ^{3}H-spiroperidol, a dopamine receptor agonist with a high receptor affinity, by either dopamine or haloperidol from striatal membranes of naive rats, did not differ from the displacement seen in membranes obtained from tolerant/dependent rats, indicating that neither the affinity nor the number of dopamine receptors had changed (14). The mechanism underlying the opiate-induced dopaminergic supersensitivity obviously differs from that involved in neuroleptic-induced supersensitivity, which has been shown to be associated with an increase in the number of dopamine binding sites (2). On the other hand, that the observed increase in binding sites after neuroleptic treatment was rather low ($\sim 20\%$), suggests that, also in the case of neuroleptic mechanisms, a factor other than an increase in the number of binding sites may be at least partly responsible for the observed increase in sensitivity to dopamine.

Recently, an increase in the number of β-adrenergic binding sites in the cortex of morphine-tolerant/dependent rats has been reported (17,24). In view of the limited extent of this increase ($\sim 20\%$), one must consider the possibility that other mechanisms contribute to the hypersensitivity to norepinephrine seen in these experiments.

Changes Beyond the Neurotransmitter Receptor

In view of the lack of—or at most the limited nature of—the adaptive changes taking place at the neurotransmitter/receptor level during the development of opiate tolerance/ dependence, alterations in the postreceptor effector system appear more important for the explanation of the observed shifts in sensitivity to neurotransmitters. It is probable that adenosine 3′, 5′-monophosphate (cyclic AMP) and guanosine 3′, 5′-monophosphate (cyclic GMP) act as "second messengers" in synaptic transmission and thus constitute the immediate link between ligand/receptor coupling and subsequent cellular processes.

Evidence suggests that changes in the cyclic AMP system may be closely related to supersensitivity phenomena. For example, opiate studies in neuroblastoma $\times$ glioma hybrid cells have demonstrated an enhanced activity of adenylate cyclase in opiate-tolerant/dependent cells undergoing withdrawal. This increased activity is manifested by an increased sensitivity to PGE_1. [There is, however, no clear shift of the dose-response curve to the left but a high increase in the maximal response: thus this does not represent supersensitivity in the strict sense (26,27).] An increased formation of cyclic AMP in response to norepinephrine and isoprenaline has also been found in cortical slices taken from morphine-tolerant/dependent as compared to placebo rats. This increased activity of adenylate cyclase is thought to reflect processes compensating for the inhibitory effects of opiates on adenylate cyclase (17,24). The observation that the adenylate cyclase system is apparently able to adapt not only to opiate-induced inhibition but also to adrenergic and cholinergic inhibitory effects suggests that this system might represent a general homeostatic principle of the cell.

Biochemical changes in the "effector system" of cells, e.g., in adenylate cyclase, may manifest themselves electrophysiologically in a change of membrane potential. This supposition is the basis of the hypothesis that opiate-induced supersensitivity phenomena may reflect a partial depolarization of neuronal membranes (7,16). Such proposed changes in the resting potential of membranes would account for the apparently unspecific nature of the sensitivity changes observed during withdrawal.

Cellular Site of Sensitivity Changes

One important aspect in this context is whether the adaptive changes leading to an increased sensitivity to excitatory neurotransmitters take place in the opiate-sensitive cell itself or in other neurons, interacting with opiate-responsive neurons. Experiments in intact animals provide little information germane to this question. Experiments in the isolated guinea pig ileum point to a change in the opiate-sensitive cell itself. The electrophysiological studies of single neurons, in addition to the biochemical studies in cell culture, clearly show that the opiate-sensitive neuron itself develops tolerance and dependence (4). On the other hand, the changes at the receptor level and in the biochemical machinery observed in the rat cortex after chronic morphine treatment (17) indicate that adaptive changes may take place downstream of the opiate-sensitive cell. This may be most easily explained by opiate-induced inhibition of neurotransmitter release, as postulated in the original theories of denervation supersensitivity (15). Thus one may conclude that there are a variety of possibilities at different levels of neuronal organization allowing for induction of compensatory changes in response to chronic opiate treatment.

ACKNOWLEDGMENT

This investigation was supported bei Deutsche Forschungsgemeinschaft, Bonn.

REFERENCES

1. Adler, M. W., Lin, C., Smith, K. P., Tresky, R., and Gildenberg, P. L. (1974): Lowered seizure threshold as a part of the narcotic abstinence syndrome in rats. *Psychopharmacologia,* 35:243–247.
2. Burt, D. R., Creese, I., and Snyder, S. H. (1977): Antischizophrenic drugs: Chronic treatment elevates dopamine receptor binding in brain. *Science,* 196:326–328.
3. Collier, H. O. J. (1968): Supersensitivity and dependence. *Nature,* 220:228–231.
4. Collier, H. O. J. (1980): Cellular sites of opiate dependence. *Nature,* 283:625–629.
5. Eibergen, R. D., and Carlson, K. R. (1975): Dyskinesias elicited by methamphetamine: Susceptibility by former methadone-consuming monkeys. *Science,* 190:588–590.
6. Eibergen, R. D., and Carlson, K. R. (1976): Behavioral evidence for dopaminergic supersensitivity following chronic treatment with methadone or chlorpromazine in the guinea pig. *Psychopharmacology,* 48:139–146.
7. Fleming, W. W. (1976): Variable sensitivity of excitable cells: Possible mechanism and biological significance. In: *Reviews of Neuroscience, Vol. 2,* edited by S. Ehrenpreis and I. J. Kopin, pp. 43–90. Raven Press, New York.
8. Fry, J. P., Herz, A., and Zieglgänsberger, W. (1980): A demonstration of naloxone-precipitated opiate withdrawal on single neurones in the morphine-tolerant/dependent rat brain. *Br. J. Pharmacol.,* 68:585–592.
9. Goldstein, A., and Schulz, R. (1973): Morphine-tolerant longitudinal muscle strip from guinea-pig ileum. *Br. J. Pharmacol.,* 48:655–666.
10. Greer, C. A., Alpern, H. P., and Collins, A. C. (1976): Increased CNS sensitivity to flurothyl as a measure of physical dependence in mice following morphine, phenobarbital, and ethanol treatment. *Life Sci.,* 18:1,375–1,382.
11. Halliwell, J. V., and Kumar, R. (1977): Influence of morphine dependence and withdrawal on circling behavior in rats with unilateral nigral lesions. *Br. J. Pharmacol.,* 59:454P.
12. Herz, A., Bläsig, J., Fry, J. P., Höllt, V., Meyer, G., and Przewłocki, R. (1978): Opiate receptors, their endogenous ligands and the development of tolerance/dependence. In: *Advances in Pharmacology and Therapeutics, Vol. 1,* edited by J. Jacob, pp. 47–56. Pergamon Press, Oxford.
13. Herz, A., and Schulz, R. (1978): Changes in neuronal sensitivity during addictive processes. In: *The Bases of Addiction,* edited by J. Fishman, pp. 375–394. Dahlem Konferenzen, Berlin.
14. Höllt, V., Bläsig, J., Dum, J., Przewłocki, R., and Herz, A. (1978): Opiate receptors and endorphins in opiate addiction. In: *Proceedings of the European Society for Neurochemistry, Vol. 1,* edited by V. Neuhoff, pp. 386–403. Verlag Chemie, Weinheim.
15. Jaffe, J. H., and Sharpless, S. K. (1968): Pharmacological denervation supersensitivity in the central nervous system: A theory of physical dependance. *Res. Publ. Assoc. Res. Nerv. Ment. Dis.,* 46:226–246.
16. Johnson, S. M., Westfall, D. P., Fleming, W. W., and Howard, S. A. (1977): Sensitivity changes in the ileal longitudinal muscle-myenteric plexus preparation of the guinea pig after chronic morphine implantation. *Fed. Proc.,* 36:1010.
17. Llorens, C., Martres, M. P., Baudry, M., and Schwartz, J. C. (1978): Hypersensitivity to noradrenaline in cortex after chronic morphine: Relevance to tolerance and dependence. *Nature (Lond.),* 274:603–605.
18. Puri, S. K., and Lal, H. (1974): Reduced threshold to pain induced aggression specifically related to morphine dependence. *Psychopharmacologia,* 35:237–241.
19. Satoh, M., Zieglgänsberger, W., and Herz, A. (1976): Supersensitivity of cortical neurones of the rat to acetylcholine and L-glutamate following chronic morphine treatment. *Naunyn Schmiedebergs Arch. Pharmacol.,* 293:101–103.
20. Schulz, R., and Goldstein, A. (1973): Morphine tolerance and supersensitivity to 5-hydroxytryptamine in the myenteric plexus of the guinea-pig. *Nature,* 244:168–170.
21. Schulz, R., and Herz, A. (1976): Aspects of opiate dependence in the myenteric plexus of the guinea-pig. *Life Sci.,* 19:1,117–1,128.
22. Schulz, R., and Herz, A. (1977): Naloxone precipitated withdrawal reveals sensitization to neurotransmitters in morphine tolerant/dependent rats. *Naunyn Schmiedebergs Arch. Pharmacol.,* 299:95–99.
23. Schulz, R., Bläsig, J., Laschka, E., and Herz, A. (1978): Site of naloxone-precipitated opiate withdrawal dissociates from that at which apomorphine reinitiates this phenomenon. *Naunyn Schmiedebergs Arch. Pharmacol.,* 305:1–4.
24. Schwartz, J. C. (1979): Opiate receptors on catecholaminergic neurones in the brain. *Trends Neurosci.,* 2:137–139.

25. Smee, M. L., and Overstreet, D. H. (1976): Alterations in the effects of dopamine agonists and antagonists on general activity in rats following chronic morphine treatment. *Psychopharmacology,* 49:125–130.
26. Sharma, S. K., Klee, W. A., and Nirenberg, M. (1975): Dual regulation of adenylate cyclase accounts for narcotic dependence and tolerance. *Proc. Natl. Acad. Sci. USA,* 72:3,092–3,096.
27. Traber, J., Gullis, R., and Hamprecht, B. (1975): Influence of opiates on the levels of adenosine 3′:5′-cyclic monophosphate in neuroblastoma × glioma hybrid cells. *Life Sci.,* 16:1,863–1,868.
28. Vasquez, B. J., Overstreet, D. H., and Russel, R. W. (1974): Psychopharmacological evidence for increase in receptor sensitivity following chronic morphine treatment. *Psychopharmacologia,* 38:287–302.
29. Yarbrough, G. G., and Phillis, J. W. (1975): Supersensitivity of central neurons—a brief review of an emerging concept. *Can. J. Neurol. Sci.,* 2:147–152.

Advances in Neurology, Vol. 33, edited by
M. Critchley et al. Raven Press, New York © 1982

Effect of Antimigraine Drugs
on Nonopioid Analgesia

A. Bartolini, P. Malmberg, R. Bartolini, and A. Giotti

Department of Pharmacology, University of Florence, Florence, Italy

Pain perception is modulated at a central level by various neuronal systems, of which the opiate one is the best known. Other systems, however, play an important role in the control of pain. It is well accepted (5,14,17,18,21) that stimulation of the muscarinic type of central cholinergic receptors induces powerful analgesia with side effects that make therapeutic application impossible. Furthermore, we have recently shown (7) that analgesia may also be induced through stimulation of a particular type of γ-aminobutyric acid (GABA) receptor, which has been described by Bowery et al. (10,11) and is stimulated solely by GABA and by baclofen, a selective agonist molecule. No antagonist molecule is yet known. The new GABAergic receptor is insensitive to both muscimol and bicuculline, the former an agonist of the classic GABA receptor and the latter an antagonist.

There are at least three types of receptors and as many neurotransmitters, such as enkephalins, acetylcholine (ACh), and GABA, involved in pain modulation. The serotoninergic-mediated system could be added, although it is less potent in inducing analgesia. Moreover, since it is activated by opioid stimulation (1), there is reason to assume an interdependence of the two systems (5).

The presence in the central nervous system (CNS) of numerous neurotransmitters for pain control is borne out by two observations: (a) The analgesia induced by electrical stimulation of specific cerebral areas and by acupuncture or electroacupuncture is never completely antagonized by pure opioid antagonists, such as naloxone (3,4,28). The same can be said for hypnotic (15) and foot-shock analgesia (22). Lewis et al. (22) showed that, depending on its temporal parameters, inescapable foot-shock can cause either an opioid or a nonopioid type of analgesia. (b) Only vertebrates possess opioid receptors (24). Invertebrates, in the absence of these receptors, control their painful sensations through some other phylogenetically older mechanism. In this connection, it could be significant that they possess both muscarinic and GABAergic receptors.

Two major agents are used throughout the world in the therapy of migraine headaches. One is ergotamine, a classic ergot alkaloid; the other is methysergide, a synthetic ergot derivative. We sought to determine how these antimigraine drugs interact with the major classes of centrally acting analgesics.

We have already demonstrated (6,23) that methysergide and cyproheptadine strongly enforce the analgesia induced by exogenous and endogenous opioid agonists, while ergotamine does not. We report here on the action of ergotamine and methysergide on the analgesia induced by both the muscarinic agonist oxotremorine and the new type of GABAergic agonist baclofen.

The most interesting finding that emerged from this research is that, while methysergide potentiates all types of analgesia, however induced, ergotamine enforces only oxotremorine and baclofen analgesia and has no action on opiate analgesia.

MATERIAL AND METHODS

Experiments were carried out on Wistar male albino rats and Swiss-Webster male mice. The following analgesic tests were used: the tail-flick test, according to D'Amour and Smith (12), utilizing a Galileo analgesimeter; the hot-plate test, according to Woolfe and Mac Donald (27); and the acetic acid writhing test, according to Koster et al. (19). In the hot-plate test, the cut-off time was fixed at 45 sec.

Analgesia was induced either by intraperitoneally or subcutaneously injecting agonists for opioid, muscarinic, or new type GABA receptors. Morphine, HCl (Erba), and eseroline salicylate were used as exogenous opioid agonists.

Eseroline is a powerful new analgetic, structurally related to physostigmine, which was recently discovered by our group (8,13). Although it has the chemical structure of physostigmine, it has completely lost the characteristic anticholinesterase activity of the latter and gained a strong agonistic effect on the opiate receptor, which is antagonized by naloxone. Oxotremorine-HCl (Fluka AG) and baclofen-HCl (CIBA-GEIGY) were used as muscarinic and new type GABA agonists, respectively.

Methysergide bimaleate (Sandoz) and ergotamine tartrate (Gynergen, Sandoz) were used as antimigraine drugs. Naloxone-HCl (Endo Laboratories) and atropine sulfate (BDH) were used as pure opioid and muscarinic antagonists. The doses of all drugs refer to their salts.

RESULTS

Analgesic Effect of Baclofen

Figures 1 and 2 show the analgesic effect of baclofen in the rat (Fig. 1) and in the mouse (Fig. 2). Analgesia resulting from subcutaneously administered baclofen reached its maximum in about 60 min. Similar results were also obtained intraperitoneally. The mouse was slightly more sensitive than the rat to the baclofen analgesic action, as may be seen from the lower doses used on the former.

($\pm$) Baclofen had largely the same analgesic potency as morphine (Fig. 3), which was, however, greatly inferior to that of oxotremorine. Baclofen analgesia, like that of both morphine and oxotremorine, manifested itself at different doses, depending on the analgesic test used. For example, in the writhing test on the mouse, baclofen analgesic action was obtained at doses as low as 1 mg/kg s.c. (see Fig. 6), while in the hot-plate test it was reached with only 2.5 mg/kg s.c. (Fig. 3). Regardless of which analgesic test was used, however, the antinociceptive action of baclofen always manifested itself at lower doses (and sometimes notably lower) than those at which baclofen induced muscular relaxation in the mouse and rat.

Figure 4 shows that baclofen analgesic action was stereospecific; it was induced only with the levoisomer. Finally, Fig. 2 shows that the baclofen action was not antagonized by naloxone, even at enormous doses, or by atropine or bicuculline.

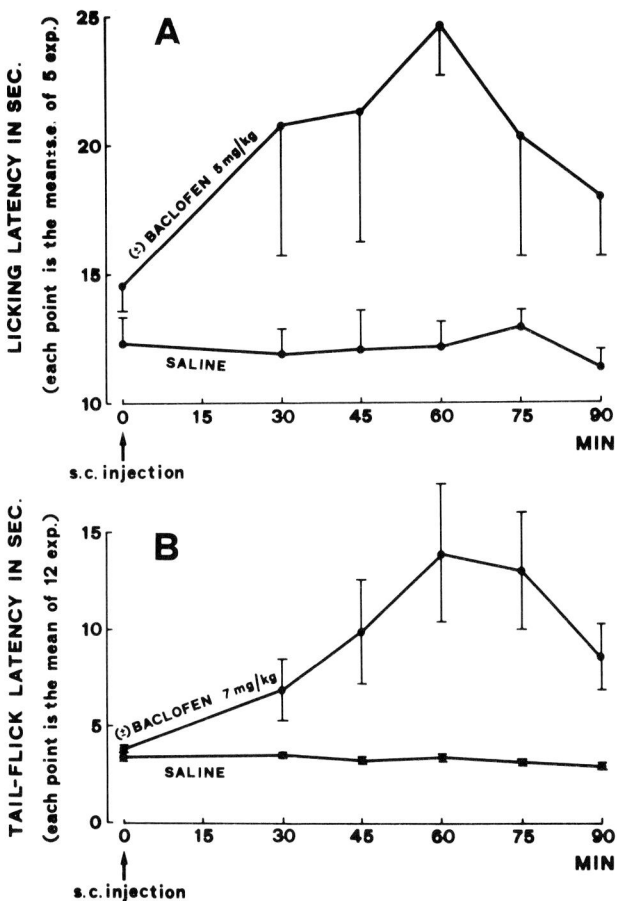

FIG. 1. Analgesia induced by (±) baclofen in rats. **A:** Hot-plate test. **B:** Tail-flick test.

Baclofen analgesia thus was not mediated by the stimulation of either the opiate, the muscarinic, or the classic GABA receptors. We hypothesize (7) that baclofen analgesic action may be attributed to the stimulation of a particular GABA receptor recently described by Bowery et al. (10,11).

Effect of Ergotamine on Baclofen Analgesia

As can be seen in Figs. 5 and 6 and Tables 1 and 2, ergotamine tartrate (Gynergen®) at doses of 0.1 to 0.5 mg/kg s.c. strongly potentiated baclofen analgesic action in the mouse. Obviously, the potentiation was much greater when baclofen was used at doses provoking only a slight degree of analgesia. Although this potentiation was extremely significant in the mouse, from preliminary experiments, it has not yet proved to be similarly evident in the rat. We are unable to explain the mechanism by which ergotamine potentiates the antinociceptive effect of baclofen. In fact, ergotamine (13 nM) does not modify the inhibition induced by baclofen of the contraction of the field-stimulated longitudinal muscle of guinea pig ileum *in vitro*.

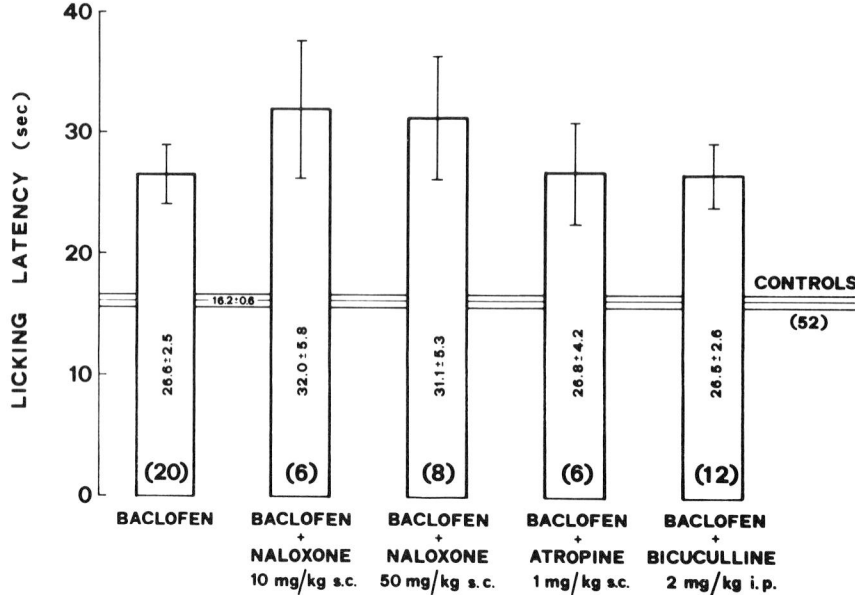

FIG. 2. Effect of naloxone, atropine, and bicuculline on baclofen analgesia in mice tested on hot-plate. (±) Baclofen (4 mg/kg s.c.) was injected 30 min prior to the analgesic test. Naloxone, atropine, and bicuculline were injected 30, 20, and 15 min, respectively, prior to the test. Number of mice in parentheses.

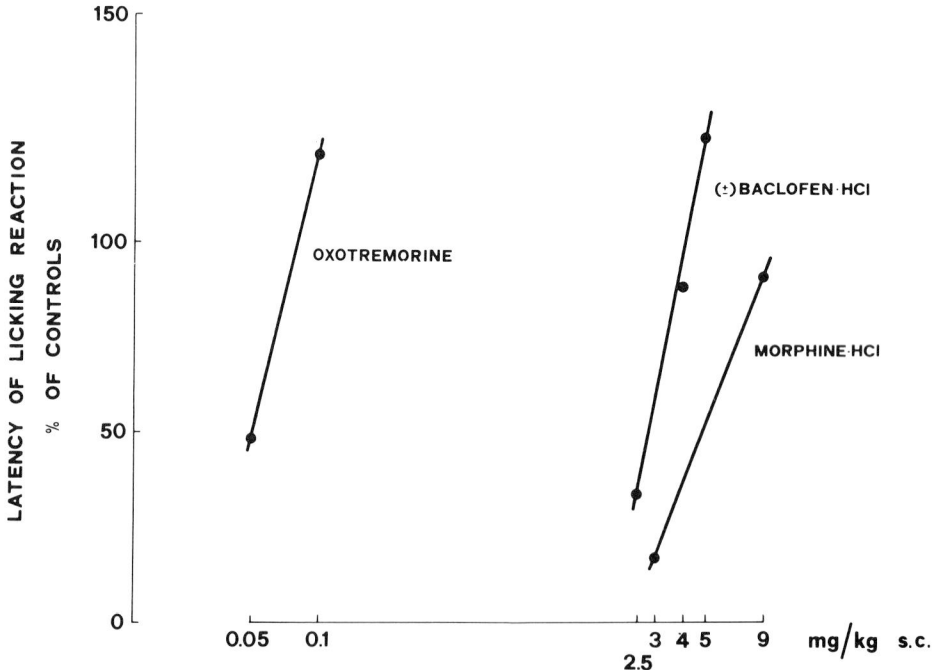

FIG. 3. Comparison of the analgesic activities of morphine, baclofen, and oxotremorine in the mouse hot-plate test. Each point represents the mean of at least seven mice.

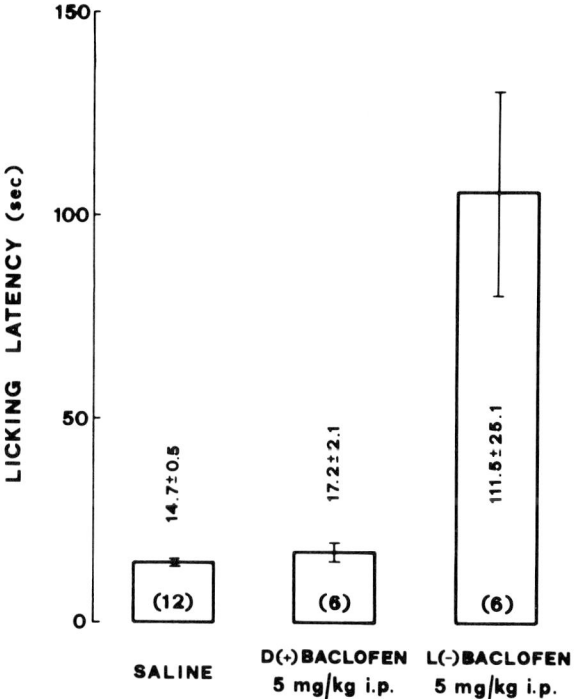

FIG. 4. Stereospecific action of baclofen on analgesia in the hot-plate test in mice. Baclofen was injected 45 min before the test. Number of mice in parentheses.

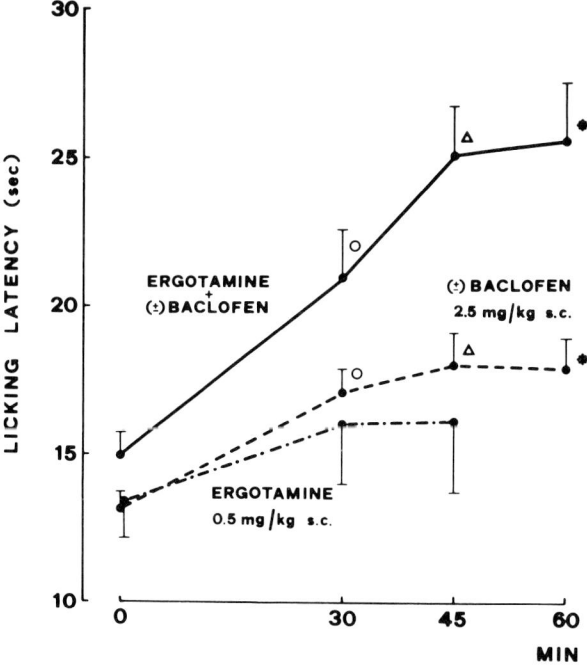

FIG. 5. Effect of ergotamine on analgesia induced by baclofen in mice tested on hot-plate. Baclofen and ergotamine were injected at 0 and 10 min, respectively. Each point is the mean $\pm$ SE of at least seven experiments. *Triangle, p < 0.001; asterisk, p < 0.001; circle, p < 0.05.*

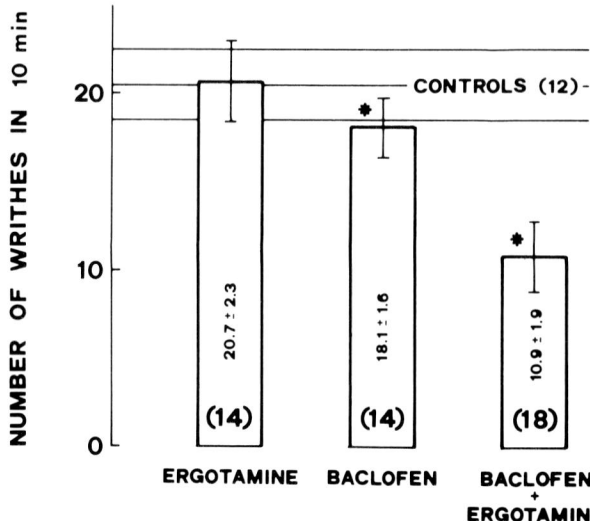

FIG. 6. Effect of ergotamine on analgesia induced by baclofen in mice tested with the acetic acid writhing procedure. (±) Baclofen (1mg/kg s.c.) and ergotamine (0.1 mg/kg s.c.) were injected 30 and 15 min, respectively, before the analgesic test. Number of mice in parentheses. *Asterisk, p* < 0.01.

Effect of Ergotamine on Oxotremorine Analgesia

As shown in Tables 1 and 2, ergotamine tartrate at doses of 0.5 mg/kg i.p. significantly potentiates oxotremorine analgesia. Here, too, oxotremorine doses were the minimum necessary for inducing a slight degree of analgesia. Thus the potentiation by ergotamine was seen more clearly.

TABLE 1. *Effect of ergotamine and methysergide on analgesia induced*
by (±) baclofen and oxotremorine in the hot-plate test in mice[a]

Agent	Saline	Baclofen (2.5 mg/kg s.c.)	Oxotremorine (20 μg/kg i.p.)
Saline	15.2 ± 0.6 (25)[b]	18.0 ± 1.1[c,d] (23)	17.4 ± 0.8[e] (25)
Ergotamine tartrate (0.5 mg/kg i.p.)	15.9 ± 0.7 (25)	25.1 ± 1.7[c] (25)	26.0 ± 1.7[e] (25)
Methysergide dimaleate (1 mg/kg s.c.)	15.6 ± 1.7 (20)	30.1 ± 3.6[d] (10)	—

[a] Results are expressed as licking reaction latency (sec). Baclofen, oxotremorine, methysergide, and ergotamine were injected 45, 30, 35, and 30 min, respectively, before the analgesic test.
[b] Number of mice in parentheses.
[c] $p < 0.001$; [d] $p < 0.01$; [e] $p < 0.001$.

TABLE 2. Effect of antimigraine drugs on analgesia induced by the opiate agonists morphine and eseroline, by the new GABA receptor agonist baclofen, and by the muscarinic agonist oxotremorine

Antimigraine drugs	Animal species	Analgesic test	Effect on analgesia induced by			
			Morphine	Eseroline	(±) Baclofen	Oxotremorine
Methysergide dimaleate (1 mg/kg s.c.)	Mouse	Writhing	Potentiated	Potentiated		Potentiated
	Mouse	Hot-plate	No effect	Potentiated	Potentiated	Potentiated
	Rat	Tail-flick	Potentiated	Potentiated		Potentiated
Ergotamine tartrate (0.5 mg/kg s.c.)	Mouse	Writhing		No effect	Potentiated	
	Mouse	Hot-plate		No effect	Potentiated	
	Rat	Tail-flick	No effect	No effect		Potentiated

Effect of Methysergide on Baclofen Analgesia

Table 1 shows that baclofen analgesia is also strongly potentiated by methysergide bimaleate administered in doses of 1 mg/kg s.c. 35 min before the analgesic test. As already pointed out (6,23) methysergide also potentiates oxotremorine analgesia in all tests in both the rat and mouse.

In Table 2, which summarizes data already partially published (6), it may be seen that, while 1 mg/kg s.c. methysergide potentiates analgesia of every type, however induced, ergotamine increases only the analgesia evoked by the stimulation of muscarinic and new type GABAergic receptors and does not modify that induced by stimulation of the opioid receptors.

DISCUSSION

Methysergide, a drug widely used in the prevention of migraine attacks, potentiates the analgesia induced not only by both endogenous and exogenous opiate agonists (6,23), but also by muscarinic agonists, such as oxotremorine (5). Ergotamine, another drug widely used in migraine attacks, does not modify opiate analgesia in either the rat or the mouse. On the other hand, the data presented here clearly show that ergotamine potentiates both baclofen- and oxotremorine-induced analgesia. In other words, ergotamine is able to potentiate analgesia produced by nonopioid, centrally acting molecules. Thus, while methysergide potentiates analgesia, however induced, ergotamine potentiates only nonopiate-stimulated analgesia.

It is well known that oxotremorine induces analgesia through stimulation of the central muscarinic receptors. This is confirmed by the fact that its antinociceptive action is completely eliminated by atropine while only partially antagonized by naloxone (5). Furthermore, baclofen induces analgesia through the stimulation of a particular GABA receptor (7), which is insensitive to both muscimol and bicuculline, an agonist and an antagonist of the classic GABA receptor, respectively. That ergotamine succeeds in potentiating only nonopioid stimulation seems to us extremely significant. In fact, apart from clarifying the difficult and multifaceted mechanism of action of ergotamine on migraine headaches, this finding also sheds light on the pathogenesis of migraine. That headache sufferers get no relief from opiate drugs is also significant here.

Although further research is still required, results point to the hypothesis that a deficiency in the nonopiate, physiological analgesic mechanisms may lie at the root of headache attacks. This hypothesis is supported by the efficacy of methysergide in migraine headaches; it potentiates not only the analgesic effect of opiate agonists but also that of nonopiate agonists.

As we have previously stated (6), basing our conclusion on data from the literature (9,16,20,25,26), methysergide action consists of the stimulation of the inhibitory 5-hydroxytryptamine (5-HT) receptors of the CNS. This action would thus amount to an activation of the serotoninergic analgesic system; it is the same action that the precursors of 5-HT (such as tryptophan and 5-hydroxytryptophan exerts.

This work was supported by Italian C.N.R. grant nos. CT 790183904 and 800039404. The authors thank CIBA-GEIGY for baclofen, Endo Laboratories for naloxone, and Sandoz for methysergide.

REFERENCES

1. Aiello Malmberg, P., Bartolini, A., Bartolini, R., and Galli, A. (1979): Effect of morphine, physostigmine and raphe nuclei stimulation on 5-hydroxytryptamine release from the cerebral cortex of the cat. *Br. J. Pharmacol.*, 65:547–555.

2. Akil, H., Madden, J., Patrick, R. L., and Barchas, J. D. (1976): Stress-induced increase in endogenous opiate peptides: concurrent analgesia and its partial reversal by naloxone. In: *Opiates and Endogenous Opioid Peptides,* edited by H. W. Kosterlitz, pp. 63–70. Elsevier, Amsterdam.

3. Akil, H., Mayer, D. J., and Liebeskind, J. C. (1976): Antagonism by stimulation-produced analgesia by naloxone, a narcotic antagonist. *Science,* 191:961–962.

4. Andersson, S. (1978): Peripheral modulation: Behavioral experiments. *Neurosci. Res. Prog. Bull.,* 16:155–160.

5. Bartolini, A., Bartolini, R., Malmberg Aiello, P., Biscini, A., and Renzi, G. (1981): New data concerning the interaction between cholinergic, enkephalinergic and serotoninergic systems during analgesia. In: *Opiate Receptors and the Neurochemical Correlates of Pain,* edited by Susanna Fürst, pp. 171–181. Pergamon Press—Akademiai Kiadò, Budapest.

6. Bartolini, A., Bartolini, R., Aiello Malmberg, P. and Renzi, G. (1981): Antinociceptive interactions between opiates and two antimigraine ergot derivatives: Clinical implications. *Int. J. Clin. Pharm. Res.,* 1:131–137.

7. Bartolini, A., Bartolini, R., Biscini, A., Giotti, A., and Malmberg, P. (1981): Investigations into baclofen analgesia: Effect of naloxone, bicuculline, atropine and ergotamine. *Br. J. Pharmacol.,* 72:156P–157P.

8. Bartolini, A., Renzi, G., Galli, A., Malmberg Aiello, P., and Bartolini, R. (1981): Eseroline: A new antinociceptive agent derived from physostigmine with opiate receptor agonist properties. Experimental in vivo and in vitro studies on cats and rodents. *Neurosci. Lett.,* 25:179–183.

9. Bourgoin, S., Artaud, F., Bockaert, J., Hery, F., Glowinski, J., and Hamon, M. (1978): Paradoxical decrease of brain 5-HT turnover by metergoline, a central 5-HT receptor blocker. *Naunyn Schmiedebergs Arch. Pharmacol.,* 302:313–321.

10. Bowery, N. G., Doble, A., Hill, D. R., Hudson, A. L., Shaw, J. S., and Turnbull, M. J. (1979): Baclofen: A selective agonist for a novel type of GABA-receptor. *Br. J. Pharmacol.,* 67:444P–445P.

11. Bowery, N. G., Hill, D. R., Hudson, A. L., Doble, A., Middlemiss, D. N., Show, J., and Turnbull, M. (1980): (⁻)Baclofen decreases neurotransmitter release in the mammalian CNS by an action at a novel GABA receptor. *Nature,* 283:92–94.

12. D'Amour, F. E., and Smith, D. L. (1941): A method for determining loss of pain sensation. *J. Pharmacol.,* 72:74–79.

13. Galli, A., Renzi, G., Bartolini, A., Bartolini, R., and Aiello Malmberg, P. (1979): Inhibition of naloxone-³H binding in homogenates of rat brain by eseroline, a new analgesic drug related to physostigmine. *J. Pharm. Pharmacol.,* 31:784–786.

14. George, R., Haslett, W. L., and Jenden, D. J. (1962): The central action of a metabolite of tremorine. *Life Sci.,* 1:361–363.

15. Goldstein, A., and Hilgard, E. R. (1975): Failure of opiate antagonist naloxone to modify hypnotic analgesia. *Proc. Natl. Acad. Sci. (USA),* 72:2,041–2,043.

16. Haigler, H. J., and Aghajanian, G. K. (1977): Serotonin receptors in the brain. *Fed. Proc.,* 36:2159.

17. Harris, L. S., Dewey, W. L., Howes, J. F., Kennedy, J. S., and Pars, H. (1969): Narcotic-antagonist analgesics: Interactions with cholinergic systems. *J. Pharmacol. Exp. Ther.,* 169:17–22.

18. Herz, A. (1962): Wirkungen des Arecolins auf das Zentralnervensystem. *Arch. Exp. Pathol. Pharmakol.,* 242:414–429.

19. Koster, R., Anderson, M., and De Beer, E. J. (1959): Acetic acid for analgesic screening. *Fed. Proc.,* 18:412.

20. Jacoby, J. H., Poulakos, J. J., and Bryce, G. F. (1978): On the central antiserotoninergic actions of cyproheptadine and methysergide. *Neuropharmacology,* 17:299–306.

21. Lenke, D. (1958): Narkosepotenzierende und analgetische Wirkung von 1,4-Dipyrrolidino-2-butin. *Arch. Exp. Pathol. Pharmakol.,* 234:35–45.

22. Lewis, J. W., Cannon, J. T., and Liebeskind, J. C. (1980): Opioid and nonopioid mechanisms of stress analgesia. *Science,* 208:623–625.

23. Malmberg, P., Bartolini, R., Bartolini, A., and Spagnesi, S. (1978): Effetto della metisergide, ciproeptadina e metergolina sull'azione analgesica ed ipotermica della eserolina. *XIX Congr. Soc. It. Farmacol.,* p. 533. *(Abstr.).*

24. Pert, C. B., Aposhian, D., and Snyder, S. H. (1974): Phylogenetic distribution of opiate receptor binding. *Brain Res.,* 75:356–361.

25. Sofia, R. D., and Vassar, H. B. (1975): The effect of ergotamine and methysergide on serotonin metabolism in the rat brain. *Arch. Int. Pharmacodyn.,* 216:40–50.

26. Weinstock, M., Weiss, C., and Gitter, S. (1977): Blockade of 5-hydroxytryptamine receptors in the central nervous system by β-adrenoceptor antagonists. *Neuropharmacology,* 16:273–276.

27. Wolfe, G., and Mac Donald, A. D. (1944): The evaluation of analgesic effect of phetidine hydrochloride. *J. Pharmacol.,* 80:300–307.

28. Yaksh, T. L., Yeung, J. C., and Rudy, T. A. (1976): An inability to antagonize with naloxone the elevated nociceptive thresholds resulting from electrical stimulation of the mesencephalic central gray. *Life Sci.,* 18:1,193–1,198.

Advances in Neurology, Vol. 33, edited by
M. Critchley et al. Raven Press, New York © 1982

On the Etiopathogenesis of Migraine: A Possible Link Between the Amines and Endorphin Hypotheses

A. Agnoli, A. Denaro, E. Ceci, and *P. Falaschi

*Department of Neurology, University of L'Aquila, L'Aquila, Italy; and *V Medical Clinic,
University of Rome, Rome, Italy*

At present, two etiopathogenetic hypotheses are most accredited in migraine: (a) the vascular or "dry," closely integrated with the "humid" aminic (7,11), and (b) the endorphinic (8). In the vascular and aminic theory, serotonin, norepinephrine, histamine, and other amines play a fundamental role in the determination of the migraine, which then is self-maintained through a mechanism that implicates humoral and tissular factors, considering the cerebral vessel, both intra- and extracranial, as a target. At the intracranial phase, vascular constriction corresponds to the prodromic phenomena of the migraine crisis; during the vascular relaxation phase, the pain appears.

The endorphinic theory attributes the occurrence of migrainous pain to the dysfunction of the endogenous opiate system as the modulator of the pain and sensitivity. A clinical observation may be useful: During the crisis of abstinence from opiates, a symptomatology partially resembling that of the migraine crisis can be seen. This feature was noted by Sicuteri (9), who interpreted it in light of the endorphinic theory. In reality, the symptomatology presents *in toto* during the critical lack of opiates and partially in the migraine crisis; it is characterized primarily by the effects of a hypertone of noradrenergic and other amines (dopamine, acetylcholine). Table 1 summarizes the main symptoms, which appear in both clinical pictures associated with the eventual role of the neurotransmitters involved.

The casual observation of the positive effect of clonidine, an α_2 selective stimulant, during withdrawal from opiates and its use in the treatment of migraine has suggested the existence of a structure common to the action involved in both clinical pictures. In effect, the clonidine seems to exercise its action principally at the central level and precisely at the level of the locus ceruleus. This structure is constantly controlled by endogenous opiates (endorphins), which modulate the release of norepinephrine and other amines with an inhibitory tone. The chronic assumption of opiates determines a reduction of the release (norepinephrine and dopamine) with consequent successive supersensitivity of the receptors due to a chemical denervation (Fig. 1). It is possible to hypothesize a theory of migraine, considering the endorphin-regulated locus ceruleus as the structure implicated in the unleashing of the migraine crisis. The successive phase is aminic, with an initial phase of vascular constriction. The diverse phases which can lead to the migraine crisis are described (Fig. 2). At the level of the locus ceruleus,

TABLE 1. *Main symptoms occurring during both withdrawal and migraine crisis and the neurotransmitters involved*

Withdrawal		Migraine
Mydriasis		Mydriasis
Increase pulse rate		Increase pulse rate
Increase respiratory rate		—
Gooseflesh		—
Perspiration		Perspiration
Hypertension	Norepinephrine	—
Spontaneous orgasm		—
Ejaculation		—
Anxiety		Anxiety
Tremor		—
Hot and cold flashes		—
Nausea		Nausea
Vomiting	Dopamine	Vomiting
Yawning		—
Lacrimation		Lacrimation
Rhinorrhea	Acetylcholine	Rhinorrhea
Diarrhea		Diarrhea
Craving		—
Aching bones and muscles	Complex	—
Anorexia	Interaction	Anorexia
Sleep disturbances		—

there is initially a sudden loss of inhibitory tone of endorphins for unknown reasons. It is demonstrated by the sudden decrease in the endorphin level in the cerebrospinal fluid (CSF) (10). The lack of inhibitory control provokes an aminic overflow, mainly of norepinephrine, which causes an intracranial vasoconstriction. In this phase, control of the evolution of the symptomatology is possible using clonidine, a selective α_2 stimulant able to counteract the norepinephrine overflow. This phase of vasoconstriction corresponds to the prodromic phase of the migraine crisis, during which pain does not appear but there is a consequent reduction of cerebral blood flow (scotoma, paresthesia, aphasia) as an effect of the vasoconstriction in the territory of the internal carotid.

The successive vascular phenomena (which lead to the painful symptomatology) depend on the liberation of vascular-activating amines and humoral factors (histamine, prostaglandins, bradykinin), which provoke vascular relaxation and perivascular edema, predominately extracranial. Moreover, a possible involvement of prolactin (PRL) has been suggested in association with the pathogenetic role of the amines and endorphins in migraine. Contrasting data exist regarding its direct action on vascular tone (3,4), in which the effect of vascular dilatation and constriction depend on its plasma levels. Alternatively, PRL could be considered as an expression of the activity of either the cerebral amines, particularly dopamine and 5-HT, and enkephalins, which are involved in the etiopathogenetic mechanisms of migraine.

The secretion of PRL is principally modulated with inhibitory tone by influences exercised by the dopaminergic tuberoinfundibular neurons (TIDA). Further proof exists that 5-HT plays a role in the release of the hormone. Enkephalins have been implicated in the control of PRL secretion by direct action on the hypophysis enkephalinergic

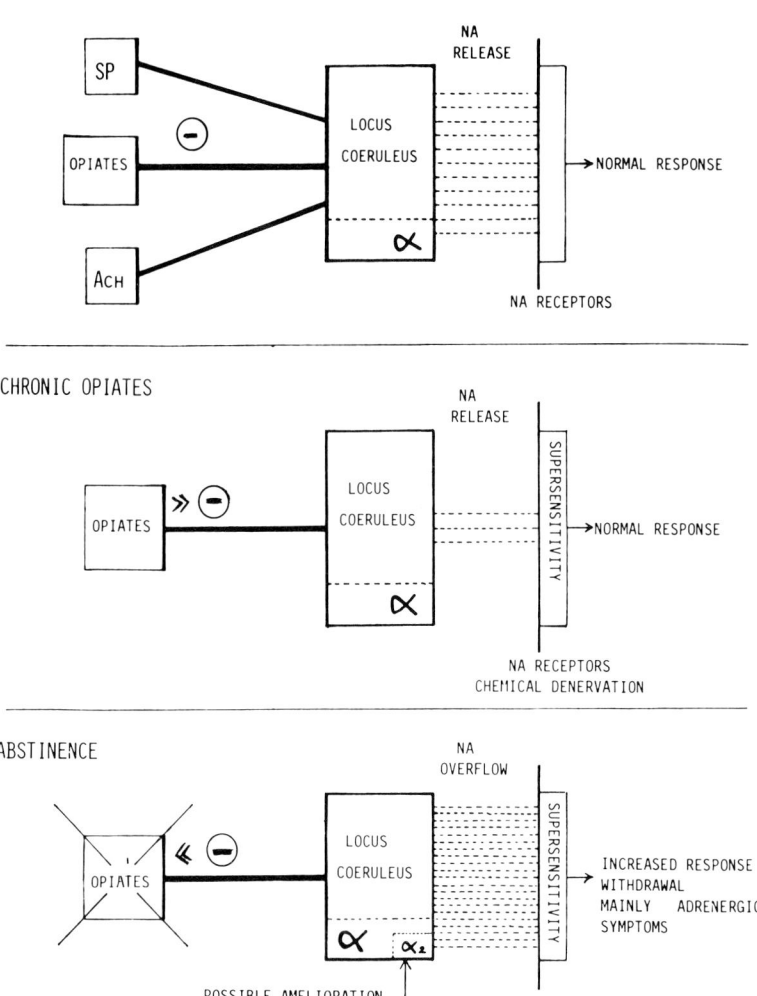

FIG. 1. Effect of the administration of opiates on norepinephrine (NA) release and the possible use of clonidine in the control of norepinephrine overflow.

receptors and by their inhibitory action on the release of dopamine, 5-HT, and norepinephrine.

Other data (5) regarding the pharmacological induction of pain with substances that involve diverse monoaminergic systems suggest that the hyperprolactinemia of itself has any pathogenetic function; the finding of a hyperprolactinemia during the migraine crisis induced with reserpine must be considered secondary. The aims of this study are (a) to verify the implications of the opiate system in the control of migraine pain, utilizing stimulants and blockers, and (b) to verify the eventual modification of PRL levels as a possible index of monoaminergic and enkephalinergic activity.

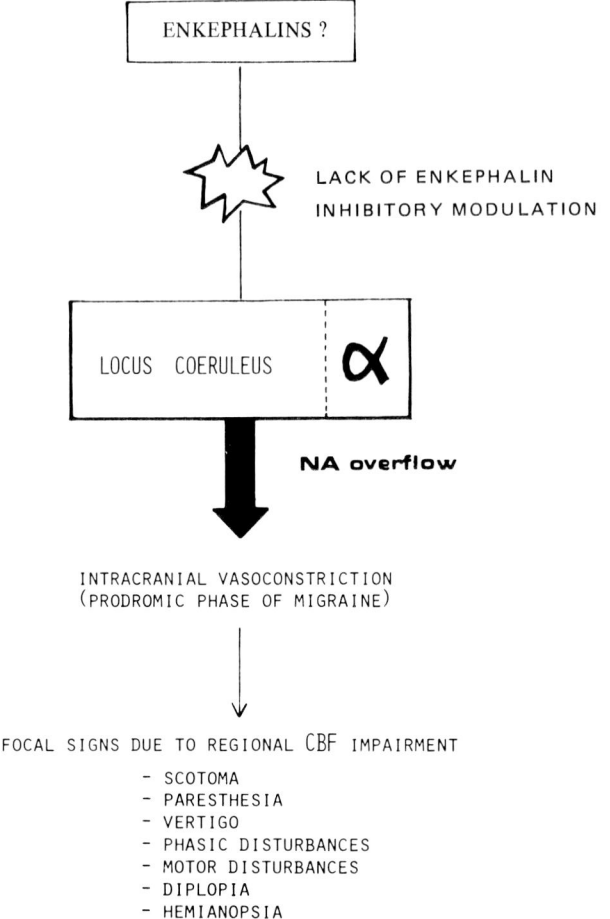

FIG. 2. A possible link between amine (norepinephrine, NA) and enkephalins in the etiopatho-genesis of migraine. The lack of inhibitory control of enkephalins at the locus ceruleus might trigger the following phases of migraine attack.

METHODS AND MATERIALS

Five subjects, four male and one female, who were affected by migraine, were studied. Their ages ranged from 32 to 45 years (mean, 35 years). The woman began the study on the sixth day of her menstrual cycle.

The study was conducted in different phases: (a) confirmation of the clinical diagnosis of migraine using the histamine threshold test; verification of the basal PRL curve; (b) quantification of the pain response to the threshold dose using a linear scale of self-evaluation (analog visual line) with points from 0 (absence of pain) to 10 (maximum intensity of pain); (c) administration of histamine at a dose 25 gammas superior to the threshold dose after pretreatment with a synthetic analog of met-enkephalin (0.5 mg i.v.); (d) evaluation of the pain response using the analog visual line; (e) administration of histamine at a dose 25 gammas inferior to the threshold dose after pretreatment with naloxone (8 mg. i.v.); (f) evaluation of the pain response using the visual analog

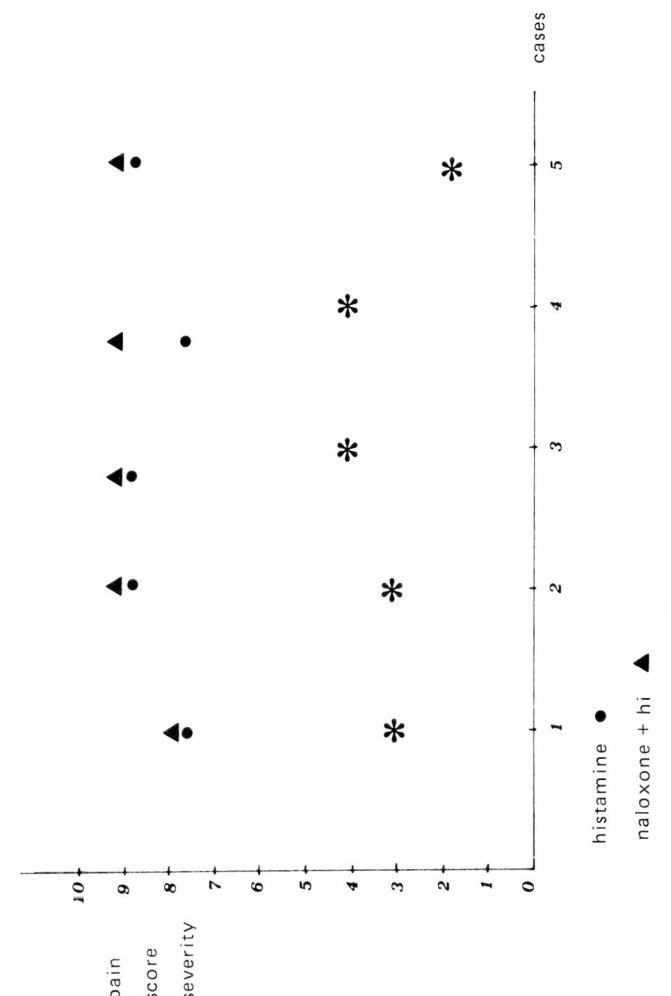

Fig. 3. Pain responses to histamine *(circles)* after pretreatment with both naloxone *(triangles)* and the synthetic analog of met-enkephalin *(asterisks)*. Note the constant protection after pretreatment with the synthetic analog of met-enkephalin.

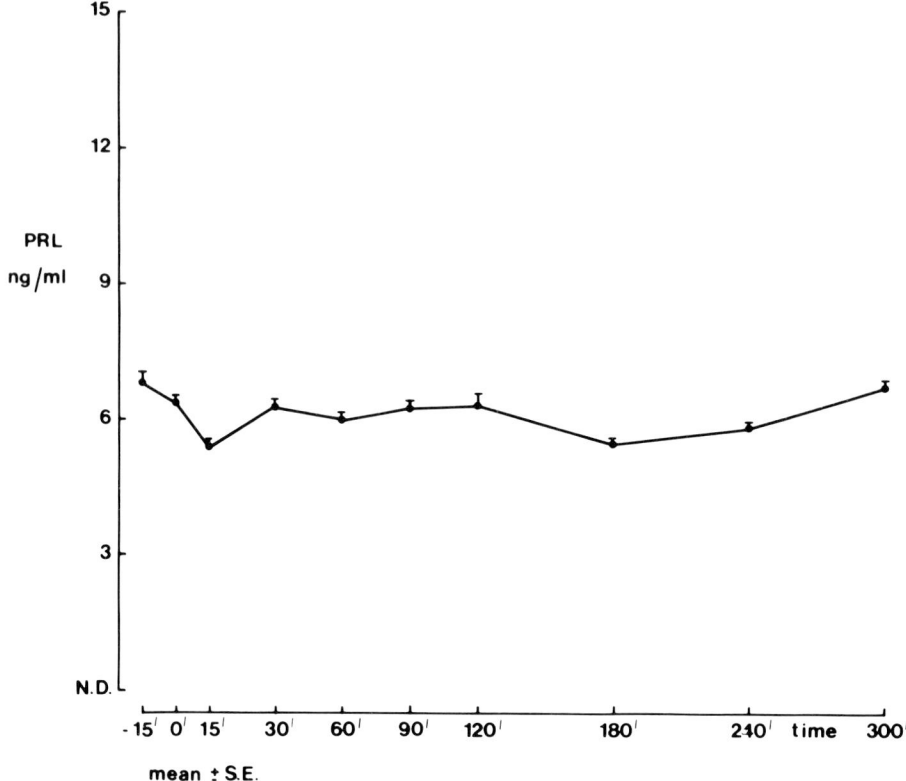

FIG. 4. PRL response to naloxone.

scale; (g) verification of the PRL curves after administration of naloxone (8 mg. i.v.); and (h) verification of the PRL curves after administration of a synthetic analog of met-enkephalin (0.5 mg. i.v.). Side effects after administration of the drugs were observed.

RESULTS

All the subjects studied showed a pain response similar to the spontaneous attack after doses of histamine inferior or equal to 150 gammas, which represents the threshold of discrimination for the vascular headache (1). After pretreatment with naloxone, an inconsistent increase in the pain response to the histaminic stimulus was observed that took place in only one patient (Fig. 3). Pretreatment with the synthetic analog of met-enkephalin was constantly able to protect against migraine attack induced by histamine (Fig. 3). Side effects were not observed, nor was the spontaneous onset of pain after administration of naloxone. Administration of the synthetic analog of met-enkephalin caused tachycardia, tachypnea, and slight muscle contraction in some patients. Examination of the curves of the plasma PRL levels showed a significant rise in values at 30, 45, and 60 min, according to published data (6) (Fig. 4). No modifications were observed after the administration of naloxone. (Fig. 5).

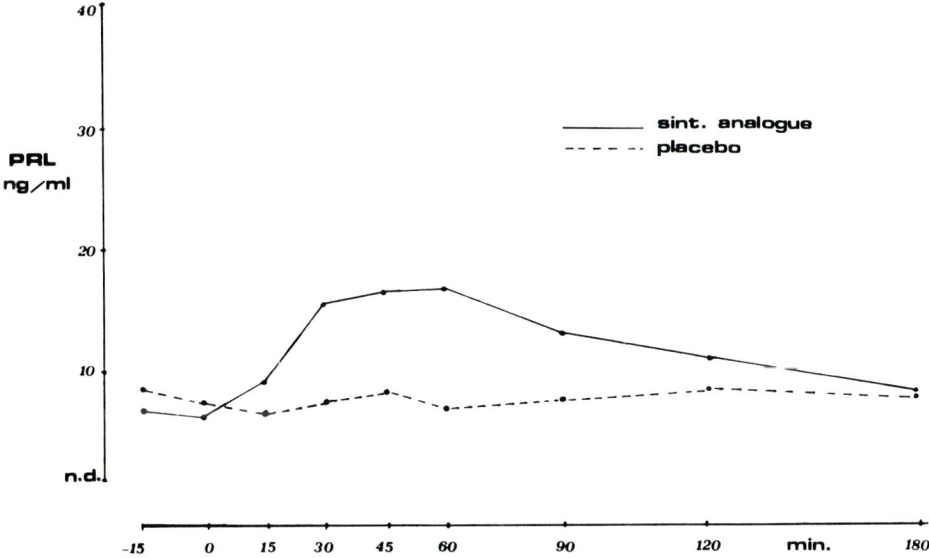

Fig. 5. PRL response to a synthetic analog of met-enkephalin *(solid line)* and placebo *(dashed line)*.

CONCLUSIONS

Our results confirm the diagnostic validity of the histamine threshold test. Naloxone was not constantly able to potentiate the effects of the administration of histamine; this confirms the results in the literature and suggests the existence of a subgroup of receptors (2) implicated in the modulation of pain which either could not be blocked or was blocked only in part by the dose of naloxone used.

The synthetic analog of met-enkephalin showed a constant protective effect on the pain stimulus, confirming reports in literature. The side effects observed after this drug suggest a possible action similar to the histaminic type. PRL showed a rise in its values at 30, 45, and 60 min, in agreement with published reports (6). The late rise of these values is tied to an action mediated by a neurotransmitter system (probably dopaminergic) and is not due to a direct action on enkephalinergic receptors. The observation of the elevated levels of PRL during protection from pain confirms the data of Savoldi and Nappi (5) on the relationship between hyperprolactinemia and migraine, and conflicts with the data of Horrobin (3) regarding a possible etiopathogenetic action of PRL in migraine.

REFERENCES

1. Agnoli, A., Ruggieri, S., Martucci, N., and Denaro, A. (1976). The histamine test in the diagnosis of vascular headache. In: *Headache: New Vistas,* edited by F. Sicuteri, Biomedical Press, Florence, pp. 163–171.
2. Della Bella, D., Casacci, F., and Sassi, A. (1978): Opiate receptors: Different ligand affinity in various brain regions. In: *Advances in Biochemical Psychopharmacology, Vol. 18,* edited by E. Costa and M. Trabucchi, Raven Press, New York.
3. Horrobin, D. F. (1973): *Lancet,* i:777.
4. Nader, S., Tulloch, R., Blair, C., Vydelingum, N., and Fraser, T. R. (1974): Is prolactin involved in precipitating migraine? *Lancet,* II:17–19.

5. Savoldi, F., and Nappi, G. (1979) : Proceedings of the Annual Meeting of the Italian Society of Neurology.
6. Shaar, C. J., Frederikson, R. C. A., Dininger, N. B., and Jackson, L. (1977): Enkefalin analogues and naloxone modulate the release of growth hormone and prolactin—Evidence for regulation by an endogenous opioid peptide in brain. *Life Sci.,* 21:853–860.
7. Sicuteri, F. (1963): Mast cells and their active substances. Their role in the pathogenesis of migraine. *Headache,* 3:86.
8. Sicuteri, F. (1976): In: *Advances in Pain Research and Therapy,* edited by J. J. Bonica and D. Albe-Fessard, pp. 871–880. Raven Press, New York.
9. Sicuteri, F. (1979): Annual meeting of Italian Society of Headache.
10. Sicuteri, F., Anselmi, B., Curradi, C., Michelacci, S., and Sassi, A. (1978): Morphine-like factors in CSF of headache patients. In: *Advances in Biochemical Psychopharmacology, Vol. 18,* edited by E. Costa and M. Trabucchi. Raven Press, New York.
11. Wolff, H. G. (1938): Headache and cranial arteries. *Trans. Assoc. Am. Phys.,* 53:193.

Advances in Neurology, Vol. 33, edited by
M. Critchley et al. Raven Press, New York © 1982

Mechanisms of Opiate Analgesia and the Role of Endorphins in Pain Suppression

Agu Pert

*Section on Biochemistry and Pharmacology, Biological Psychiatry Branch, National Institute of
Mental Health, National Institutes of Health, Bethesda, Maryland 20205*

MECHANISMS OF OPIATE ANALGESIA

Undoubtedly, the most efficacious drugs to alleviate acute and chronic pain are the opiate analgesics. Two recent discoveries have advanced our understanding of opiate actions in the central nervous system (CNS). The first was the discovery of opiate receptors in brain tissue (137,156,163); second was the isolation and characterization of endogenous opioid peptides from brain (81). Collectively, both these discoveries prompted the exciting proposal that the brain may contain its own pain suppression mechanism.

Opiate receptors are simply neuronal membrane binding sites through which all opiate agonists exert their pharmacological actions. These binding sites are thought to be related to the sodium ionophore (135), and opiate agonists are thought to produce their effects by preventing the influx of sodium ions into the neuron (179). Opiate antagonists (such as naloxone and naltrexone), on the other hand, are able to reverse and block the pharmacological effects of opiate agonists by competitive inhibition at the receptor.

Opioid peptides, termed methionine and leucine enkephalin, were first isolated from calf brain in 1975 by Hughes (81). Methionine enkephalin was composed of the amino acid sequence Tyr-Gly-Gly-Phe-Met, while leucine enkephalin had a similar sequence, with leucine instead of methionine in the terminal position. Subsequent to the discovery of enkephalins, it was found (82) that the methionine enkephalin amino acid sequence also appeared in β-lipotropin and its COOH-terminal 31 amino acid residue (called β-endorphin), which had been isolated in 1965 by Li et al. (105) from sheep pituitaries. β-Endorphin has also been found to be present in the brain as well as pituitary of a number of species. The pituitary presence suggests a hormonal function for this opioid peptide.

Both enkephalins and β-endorphin have been reported to produce analgesia in animals (20,36,108) and in man (72) following intracerebral injections. The analgesic effects of enkephalins, however, were found to be relatively weak and short lasting due to their rapid enzymatic destruction in brain by specific peptidases (36). Synthesis of compounds resistant to enzymatic destruction by substitution in D-amino acids in the number two position of enkephalin has resulted in potent and long-lasting analgesics (138,169), some of which are effective even following oral administration (142). Pharmacologically, the opioid peptides have a spectrum of action relatively similar to that of the opiate alkaloids (126).

Endogenous opioid peptides and opiate alkaloids, which simply mimic the endogenous opioids, could induce analgesia by (a) inhibiting primary afferents in the dorsal horn, (b) inhibiting somatosensory pathways at supraspinal levels, and (c) activating descending inhibitory pathways.

Direct Spinal Actions of Opiates

Substantial evidence indicates that one important focus for the analgesic effects of opiates is the spinal cord. A number of investigators have reported direct effects of morphine on dorsal horn cells, especially those that have been implicated in processing and transmitting nociceptive information (laminae I and V cells), and on axons in the anterolateral pathways. Grossman and Jurna (65) reported that morphine, in a dose as low as 0.5 mg/kg, depressed the spontaneous and evoked activity in axons in the ventrolateral tract of the spinal cord (T 10 level) by stimulation of Aδ fibers in the sural nerve. Koll et al. (94) also reported that the ipsilateral nociceptive reflex discharge recorded from the ventral root following C-fiber stimulation was thoroughly depressed by 0.3 to 0.4 mg/kg morphine in decerebrated and spinalized cats at L1. Iwata and Sakai (85) likewise reported that fentanyl suppressed the discharge of spinal interneurons in the dorsal horn evoked by stimulation of Aδ fibers in spinal cats.

A spinal action of opiates is also suggested by recent electrophysiological evidence. Besson et al. (25) found that phenoperidine inhibited spontaneous activity of nociceptive responses induced by natural or electrical stimulation of lamina V cells in spinal cats. More recently, LeBars et al. (99) reported that morphine suppressed lamina V neurons activated by C and Aδ fiber stimulation (pain) but had no effect on neuronal activation by Aα stimulation (nonpain). Similar findings have been reported by other laboratories. Kitahata et al. (93) found that morphine in decerebrate cats suppressed spontaneous and evoked activity in laminae I and V cells, which are known to respond primarily to noxious input, but had no effect on laminae IV and VI cells, which are known to respond predominantly to nonnoxious stimuli.

Direct microiontophoretic applications of opiates and opioid peptides to dorsal horn cells have been found to depress activity. Zieglgänsberger and Bayerl (178), employing both extra- and intracellular recording techniques, found that phoretically applied morphine and levorphanol inhibited the spontaneous activity of laminae V and IV cells as well as their induced activation by glutamate or tactile stimulation. Furthermore, both morphine and levorphanol depressed the activity of spinal neurons without influencing the resting membrane resistance or potential. The authors postulated that opiates block neuronal depolarization by impairing the sodium ion influx mechanism at the postsynaptic membrane. They further suggested that this effect is translated to an inhibitory action on neurons which predominantly discharge repetitively under physiological conditions.

There is some disagreement among other investigators regarding the precise mechanisms and loci of action of opiate agonists in modifying spinal cord activity. Calvillo et al. (33), as well as Henry and Newman (25), found that in anesthetized cats, morphine selectively depressed the firing of dorsal horn neurons excited by noxious heat but had no effect on neurons activated by nonnoxious input. These depressant actions were antagonized to some extent by naloxone. Dostrovsky and Pomeranz (43) found that morphine applied iontophoretically to laminae IV, V, and VII cells in the cat blocked both excitatory and inhibitory amino acid effects. In this study, the spontaneous rate was usually unaffected by morphine, and morphine did not depress responses elicited by cutaneous stimulation.

Belcher and Ryall (16) suggested that the analgesic effects of opiates in the dorsal horn may also involve the excitation of nonnociceptive neurons. These investigators found that phoretically applied morphine excited nonnociceptive cells and depressed nociceptive cells. Only the excitatory effects, however, were consistently antagonized by naloxone. Duggan et al. (44) reported that iontophoretic applications of morphine are more effective and selective in inhibiting laminae IV and V cells activated by noxious input when the recording electrode is in laminae IV or V and the iontophoresis is made in the substantia gelatinosa. These authors suggest that only the opiate effects in the substantia gelatinosa are relevant to the analgesic actions. This hypothesis is consistent with the high concentration of opiate receptors (11) and enkephalin (47) in this region of the dorsal horn.

Zieglgänsberger et al. (181) proposed a model of the dorsal horn in which intrinsic enkephalinergic neurons are thought to tonically inhibit laminae IV and V cells through axodendritic connections in the substantia gelatinosa. C-fiber afferents are assumed to activate inhibitory interneurons in the substantia gelatinosa, which in turn depress activity of the enkephalinergic interneurons and release laminae IV and V cells from tonic inhibition. In this scheme, enkephalinergic neurons are not part of an endogenous pain suppression mechanism but simply provide tonic inhibition to laminae IV and V cells concerned in the transmission of nociceptive information. In addition, the model provides for the direct activation of enkephalinergic neurons by spinopetal pathways, as well as for the inhibition of primary afferent terminals.

While opiates clearly suppress the spontaneous and pain-induced activation of dorsal horn cells, there is still some uncertainty concerning whether these effects are pre- or postsynaptic to primary afferents. Zieglgänsberger and Bayerl (178), on the basis of their findings regarding the inhibition of glutamate-induced activation by morphine, have proposed that the predominant actions of opiates in the dorsal horn are postsynaptic on laminae IV and V cells. Presynaptic actions, however, are supported by the decrease in opiate receptors in the dorsal horn following rhizotomy, suggesting the presence of opiate receptors on primary afferent terminals (96). The possibility that opiates act presynaptically in the dorsal horn is also supported by the finding that substance P release is inhibited by morphine in slices of spinal trigeminal nuclei (90). Substance P has been proposed to be an excitatory neurotransmitter utilized by primary afferents to the dorsal horn (74). Mudge et al. (117) have also reported that morphine inhibits substance P release in dorsal root ganglia cell cultures.

Direct spinal actions of opiates have also been suggested by recent behavioral data. Yaksh and Rudy (173) reported that injections of morphine into the subarachnoid space of the spinal cord produces analgesia in the rat. While tolerance did develop after repeated administration of morphine by this route, many of the common withdrawal signs were absent in tolerant animals when they were challenged with naloxone. This method of inducing analgesia may have a number of advantages over systemically induced analgesia and may be useful as an obstetric analgesic intervention.

Supraspinal Sites of Opiate Analgesia

Tsou and Jang (166) were the first to report that direct microinjections of minute quantities of morphine into brain regions surrounding the third ventricle (periventricular gray matter) of rabbits produce analgesia. Injections into the midbrain reticular formation, ventrobasal complex, dorsomedial thalamic nucleus, caudate nucleus, septum, tectum, and cortex were found to be ineffective. Subsequent microinjection studies (89,102,176) in the rat have revealed that the morphine responsive region in the midbrain extends further caudally than suspected by Tsou and Jang (166). Analgesia has been elicited by microinjections of morphine from the posterior hypothalamus to the caudal periaqueductal gray (PAG). The most responsive region seems to be located in the ventrolateral PAG (176).

Pert and Yaksh (130) reported two different brain regions in the rhesus monkey in which direct injections of morphine were found to increase thresholds to electrical foot shock. The first and most significant region in terms of latency and magnitude of response was located in the periventricular-PAG matter. It extended from the lower portion of the third ventricle along the aqueduct and into the floor of the fourth ventricle. Several sites were also found in the region of the subthalamic nucleus and in the vicinity of the thalamic intralaminar nuclear group. The second morphine-responsive brain region followed a more lateral distribution. These sites were distributed in a pattern that passed in the vicinity of the lateral reticular nucleus, up through the substantia nigra, dorsolateral to the red nucleus, and into the most lateral aspects of the intralaminar thalamic nuclei.

Herz and his colleagues (77), in a novel series of experiments, have presented compelling evidence for the participation of structures more caudal to the aqueduct in morphine analgesia. By blocking the aqueduct, as well as other parts of the ventricular system, with injections of eucerine, these investigators (77) were able to inject morphine into restricted and defined parts of the ventricular system of rabbits. Only a slight analgesic response was seen when morphine was restricted to the ventricular system rostral to the aqueduct. Applications of opiates into the aqueduct and fourth ventricle, however, induced a complete inhibition of nociceptive reactions. The same investigators reported that marked antinociceptive effects could also be elicited following injections of morphine into the hypothalamus, subthalamus, and PAG. The interpretation of these findings was difficult, however, considering the possibility that morphine could have diffused into the ventricular system from structures close to the ventricular wall. Few of the rodent microinjection studies have presented adequate controls for diffusion. Subsequent autoradiographic studies by the same group (164) further confirmed the contention that an important region for mediating opiate analgesia is located in the brainstem caudal to the aqueduct.

The importance of caudal brainstem structures in opiate analgesia has received direct confirmation from a series of microinjection studies. Takagi et al. (159) reported that microinjections of rather small quantities of morphine into the nucleus reticularis gigantocellularis (nRGC) in the medulla produce profound analgesia in the rat. Similarly, long-lasting analgesia was reported by the same group (160) following injections of either methionine enkephalin or leucine enkephalin into the nRGC or the nucleus reticularis paragigantocellularis (nPGC) just ventral to the nRGC. This is surprising in light of the transient analgesic effects that have been reported by others following intraventricular and intracerebral (53) injections of much greater quantities of the rapidly degradable enkephalins. The same group has reported that the nPGC appears to be more sensitive to the direct application of morphine than the nRGC. In that study, it was found that direct electrical stimulation of the nPGC but not the nRGC would suppress nociceptive reactions in the rat. Pert and Mitchell (127) and Pert et al. (134) confirmed some of these findings and found that the nRGC is a rather responsive site for the induction of morphine analgesia. However, while Takagi et al. (159) found morphine to be 30 to 40 times more efficacious in eliciting analgesia in the pontine reticular formation than the PAG, Pert and Mitchell (127) observed only a three- or fourfold difference.

One important observation concerning brain regions that appear to mediate opiate analgesia (i.e., PAG, reticular formation, and medial thalamus) is the fact that they all receive input from the anterolateral spinal pathways that presumably carry pain information (see above). This correspondence prompted Pert and Yaksh (130) to suggest that opiates may induce analgesia, at least in part, by specifically interfering with the processing of pain in these terminal areas of the pain pathway and by preventing the access of pain information into limbic structures that mediate the affective and emotional components of the pain experience.

The PAG-periventricular gray matter, medial thalamus, and nRGC have all been implicated in the appreciation of the aversive quality of pain by a number of findings. Single cells in all these regions have been found to be selectively activated by noxious stimulation (34,46). Electrical stimulation of the central gray region (118,158), hypothalamus (83), medial, and intralaminar thalamic nuclei, as well as the nRGC (35), has produced aversive reactions indicative of pain in a number of species, including man (118). Lesions in these regions, on the other hand, produced moderate analgesia or attenuated aversive responses to nociception input (7,8,69,115). Recent electrophysiological studies support an inhibitory role for morphine in these brain regions for both spontaneous and pain-induced activation of neurons (31,54,59,67).

Another observation concerning the brain sites that are responsive to the direct application of morphine or enkephalin is that they appear to be relatively high in opiate receptors (97), enkephalin (78), and enkephalin terminals (149). The medial thalamus, PAG, and surrounding tegmentum are among the highest in opiate receptor content in brain. While autoradiography (10) has not shown the medullary region to be very high in opiate receptors in the rat, the analogous region in the monkey is as high in receptors as the PAG (97). Sar et al. (149) have demonstrated the presence of enkephalin terminals in the nRGC of the rat. β-Endorphin, on the other hand, cannot be important for modulating pain at this level of the brain or in the spinal cord since none is found caudal to the locus ceruleus (26). The presence of opiate receptors as well as enkephalin in regions of the brain that mediate opiate analgesia suggests the existence of an endogenous pain suppression mechanism.

Descending Inhibitory Mechanisms

Although the inhibition of neuronal activity at the terminal regions of the ascending pain pathways may contribute to opiate analgesia, evidence shows that the actions of opiates on supraspinal structures may also activate descending spinal pathways that interfere with pain processing by inhibiting dorsal horn cells.

Irwin et al. (84) compared the effects of morphine and methadone on the nociceptive tail-flick reflex (reflexive removal of the tail from radiant heat) in intact rats and rats that had spinal cord transections at the midthoracic level. Both opiate analgesics were found to be much less efficacious in inhibiting the tail-flick response in spinal than in intact animals. These results suggested that morphine inhibits nociceptive spinal reflex activity by at least two mechanisms: (a) by a direct action on the reflex arc at the spinal levels, and (b) by enhancing descending supraspinal inhibitory mechanisms that regulate nociceptive reflexes. Satoh and Takagi (150), on the other hand, state that the analgesic effects of opiates are determined solely by their effects on descending supra-spinal inhibitory mechanisms. These authors found that splanchnic afferent impulses recorded from the ventrolateral funiculus, which carries ascending nociceptive informa-tion, were inhibited 37% in amplitude by morphine in intact but not in spinal cats. Furthermore, the origin of the descending influences appeared to be limited to a region caudal to the inferior olive, since the only brain transactions that were effective in abolish-ing the opiate effects were caudal to this structure. In a further series of studies, Satoh et al. (152) and Takagi et al. (161) presented additional support for the role of descending supraspinal mechanisms in opiate analgesia by demonstrating that bradykinin-induced increases in firing rates of dorsal horn cells were inhibited by 2 mg/kg morphine in intact but not in spinal rabbits.

Role of Descending Serotonergic Pathways in Morphine Analgesia

Although serotonin (5-HT) had been postulated to mediate some aspects of opiate analgesia for a number of years (116,148,162), it was only recently that Proudfit and Anderson (141) suggested the direct involvement of spinopetal 5-HT pathways originating from the bulbar serotonergic nuclei (e.g., nucleus raphe magnus) in this opiate effect. This proposal was based on the observation that electrolytic lesions of the nucleus raphe magnus (nRM) were effective in reducing morphine analgesia in the rat. Interestingly, the lesions were also accompanied by hyperalgesia, suggesting a tonic inhibitory function for 5-HT in pain-induced reflex behavior. Yaksh et al. (175) reported similar findings. Vogt (168) also stressed the importance of spinal 5-HT in morphine analgesia based on her finding that depletion of spinal 5-HT with 5,6-dihydroxytryptamine (a specific 5-HT neuronal neurotoxin) decreases the analgesic efficacy of morphine. While raphe magnus (RM) lesions have been reported to partially antagonize morphine analgesia and to induce hyperalgesia, electrical stimulation of this structure has been found to elicit analgesia in the rat (141) and cat (121,122). Analgesia elicited by RM stimulation in the cat is antagonized by naloxone (80), suggesting an enkephalinergic link in the descending system, possibly in the dorsal horn.

Recent electrophysiological and neuroanatomical findings are consistent with the no-tion that descending 5-HT pathways may modulate pain transmission in spinal cord. LeBars et al. (98) reported that stimulation of the RM inhibits spinal neurons responding to noxious stimulation. Fields et al. (52) and McCreery et al. (110) reported similar findings. In addition, Fields et al. (52) also found that lesions of the dorsolateral funiculi (DLF) in the spinal cord abolished this inhibition. The latter finding suggested that 5-HT pathways descend in the DLF and terminate in the dorsal horn to modulate nocicep-tive input. This possibility is consistent with recent neuroanatomical studies that have described the presence of spinopetal pathways in the DLF originating from the NRM (14). Dahlström and Fuxe (40) reported the presence of spinopetal 5-HT pathways in the DLF that terminate, at least in part, in the dorsal horn.

In the dorsal horn, iontophoretically applied 5-HT has been shown to inhibit the spontaneous as well as pain-induced activation of neurons (145). In addition, Benelli (21) demonstrated that 5-hydroxytryptophan (5-HTP, a precursor for 5-HT) inhibits the activation of lamina V cells by stimulation of peripheral nerves. Belcher et al. (18) compared the effects of bulbar raphe stimulation and iontophoretic applications of 5-HT on neurons in the spinal cord dorsal horn which were activated by noxious input; both were effective in inhibiting these cells. Surprisingly, however, the depressant effects of 5-HT were not antagonized by methysergide (a putative 5-HT antagonist), which brings into question the use of this compound to test for specific 5-HT effects. Recent behavioral evidence supports the notion that 5-HT may be involved in pain suppression at the spinal level and in the analgesic actions of morphine. Wang (170) reported that intrathecal applications of 5-HT will produce analgesia in the rat, while Yaksh et al. (174) found that intrathecal methysergide partially antagonizes analgesia induced by microinjections of morphine into the PAG. The significance of this finding, however, awaits clarification regarding the specificity of methysergide.

For morphine to induce analgesia through descending 5-HT pathways, it must activate the RM neurons. Systemically administered opiates have been shown to increase the spontaneous activity of RM neurons in several studies (9,107). This activation, however, is not determined by a direct effect of morphine, since iontophoretic application of opiates to neurons has not been found to change their spontaneous activity (68,107). Opiates, therefore, must induce their effects on RM neurons by their primary actions on other structures. Since microinjection studies in rats have shown the PAG and the nRGC to be the primary analgesic foci for opiates in brain, morphine must exert its effects on Rm neurons through either of these two structures. The PAG and surrounding tegmentum, as well as the nRGC, do, in fact, send afferents to the RM (58,147). Evidence suggests that the effects of opiates in the PAG activate RM neurons. Fields and Anderson (51) reported that microinjections of morphine or etorphine into the PAG increased spontaneous activity of neurons in the RM. Electrical stimulation of the PAG produced similar effects. Behbehani and Pomeroy (15) also reported excitatory effects in the RM after either iontophoretic applications or direct microinjections of morphine into the PAG. The effects were not as pronounced or consistent if morphine was indeed exerting its full analgesic effects through the RM. Of 37 cells in the nRM, only 12 were excited, and five were inhibited by iontophoretic applications of morphine into the PAG. The effects seen following microinjections of morphine were no more convincing, since of 32 cells studied, 11 were excited and 10 were inhibited. This study brings into question the critical importance of the PAG-RM link in morphine analgesia.

Lorens (109) questioned the involvement of 5-HT in morphine analgesia. He found that while electrolytic lesions to the RM area partially antagonize morphine analgesia, they are not accompanied by significant changes in 5-HT levels. The same lesions, however, did decrease norepinephrine in the cord, suggesting the presence of pathways in the vicinity of the RM coded by other neurotransmitters (e.g., norepinephrine) that may be involved in descending modulation of pain transmission and opiate analgesia. Pert et al. (133) evaluated morphine analgesia after 5,7-dihydroxytryptamine (a serotonergic neuronal neurotoxin) lesions to the RM. Although the lesion decreased 5-HT in the dorsal horn by 50%, it had only a relatively slight antagonistic effect on morphine analgesia. Lorens (109) also reported similar effects following 5,7-dihydroxytryptamine lesions. Thus, while the descending 5-HT pathways may play some role in opiate analgesia, not all opiate analgesic effects (even those determined by descending inhibitory pathways) can be accounted for by the simple activation of these pathways by morphine. The spinopetal 5-HT pathways may be involved in opiate analgesia; but other pathways and mechanisms are also critical.

Since iontophoretic applications of morphine to PAG neurons are inhibitory (55,60), one must postulate the existence of inhibitory intervening neurons in the PAG between enkephalinergic neurons and other inhibitory neurons that descend from the PAG to the RM. In this scheme, morphine (mimicking enkephalin) in the PAG produces activation of RM neurons through disinhibition. At the same time, of course, opiates also probably inhibit the transmission of pain information through this structure by inhibiting the nociceptive relay neurons in the PAG.

Noradrenergic Descending Pathways and Morphine Analgesia

Emphasis has been placed on the importance of descending 5-HT pathways in morphine analgesia. It has recently become evident, however, that other descending pathways are also involved. Shiomi and Takagi (153) proposed that the analgesic effects of opiates in the brainstem are mediated by the activation of descending noradrenergic pathways, presumably originating from the catecholamine nuclei in the vicinity of the lateral reticular nucleus (A-1). These investigators found that morphine administered systemically increased the concentration of the norepinephrine metabolite normetanephrine selectively in the dorsal horn. This effect was abolished following a spinal transection at C-1 but not following a brainstem transection at the intercollicular level. Kuraishi et al. (95) reported that injections of morphine or enkephalin into the nRGC of rats also increased normetanephrine in the spinal cord. Injections of morphine into the PAG, on the other hand, were without effect. These findings suggest that the analgesic actions of morphine in the nRGC may be partially mediated by the activation of descending norepinephrine pathways in the more lateral A-1 nuclei. Pert et al. (133) found that lesions to A-1 nuclei with 6-hydroxydopamine (6-OHDA, a catecholamine neuronal neurotoxin) were somewhat more effective in antagonizing morphine analgesia than 5,7-dihydroxytryptamine lesions to the RM. A-1 lesions also partially antagonized analgesia (only in one analgesic measure) following microinjections of morphine into the nRGC.

Spinopetal norepinephrine pathways innervating the dorsal horn descend in the dorsolateral funiculi of the spinal cord (41); iontophoretic application of norepinephrine to dorsal horn nociceptive neurons has been found to inhibit both spontaneous and pain-induced activation (17). Both norepinephrine and 5-HT spinopetal pathways are involved in opiate analgesia, at least to some degree. In this regard, Yaksh (172) recently reported that while neither phentolamine (an α-adrenergic blocker) nor methysegide (a putative 5-HT antagonist) administered intrathecally was as able to completely antagonize morphine analgesia in the tail-flick test following PAG injections, the combination of the two compounds was more efficacious.

Recent evidence indicates that morphine may activate other spinopetal inhibitory pathways besides those coded by norepinephrine and 5-HT. Akaike et al. (1) reported that both electrical stimulation of the nPGC and morphine microinjections into this nucleus produce analgesia in rats. Furthermore, Satoh et al. (151) found that iontophoretic applications of morphine and enkephalin to the nRPG produced excitation. The same neurons were also activated by noxious stimulation. It is not clear whether the excitation found in this region following phoretic application of opiates is due to a direct effect or to a disinhibition of inhibitory interneurons as in the hippocampus (180). Basbaum and Fields (113) also demonstrated the presence of descending pathways from the nRPC in the DLF.

ENDOGENOUS OPIOID PAIN SUPPRESSION SYSTEM

The presence of enkephalinergic terminals and opiate receptors in CNS regions involved in processing pain information suggests that the brain contains an endogenous pain suppression mechanism. There are two possible functions for such a mechanism: (a) it may simply be part of a tonically active inhibitory system, possibly part of a negative feedback loop; or (b) enkephalinergic neurons may be phasically activated by certain environmental conditions or endogenous factors. If the endorphin mechanism is phasically active, what kind of input is sufficient to increase its output? One way in which the CNS endorphin system can be activated is by direct electrical stimulation.

Mayer and Liebeskind (113) demonstrated that potent analgesia could be induced in rats during electrical stimulation of the PAG—the enkephalin-rich area that is a critical focus for opiate-induced analgesia. Analgesia induced by focal brain stimulation (SPA) has been subsequently demonstrated by other investigators in a number of species (12,103,106,124). Most important, however, is the finding that naloxone partially antagonizes SPA in laboratory animals (2,123) although not invariably (128,177). More recently, Hosobuchi et al. (79) reported that electrical stimulation of the periventricular gray matter in six human patients produced long-lasting relief from intractable pain. This effect was also significantly antagonized by the administration of 0.2 to 1 mg naloxone. The antagonism of SPA by naloxone led a number of investigators to conclude that SPA is mediated by the release of enkephalin in the midbrain, which presumably activates descending inhibitory pathways to the dorsal horn of the spinal cord. Several investigators have reported increases in cerebrospinal fluid (CSF) endorphins concomitant with analgesia following electrical stimulation of periventricular brain structures in man (3,4,80).

Manipulations other than direct electrical stimulation of the enkephalinergic-rich brain regions have been postulated to induce analgesia by the release of enkephalin on the activation of enkephalinergic pathways. Hayes et al. (73) found that acute stress produces analgesia in rats. Madden et al. (112) reported that acute stress induced by electrical shock to the feet increased levels of opioid peptides in brain (as measured by the opiate receptor assay) with concurrent decreases in pain responsiveness in the rat. These authors concluded that stressful stimuli may recruit pain-inhibitory mechanisms in the CNS, bringing about alterations in enkephalins with concurrent or subsequent changes in responses to pain. This hypothesis was particularly attractive, considering the fact that both β-endorphin and ACTH are contained in the same prohormone and are released concomitantly into the blood from the pituitary during stress (66). Subsequent studies using more specific radioimmunoassays failed to find increases in either enkephalin (57) or β-endorphin (146) levels in whole brain following stress. Pert et al. (131), on the other hand, found decreases in endorphin levels in the basomedial hypothalamus, medial thalamus, and PAG following foot-shock stress. These decreases in tissue levels were also accompanied by increases in CSF levels. Such findings indicate that stress is capable of activating CNS endorphin mechanisms.

While the findings above suggest a role for CNS endorphins in stress-induced analgesia, there is also evidence for the participation of pituitary endorphins in this phenomenon. For example, both hypophysectomy and the administration of dexamethasone (a synthetic corticosteroid which decreases the release of β-endorphin and ACTH) have been found to partially reverse the analgesic effects of stress (28,104,131). Although stress activates both central and peripheral endorphin systems, it is unlikely that the analgesic effects of stress are mediated by endorphins alone. This notion is supported by findings that stress-induced analgesia is relatively resistant to antagonism by naloxone (28,29,131).

It has been proposed that acupuncture may also produce its analgesic effects by releasing enkephalins and endorphins. This proposal was originally based on the observation that acupuncture analgesia is partially antagonized by naloxone in man (114). Other investigators have also reported antagonism of acupuncture analgesia in mice by naloxone (37,139). Pomeranz and Chiu (139) reported antagonism of acupuncture analgesia by hypophysectomy, suggesting the involvement of pituitary β-endorphin. McLennan et al. (111), on the other hand, were not able to antagonize acupuncture analgesia in rabbits with naloxone. The most intriguing study linking acupunture analgesia to endorphins has been reported by Sjölund et al. (157), who found an increase in an opiate-like substance in the CSF of chronic pain patients following acupuncture. Pert et al. (132) also reported that auricular electroacupuncture in rats increases CSF levels of endorphins. The same investigators also found a concomitant decrease in endorphin levels in the basomedial hypothalamus, medial thalamus, and PAG.

Transcutaneous stimulation and placebo effects have been related to endogenous opioid involvement. Chapman and Benedetti et al. (39) reported that naloxone was effective in antagonizing transcutaneous electrical stimulation-induced analgesia during tooth pulp stimulation. Likewise, Woolf et al. (171) found that inhibition of the tail-flick reaction in rats by electrical stimulation of the base of the tail was also antagonized by naloxone. Levine et al. (100) proposed that placebo-induced analgesia might also involve the endorphins. These investigators reported that placebo responders were less responsive to subsequent placebo-induced analgesia when given naloxone. Their paper, however, has been severely criticized on methodological grounds by Karczyn (92).

Naloxone has been reported to antagonize antinociceptive effects induced by other drugs and manipulations not directly related to opiates, such as physostigmine (70), cannabinol analogs (27), nitrous oxide (23), intracerebral acetylcholine (125), intracerebral lanthanum ions (71), and phenoxybenzamine (48), an α-adrenergic blocker. Since it is unlikely that the analgesic actions of these compounds are mediated through opiate receptors which are highly specific (136), there are only two possibilities: (a) these compounds release enkephalin, or (b) the apparent antagonism is related to decreased nociceptive thresholds per se produced by naloxone. There is considerable evidence, in fact, that under proper conditions, naloxone is a weak hyperalgesic (see below). This makes interpretation of studies in which naloxone has been observed to reverse a particular analgesic manipulation extremely difficult. It is not known whether one is dealing with pharmacological (competitive inhibition of released endorphins) or physiological (induction of hyperalgesia) antagonism by naloxone. Thus antagonism by naloxone is only a necessary but clearly not sufficient condition to conclude that one is dealing with an opiate mechanism.

DOES NALOXONE INDUCE HYPERALGESIA?

If an endogenous opioid pain suppression system exists that is tonically active or that is part of a negative feedback system, then opiate antagonists should be effective hyperalgesic agents. An early report by Jacob et al. (88) suggested that under certain conditions, opiate antagonists may enhance pain in laboratory animals. These investigators found that naloxone-pretreated rats exposed to a hot-plate exhibited shorter escape latencies than saline-pretreated rats. The same laboratory has extended this finding to other opiate antagonists and demonstrated that opiate antagonist hyperalgesia appears to be stereospecifically elicited (86,143). Similar effects have been reported by others using the hot-plate to measure nociception (6,63,165). In all these studies, only the escape reactions are affected by naloxone and not the paw-lick reactions, which have a more rapid onset. Frederickson et al. (56) reported a diurnal rhythm in the responsiveness of mice to nociceptive stimuli and in the hyperalgesic activity of naloxone, with mice being more sensitive to naloxone during the dark phase of the cycle. The authors suggested that these oscillations in sensitivity may reflect a diurnal rhythmicity in the activity of endogenous opioid peptides. Thus time of testing may be an important variable to consider in evaluating the hyperalgesic actions of opiate antagonists.

Whereas there is good agreement concerning the effects of naloxone on escape latencies in the hot-plate test, the results regarding the hyperalgesic effects of opiate antagonists from studies employing other nociceptors are more equivocal. For example, naloxone has uniformly failed to decrease nociceptive thresholds in electrical shock-motivated tasks (30,62,129). In the tail-flick task, which measures a nociceptive reflex, naloxone has been found either to have no effect (129,167) or to produce a decrease in reaction latencies (24). The authors of the latter study, however, were not able to extend their observations regarding naloxone to the tail-pinch test. Conflicting findings have also been reported regarding the hyperalgesic effects of naloxone in tests in which nociception is induced by abdominal injections of various irritants (e.g., acetic acid, formalin, prostaglandins, phenylquinone) and assessed by counting the number of writhing reactions. Naloxone has not been found to change writhing reactions induced by either acetic acid (49), phenylquinone (22), or formalin (22,119). Ramabadran and Jacob (144) and Kokka and Fairhurst (91), on the other hand, reported that naloxone enhances writhing reactions. Finally, Chesher and Chou (38) found that naloxone actually decreased writhing induced by prostaglandin E_1, suggesting analgesic activity.

Naloxone has been found to enhance both monosynaptic and polysynaptic reflexes in spinal cats (61) and the ventral root reflex in cats evoked either electrically or by radiant heat (19). These effects, however, may not be related to hyperalgesia since systemically administered naloxone has no significant effect on the spontaneous activity or the nociceptive and nonnociceptive responses of neurons in the dorsal horn (45).

The effects of naloxone on pain thresholds in humans are conflicting. Grevert and Goldstein (64) reported that experimental pain produced by either ischemia or cold-water immersion was not affected by naloxone. El-Sobky et al. (50) confirmed these findings in another paradigm. Levine et al. (101), on the other hand, evaluated the effects of naloxone on clinical pain (extraction of impacted wisdom teeth) and found that naloxone enhanced pain in this situation. Buchsbaum et al. (32) reported that the effects of naloxone depend on the pain sensitivity of the subject. Pain-insensitive subjects found electrical shock more painful after naloxone, while pain-sensitive subjects experienced less pain to shock. The authors suggest that individual differences in pain sensitivity may relate to differences in the activity of endogenous opioid systems.

In conclusion, the hyperalgesic effects of naloxone are subtle and seem to depend on a multitude of factors, including the diurnal rhythm, test situation, nociceptive stimuli, dosage of naloxone (87), and the subject's pain sensitivity or insensitivity. Such subtle and variable effects preclude the possibility that enkephalins exert a critical tonic inhibitory influence on pain transmission; rather opioid peptides likely are involved in a phasically active pain suppression system.

ENDORPHINS IN PATHOLOGICAL PAIN STATES

Several recent studies suggest changes in endorphin activity associated with pathological pain states. Almay et al. (5), using the radioreceptor assay, found lower opioid-like substances in the CSF of patients suffering from organic pain syndromes than in patients suffering from psychogenic pain. In the same study, there was a significant correlation between CSF endorphin levels and the depth of depressive symptomatology. The same group of investigators reported that patients with high levels of CSF endorphins had higher pain thresholds and pain tolerance levels than patients with low levels of endorphins. Finally, Dehen et al. (42) compared the effects of naloxone and placebo in several normal patients and in one with congenital insensitivity to pain. They found that naloxone had no effect on nociceptive flexar reflexes in normals, whereas it decreased the threshold by 67% in the patient with congenital pain.

Sicuteri et al. (155) recently advanced the intriguing hypothesis that idiopathic headaches, including migraine, may be caused in part by disturbances in the endogenous analgesic mechanisms encoded in part by endorphins. These investigators proposed that a migraine attack could be considered as an intermittent failure of the endogenous analgesic system caused by a periodic lowering of endorphins. This deficiency could also produce an intermittent morphine abstinence syndrome, with consequent supersensitivity of the venous muscles to 5-HT and norepinephrine. The same investigators presented preliminary evidence that suggests that the CSF endorphin content of migraine sufferers is drastically lowered during an attack (154). Herkenham and Pert (76), using autoradiographic techniques, demonstrated a high density of opiate receptors in the marginal gelatinous layers of the nucleus caudalis of the spinal trigeminal complex. Dysfunctions of endogenous opiate mechanisms at this level may indeed contribute to the idiopathic headaches.

REFERENCES

1. Akaike, A., Shibota, T., Satoh, M., and Takagi, H. (1978): *Neuropharmacology* 17:775–778.
2. Akil, H., Mayer, D. J., and Liebeskind, J. C. (1976): *Science* 191:961–962.
3. Akil, H., Richardson, D. E., Barchas, J. D., and Li, C.-H. (1978): *Proc. Natl. Acad. Sci. USA* 75:5,170–5,172.
4. Akil, H., Richardson, D. E., Hughes, J., Barchas, J. D. (1978): *Science* 201:463–465.
5. Almay, B. G. I., Johansson, F., Von Knarring, L., Terenius, L., and Wahlström, A. (1978): *Pain* 5:153–162.
6. Amir, S., and Amit, Z. (1978): *Life Sci.* 23:1,143–1,152.
7. Anderson, K. V., and Mahan, D. E. (1971): *Psychon. Sci.* 23:113–114.
8. Anderson, K. V., and Pearl, G. S. (1977): In: *Proceedings of the First World Congress on Pain (Advances in Pain Research and Therapy, Vol. I),* edited by J. J. Bonica and D. Albe-Fessand. Raven, New York, 1977.
9. Anderson, S. D., Basbaum, A. I., and Fields, H. L. (1977): *Brain Res.* 123:363–368.
10. Atweh, S. F., and Kuhar, M. J. (1977): *Brain Res.* 124:53–67.
11. Atweh, S. F., and Kuhar, M. J. (1977): *Brain Res.* 124:53–67.
12. Balagura, S., and Ralph, T. (1973): *Brain Res.* 60:369–379.
13. Basbaum, A. I., and Fields, H. L. (1981): *J. Comp. Neurol. (in Press).*
14. Basbaum, A., Clanton, C. H., and Fields, H. L. (1978): *J. Comp. Neurol.* 178:209–224.
15. Behbehani, M. M., and Pomeroy, S. L. (1978): *Brain Res.* 149:266–269.
16. Belcher, G., and Ryall, R. W. (1978): *Brain Res.* 145:303–314.
17. Belcher, G., Ryall, R. W., and Schaffner, R. (1978): *Brain Res.* 151:307–321.
18. Belcher, G., Ryall, R. W., and Schaffner, R. (1978): *Brain Res.* 151:307–321.
19. Bell, J. A., and Martin, W. R. (1977): *Eur. J. Pharmacol.* 42:147–154.
20. Belluzzi, J. D., Grant, N., Garsky, V., Sarantokis, D., Wise, C. D., and Stein, L. (1976): *Nature* 260:625–626.
21. Benelli, G. (1978): In: *Factors Affecting Actions of Narcotics,* edited by M. L. Adler, L. Manara, and R. Samanin, pp. 579–588. Raven, New York, 1978.
22. Berkowitz, B. A., Finch, A. D., and Ngai, S. H. (1977): *J. Pharmacol. Exp. Ther.* 203:539–547.
23. Berkowitz, B. A., Finck, D. A., and Ngai, S. H. (1977): *J. Pharmacol. Exp. Ther.* 203:539–547.
24. Berntson, G. G., and Walker, J. M. (1977): *Brain Res. Bull.* 2:157–159.
25. Besson, J. M., Wyon-Maillard, M. C., Benoist, J. M., Conseiller, C., and Hamann, K. F. (1973): *J. Pharmacol. Exp. Ther.* 187:239–245.

26. Bloom, F., Battenberg, E., Rossier, J., Ling, N., and Guillemin, R. (1978): *Proc. Natl. Acad. Sci. USA* 75:1,591–1,595.
27. Bloom, A. S., Dewey, W. L., Harris, L. S., and Brasins, K. (1975): *Neurosci. Abst.* 1:375.
28. Bodnar, R. J., Glusman, M., Brutus, M., Spiaggia, A., and Kelly, D. D. (1979): *Physiol. Behav.* 23:53–62.
29. Bodnar, R. J., Kelly, D. D., Spiaggia, A., Ehrenberg, C., and Glusman, M. (1978): *Pharmacol. Biochem. Behav.* 8:667–672.
30. Bodnar, R. J., Kelly, D. D., Spiaggia, A., Ehrenberg, C., and Glusman, M. (1978): *Pharmacol. Biochem. Behav.* 8:667–672.
31. Bradley, P. B., Briggs, I., Gayton, R. J., and Lambert, L. A. (1976): *Nature* 261:425–426.
32. Buchsbaum, M. S., Davis, G. C., and Bunney, W. E., Jr. (1977): *Nature* 270:620–622.
33. Calvillo, O., Henry, J. L., and Newman, R. S. (1974): *Can. J. Physiol. Pharmacol.* 52:1,207–1,211.
34. Casey, K. L. (1971): *Int. J. Neurosci.* 2:15–28.
35. Casey, K. L. (1971): *Int. J. Neurosci.* 2:29–34.
36. Chang, J-K., Fong, T. W., Pert, A., and Pert, C. B. (1976): *Life Sci.* 18:1,473–1,481.
37. Cheng, R. S. S., and Pomeranz, B. (1978): In: *Characteristics and Function of Opioids,* edited by J. M. Van Ree and L. Terenius, pp. 161–166. Elsevier/North Holland, Amsterdam.
38. Chesher, G. B., and Chou, B. (1977): *Life Sci.* 21:1,569–1,574.
39. Chapman, C. R., and Benedetti, C. (1977): *Life Sci.* 21:1,645–1,648.
40. Dahlström, A., and Fuxe, K. (1965): *Acta Physiol. Scand.* 64:Suppl. 247.
41. Dahlström, A., and Fuxe, K. (1965): *Acta Physiol. Scand.* 64:Suppl. 247.
42. Dehen, H., Willer, J. C., Prier, S., Boureau, F., and Cambier, J. (1978): *Pain* 5:351–358.
43. Dostrovsky, J., and Pomeranz, B. (1973): *Nature* 246:222–224.
44. Duggan, A. W., Hall, J. G., and Headley, P. M. (1977): *Br. J. Pharmacol.* 61:65–76.
45. Duggan, A. W., Hall, J. G., Headley, P. M., and Griersmith, B. T. (1977): *Brain Res.* 138:185–189.
46. Eickhoff, R., Handinerku, H. O., McQueen, D. S., and Schick, E. (1978): *Pain* 5:99–113.
47. Elde, R., Hokfelt, T., Johansson, O., Ljungdahl, A., Nilsson, G., and Jeffcoate, S. L. (1976): In: *Centrally Acting Peptides,* edited by J. Hughes, pp. 17–35. Macmillan, London.
48. Elliott, H. W., Spiehler, V., and Navarro, G. (1976): *Life Sci.* 19:1,637–1,644.
49. Elliott, H. W., Spiehler, V., and Navarro, G. (1976): *Life Sci.* 19:1,637–1,644.
50. El-Sobky, A., Dothavsky, J. O., and Wall, P. D. (1976): *Nature* 263:783–784.
51. Fields, H. L., and Anderson, S. D. (1978): *Pain* 5:333–349.
52. Fields, H. L., Basbaum, A. I., Clanton, C. H., and Anderson, S. D. (1977): *Brain Res.* 126:441–453.
53. Frederickson, R. C. A. (1977): *Life Sci.* 21:23–42.
54. Frederickson, R. C. A., and Norris, F. H. (1976): *Science* 194:440–442.
55. Frederickson, R. C. A., and Norris, F. H. (1976): *Science* 194:440–442.
56. Frederickson, R. C. A., Burgis, V., and Edwards, J. D. (1977): *Science* 198:756–758.
57. Fratta, W., Yang, H. Y. T., Hong, J., and Costa, E. (1977): *Nature* 268:452–453.
58. Gallager, D. W., and Pert, A. (1978): *Brain Res.* 144:257–275.
59. Gent, J. P., and Wolstencroft, J. H. (1976): *Nature* 261:426–427.
60. Gent, J. P., and Wolstencroft, J. H. (1976): *Nature* 261:426–427.
61. Goldfarb, J., Kaplan, E. I., and Jenkins, H. R. (1978): *Neuropharmacology* 17:569–575.
62. Goldstein, A., Pryor, G. T., Otis, L. S., and Larsen, F. (1976): *Life Sci.* 18:599–604.
63. Grevert, D., and Goldstein, A. (1977): *Psychopharmacology* 53:111–113.
64. Grevert, P., and Goldstein, A. (1978): *Science* 199:1,093–1,095.
65. Grossman, W., and Jurna, I. (1974): *Eur. J. Pharmacol.* 29:171–174.
66. Guillemin, R., Vargo, T., Rossier, J., Minick, S., Ling, N., Rivier, J., Vale, W., and Bloom, F. (1977): *Science* 197:1,367–1,369.
67. Haigler, H. J. (1976): *Life Sci.* 19:841–858.
68. Haigler, H. J. (1978): In: *Iontophoresis and Transmitter Mechanisms in the Mammalian Central Nervous System,* edited by R. W. Ryall and J. S. Kelly, pp. 326–328. Elsevier/North Holland, Amsterdam.
69. Halpern, M. (1978): *Physiol. Behav.* 3:171–178.
70. Harris, L. S., Dewey, W. L., Homes, J. F., Kennedy, J. S., and Parr, H. (1969): *J. Pharmacol. Exp. Ther.* 169:17–22.
71. Harris, R. A., Loh, H. H., and Way, E. L. (1975): *J. Pharmacol. Exp. Ther.* 196:288–297.
72. Hasabuchi, Y., and Li, C. H. (1978): *Comm. Psychopharmacol.* 2:33–37.
73. Hayes, R. L., Bennett, G. J., Newton, P. G., and Mayer, D. J. (1978): *Brain Res.* 155:69–90.
74. Henry, J. L. (1977): In: *Substance P,* edited by U. S. Von Euler and B. Pernow, pp. 231–240. Raven Press.
75. Henry, J. L., and Newman, R. S. (1974): *Can. Fed. Biol. Soc.* 17:632 (abstr).
76. Herkenham, M., and Pert, C. B. (1980): *Proc. Natl. Acad. Sci. USA* 77:5,532–5,536.
77. Herz, A., Albus, K., Metys, T., Schubert, P., and Teschenmacher, H. J. (1970): *Neuropharmacology* 9:539–551.
78. Hong, J. S., Yang, H.-Y. T., Fratta, W., and Costa, E. (1977): *Brain Res.* 134:383–386.

79. Hosobuchi, Y., Adams, J. E., and Linchitz, R. (1977): *Science* 197:183–186.
80. Hosobuchi, Y., Rossier, J., Bloom, F. E., and Guillemin, R. (1979): *Science* 203:279–281.
81. Hughes, J. (1975): *Brain Res.* 88:295–308.
82. Hughes, J., Smith, T. W., Kosterlitz, H. W., Fothergill, L. A., Morgan, B. A., and Morris, H. R. (1975): *Nature* 258:577–579.
83. Hunsperger, R. W. and Bucher, V. M. (1967): In: *Structure and Function of the Limbic System,* edited by W. R. Adey and T. Takizane, pp. 103–127. Elsevier, Amsterdam.
84. Irwin, S., Houde, R. W., Bennett, D. R., Hendershot, L. C., and Seevers, M. H. (1951): *J. Pharmacol. Exp. Ther.* 101:132–143.
85. Iwata, N., and Sakai, Y. (1971): *Jpn. J. Pharmacol.* 21:413–416.
86. Jacob, J. J. C., and Ramabadran, K. (1978): *Br. J. Pharmacol.* 64:91–98.
87. Jacob, J. J. C., and Ramabadran, K. (1978): *Br. J. Pharmacol.* 64:91–98.
88. Jacob, J. J., Trembloy, E. C., and Colombel, M. C. (1974): *Psychopharmacologia* 37:217–223.
89. Jacquet, Y., and Lajtha, A. (1974): *Science* 185:1,055–1,057.
90. Jessell, T. M., and Iversen, L. L. (1977): *Nature* 268:549–551.
91. Kokka, N., and Fairhurst, A. S. (1977): *Life Sci.* 21:975–980.
92. Karczyn, A. D. (1978): *Lancet* 2:1,304–1,305.
93. Kitahata, L. M., Kosaka, Y., Taub, A., Bonikos, K., and Hoffert, M. (1974): *Anesthesiology* 41:39–48.
94. Koll, W., Hasse, J., Block, G., and Mühlberg, B. (1963): *Int. J. Pharmacol.* 2:57–65.
95. Kuraishi, Y., Fukui, K., Shiomi, H., Akaike, A., and Takagi, H. (1978): *Biochem. Pharmacol.* 27:2,756–2,758.
96. LaMotte, C., Pert, C. B., and Snyder, S. H. (1976): *Brain Res.* 112:407–412.
97. LaMotte, C. C., Snowman, A., Pert, C. B., and Snyder, S. H. (1978): *Brain Res.* 155:374–379.
98. LeBars, D., Menetrey, D., Consisller, C., and Besson, J. M. (1974): *C.R.H. Acad. Sci.* 279:1,369–1,371.
99. LeBars, D., Guilbaud, G., Jurna, I., and Besson, J. M. (1976): *Brain Res.* 115:518–524.
100. Levine, J. D., Gordon, N. C., and Fields, H. L. (1978): *Lancet* 2:654–657.
101. Levine, J. D., Gordon, N. C., Jones, R. T., and Fields, H. L. (1978): *Nature* 272:826–827.
102. Lewis, V. A., and Gebhart, G. F. (1977): *Brain Res.* 124:283–303.
103. Lewis, V. A., and Gebhart, G. F. (1977): *Brain Res.* 124:283–303.
104. Lewis, J. W., Cannon, J. T., and Liebeskind, J. C. (1980): *Science* 208:623–625.
105. Li, C. H., Barnafi, L., Chretien, M., and Chung, D. (1965): *Nature* 208:1,093–1,094.
106. Liebeskind, J. C., Guilbaud, G., Besson, J. M., and Oliveras, J.-L. (1973): *Brain Res.* 50:441–446.
107. Lobatz, M. A., Proudfit, H. K., and Anderson, E. G. (1976): *Pharmacologist* 18:213.
108. Loh, H. H., Tseng, L. F., Wei, E., and Li, C. H. (1976): *Proc. Natl. Acad. Sci. USA* 73:3,895–3,898.
109. Lorens, S. A. (1978): *Ann. N.Y. Acad. Sci.* 305:532–535.
110. McCreery, D. B., Bloedel, J. R., and Hames, E. G. (1979): *J. Neurophysiol.* 42:166–182.
111. McLennan, H., Gilfillan, K., and Heap, Y. (1977): *Pain* 3:229–238.
112. Madden, J., Akil, H., Patrick, R. L., and Barchas, J. D. (1977): *Nature* 265:358–360.
113. Mayer, D. J., and Liebeskind, J. C. (1974): *Brain Res.* 68:73–93.
114. Mayer, D. J., Price, D. D., and Rafii, A. (1977): *Brain Res.* 121:368–372.
115. Melzack, R., Stotler, W. A., and Livingston, W. K. (1958): *Neurophysiology* 21:353–367.
116. Messing, R. B., Phebus, L., Fisher, L. A., and Lytle, L. D. (1975): *Psychopharmacol. Comm.* 1:511–521.
117. Mudge, A. W., Leeman, S. E., and Fischbach, G. D. (1979): In: *Endorphins and Mental Health Research,* edited by E. Usdin, W. E. Bunney, Jr., and N. S. Kline, pp. 344–351. Macmillan Press, New York, 1979.
118. Nashold, B. S., Wilson, W. P., and Slaughter, D. G. (1969): *J. Neurosurg.* 30:14–24.
119. North, M. A. (1978): *Life Sci.* 22:295–302.
120. Oleson, T., Twambly, D. A., and Liebeskind, J. C. (1978): *Pain* 4:211–230.
121. Olivaras, J. L., Besson, J. M., Guilband, G., and Liebeskind, J. C. (1974): *Exp. Brain Res.* 20:32–44.
122. Oliveras, J. L., Hasobuchi, Y., Redjemi, F., Guilband, G., and Besson, J. M. (1977): *Brain Res.* 120:221–229.
123. Oliveras, J. L., Hosobuchi, Y., Redjemi, F., Guilbaud, G., and Besson, J. M. (1977): *Brain Res.* 120:221–229.
124. Oliveras, J. L., Redjemi, F., Guilbaud, G., and Besson, J. M. (1975): *Pain* 1:136–145.
125. Pedigo, N., Dewey, W. L., and Harris, L. S. (1975): *J. Pharmacol. Exp. Ther.* 193:845–852.
126. Pert, A. (1976): In: *Opiates and Endogenous Opioid Peptides,* edited by H. W. Kosterlitz, pp. 87–94, Elsevier/North Holland, Amsterdam.
127. Pert, A., and Mitchell, J. (1978): *Pain Abst.* 1:261.
128. Pert, A., and Walter, M. (1976): *Life Sci.* 19:1,023–1,032.
129. Pert, A., and Walter, M. (1976): *Life Sci.* 19:1,023–1,032.

130. Pert, A., and Yaksh, T. (1974): *Brain Res.* 80:135–140.
131. Pert, A., Bragin, E., and Pert, C. B. (1981): *(in preparation).*
132. Pert, A., Dionne, R., Ng, L., Bragin, E., Moody, T. W., and Pert, C. B. (1981): *Brain Res. (in press).*
133. Pert, A., Massari, V. J., Tizabi, Y., O'Donohue, T. L., and Jacobowitz, D. (1980): In: *Endogenous and Exogenous Opiate Agonists and Antagonists,* edited by E. L. Way, pp. 151–154. Pergamon, New York.
134. Pert, A., Massari, V. J., Tizabi, Y., O'Donohue, T. L., and Jacobowitz, D. (1980): In: *Endogenous and Exogenous Opiate Agonists and Antagonists,* edited by E. L. Way, pp. 151–154. Pergamon, New York.
135. Pert, C. B., and Garland, B. L. (1978): In: *Receptors and Hormone Action,* edited by B. W. O'Malley and L. Birnbaumer, pp. 535–551. Academic Press, New York, 1978.
136. Pert, C. B., and Snyder, S. H. (1973): *Proc. Natl. Acad. Sci. USA* 70:2,243–2,247.
137. Pert, C. B., and Snyder, S. H. (1973): *Science* 179, 1,011–1,014.
138. Pert, C. B., Pert, A., Chang, J-K., and Fong, B. T. W. (1976): *Science* 194:330–332.
139. Pomeranz, B., and Chiu, D. (1976): *Life Sci.* 19:1,757–1,762.
140. Pomeranz, B., Cheng, R., and Law, P. (1977): *Exp. Neurol.* 54:172–178.
141. Proudfit, H. K., and Anderson, E. G. (1975): *Brain Res.* 98:612–618.
142. Raemer, D., Buescher, H. H., Hill, R. C., Pleis, J., Bauer, W., Cardinaux, F., Classe, A., Hauser, D., and Huguenin, R. (1977): *Nature* 268:547–549.
143. Ramabadran, K., and Jacob, J. J. C. (1979): *Life Sci.* 24:1,959–1,970.
144. Ramabadran, K., and Jacob, J. J. C. (1979): *Life Sci.* 24:1,959–1,970.
145. Rancic, M., and Yu, H. H. (1976): *Brain Res.* 111:197–203.
146. Rossier, J., French, E. D., Rivier, C., Ling, N., Guillemin, R., and Bloom, F. E. (1977): *Nature* 270:618–620.
147. Ruda, M. (1975): Autoradiographic study of the efferent projections of the midbrain central gray of the cat. Ph.D. Dissertation, University of Pennsylvania, Philadelphia.
148. Samanin, R., Gumulka, W., and Valzelli, L. (1970): *Eur. J. Pharmacol.* 10:339–343.
149. Sar, M., Stumpf, W. E., Miller, R. J., Chang, K-J., and Cuatrecasas, P. (1978): *J. Comp. Neurol.* 182:17–38.
150. Satoh, M., and Takagi, H. (1971): *Eur. J. Pharmacol.* 14:60–65.
151. Satoh, M., Akaike, A., and Takagi, H. (1979): *Brain Res.* 169.
152. Satoh, M., Nakamura, N., and Takagi, H. (1971): *Eur. J. Pharmacol.* 16:245–247.
153. Shiomi, H., and Takagi, H. (1974): *Br. J. Pharmacol.* 52:519–526.
154. Sicuteri, F., Anselmi, B., Curradi, C., Smchelocci, S., and Sassi, A. (1978): In: *Advances in Biochemical Psychopharmacology, Vol. 18,* edited by E. Costa and M. Trabucchi, pp. 363–366. Raven Press, New York.
155. Sicuteri, F., Del Bianco, D. L., and Anselmi, B. (1979): *Psychopharmacology* 65:205–209.
156. Simon, E. J., Hiller, J., and Edelman, I. (1973): *Proc. Natl. Acad. Sci. USA* 72:2,404–2,407.
157. Sjölund, B., Terenius, L., and Eriksson, M. (1977): *Acta Physiol. Scand.* 100:382–384.
158. Skultety, F. M. (1963): *Arch. Neurol.* 8:608–620.
159. Takagi, H., Satoh, M., Akaike, A., Shibata, T., and Kuraishi, Y. (1977): *Eur. J. Pharmacol.* 45:91–92.
160. Takagi, H., Satoh, M., Akaike, A., Shibata, T., Yajima, H., and Ogawa, H. (1978): *Eur. J. Pharmacol.* 49:113–116.
161. Takagi, H., Satoh, M., Doi, K., Kamasaki, K., and Akaike, A. (1976): *Arch. Int. Pharmacodyn.* 221:96–104.
162. Tenan, S. S. (1968): *Psychopharmacologia* 12:278–285.
163. Terenius, L. (1973): *Acta Pharmacol. Toxicol.* 33:377–384.
164. Teschemacher, H., Schubert, P., and Herz, A. (1973): *Neuropharmacology* 12:123–131.
165. Trembloy, E., Colombel, M. C., and Jacob, J. J. (1976): *Psychopharmacology* 49:41–48.
166. Tsou, K., and Jang, C. S. (1964): *Sci. Sin.* 13:1,099–1,109.
167. Tulmay, F. C., Sparker, S. B., and Takemou, A. E. (1975): *Eur. J. Pharmacol.* 33:65–70.
168. Vogt, M. (1974): *J. Physiol.* 236:483–498.
169. Walker, J. M., Berntson, G. G., Sandman, C. A., Coy, D. H., Schally, A. V., and Kastin, A. J. (1977): *Science* 196:85–87.
170. Wang, J. K. (1977): *Anesthesiology* 47:269–271.
171. Woolf, C. J., Barrett, G. D., Mitchell, D., and Myers, R. A. (1977): *Eur. J. Pharmacol.* 45:311–314.
172. Yaksh, T. L. (1979): *Brain Res.* 160:180–185.
173. Yaksh, T. L., and Rudy, T. A. (1976): *Science* 192:1,357–1,358.
174. Yaksh, T. L., DuChateau, J. C., and Rudy, T. A. (1976): *Brain Res.* 104:367–372.
175. Yaksh, T. L., Plant, R. L., and Rudy, T. A. (1977): *Eur. J. Pharmacol.* 41:399–408.
176. Yaksh, T. L., Yeung, J. C., and Rudy, T. A. (1976): *Brain Res.* 14:83–103.
177. Yaksh, T. L., Yeung, J. C., and Rudy, T. A. (1976): *Life Sci.* 18:1,193–1,198.

178. Zieglgänsberger, W., and Bayerl, H. (1976): *Brain Res.* 115:111–128.
179. Zieglgänsberger, W., and Bayerl, H. (1976): *Brain Res.* 115:111–128.
180. Zieglgänsberger, W., Siggins, G., French, E., and Bloom, F. (1978): In: *Characteristics and Functions of Opioids,* edited by J. M. Van Ree and L. Terenius, pp. 75–86. Elsevier/North Holland, Amsterdam.
181. Zieglgänsberger, W., Siggins, G., French, E., and Bloom, F. (1978): In: *Characteristics and Functions of Opioids,* edited by J. M. Van Ree and L. Terenius, pp. 75–85. Elsevier/North Holland, Amsterdam.

Advances in Neurology, Vol. 33, edited by
M. Critchley et al. Raven Press, New York © 1982

Personality Aspects of Headache Patients

S. Gori-Savellini, *L. Lisci, *M. Marini, and M. Martorana

*Departments of Experimental Psychology, and *Clinical Pharmacology, Headache Center,
University of Florence, Florence, Italy*

Previous studies (3,7) have shown significant correlations between certain personality traits and specific symptomatic patterns. Nevertheless, caution should be exerted when approaching this subject (1,2). This chapter discusses those psychological characteristics that differentiate headache patients.

A testing device that reveals eventual difficulties in memory (5) was administered to 26 inpatients and 16 outpatients at the Headache Center of Florence. The resulting data, when compared with those from a group of 19 control subjects, indicate significant differences (Fig. 1). This chapter attempts to provide answers regarding the classification of these phenomena into a personality picture. It is important to investigate the nature of pain in idiopathic headache. The results have confirmed the neuroticizing effect (6). Therefore, we administered the Eysenck Personality Inventory (EPI) (Fig. 2) to subjects previously studied in order to isolate other eventual neurotic or psychotic dimensions related to a propensity (or disinclination) toward interpersonal relationships (socializa-

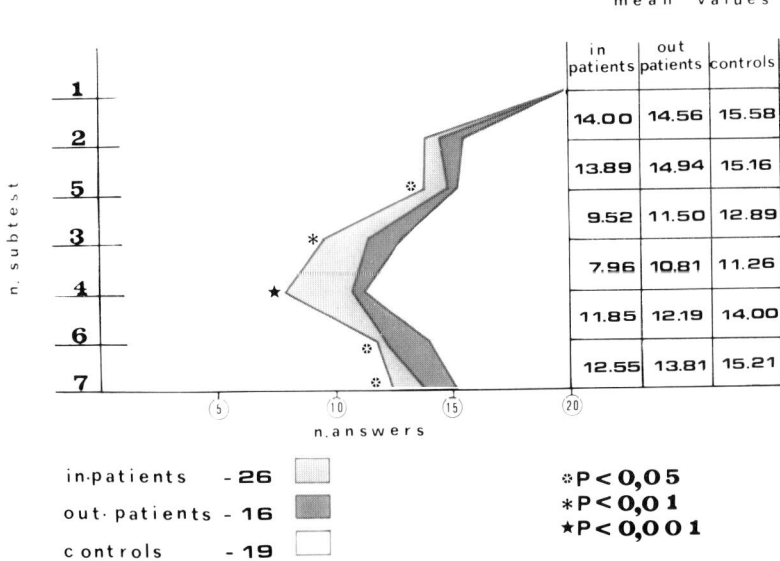

FIG. 1. Mnestic output curves in inpatients, outpatients, and controls. Results obtained by the three groups of subjects in Rey's different subtests emphasizing memory difficulties.

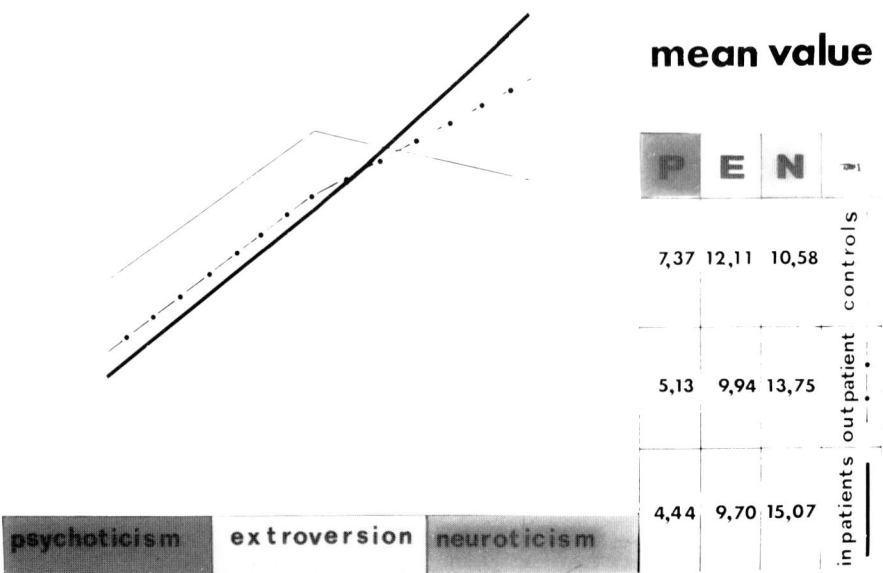

FIG. 2. Personality patterns: EPI. Average pattern for the three groups of subjects as seen from the three personality dimensions (psycoticism, extraversion, and neuroticism).

tion). A comparison among the results provided by the inpatients, outpatients, and control subjects reveals differences in the three dimensions examined, with particular reference to the psychotic and the neurotic. In fact, in the psychotic dimension, the inpatients seem to be more controlled then the outpatients, especially when compared to the control group. On the other hand, in the neurotic dimension, the highest data issue from the inpatients, followed by the outpatients; the control group is far less neurotic; the tested headache patients, therefore, appear to have a neurotic personality

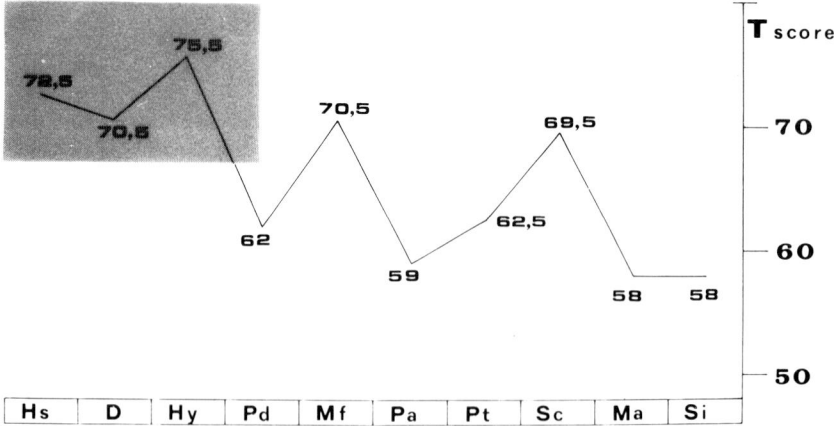

FIG. 3. Personality patterns: MMPI. Average personality pattern for a group of outpatients. The results obtained in hysteria, depression, and hypochondriasis scales (neurotic triad) are emphasized.

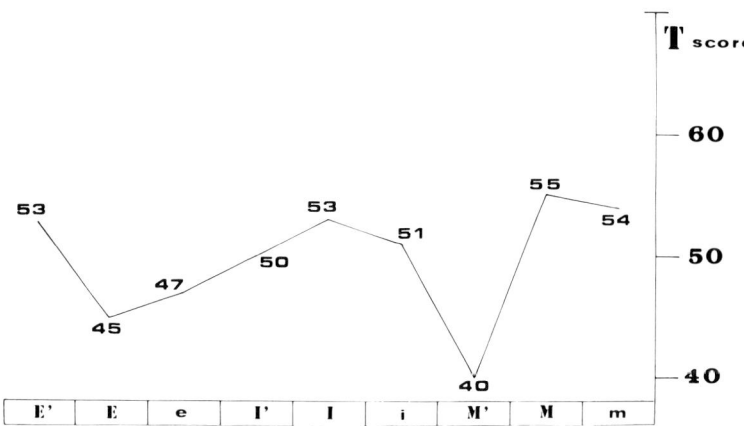

FIG. 4. Personality patterns: PFS. Average personality pattern for outpatients. This pattern shows the different aggressive answers to frustrating situations (extra-, intra-, impunitive answers).

structure. To confirm these results and to hypothesize a more defined personality picture, another small group of headache outpatients was subjected to a battery of tests, including Rosenzweig's Picture Frustration Study (PFS), the Minnesota Multiphasic Personality Inventory (MMPI), and the Cattell's Anxiety Scale (AS), as well as the EPI.

A comparison of the results of the headache patients with those of the normal subjects shows certain typical personality traits of the headache sufferers. Specifically, the results of the MMPI (Fig. 3) indicate the neurotic triad, that is, high degrees in the hysteria, depression, and hypochondriasis scales. The PFS results (Fig. 4) indicate a profile characterized by intrapunitive and, above all, impunitive traits. These elements, together with other results, present a picture fundamentally characterized by anxiety (results of AS IPAT) and by neurotic traits (the results of the N scale of EPI are confirmed), which can be of the obsessive type (4) (Fig. 5).

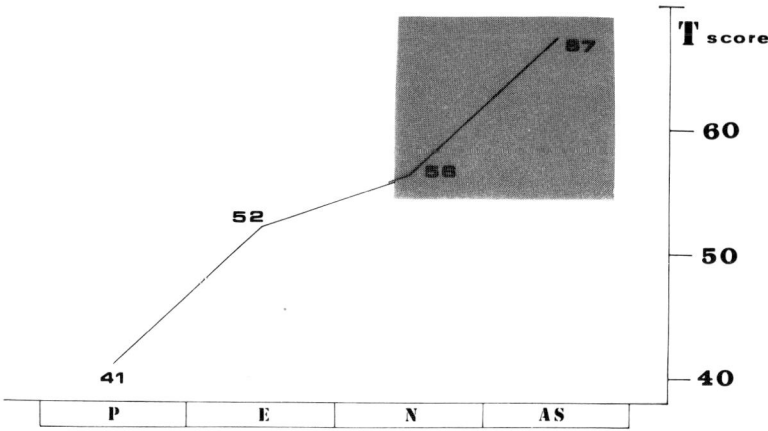

FIG. 5. Personality patterns: EPI-AS. Average personality pattern for outpatients. Note the high scores on the neuroticism and anxiety subscales.

These data constitute only one of many aspects of the complex problem of idiopathic headache. With respect to present research, they can be comparated with data relative to certain aspects of child sufferers. We examined 25 children who had come to the Headache Center of Florence and found traits of introversion, inhibition of aggressivity, and difficulty in finding a place for themselves within the family group. These results indicate that a great deal of further research is required but leave no doubt as to the social repercussions of headache.

ACKNOWLEDGMENT

We thank Dr. M. G. Nardelli for her help in presenting the work.

REFERENCES

1. Biondi, M. (1979): Recenti modelli patogenetici in medicina psicosomatica. *Med. Psicosom.,* 24:287–309.
2. Canestrari, R., and Fava, G. (1979): La concezione psicosomatica della colite ulcerosa. *Med. Psicosom.,* 24:225–250.
3. Gori-Savellini, S., and Martorana, M. (1977): Personalità e cardiopatie. *Rass. Stud. Psichiatr.,* 66:4.
4. Nencini, R., and Belcecchi, M. V. (1979): Il P.F.S. di Rosenzweig nelle malattie mentali. *Boll. Psicol. Appl.,* 149:57–110.
5. Rey, A. (1966): *Les Troubles de la Memoire et leur Examen Psychometrique.* Charles Dessart, Bruxelles.
6. Sicuteri, F., and Fonda, C. (1976): Sulla natura centrale o periferica del dolore nelle cefalee essenziali. *Min. Med.* 67:1,826–1,833.
7. Sirigatti, S., Ieri, A., Gori-Savellini, S., Corchia, F., Frintino, A., Martorana, M., Maggi, L., and Zipoli, A. (1979): Study of the structure of personality in various groups of patients with heart disease and in normal subjects. *International Congress Series no. 491. Florence International Meeting on Myocardial Infarction,* edited by D. T. Mason, G. G. Neri Serneri and M. F. Oliver, pp. 436–438. Excerpta Medica, Amsterdam.

Advances in Neurology, Vol. 33, edited by
M. Critchley et al. Raven Press, New York © 1982

Mechanisms of Fever Occurring in Migraine

J. Jacob

Pharmacological Laboratory, Pasteur Institute, Paris, France

High fever, a rare event in migraine, is observed regularly only in familial hemiplegic migraine and sometimes in migraine complicated by neurologic disturbances (4). Moderate rises in temperature, however, are not uncommon, especially in children and in thermolabile patients (7). Because it is not considered important, it is rarely recorded and thus few statistics, except those of Michelacci (29), are available. Conversely, high fever is often accompanied by headache. Some common factors exist in the mechanism of hyperthermia and of migraine but they are generally located or modulated differently so that disturbance of temperature regulation predominates in the first case, pain in the second.

Many biogenic substances have been suggested to be involved in both temperature regulation or disorders and migraine pathogenesis; only four—5-hydroxytryptamine (5-HT), norepinephrine (NE) and related amines, prostaglandins (PGs), and endogenous morphine (EM)—are considered here. Presentation or discussion will allow consideration of other relevant products. Their possible role in fever accompanying migraine is discussed.

EFFECTS OF 5-HT, NE, PGS, AND EM ON BODY TEMPERATURE

5-HT

5-HT is slightly effective on body temperature when injected systemically, by the subcutaneous or intravenous route, and doses of the order of magnitude of 1 mg/kg are necessary to produce moderate modifications in, e.g., the rabbit and rat. On the contrary, micrograms or still smaller doses are effective when injected into the cerebrospinal fluid (lateral central ventricle or cisterna magna) (21). The dominant central effect of 5-HT varies according to species (18). For instance, in the rabbit, lower doses produce a small but distinct hypothermia followed by a late (2 to 3 hr) moderate rise in temperature. This latter effect is probably mediated by PGs, as it is antagonized by inhibitors of their synthesis (indomethacin, ketoprophen). When the dose is increased, the early fall in temperature decreases and merges into an opposite effect, which becomes very important (2 to 3°C). The late rise develops somewhat but never becomes as great as the early one (21).

Some other components probably also exist. Pharmacological analysis indicates that different receptors are triggered as selective antagonists have been found (14). Using an intermediate dose of 5-HT, cinanserin inhibits selectively the early rise in temperature, unmasking an important early fall; it does not affect the late rise. On the contrary, bromlysergamide potentiates the early rise. With antagonistic doses, cinanserin has almost no thermic effect, indicating that the early rise has no physiological significance in the rabbit. On the contrary, bromlysergamide induces a moderate but definite rise in temperature. This action might be related to an antagonism of the early fall and thus represents an argument in favor of a physiological role of 5-HT in keeping the normal temperature low. Such a hypothermic function also appears in fever induced by pyrogen, which is clearly decreased by 5-HT, even with high doses (36), and increased by parachlorophenylalanine (pCPA), a 5-HT depletor (18). This does not mean that the early rise produced by 5-HT might not have a pathological or a toxic role as various hyperthermia produced by, e.g., association of reserpine with other drugs can be reduced with 5-HT antagonists. Cyproheptadine resembles cinanserin in antagonizing the early rise but is not as selective, being able to depress partly the two other components. Increasing doses of methysergide antagonize successively the early fall, the early rise, and the late rise; methysergide itself is moderately but definitely hyperthermic.

These selective antagonisms indicate that distinct receptors might be involved. If so, they would themselves be different from the H_1 and H_2 receptors of Haigler (this volume) for which the cited antagonists have no affinity; they might be of the H_3 type. Intracerebroventricular 5-HT may reach receptors not innervated by serotoninergic terminals, or the receptors of the hypothalamus (which is the site of action of 5-HT) may be of a class not yet observed by Haigler. Also, it is not known if one or another effect of intracerebroventricular 5-HT is caused by an action of the amine on the vessel of the thermoregulatory center(s). Such indirect effects of vascular origin, however, could not account for the entire phenomenon, as 5-HT applied by microelectrophoresis has been shown to modify thermosensitive neurons.

Cinanserin, cyproheptadin, and methysergide are not absolutely specific for 5-HT; they are able to depress with somewhat higher doses the early hyperthermia induced by dopamine, probably by acting on dopamine receptors (14); this must be kept in mind when interpreting the effect of one of these substances in human hyperthermia, which might thus be serotoninergic or dopaminergic or mixed. Furthermore, cyproheptadin has a fleeting antagonistic action on the hyperthermia induced by PGE_1 (24).

In the human, the effects of 5-HT itself are not known, but those of precursors and of an inhibitor of its synthesis, pCPA, have been described. The actions of high doses of precursors indicate that peripheral and (or) central excesses of 5-HT produce rises in temperature. Hyperthermias were observed after administration of tryptophan administered with an inhibitor of amine oxidase (26) and of 5-hydroxytryptophan ethylester with an inhibitor of peripheral carboxylase (25). In the latter case, however, the initial rise was followed by a fall in men and by a rise in women. The effects described for pCPA are apparently contradictory: rises were observed in normal humans (38), falls in patients with carcinoid tumors (41). The rises might correspond to the inhibition of the normal function of 5-HT, which is to keep the temperature low, as mentioned above for the rabbit. The situation might be quite different in patients with carcinoid tumors, in whom concentrations of 5-HT are increased. The results might be comparable to those obtained in the rabbit, keeping in mind that the direction of the effects of 5-HT—increase or decrease in temperature—depends on the dose.

NE

NE, like 5-HT, is much less effective by peripheral route than by central administration. Nevertheless, hyperthermic effects appear, especially by the subcutanous route, which probably relate to its calorigenic action (15). The dominant central effect of NE varies from species to species. In the rabbit, it is hyperthermic by the intracerebroventricular route, as is the action of epinephrine, dopamine (DA), and isopropyl NE. The study of many doses did not show various components, as if no distinct α and β effects exist. This conclusion is not true because the use of specific antagonists demonstrates clearly that the hyperthermia is an α effect, antagonized by phenoxybenzamine, which unmasks a β hypothermic effect. Conversely, propanolol increases the hyperthermic action by antagonizing the hypothermic component. With antagonistic doses, pnenoxybenzamine has no important effect on its own, but β inhibitors produce a moderate rise, indicating a possible physiological role of NE in maintaining a relatively low temperature in the rabbit. With respect to 5-HT, part of the rise of temperature produced by central NE is mediated by PG, as shown par partial antagonism with nonsteroid, antiinflammatory drugs (24).

In the rat, the principal peripheral effect is hyperthermia; the central one is hypothermia. The situation is complex, as several effects have been described (22). In the human, *l*-dioxyphenylalanine, the precursor of the catecholamines, produced a fall of temperature (5).

PGs

The PGs, like the amines, are effective when administered by central (intracisternal, intracerebroventricular, intrahypothalamic) but not by systemic routes. They differ from the amines in being much more potent (nanogram rather than microgram doses can be sufficient) and in inducing rises in temperature in all animal species tested. Temperature rises have also been described in the human (12).

The PGs of the E series are the most effective; those of the F, G, I, and D series are less. The same holds true for the corresponding endoperoxide analogs. Thromboxane is seemingly not effective because imidazole, an inhibitor of thromboxane synthetase, has no effect on the increase in temperature produced by arachidonic acid (31). This action is not mediated by 5-HT nor by NE in the species in which these latter substances are hyperthermic, e.g., the rabbit. The effect of PG_1 injected into the lateral central ventricle is not antagonized by cinanserin or phentolamine but it is by cyproheptadine, which probably owes this effect to a property other than its anti-5-HT activity (24). This property might have some relevance for the effectiveness of cyproheptadine in the prophylactic treatment of migraine. PGE fever might be mediated by cAMP, but the problem is complex and cannot be discussed here.

PGs are considered the mediators of the temperature increases produced by many substances. 5-HT and NE have already been mentioned; substances that result from lesioned brain tissue also produce fever by an increase of PG synthesis, as their effect is prevented by nonsteroid antiinflammatory drugs (37). PGEs mediate the fever produced by endogenous pyrogen, which is itself the mediator of endotoxins, lipid A, virus, various antigens or mitogens, lymphokins, antigen-antibody complexes, progesterone metabolites, and LHRH (2,12,13,30,42). The endogenous pyrogen is released not only from granulocytes and macrophages but also from glials cells of the brain.

Exogenous and Endogenous Morphines

Morphine exerts various effects on body temperature, depending on both species and dose. In the rat, low doses of morphine induce increases and higher doses decreases.

The rise has been considered to be essentially of cholinergic (35) or noradrenergic (6) origin. In the human, therapeutic doses of morphine have irrelevant action; somewhat higher doses produce decreases in temperature. In the rat, repeated doses of morphine induce tolerance, i.e., diminution of the effectiveness, and dependence. Abstinence is characterized by a fall in temperature in the rat (35) and monkey (17) and by a rise in the dog (19) and human (16). Tolerance and dependence can also follow a single dose, as shown in the rat (1,20), dog (28), and human (23).

In the tolerant rat, the responses to the amines are modified. Whether these are administered by the subcutaneous or intracerebroventricular route, their hyperthermic component is increased moderately. This occurs with 5-HT, NE, DA, and acetylcholine, indicating a nonspecific increase in peripheral and central excitability (20).

Endogenous morphines are slightly effective by systemic routes; when administered centrally, they mimic the effect of morphine. According to Bläsig et al. (3), various enkephalin analogs and β-endorphin produced rises in temperature with doses lower than those necessary for inducing antinociceptive effects. Handling of the animals is followed by small rises, which were antagonized by high doses of naloxone.

POSSIBLE MECHANISMS OF FEVER OCCURRING IN MIGRAINE

Slight to moderate rises in temperature are common in migraine, whereas high fever is a rare event observed regularly only in familial hemiplegic migraine and sometimes in migraine complicated by severe neurologic disturbances (8,9,27,32). A mechanism hypothesized for migraine itself (4) might account for the slight to moderate fever.

First, peripheral releases of 5-HT from the platelets or of PGEs from the pulmonary bed, or increases in NE blood levels are not liable to produce hyperthermias by their own right. All these substances are almost inactive by systemic routes unless massive doses are administered. Possible exceptions are the nonphenolic amines (phenylethylamine, tryptamine), which more easily cross the blood-brain barrier and have been suspected to be involved in migraines caused or enhanced by some nutrients. The increases in the blood levels of these substances may reflect similar central phenomena, in which case hyperthermia could be expected, as 5-HT, NE, and PGs all are able to induce fever by intracerebral routes.

Another possibility is that the blood-brain barrier might be altered and allow for a greater permeation of the substances cited above. Recent work by Dascombe (10) indicates that the permeability of the blood-brain barrier to PGs can be altered, but the relevance of this observation for the hyperthermias of migraine is still obscure.

A third possibility is supersensitivity to hyperthermic material. 5-HT supersensitivity has been observed by Sicuteri et al. (38) at peripheral levels in volunteers suffering from intractable migraine following treatment with PCPA. These authors postulated that a similar supersensitivity at brain levels would explain several signs of migraines. Experimentally, 5-HT supersensitivity can be produced by chemical denervation e.g., with 5,7-dihydroxytryptamine, or after treatment with antagonists, such as methiothepine. In both cases, it coexists with an increase in the number of serotoninergic binding sites (33,34). Moderate but definite supersensitivity to the hyperthermic effects of 5-HT, NE, or DA administered either into the lateral ventricle or by the subcutaneous route has also been observed in rats rendered morphine dependent (20). This might also be related to increases in the number of receptors. This observation supports the provocative proposal of Sicuteri et al. (39,40), who stressed the similarities existing between migraine and the abstinence syndrome in patients dependent on opiates. Hyperthermia is one sign of this syndrome, being one of the items of the classic Hasselbach scale for the evaluation of the dependence potential; its intensity varies from patient to patient.

Another pathogenic hypothesis of migraine advocates some deficiency of 5-HT resulting possibly from sequestration of the amine (11). If it occurs in the vicinity of or at the thermoregulatory center, it might cause moderate hyperthermia. It has been indicated that the normal central function of 5-HT in the rabbit, and possibly in the human, is to keep the temperature low. A deficiency would produce moderate fever. The same result would also follow a local deficiency in catecholamines acting as β-agonists.

Further hypotheses involving biogenic amines and PGEs rest on constriction of the cerebral blood vessels and increase of the permeability of capillaries, resulting in edema. Constriction of the blood vessels is produced in the human by 5-HT, NE, and PGEs and perivascular inflammation by 5-HT and PGEs. These two processes might create local ischemia, resulting in the release of pyrogenic factors. Furthermore, perivascular inflammation is characterized by local accumulation of pyrogenic material, including 5-HT, PGEs, and kinins, the latter being able to release endogenous pyrogen.

Finally, the influences of allergic factors and of the hormonal cycle might be traced to the ability of antigens, antigen-antibody complexes, and various kinins on one side and of LHRH and progesterone metabolites on the other to release endogenous pyrogens.

Some reasons for the slight to moderate character of the hyperthermia accompanying migraine have already been considered for the sensitization and deficiency hypotheses. Another reason might be that 5-HT, NE, and EMs, even when administered by cerebral routes, are only slightly effective when compared to PGEs: the first are hyperthermic in the range of micrograms, the second in the range of nanograms. Thus fever caused by 5-HT, NE, or EM may result from a critical localization of the phenomenon and (or) from an abnormally high sensitization of relevant receptor systems. The synthesis of PGEs would be only moderately increased not only by 5-HT or NE but also by physiological levels of LHRH or metabolites of progesterone.

Severe edema and (or) vasoconstriction, localized at or in the vicinity of the thermoregulatory center, should be at the origin of high fever. Such mechanisms have been evoked for the high fever observed regularly in familial hemiplegic migraine. Indeed, intense perivascular edema, ischemic lesions, and (or) microinfarcts have been found at autopsy. Important lesions have also been observed in migraine complicated by severe neurologic disturbance. Intense perivascular edema implies accumulation of pyrogenic material. Local lesions, whether or not hemorrhagic, are also able to produce fever. Rudy (37) has shown that injection of blood into the third ventricle of the cat was followed by high fever. The active substance was not characterized; it was seemingly produced not by clotting itself but by a subsequent process. The same author demonstrated that destruction of the preoptic anterior hypothalamic area (site of the thermoregulatory center) on one side also produced a high fever. This was prevented or abolished by indomethacin. Rudy postulated that the lesions produced, directly or indirectly, high amounts of PG or PG-like substances. Strict localization at the thermoregulatory center of the various indicated perturbations may account for the so-called hyperthermic equivalents of migraine.

REFERENCES

1. Ary, M. L., and Lomax, P. (1977): Changes during morphine dependence and withdrawal in the rat. In: *Drugs, Biogenic Amines and Body Temperature,* edited by K. E. Cooper, P. Lomax, and E. Schönbaum, pp. 188–195. Karger, Basel.

2. Atkins, E., and Francis, L. (1977): Additional studies on the role of a lymphokine in the genesis of antigen-induced fever in delayed hypersensitivity. In: *Drugs, Biogenic Amines and Body Temperature,* edited by K. E. Cooper, P. Lomax, and E. Schönbaum, pp. 118–121. Karger, Basel.

3. Bläsig, J., Höllt, V., Bäuerle, U., and Herz, A. (1978): Involvement of endorphins in emotional hyperthermia of rats. *Life Sci.,* 23:2,525–2,532.

4. Bousser, M. G., and Baron, J-C. (1979): *Migraines et Algies Vasculaires de la Face.* Sandoz, Paris.

5. Boyd, A. E., III, Mager, M., Angoff, G., and Lebovitz, H. E. (1974): Effect of acute administration of l-dopa on body temperature in man. *J. Appl. Physiol.,* 37:675–678.

6. Burks, T. F., and Rosenfeld, G. C. (1979): Neurotransmitter mediation of morphine hypothermia in rats. *Life Sci.,* 24:1,067–1,074.

7. Cernibori, A., and Rovetta, P. (1969): Sull'emicrania febbrile e sull'equivalente febbrile dell'emicrania. *Ross. Neurol. Veg.,* 23:194–201.

8. Codina, A., Acarin, P. N., Miquel, F., and Noguera, M. (1971): Migraine hémiplégique associée à un nystagmus. *Rev. Neurol.,* 124:526–530.

9. Conner, R. C. (1962): Complicated migraine. *Lancet,* 2:1072–1075.

10. Dascombe, M. J. (1980): Prostaglandin E$_2$ from the cerebral circulation: A possible mediator of pyrexia. In: *Thermoregulatory Mechanisms and Their Therapeutic Implications,* edited by E. Cox, P. Lomax, A. S. Milton, and E. Schönbaum, pp. 93–94. Karger, Basel.

11. Fanchamps, A. (1979): *Recepteurs Sérotoninergiques et Vasomotricité extra- et intracrânienne. Mécanisme dAction de l'Ergotamine.* Extrait de Colloque du GREC, Geneva.

12. Feldberg, W., and Milton, A. S. (1978): In: *Inflammation,* edited by J. R. Vane and S. H. Ferreira, pp. 617–656. Springer Verlag, Berlin.

13. Gander, G. W., and Kenny, M. (1977): Characteristics of a leukocyte activator for pyrogen production isolated from rabbit peritoneal exudate fluid. In: *Drugs, Biogenic Amines and Body Temperature,* edited by E. Cooper, P. Lomax, and E. Schönbaum, pp. 111–117. Karger, Basel.

14. Girault, J. M., and Jacob, J. (1979): Serotonin antagonists and central hyperthermia produced by biogenic amines in conscious rabbits. *Eur. J. Pharmacol.,* 53:191–200.

15. Girault, J-M., Kandasamy, B., and Jacob, J. (1974): Actions centrales des amines catéchiques sur la température du Lapin éveillé. Antagonismes par des adrénolytiques α et β. *J. Pharmacol.,* 5:343–362.

16. Halbach, H., and Eddy, N. B. (1963): Tests for addiction (chronic intoxication) of morphine type. *Bull. Org. Mond. Santé,* 28:139–173.

17. Holzman, S. G., and Villarreal, J. E. (1969): Reversal of morphine withdrawal hypothermia as an adjunctive criterion for morphine-like physical dependence liability. *Proceedings of the Annual Scientific Meeting of the Committee on the Problem of Drug Dependence. Natl. Acad. Sci. Natl. Res. Council.,* pp. 6,029–6,038.

18. Jacob, J., and Girault, J-M. (1979): 5-Hydroxytryptamine. In: *Body Temperature: Regulation, Drug Effects and Therapeutic Applications,* edited by P. Lomax and E. Schönbaum, pp. 183–230. Marcel Dekker, New York.

19. Jacob, J., and Michaud, G. (1976): Production par la naloxone d'effets inverses de ceux de la morphine chez le Chien éveillé. *Arch. Int. Pharmacodyn.,* 222:332–340.

20. Jacob, J., and Suaudeau, C. (1977): Temperature effects of morphine, naloxone and biogenic amines in morphine-treated rats. In: *Drugs, Biogenic Amines and Body Temperature,* edited by K. E. Cooper, P. Lomax, and E. Schönbaum, pp. 196–203. Karger, Basel.

21. Jacob, J., Girault, J-M., and Peindaries, R. (1972): Actions of 5-hydroxytryptophan injected by various routes on the rectal temperature of the rabbit. *Neuropharmacology,* 11:1–6.

22. Jacob, J., Suaudeau, C., and Michaud, G. (1971): Actions de la noradrenaline, de la dopamine, de l'isopropylnoradrénaline et de la 5-hydroxytryptamine administrées par voie intracisternale et sous-cutanée sur la température du rat éveillé. *J. Pharmacol.,* 2:401–422.

23. Jones, R. T. (1980): Dependence in non-addict humans after a single dose of morphine, In: *Endogenous and Exogenous Opiate Agonists and Antagonists,* edited by E. L. Way, pp. 557–560. Pergamon Press, New York.

24. Kandasamy, B., Girault, J-M., and Jacob, J. (1975): Central effects of a purified bacterial pyrogen, prostaglandin E$_1$ and biogenic amines on the temperature in the awake rabbit. In: *Temperature Regulation and Drug Action,* edited by P. Lomax, E. Schönbaum, and J. Jacob, pp. 124–132. Karger, Basel.

25. Lacoste, V., Wirz-justice, A., Gastpar, M., and Da Prada, M. (1977): Induction of hypothermia in men and hyperthermia in women after 200 mg i.v. l-5HTP. *Experientia,* 33:807.

26. Lovett-Doust, J. W., Huszka, L., and Little, M. H. (1973): Metabolic control of body temperature in man. *Int. Pharmacopsychiatry,* 8:239–244.

26. Lovett-Doust, J. W., Huszka, L., and Little, M. H. (1973): Metabolic control of body temperature in man. *Int. Pharmacopsychiatry,* 8:239–244.

27. Mallet, R., Sterba, S., Ribierre, M., and Labrune, B. (1968): Migraine hemiplegique familiale. *Ann. Pediatr.,* 519–525.

28. Michaud, G., and Jacob, J. (1973): Interactions between morphine and naloxone in the intact dog. A contribution to the problem of acute dependence. *Proceedings of the 35th Annual Scientific Meeting of*

the Committee on the Problem of Drug Dependence. Natl. Acad. Sci. Natl. Res. Council, pp. 535–548.

29. Michelacci, S. (1964): Alcuni rilievi statistici su 800 casi di emicrania. In: *L'Emicrania, Motivi di Fisiopatogenesi e di Terapia*, edited by E. Greppi, and F. Sicuteri. Pozzi, Roma.

30. Milton, A. S., and Dascombe, M. J. (1977): Cyclic nucleotides in thermoregulation and fever. In: *Drugs, Biogenic Amines and Body Temperature*, edited by K. E. Cooper, P. Lomax, and E. Schönbaum, pp. 129–135. Karger, Basel.

31. Milton, A. S., Crenades-Campos, A., Sawhney, V. K., and Bichard, A. (1980): Effects of prostacyclin, 6-oxo-$PGE_{1\alpha}$ and endoperoxide analogues on the body temperature of cats and rabbits. In: *Thermoregulatory Mechanisms and Their Therapeutic Implications*, edited by E. Cox, P. Lomax, A. S. Milton, and E. Schönbaum, pp. 87–92. Karger, Basel.

32. Neligan, P., Harriman, D. G., and Pierce, J. (1977): Respiratory arrest in familial hemiplegic migraine: A clinical and neuropathological study. *Br. Med. J.*, 11:732–734.

33. Nelson, L., Herbet, A., Bourgoin, S., Glowinski, J., and Hamon, M. (1978): Characteristics of central 5HT receptors and their adaptive changes following intracerebral 5,7-dihydroxytryptamine administration in the rat. *Mol. Pharmacol.*, 14:983–995.

34. Nelson, D. L., Herbet, A., Pichat, L., Glowinski, J., and Hamon, M. (1979): In vitro and in vivo disposition of ^{3}H-methiothepin in brain tissues. Relationship to the effects of acute treatment with methiothepin on central serotoninergic receptors. *Naunyn Schmiedebergs Arch. Pharmacol.*, 310:25–33.

35. Oka, T., Nozaki, M., and Hosoya, E. (1972): Effects of p-chlorophenylalanine and cholinergic antagonists on body temperature changes induced by the administration of morphine to non-tolerant and morphine-tolerant rats. *J. Pharmacol. Exp. Ther.*, 180:136–143.

36. Peindaries, R., and Jacob, J. (1971): Interactions between 5-hydroxytryptamine and a purified bacterial pyrogen when injected into the lateral cerebral ventricle of the wake rabbit. *Eu. J. Pharmacol.*, 13:347–355.

37. Rudy, T. A. (1980): Pathogenesis of fever associated with cerebral trauma and intracranial hemorrhage. In: *Thermoregulatory Mechanisms and Their Therapeutic Implications*, edited by B. Cox, P. Lomax, A. S. Milton, and E. Schönbaum, pp. 75–81. Karger, Basel.

38. Sicuteri, F., Anselmi, B., and Del Bianco, P. L. (1973): 5-Hydroxytryptamine supersensitivity as a new theory of headache and central pain: A clinical pharmacological approach with p-chlorophenylalanine. *Psychopharmacology*, 29:347–356.

39. Sicuteri, F., Del Bianco, P. L., and Anselmi, B. (1979): Morphine abstinence and serotonin supersensitivity in man: Analgesics with the mechanismal migraine. *Psychopharmacology*, 65:205–209.

40. Sicuteri, F., Anselmi, B., Curradi, C., Michelacci, S., and Sassi, A. (1978): Morphine-like factors in CSF of headache patients. In: *Advances in Biochemical Psychopharmacology, Vol. 18*, edited by E. Costa and M. Trabucchi, pp. 363–366. Raven Press, New York.

41. Vaidya, A. B., and Levine, R. J. (1971): Hypothermia in a patient with carcinoid syndrome during treatment with parachlorophenylalanine. *N. Engl. J. Med.*, 284:255–257.

42. Woolf, C. J., Willies, G. H., and Rosendorff, C. (1977): Pyrogen, prostaglandin and cyclic AMP fevers in the rabbit. In: *Drugs, Biogenic Amines and Body Temperature*, edited by K. E. Cooper, P. Lomax, and E. Schönbaum, pp. 136–139. Karger, Basel.

Advances in Neurology, Vol. 33, edited by
M. Critchley et al. Raven Press, New York © 1982

Pain and Emotion: Their Correlation In Headache

H. Merskey

*Department of Psychiatry, University of Western Ontario, and Department of Education and
Research, London Psychiatric Hospital, London, Ontario, Canada*

Medical practitioners who become known for their skill in the diagnosis and management of particular illnesses are subjected to a special fate. They must care for patients who do not get better, who are especially persistent in looking for help, and who are, usually, different psychologically from more ordinary people who have illnesses. Two items of evidence clearly demonstrate how this may occur. The first is from a general practice study (4) in which patients were asked to keep a regular sickness diary. Analysis of the diaries showed that the patients consulted doctors only for a small proportion of the symptoms recorded. Headaches, vomiting, colds, sore throats, gastrointestinal disturbances, dizziness, and the banal complaints from which we all suffer were plentifully recorded. Only 3% of all the symptoms or sickness episodes led to a medical consultation. Certain symptoms, such as upper respiratory tract infections, generated proportionately more consultations. It follows that those who take their headache to a doctor belong to a special group, one which perhaps places increased emphasis on the value of medical care or is particularly concerned about physical symptoms, or possibly has more severe complaints.

The second item of evidence deals with the process of secondary medical referral. The primary practitioner may suffice for the patient with somatic symptoms. If not, the patient will be referred further, in many countries to a specialist; thus patients with epilepsy are referred to neurologists. It has been shown, however, that patients with psychological problems and epilepsy were twice as likely to be referred from general practice to neurologists as when they had epilepsy uncomplicated by such psychological problems (49). The neurologist may have been asked to manage the emotional problem rather than organic disease. When we consider not merely the first specialist or second doctor whom the patient sees but the third, fourth, or fifth, we can expect the patient to be still more highly selected for specific psychiatric characteristics.

In pain clinics, one of the predominant patterns has been characterized as abnormal illness behavior (48). In migraine studies, the migraine clinic patient is more abnormal psychologically than the patient found by survey techniques (25). It is not surprising that a respected physician (67,68) was impressed by the special characteristics of the migraine personality. Some patients have these special features, but so far only one study (13) provides evidence that migraineurs, or people with low back pain, are emotionally different from other people. Most studies show that the further we get from examining truly unselected patients, the more abnormal psychologically the individual appears.

135

Many reports from pain clinics and from special studies of pain indicate the psychological abnormalities of pain patients (12). The question of selection is one that confounds almost all studies of pain and personality and probably most studies of psychosomatic illness as well. Nevertheless, there is good reason to assume that pain and emotion are intimately related. Some of the reasons are discussed below.

ACUTE PAIN AND EMOTION

For many years, the classic reference to the suppression of pain by emotion was that of Beecher's (9) studies of soldiers wounded at Anzio. Beecher held that the significance of the wound in soldiers or civilians influenced the severity of pain and determined the demand for analgesics. Wall (63) has recently expressed doubts about the part played by the significance of the wound and indicated that other psychological conditions, such as expectation and attention, may be more relevant. Nevertheless, while high arousal reduces pain, moderate arousal increases it (39). Patients with anxiety have relatively more pain, patients with schizophrenia relatively less (15,36). Experimental investigations indicate that anxiety and anticipation increase the pain from a stimulus, and measures that induce confidence abate pain (5,10,44,58). There is some connection between emotion and the threshold at which pain is noticed from a noxious stimulus, but the relationship is clearer and more definite if the subject is asked to tolerate pain above threshold (18,43,65,66). With unselected samples of subjects, the severity of pain reported for a given stimulus or lesion and the frequency with which pain is reported are correlated with anxiety (21,24). Even if the samples are selected, it still holds true within the group that those who have more pain are those with more evidence of anxiety. The studies that in different ways demonstrate a connection between pain and anxiety either experimentally or in clinical comparisons are accordingly numerous (44).

We have learned that emotional factors are enough to relieve or exacerbate acute pain. Elsewhere I have noted anecdotal reports that demonstrate that pain at times may be wholly due to thought processes (41). One given by Beck (8) describes an intern who, while engaged in puncturing a patient to withdraw sternal marrow, experienced a sharp pain in his own sternum. Another example of the relatively acute induction of pain by thought processes in susceptible subjects is provided by the Couvade syndrome, in which the husbands of pregnant women experience labor pains, other abdominal pains, or pains elsewhere in the body (6,7,14,51,62).

Despite the problem of selection, there is reason to believe that certain chronic psychiatric states cause patients to experience pain located in the body. A significant number of chronic psychiatric patients have chronic pain attributable only to their emotional state or personality. The characteristics of these patients have been described by many authors. The studies of Gidro-Frank et al. (19), Gittleson (20), Spear (57), and Merskey (36,37) were among the first controlled comparisons of these groups with other patients, but the characteristics of pain patients have been reported by numerous authors, and their psychological features are generally agreed. A small proportion, 1 or 2%, have schizophrenia; up to 24% have significant depressive illness; and the remainder have syndromes of anxiety of hysterical complaints. The Minnesota Multiphasic Personality Inventory (MMPI) often shows the well-known conversion V triad, in which the scale for depression is elevated, but the scales for hysteria and hypochondriasis are elevated even more (47). This is true for low back pain (59) and for headache of various types (23). It is accepted that those who have chronic pain often do so for reasons related more to their psychological state than their physical condition.

PSYCHOLOGICAL FACTORS RELIEVING PAIN

Both acute and chronic pain are relieved by a variety of means. Much pain is eased by specific remedies (antibiotics for the headache of meningitis, ergot preparations for migraine) and by recognized analgesics. Numerous psychological techniques, however, are also effective in relieving pain, regardless of its cause (5,10,26,44). Two observations may be made. First, chronic painful conditions are almost always harder to relieve than acute ones. Second, if the pain has an organic cause, there is reason to believe that slowly rising pain of mild or moderate intensity usually responds better to psychological techniques than does abrupt, severe pain (34). On the other hand, severe pain with abrupt onset associated with sudden panic, or at least with rapid increase of anxiety, may be substantially relieved by procedures or agents that calm the individual.

PSYCHIATRIC CONDITIONS AND HEADACHE

Headache is the most common form of pain seen by the psychiatrist or neurologist (15,36,64). Even in general practice, headache is more common than other pains (3). In some pain clinics, the low back is the most common site of pain (60). The association of headache with psychological illness, however, is common and undisputed. Gittleson (20) noted that the description of headache by psychiatric patients was usually of a constant bilateral frontal pressure. This is in accordance with other reports that pain in psychiatric patients is not usually bizarre (1,16).

It is commonly said that tension headache is described by English-speaking patients as gripping or like a tight band. It is doubtful that this occurs with great frequency. One or two observational studies should settle the matter.

The characteristics of the psychiatric patients with headache are like those of other psychiatric patients with pain. There is a mixture of anxiety and hysterical features, the exact proportion depending on the sample. In perhaps 50% of chronic headache patients, hysterical features appear to be the predominant aspect. If the patients are not selected for chronicity, the frequency of hysterical features is reduced. Spear (56), in a random psychiatric sample, tentatively considered that of 72 patients with headache, 42 could be regarded as due to muscle tension, 11 to vascular mechanisms, and eight (11%) to conversion. In family practice, the proportion with hysterical mechanisms may be still smaller; in neurological and in other specialist practice, the numbers with conversion mechanisms will be like those in Spear's series and, if the pain is chronic, may be greater.

Headache due to a hallucinatory mechanism in association with schizophrenia or endogenous depression is extremely rare. One of the few possible cases found by my colleagues and myself is of a woman with a schizoaffective psychosis rather than an ordinary schizophrenic illness who believed she was Jesus and had a tight, band-like headache which she attributed to her crown of thorns.

The trend of results with psychological testing and headache suggests that what is found for other disorders is also relevant for headache. The more clear the organic syndrome, the less evidence there will be of psychological disturbance, unless the organic syndrome is one which is prolonged or difficult to bear without suffering. Kudrow and Sutkus (28) defined six groups of patients: migraine, cluster headache, scalp muscle contraction headache alone, scalp muscle contraction headache with migraine, posttraumatic headache, and conversion headache. They found an increasing degree of abnormality in MMPI responses of these groups starting with migraine. Their definitions of some of these groups are broad, but the trend in their material shows how the more a patient had continuous and persistent headache without a distinct "organic" basis, the more the psychological disturbance was evident. Only in the groups that were most abnormal emotionally did the conversion V pattern appear.

TENSION HEADACHE AND HYSTERICAL HEADACHE

In the last 5 years, one of the most significant developments concerning headache has been the increasing study of electromyographic findings in relation to diagnosis, personality, and treatment. It was a disconcerting initial finding that there was more frontal muscle contraction in migraine sufferers between attacks than in so-called tension headache (2,46,50). Although significant statistically, the early correlations between muscle tension and anxiety were low, of the order of $r = 0.3$ (30), thus accounting for only about 9% of the variance. In another study, the best correlation achieved between subjective discomfort and anxiety and muscle tension was $r = 0.49$ (52), accounting for approximately 25% of the variance.

In the studies cited, it was confirmed that muscle tension was more pronounced in the parts to which the complaint was referred, but the correlation was insufficient for pain to be attributed wholly or even for the most part to the muscle tension mechanism. It must be taken into account that in the early studies, the instrumentation was not as sophisticated as today. Perhaps better measures might show a higher correlation. It remains, however, that a significant proportion of the pain experienced by people who have so-called anxiety-tension symptoms cannot be quantitatively related to muscular overactivity. Furthermore, it is common experience that many so-called tension headaches do not respond to measures that are normally excellent in the treatment of anxiety. Relaxation exercises, psychotherapy, and minor tranquilizers are all helpful but leave a significant number of patients without adequate relief. If the patients studied are more chronic, the relationship of frontalis muscle tension to headache may account for an even smaller proportion of the variance, as little as 5% (22,32).

There are a number of pains in the chest and limbs for which it is hard to show evidence of muscular tension; indeed, there are some pains of psychological origin whose time course is incompatible with the usual rate of development of pain from muscle tension. In addition, measures of headache intensity correlate with a hysterical pattern of responses in psychological testing (22). This is true also for facial pain (54) and pain in general (57). Thus we reach the position that "tension headache" is likely to be best understood as a reflection of those types of personality disorder that have traditionally been called hysterical.

MIGRAINE

Touraine and Draper (61), by describing the migraine personality, were developing ideas that were found in 19th and early 20th century writers (38). Wolff (68) echoed their views by suggesting that the typical migraine patient had a rigid, ambitious, perfectionist personality. Furmanski (17) summarized the various opinions offered about the personality of the sufferers and the causes of migraine and reached conclusions more or less as follows: It occurs in obsessional, anxious people who cannot express some feeling of resentment or hostility, of which they are unconscious. The personality also may be masochistic or narcissistic, and the inability to express hostility may be due to guilt because the object of the hatred is also a close and loved relative. The attack itself is held by some to be a "psychological vasomotor manifestation of suppressed or repressed hostility." Even if the description is true, however, it applies only to a selected sample. The suggestion that a vasomotor change is a symbolic manifestation of hostility is found in some writers but represents a logical confusion. Vasodilation or contraction may occur as a psychophysiological response, or a headache, or pain may be experienced as a symbolic symptom. To confuse the two only makes clinical discussion more difficult.

Suggestions that narcissistic or masochistic personalities are involved have not been proved in comparative studies and suffer from the problems of selection. There are important observations about masochistic and narcissistic personalities which are relevant to the psychiatric understanding of patients in psychotherapy. However, we have no evidence that any of this applies specifically to migraine or indeed to pain syndromes in general, except possibly for a small group of patients with persistent pain, not necessarily migraine. Nevertheless, these objections do not preclude an association between migraine and emotional stress. A link appears so often in clinical practice with the onset or exacerbation of migraine that we are bound to suspect a connection, even though we do not attribute that connection principally to a special personality disorder. Liveing (29) considered emotional disturbance to be one of three important etiological factors in causing migraine, the other two being gastric and menstrual disturbances. Lance *(this volume)* provides an example of how the frequency of attacks of migraine in one patient is related to changes in mood.

Two comparative studies in the literature relate to patients with migraine. One, by Maxwell (33), compares 32 migraine patients with 32 nonmigraine patients who rarely attended their doctors' surgery (office). Seventy-five percent of each of the first two groups considered themselves to be highly strung or had nervous trouble; only 22% of the third group took such a view. On the neuroticism (N) scale of the Maudsley Personality Inventory (MPI), the migraine group was found to be more neurotic than the other frequent attenders. These others had the same average score as the general population, while the population of patients who avoided their doctors was less neurotic than the general population. This study suggests that migraine patients in general practice are relatively liable to neurotic symptoms, perhaps somewhat more so than other persistent attenders. The limitations of this study are the small numbers, the use of the short form of the MPI questionnaire, and the fact that it has not been replicated directly.

The second comparative study is by Bihldorff et al. (11), who compared 88 patients with various types of headaches with 27 controls who had no history of headache; 33 of the 88 had migraine, and 41 had tension headaches. Each of these groups was examined separately. The results depended on the return of the questionnaire by mail. Only 115 of a total of 200 questionnaires sent were available for analysis. In these authors' findings, the migraine patients were thought to exemplify the inhibited and the tension headache patients the compulsive personality type. No differences were found between the groups in regard to childhood expressions of anger, e.g., temper tantrums, and a relatively "happy" picture was provided by the control patients, who had neither migraine nor tension headache. In contrast, the migraine and tension headache groups gave similar answers. Thus there are hints that patients who have chronic migraine may indeed have something of the personality described in the uncontrolled studies, but the evidence is still insufficient.

Pure migraine and cluster headache patients show less evidence of emotional abnormality than do patients with other types of chronic headache or mixed types, of which migraine is only one component. In the study by Crisp et al. (13), a truly random sample of patients with migraine was tested for evidence of emotional disorder. The workers tested 82% of eligible subjects from a population of approximately 1,000 surveyed and showed that female patients with a history of migraine in the past 2 years were significantly more anxious than controls ($p < 0.005$). The migraine patients were significantly more prone to complaints of somatic symptoms and depression and were more liable to be extroverted. In addition, both male and female migraine patients reported tension to be the most common precipitant of an attack; the menstrual period and mood change in women and alcohol in men were the next most common precipitant.

Other evidence indicates that stress may be related to the precipitation of migraine. Selby and Lance (53), in a study of 500 patients, found that emotional factors become increasingly significant as the frequency of migraine attacks increased. Klee (27) observed emotional precipitants in at least 72% of individuals with severe attacks of migraine. Marcussen (31) has provided experimental support for the view that emotional change may precipitate migraine by the demonstration that a response could be provoked in susceptible individuals under conditions of increasing tension and fatigue when they were presented with stress-producing situations.

Migraine likely is precipitated by stress. Patients under stress for long periods tend to be somewhat more anxious than others. It remains uncertain whether the emotional changes cause or result from migraine; probably both explanations are relevant.

Perhaps the most effective way to explore the relationship between migraine and stress in the future would be by studies of life events in patients with migraine in other random samples of the population. Biochemistry and affect may be causally related. If we consider that a serotoninergic effect is relevant to migraine, then it is indeed likely that affective disturbances, such as anxiety or depression, will have a bearing on the occurrence of attacks. A variety of cinvincing reasons show that much depression and some anxiety are related to disturbances of serotoninergic pathways. While there is no specific migraine personality, there may be a relationship between migraine and anxiety and depression. Evidence related to chronic pain suggests that only a minority of patients with psychological illness and chronic severe migraine headache can be expected to respond to antidepressants.

EFFECTS OF PAIN

Obviously, pain can cause emotional changes. Physical lesions or severe noxious input may cause great pain, which debilitates the individual. Mitchell (45) recognizes this in regard to causalgia. The apprehension and misery that develop in patients with trigeminal neuralgia on recurring attacks of cluster headache is well recognized. Discussion can be found in the literature of the evidence that pain from physical lesions may produce anxiety and depression (40,59,69). One of the most notable pieces of evidence is from Crown and Crown (13a), who showed more neurotic features in patients with chronic than acute rheumatoid arthritis. In the field of migraine, Klee (27) demonstrated more affective change in patients with chronic severe migraine than in those without. Snow (55) has described the intolerable distress provoked by migraine:

> . . . they were such a misery that I suppose I did not expect to get through three weeks without one; and when it occurred it would last for something like five days of slowly diminishing pain and general misery . . . I have been lucky enough in the last four years to have found a proprietary drug which works for me. It has more or less transformed my life though it may not do much for many other people.

In conclusion, on the basis of more extensive discussion in the sources quoted, pain due to organic lesions or dysfunction is a significant cause of emotional change.

DEFINITION OF PAIN

Pain is most often due to emotional causes, even though the effects of selection of patients make this hard to prove. Anxiety, depression, and hysterical mechanisms are the principal psychiatric factors in the causation of headache. The more chronic the pain, the more hysterical factors will be evident. There is no good evidence for a migraine personality, but adequate studies will ultimately show some causal relationship between stress and migraine, especially if there is a predisposition toward anxiety. All chronic pain from organic lesions or dysfunction can be expected to produce emotional changes. It remains to note how we should define pain.

Paradoxically, the acceptance of a definition is stronger after some exposure to the topic to be defined. Placing a definition at the beginning may provide an obstacle to the discussion. Pain has been defined recently by the Subcommittee on Taxonomy of the International Association of the Study of Pain (42) as: "An unpleasant sensory and emotional experience associated with actual or potential tissue damage, or described in terms of such damage"; this is close to one proposed in 1964 (35). One of its purposes is to emphasize that pain is a subjective experience, about which we learn from our patients' descriptions.

REFERENCES

1. Agnew, D. C., and Merskey, H. (1976): Words of chronic pain. *Pain*, 2:73–81.
2. Bakal, D. A., and Kaganov, J. A. (1977): Muscle contraction and migraine headache; psychophysiologic comparison. *Headache*, 17(5):208–215.
3. Baker, J. W., and Merskey, H. (1967): Pain in general practice. *J. Psychosom. Res.*, 10:383–397.
4. Banks, M. H., Beresford, S. H. A., Morrell, D. C., Waller, J. J., and Watkins, C. J. (1975): Factors influencing demand for primary medical care in women age 20–40 years; a preliminary report. *Int. J. Epidemiol.*, 4:189–255.
5. Barber, T. X. (1959): Toward a theory of pain: Relief of chronic pain by prefrontal leucotomy opiates, placebos and hypnosis. *Psychol. Bull.*, 56:430–460.
6. Bardhan, P. N. (1965): The fathering syndrome. *Ind. Armed Forces Med. J.*, 20:200–208.
7. Bardhan, P. N. (1965): The couvade syndrome. *Br. J. Psychiatry*, 111:908–909.
8. Beck, A. T. (1976): *Cognitive Therapy and the Emotional Disorders.* International Universities Press, New York.
9. Beecher, H. K. (1956): Relationship of significance of wound to the pain experienced. *JAMA*, 161:1609–1613.
10. Beecher, H. K. (1959): *Measurement of Subjective Responses. Quantitative Effects of Drugs.* Oxford University Press, New York.
11. Bihldorff, J. P., King, S. H., and Parnes, L. R. (1971): Psychological factors in headache. *Headache*, 11:117–127.
12. Bonica, J. J., and Albe-Fessard, D. G. (1976): *Advances in Pain Research and Therapy, Vol. 1.* Raven Press, New York.
13. Crisp, A. H., Kalucy, R. S., McGuinness, B., Ralph, P. C., and Harris, G. (1977): Some clinical, social and psychological characteristics of migraine subjects in the general population. *Postgrad. Med. J.*, 53:691–697.
13a. Crown, S., and Crown, J. M. (1973): Personality in early rheumatic disease. *J. Psychosom. Res.*, 17:189–196.
14. Curtis, J. L. (1965): A psychiatric study of 55 expectant fathers. *U.S. Armed Forces Med. J.*, 6:937–950.
15. Delaplaine, R., Ifabumuyi, O. I., Merskey, and Zarfas, J. (1978): Significance of pain in psychiatric hospital patients. *Pain*, 4:361–366.
16. Devine, R., and Merskey, H. (1965): The description of pain in psychiatric and general medical patients. *J. Psychosom. Res.*, 9:311–316.

17. Furmanski, A. R. (1952): Dynamic concepts of migraine. *Arch. Neurol. Psychiatry,* 67:23–31.
18. Gelfand, S. (1964): The relationship of experimental pain tolerance to pain threshold. *Can. J. Psychol.,* 18:3642.
19. Gidro-Frank, L., Gordon, T., and Taylor, H. C. (1960): Pelvic pain and female identity. *Am. J. Obstet. Gynecol.,* 79:1184–1202.
20. Gittleson, N. L. (1961): Psychiatric headache: A clinical study. *J. Ment. Sci.,* 107:403–416.
21. Hall, K. R. L., and Stride, E. (1954): The varying response to pain in psychiatric disorders. A study in abnormal psychology. *Br. J. Med. Psychol.,* 27:48–60.
22. Harper, R. G., and Steger, J. C. (1978): Psychological correlates of frontalis EMG and pain in tension headache. *Headache,* 18(4):215–218.
23. Harrison, R. H. (1975): Psychological testing in headache: A review. *Headache,* 13:177–185.
24. Hemphill, R. D., Hall, K. R. L., and Crookes, T. G. (1952): A preliminary report on fatigue and pain tolerance in depressive and psychoneurotic patients. *J. Ment. Sci.,* 98:433–440.
25. Henryk-Gutt, R., and Rees, W. L. (1973): Psychological aspects of migraine. *J. Psychosom. Res.,* 17:141–153.
26. Jellinek, E. M. (1946): Clinical tests on comparative effectiveness of analgesic drugs. *Biomet. Bull.,* 2:87–91.
27. Klee, A. (1968): *A Clinical Study of Migraine with Particular Reference to the Most Severe Cases.* Munksgaard, Copenhagen.
28. Kudrow, L., and Sutkus, B. J. (1979): MMPI pattern specificity in primary headache disorders. *Headache,* 19:18–24.
29. Liveing, E. (1873): *On Migraine, Sick Headache and Some Allied Disorders.* Churchill, London.
30. Malmo, R. B., and Shagass, C. (1949): Psychologic study of symptom mechanisms in psychiatric patients under stress. *Psychosom. Med.,* II:25–29.
31. Marcussen, R. M. (1950): Vascular headache experimentally induced by presentation of pertinent life experiences: Modification of the course of vascular headache by alterations of situations and reactions. *Res. Publ. Assoc. Nerv. Ment. Dis.,* 29:609.
32. Martin, P. R., and Mathews, A. M. (1978): Tension headaches: Psychophysiological investigation and treatment. *J. Psychosom. Res.,* 22:389–399.
33. Maxwell, H. (1965): *Migraine.* John Wright, Bristol.
34. Melzack, R., Weisz, A. Z., and Sprague, L. T. (1963): Stratagems for controlling pain: Contributions of auditory stimulation and suggestion. *Exp. Neurol.,* 8:239–247.
35. Merskey, H. (1964): *An Investigation of Pain in Psychological Illness.* Doctoral dissertation. Oxford University.
36. Merskey, H. (1965): The characteristics of persistent pain in psychological illness. *J. Psychosom. Res.,* 9:291–298.
37. Merskey, H. (1965): Psychiatric patients with persistent pain. *J. Psychosom. Res.,* 9:299–309.
38. Merskey, H. (1975): Psychiatric aspects of migraine. In: *Modern Topics in Migraine,* edited by J. Pearce, pp. 52–63. Heinemann, London.
39. Merskey, H. (1976): Psychiatric aspects of the control of pain. In: *Advances in Pain Research and Therapy,* vol. 3, edited by J. J. Bonica and D. G. Albe-Fessard, pp. 711–716. Raven Press, New York.
40. Merskey, H. (1978): Pain and personality. In: *The Psychology of Pain,* edited by R. A. Sternbach, pp. 111–127. Raven Press, New York.
41. Merskey, H. (1979): *The Analysis of Hysteria.* Baillière, Tindall, London.
42. Merskey, H., Albe-Fessard, D. G., Bonica, J. J., Carmon, A., Dubner, R., Kerr, F. W. L., Lindblum, U., Mumford, J. M., Nathan, P. W., Noordenbos, W., Pagni, C. A., Renaer, M. J., Sternbach, R. H., and Sunderland, S. (1979): Pain terms: A list with definitions and notes on usage. *Pain,* 6:249–252.
43. Merskey, H., and Spear, F. G. (1964): The reliability of the pressure algometer. *Br. J. Soc. Clin. Psychol.,* 3:130–136.
44. Merskey, H., and Spear, F. G. (1967): *Pain: Psychological and Psychiatric Aspects.* Baillière, Tindall and Cassell, London.
45. Mitchell, S. W. (1872): *Injuries of Nerves and Their Consequences.* Dover, New York.
46. Phillips, H. C. (1975): Migraine trust symposium meeting. *The Migraine Trust,* 19 September, pp. E1–E17. London.
47. Pilling L. F., Brannick, T. L., and Swanson, W. M. (1967): Psychological characteristics of patients having pain as a presenting symptom. *Can. Med. Assoc. J.,* 97:387–394.
48. Pilowsky, I., and Spence, N. D. (1976): Pain and illness behaviour: A comparative study. *J. Psychosom. Res.,* 20:131–134.
49. Pond, D. A., and Bidwell, B. H. (1959): A survey of epilepsy in 14 general practices. II, Social and psychological aspects. *Epilepsia,* 1:285–299.
50. Pozniak-Patewicz, E. (1976): "Cephalgic" spasm of head and neck muscles. *Headache,* 4(15):261–266.
51. Reik, T. (1914): *Ritual: Psychoanalytical Studies.* Hogarth Press, London.
52. Sainsbury, P., and Gibson, J. G. (1954): Symptoms of anxiety and tension and the accompanying physiological changes in the muscular system. *Psychosom. Med.,* 17:216–224.

53. Selby, G., and Lance, J. W. (1960): Observations on 500 cases of migraine and allied vascular headache. *J. Neurol. Neurosurg. Psychiatry,* 23:23–32.
54. Smith, D. P., Pilling, L. F., Pearson, J. S., Rushton, J. G., Goldstein, N. P., and Gibilisco, J. A. (1969): The psychiatric study of atypical facial pain. *Can. Med. Assoc. J.,* 10:286–291.
55. Snow, P. (1963): The consumer's end. *J. Coll. Gen. Practit. [Suppl.],* 6:4.
56. Spear, F. G. (1964): *A Study of Pain as a Symptom in Psychiatric Illness.* Doctoral dissertation, Bristol University.
57. Spear, F. G. (1967): Pain in psychiatric patients. *J. Psychosom. Res.,* 11:187–193.
58. Sternbach, R. A. (1968): *Pain: A Psychological Analysis.* Academic Press, New York.
59. Sternbach, R. A. (1974): *Pain Patients. Traits and Treatment.* Academic Press, New York.
60. Swanson, D. W., Floreen, A. O., and Swenson, W. M. (1976): Program for managing chronic pain. II. Short-term results. *Proc. Mayo Clinic,* 51:409–411.
61. Touraine, G. A., and Draper, G. (1934): The migrainous patient. *J. Nerv. Ment. Dis.,* 80:1–23, 182.
62. Trethowan, W. H., and Conlon, M. F. (1965): The couvade syndrom. *Br. J. Psychiatry,* III:57–66.
63. Wall, P. D. (1979): On the relation of injury to pain. *Pain,* 6.253–264.
64. Walters, A. (1961): Psychogenic regional pain alias hysterical pain. *Brain,* 84:1–18.
65. Wolff, B. B., Kantor, T. G., Jarvik, M. E., and Laska, E. (1966): Response of experimental pain to analgesic drugs. I. Morphine, aspirin and placebo. *Clin. Pharmacol. Ther.,* 7:224–238.
66. Wolff, B. B., Kantor, T. G., Jarvik, M. E., and Laska, E. (1966): Response of experimental pain to analgesic drugs. II. Codeine, and placebo. *Clin. Pharmacol. Ther.,* 7:323–331.
67. Wolff, H. G. (1937): Personality factors and reactions of subjects with migraine. *Arch. Neurol. Psychiatry,* 37:895.
68. Wolff, H. G. (1948): *Headache and Other Head Pain.* Oxford University Press, London.
69. Woodforde, J. M., and Merskey, H. (1972): Personality traits of patients with chronic pain. *J. Psychosom. Res.,* 16:167–172.

Advances in Neurology, Vol. 33, edited by
M. Critchley et al. Raven Press, New York © 1982

Prolonged Benign Exertional Headache: Clinical Characteristics and Response to Indomethacin

Seymour Diamond and Jose L. Medina

Diamond Headache Clinic and Department of Neurology, Chicago Medical School, Chicago, Illinois 60625

The occurrence of headaches during exertion was first observed in 1932, when Tinel (10,11) reported on patients who developed severe pains with maneuvers that increased the intrathoracic pressure:

> The patient cannot cough, blow his nose, hold his breath, laugh, cry, bend his head, nor could he make any minor muscular effort without feeling pain.

The headache was described (3,6) as brief, lasting for a few seconds or minutes, sharply localized, with its intensity compared to a hammer blow. This type of headache may be seen with intracranial lesions (3,5,6,9–11), such as posterior fossa cerebral tumors, foramen magnum syndromes, or other intracranial disorders, or without any apparent cause. The headaches reported here are different because of their long duration, vascular qualities, and occurrence accompanying a frequent background of spontaneous migraine or muscle contraction headaches. Their prevalence in clinical practice and their response to indomethacin are discussed.

CLINICAL CHARACTERISTICS

The type of headache described here is best illustrated by the following two cases.

Case 1

A 28-year-old woman, without any apparent precipitating cause, started to suffer from headaches in 1974. She had a constant dull ache affecting both occipital and temporal areas on either side, or bilaterally. It was sometimes associated with nausea and ringing in the ears. A different headache developed 2 years later; it was throbbing and could become severe enough to incapacitate her. The headache affected the entire head and was associated with lightheadedness, photosensitivity, and audiosensitivity. The pair was triggered by exertion and, once it occurred, would remain until she went to sleep.

Review of the systems revealed only occasional difficulty in falling asleep. Physical examination was completely normal. Routine laboratory tests (skull and cervical X-rays, computerized tomographic (CAT) scan with contrast enhancement, and CAT of the foramen magnum) were all normal. She had tried different medications in the past, including Dilantin and Darvon, without any relief. She had some relief with aspirin, however, and consumed 6 to 8 tablets daily.

Initial treatment with indomethacin (25 mg 3 times/day) completely controlled her exertion-related headaches in 2 weeks. After 1 month, amitriptyline, in 25-mg increments gradually increased to 100 mg) was added to her treatment with disappearance of the daily headache. She was kept on both for 2 years without return of the headaches. Recently, we stopped indomethacin and the exertion-related headaches returned in 1 week. She resumed indomethacin, and the headaches were again completely controlled.

Case 2

A 41-year-old man was completely well before he had an accident in April of 1978. His car was struck from behind by an 18-wheel semitruck. Upon impact, he hit the back of his head but did not lose consciousness. He was taken to a local hospital, where skull and cervical X-rays were negative for any fracture. Since the accident, he complained of a continuous, steady, dull headache in the vertex area. Any efforts, such as lifting or moving objects with his arms, would trigger a different headache. This headache was localized in the left occipital area and radiated to the left parietal area. It was a sharp pain, and its duration varied depending on the extent of activity before its onset, ranging from 12 hr to 1 week. It was frequently accompanied by nausea, blurred vision, or diplopia. His family history was negative for headaches. Review of systems revealed poor concentration, occasional sexual impotence, and difficulty falling asleep. The headaches completely incapacitated him. Physical examination was completely normal. Routine laboratory tests [skull and cervical X-rays, brain scan, CAT scan with special views of the foramen magnum, and electroencephalogram (EEG)] were normal.

He had tried many different medications but could not remember their names, and also had transcutaneous stimulation; none of these remedies helped. He was taking 4 aspirin tablets daily with some relief. Initial treatment with indomethacin (25 mg 3 times/day) completely controlled the exertional headaches in 1 week. The daily, constant headaches became much less severe and sporadic. This improvement has remained unchanged for the past 10 months. He has returned to full employment. Indomethacin was stopped for about 1 week with the return of the headaches; resumption of the medication controlled the headaches.

Both these cases illustrate prolonged benign exertional headache. It should be diagnosed only after neurological examination and tests are completely normal. The neurological tests should include a neurological examination, cervical and skull X-rays, and CAT with contrast enhancement and special views of the foramen magnum.

We have observed 15 patients (eight women and seven men) with this type of headache. Their ages ranged from 22 to 74 years (mean, 44.6 years). The headaches occurred only during physical effort in five patients (football, one; bowling, one; weight lifting, two; dancing, one; and digging, two). The others had headaches with both physical effort and diverse maneuvers that increased intrathoracic pressure (coughing, shouting, sneezing, stooping).

The location of the headache was variable but consistent in each patient. In one patient, the headache shifted sides from time to time. The headaches were bilateral in nine patients (generalized, two; bitemporal, one; bifrontal, three; biparietooccipital, two; occipital, two). The other five patients had unilateral headaches in the following locations: temporal, one; periorbital, two; temporofrontal, one; and occipitoparietal, one. The duration of the headache varied between 15 min and 16 hr (mean, 4 hr). The quality of the pain was throbbing in eight, stabbing in six, and pressure-like in one. The headaches were extremely severe with activity in three patients; when the activity ceased, the severity modified and gradually diminished. The headaches in six of the patients were unrelated to exertion but of identical characteristics to those that occurred during effort. Two patients had cluster headaches, and four had nonclassic migraine. Two patients also had muscle-contraction headaches that were quite distinct from those they had during exertion.

TABLE 1. *Results of treatment with indomethacin*

Patient no.	Daily dose (mg)	Headache response[a]	Improvement (week)	Side effect
1	25	+	1	None
2	75	+++	2	None
3	75	++	1	None
4	100	+++	3	Heartburn
5	100	0	—	Gastrointestinal distress
6	150	+	4	Heartburn
7	100	++	3	None
8	150	++	4	None
9	75	+++	1	None
10	75	0	—	None
11	75	+++	1	None
12	100	++	2	Heartburn
13	75	++	1	Heartburn
14	150	++	1	Heartburn
15	75	++	1	Heartburn

[a] +++, Complete control; ++, partial control; +, some improvement; 0, no improvement.

THERAPY WITH INDOMETHACIN

All the patients received 25 mg indomethacin 3 times/day. This amount was increased depending on the response to treatment; no other preventive medication was given. Table 1 shows the results of treatment; 13 of 15 patients improved; four were completely free of headache while on indomethacin (3+); seven patients had a 75% more production in the frequency of the headaches during exertion (2+); and two patients had some improvement with a 50 to 75% decrease in the frequency of headaches during exertion (1+). Improvement of the headache with indomethacin occurred within 2 weeks. Medication was stopped 3 to 12 months after the headaches were controlled; but in all these patients, except one, the headaches returned to pretreatment intensity in 1 to 7 days.

COMMENTS

Benign exertional headaches occur during one or several of the following maneuvers: (a) those that raise intrathoracic pressure, such as coughing, sneezing, laughing, defecating, stooping, lifting, shouting, crying, and breathholding; (b) other circumstances that may suddenly raise blood pressure, such as excessive exercise and orgasm; and (c) maneuvers that cause traction of intracranial content, such as head rotation and jumping. In some patients, headaches are brought on only by various specific circumstances, for example, exercise or orgasm (2–4). Most authors (9–11) described benign exertional headache as being short lasting. Our patients, however, belong to a different group, with long duration exertional headache. The duration of the headache varied from 15 min to 16 hr (mean, 4 hr). Other authors (4) have also reported long duration exertional headaches.

Rooke (6) collected data on 103 patients with benign exertional headaches in 14 years. He showed that they were four times more frequent in males than in females and twice as frequent in patients over the age of 40. We found no such difference, but we also observed the headaches occurring more often after the age of 40: eight of 13 patients were older than 40 years. Rooke (6) also pointed out that exertional headaches associated with intracranial disease are about two times more frequent than benign exertional headaches, and that about 10% of the cases will be misdiagnosed as benign exertional headaches. In fact, when he followed the 103 patients for 14 years, he missed Arnold-Chiari deformity in three, platybasia in two, basilar impression in one, subdural hematoma in two, and brain tumor in two. The prognosis of short duration benign exertional headaches is fairly good: 30% of Rooke's patients improved within 4 years and 73% in 10 years (6). Many patients, however, are bothered with these headaches for long periods of time and, in some cases, with great hardship.

It is obvious that all these patients have been exposed to all the physiological stimuli that provoke these headaches. Therefore, it is a change in these patients that makes these maneuvers painful. The history points toward a minor respiratory illness at the onset in seven of 31 patients (6), a seemingly inconsequential head injury in one of our patients and in some of Nick's (3) patients, or an unexplained and unexpectedly low cerebrospinal fluid (CSF) pressure (5). In many patients with long duration exertional headache, exertion behaves as a nonspecific trigger of a regular type of headache that also occurs under other nonexertional circumstances, such as in our patients with migraine and cluster headaches. Our two patients with chronic cluster headaches typify this argument; their spontaneous headaches and those provoked by exertion were identical. Many of the patients reported by Paulson and Klawans (4) also belonged to this category of benign exertional headaches associated with vascular headaches. Obviously, in many of these patients no explanation is found for their headaches. The speculative mechanisms have ranged from adhesive arachnoiditis to herniation of pachonian granulations (1) in the intracranial sinuses.

In the present study, indomethacin improved long duration exertional headaches in 13 of 15 patients (86%) in 1 to 4 weeks, an excellent response in view of the fact that these patients suffered from these headaches for 1 to 35 years (mean, 6.6 years). The medication was well tolerated in most patients. They were instructed to take indomethacin in the middle of their meals to minimize gastrointestinal distress. It is apparent that prolonged exertional headaches responded to indomethacin. In a recent report, indomethacin was found to be effective in a type of cluster headache that can be precipitated by flexion or rotation of the head (8). One would be tempted to speculate that the same vasoactive chemicals may be involved in all mechanical precipitation of headaches. During exertion, there might be an excessive liberation of prostaglandins, and indomethacin may work by decreasing the synthesis of this substance. However, indomethacin has two properties that could also explain its effectiveness in benign exertional headache: (a) it is a vasoconstrictor agent, and (b) it decreases CSF pressure (7). Unfortunately, indomethacin has only a suppressing action, and the headaches reappear soon after the drug is discontinued.

All patients with prolonged exertional headaches should have a complete neurological examination, cervical spine and skull X-rays, with special attention to the craniospinal junction, and CAT scan with infusion. Hypertensive patients should have catecholamine studies to rule out pheochromocytoma. After these examinations have been proved negative, a trial with indomethacin should be instituted.

REFERENCES

1. Lichtenstein, B. (1961): So-called cough headache. *Arch. Neurol.,* 4:112–113.
2. Lundberg, P. O., and Osterman, P. O. (1974): The benign and malignant forms of orgasmic cephalgia. *Headache,* 14:164–165.

3. Nick, J. (1976): Cephalee d'effort, migraines et cephalees, Collogue at Nantes. *Sandoz Edition,* April 24:97–113.
4. Paulson, G. W., and Klawans, H. L. (1974): Benign orgasmic cephalgia. *Headache,* 13:181–187.
5. Paulson, G. W., Zipf, R. E., and Beekman, J. F. (1974): Pheochromocytoma causing exercise-related headache and pulmonary edema. *Ann. Neurol.,* 5:96–99.
6. Rooke, D. E. (1968): Benign exertional headache. *Med. Clin. North. Am.,* 52:801–808.
7. Sicuteri, F., Michelacci, S., and Anselmi, B. (1965): Termination of migraine headache by a new anti-inflammatory vasoconstrictor agent. *Clin. Pharmacol. Ther.,* 6:336–344.
8. Sjaastad, O., Eggek, Horven, I., Kayed, K., Lund-Roland, L., Russel, D., and Slordahl, C. (1979): Chronic paroxysmal hemicrania: Mechanical precipitation of attacks. *Headache,* 19:31–36.
9. Symonds, C. (1956): Cough headache. *Brain,* 79:557–568.
10. Tinel, J. (1932): La cephalee à l'effort, syndrome de distension des veines intracranienes. *La Med.,* 13:113–118.
11. Tinel, J. (1932): Un syndrome dialgie veineuse intracraniene: la cephalee à l'effort. *La Prat. Med. Fr.,* 13:113–119.

Advances in Neurology, Vol. 33, edited by
M. Critchley et al. Raven Press, New York © 1982

Cerebral Cortex and Migraine

G. W. Bruyn

Department of Neurology, Academic Hospital, State University, Leyden, The Netherlands

The title of this chapter was suggested by Dr. Sicuteri; it implies a reserved attitude vis-à-vis the idea (a) that migraine and certain cerebral areas are related in some as yet not precisely defined way, and, if indeed they are, (b) that the cerebral areas passively play the second violin.

At present, the pathophysiological concept of migraine asserts that it is a paroxysmal and transient dysfunction (induced by a humoral factor, such as a biogenic amine) of the craniocerebral arterial tree. It is characterized by a stage of vasoconstriction followed by one of vasodilatation, associated with headache of rather specific features, and associated (or not) with autonomic and/or somatic neurological symptoms of excitation or deficit. The carotid and vertebrobasilar beds are thought to resound from the humoral déclenchement; following this, the brain or certain parts of it are thrown out of kilter. In other words, it is a humorally induced melodrama played on a vascular stage with a variable cast of hyper- or akinetic actors and a rather stereotyped constant plot.

Classic or complicated migraine constitutes the cornerstone of the thesis that the brain is (secondarily) involved. In common migraine, there is no *a prima facie* evidence that the brain is involved, other than the throbbing pain in the head, an associative type of reasoning, as shown by a 13th century manuscript of this city's Bibliotheca Laurenziana (Fig. 1). A minority group of neurologists (Sjaastad, Sicuteri, Blau, and I) argue that the brain is the δημιουργός of migraine, but that is not the issue *hic et nunc*.

Our critical analysis begins with a consideration of the scintillating scotoma first reported by Abernethy (1) in 1826 and sketched by Sir George Biddell Airy, astronomer royal, and his son Hubert Airy, physician, in 1865. It manifests as an augury in many patients, in the form of the well-known $\pm$ 10 cps shimmering fortification spectrum, but certainly as frequently as flashes, shooting-stars, lightning balls, nonmoving fiery streaks or spots, dimness of vision, or looking through heated air or through a windowpane beaten by the rain. Doubtless this phosphene should be localized to the striate cortex. The duration of about 30 min, the centrifugal march of the scotoma, the ameliorative or abolishing effect of either oral amylnitrite or the β-receptor stimulant isoproterenol, or 10% CO_2 inhalation, as well as the spuriously speculative similarity-reference to Leâo's spreading cortical depression phenomenon by the nonclinical psychologist Milner (41) suggest that the teichopsia results from temporary deprivation of the striate cortex from its blood-supply by spasm of either the calcarine artery or pial-arteries (Figs. 2–4). This presumably produces a toxin slowly diffusing through the cortex by a hypothetical self-propagating ischemia or extracellular K^+ increase, which entails an excitation wave followed by an exhaustion or depression wave, progressing in a caudorostral direction

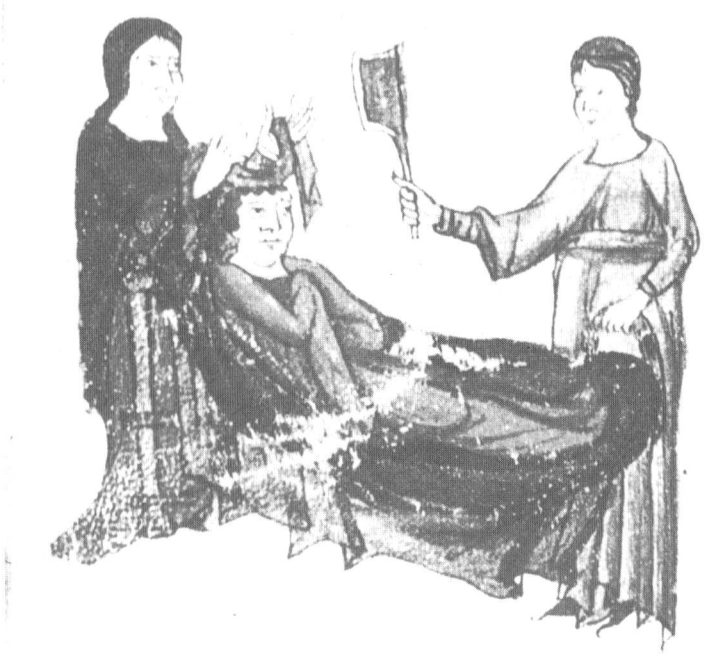

ii. Jo imicrania ut capitif dolorem.
Dciu papaucr filuaticu contrum cum aceto
impono feo habuit dolor.
iii. ao fomnu qui no cormiunt
Ieitu papaucr cu oleo arta a fronti inbucta f
omni corpi mire fomnum egro abouicit.

For migraine or headache the herb poppy (*papaver silvaticum*), bruised with vinegar and bound on the forehead will alleviate the pain. To make a sleepless person sleep: an anointing with juice of *papaver silvaticum* will bring sound sleep.

FIG. 1. From: *Medical Illustrations in Medieval Manuscripts.* Loren Mackinney, Wellcome Historical Medical Library, 1965. 13th century, Florence, Laurentian ms 73; 16, folio 63.

(Fig. 5). Variations in the phenomenological modus of the teichopsia are said to derive from variations in the calcarine artery branches supplying various parts of Brodmann's area 17.

This interpretation is based on the paradigm of the classic scintillating scotoma's march of ± 2 mm of cortical surface per minute. This interpretation disregards the other forms or modi of the phosphene, for which it is incapable to provide a rationally satisfying spatial explanation. Furthermore, Leão's (37) original report (1944) *expressis verbis* stated that as cortical electric activity becomes depressed, a conspicuous arterial dilatation occurs with a striking increase of flow-rate so that the veins turn scarlet. Leão's first figure illustrates this, refuting the presumed ischemia. Of course, the red veins provide the dogged "spreading-depressionist" with the escape to save his first

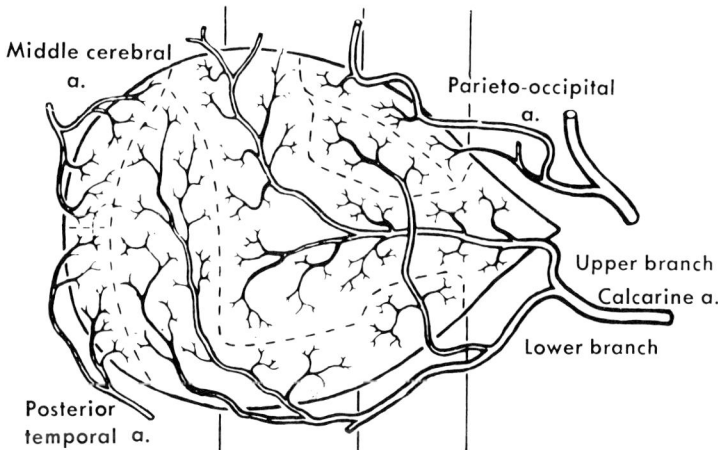

FIG. 2. From: Newton, Th., and Potts, D. G., editors (1974): *Radiology of the Skull and Brain-Angiography,* Vol. 2, Book 2. The C. V. Mosby Co., St. Louis.

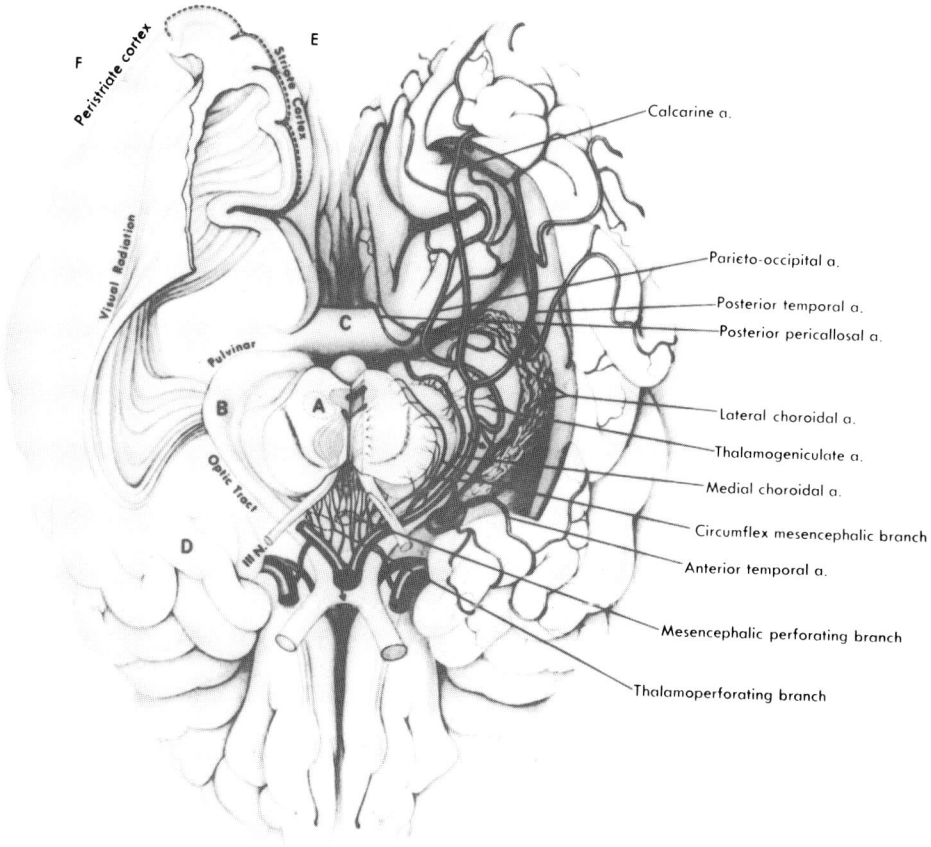

FIG. 3. From: Newton, Th., and Potts, D. G., editors (1974): *Radiology of the Skull and Brain-Angiography,* Vol. 2, Book 2. The C. V. Mosby Co., St. Louis.

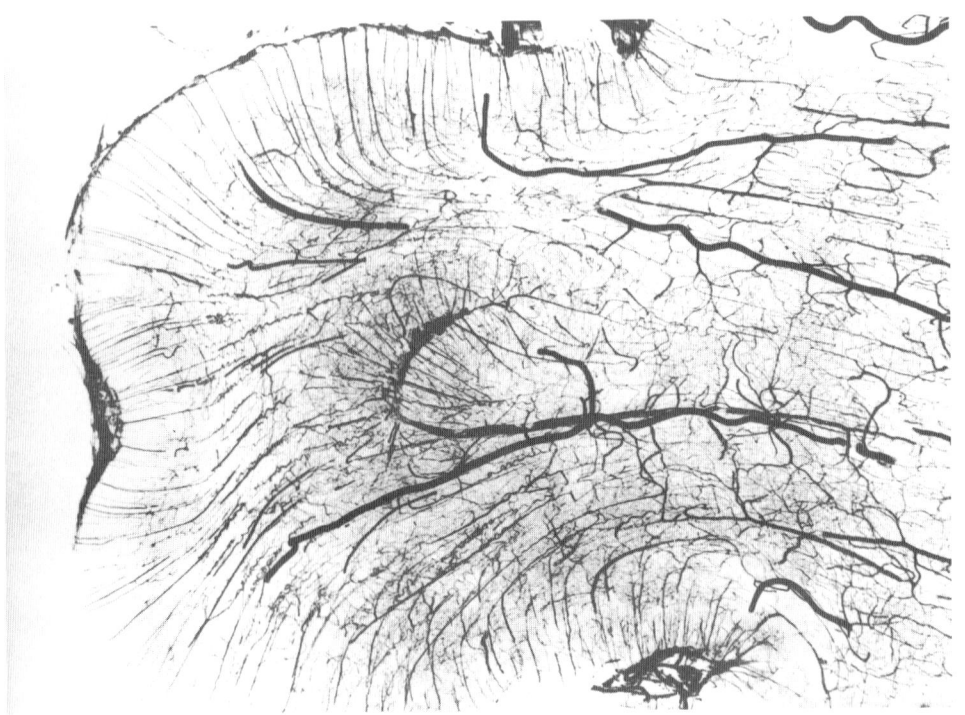

FIG. 4. From: Salamon, G., editor (1971): *Atlas of the Arteries of the Human Brain.* Sandoz.

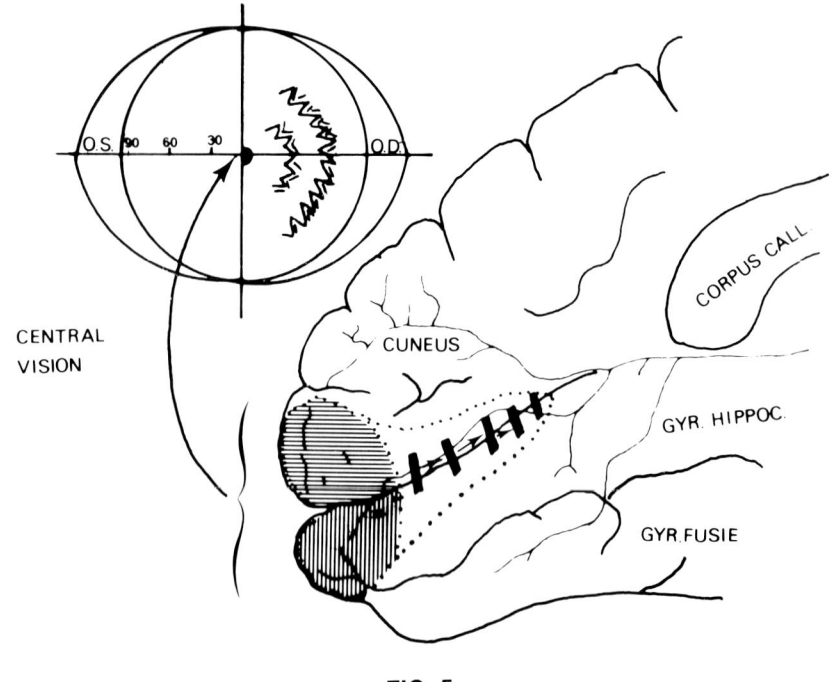

FIG. 5.

assumption from perdition by postulating another assumption, i.e., opening of arteriove-nous anastomoses with resultant tissular ischemia. In addition, Marshall's (39) fundamen-tal review of the phenomenon (1959) emphasized that the spreading depression reaction occurs only in the presence of pathology, such as exposure of the cortex. The fourth difficulty for the traditional hypothesis is to explain why this scotoma is never seen in patients with posterior cerebral artery occlusive or stenotic disease, a deliberation all the more cogent as Leâo and others reported that spreading depression invariably occurs 2 to 2.5 min after arterial occlusion. A fifth difficulty is how to visualize a biochemical process (whether based on GABA loss or K^+ release) marching along the calcarine cortex in a perfectly caudorostral direction (this follows forcibly from the centrifugal movement of the phosphene; see Fig. 5). In addition, nothing is known with certitude about macular (Brodmann's area 17 tip) sparing or involvement in hemianopic migraine. Sixth, the patient is aware of the subsequent visual field defect; classic clinical neurology teaches that cortical functional deficit remains nonsentient, whereas subcortical deficit is consciously perceived data that are pertinent to localization. Finally, the 5-arc-degree area of central vision occupies the major (caudal) portion of the striate cortex and invariably should be involved in ischemia of that area; nonetheless, the phosphenes hardly ever start in the central vision area but nearly always paracentrally. The positive-negative-positive wave front passing over the cortical lattice of orientation columns cannot explain the angles, lines, and spots of the scotoma, such as has been attempted by Richards (51).

The concept of the cortex as a six-layered "club sandwich," a delight of cytoarchitec-tonics, is outdated. From the point of view of connectivity, it *grosso modo* has three layers: the specific sensory thalamic afferents terminating in layer IV, the crossed (callosal) and uncrossed association-field afferents terminating in layers I–III, and the efferents originating from layers V and VI (Fig. 6). Work by Hubel et al. (26–28) and Szentagothai (57,58) showed that the cortex is fundamentally organized in millions of individual columnar units, modules, in which the incoming information is processed (Fig. 7). The cortex is an information processor. The retinal halves project to the lateral geniculate bodies on "center-surround" cells, which in turn project to simple center-surround cells

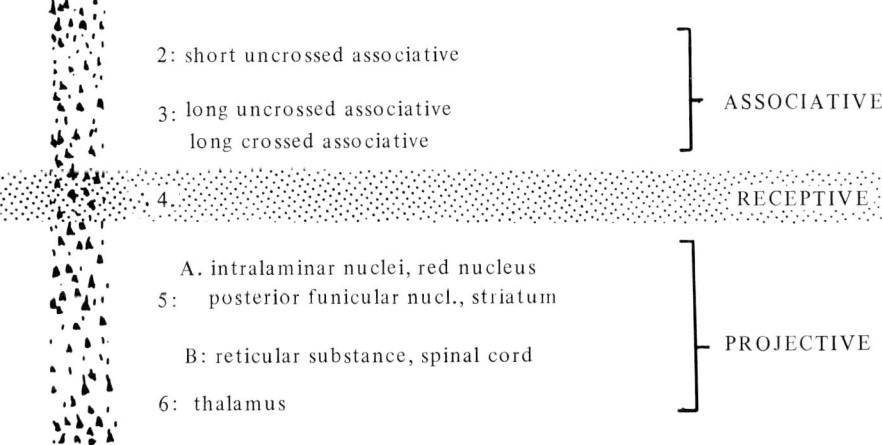

2: short uncrossed associative

3: long uncrossed associative
   long crossed associative

⎫
⎬ ASSOCIATIVE
⎭

4: RECEPTIVE

A. intralaminar nuclei, red nucleus
5:   posterior funicular nucl., striatum

B: reticular substance, spinal cord

6: thalamus

⎫
⎬ PROJECTIVE
⎭

FIG. 6.

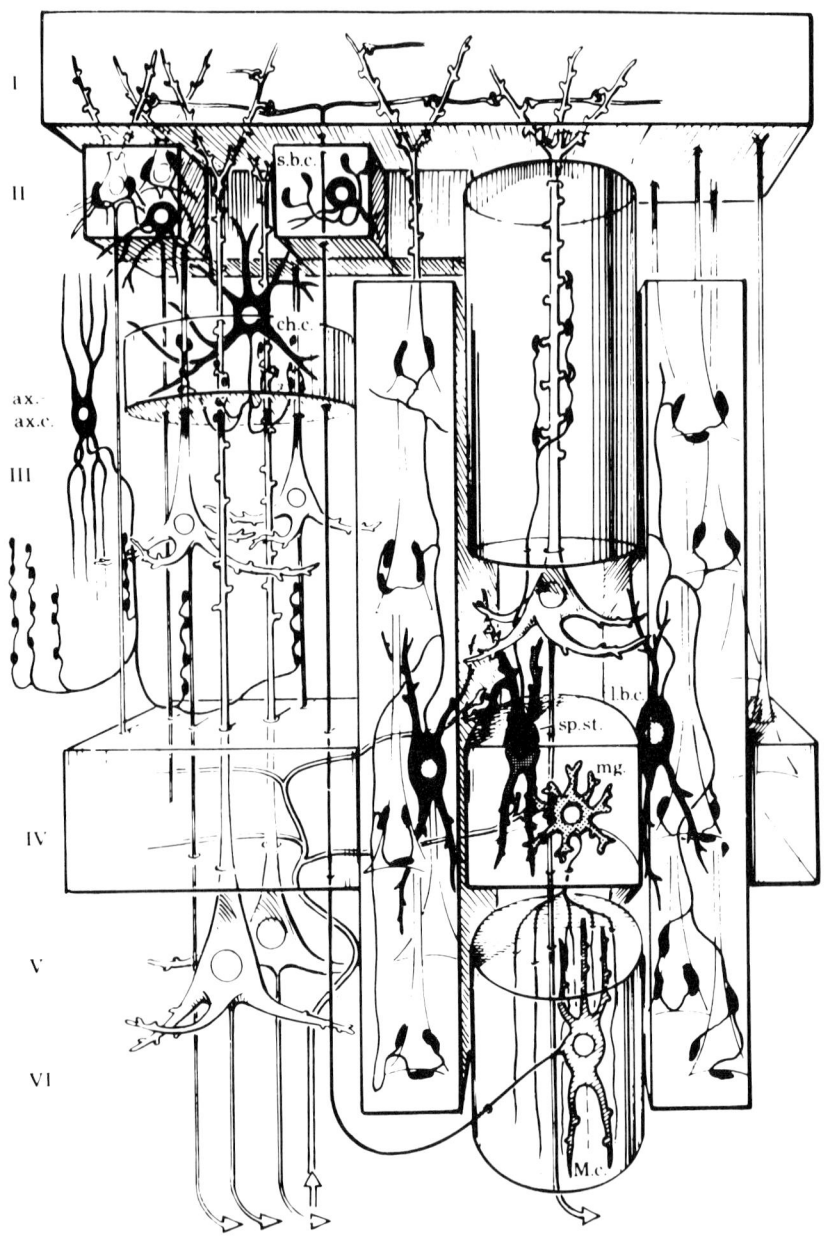

FIG. 7. From: Szentagothai, J., editor (1977): The Ferrier lecture. *Proc. R. Soc. London B* 201:219–248.

in the lower striate layer IV, arranged in alternating monocular right-left dominance columns. This arrangement is not easily reconciled with a bilateral hemifield scotoma. The orientation columns in layers I to III become visualized (as well as the whole, uninterrupted layer IV) if one uses the 2-deoxyglucose method in monkeys looking at a pattern. Accordingly, if the scintillating scotoma originates and resides in the striate cortex, its game must be played only in the upper three layers of this cortex. How calcarine artery spasm should exclusively affect these layers is an intellectual challenge only those with mental torsion-dystonia will be able to meet.

In repeated self-observations, Jung (32) recorded transgression of his phosphenes over the midline upon contralateral gaze; upon vestibular stimulation, they moved in a direction opposite to the acceleration, i.e., identical to the slow nystagmus phase. This is another worthy challenge for the striate cortex ischemia protagonists to meet. In addition, posterior occipital involvement during scintillating scotoma has been documented only in the report by Engel et al. (20) on three cases. The second case had a superior homonymous quandrantanopia, which indicates involvement of the temporal Wernicke field or of Meyer-Archambault loop, and not a striate cortex lesion. Finally, electrostimulation of the striate cortex gives rise to stationary star-like phosphenes. Wollaston, the discoverer of the optic decussation, suffered from hemianopic migraine on the right side in 1804 and on the left side in 1823. Autopsy 5 years later revealed an old malacia in the Wernicke field near the right lateral geniculate body and an egg-sized tumor in the left thalamus.

Most if not all the characteristics of scintillating scotoma can, in spite of the opinion of Hoyt/Walsh's neuroophthalmology text, be localized equally well in the lateral geniculate body, of which the magno- and parvicellular alternate layers project to the stellate cells in two very distinct regions of layer IV of striate cortex. This implies only a spatial displacement of the problem, but with the virtue of a reduced surface area of the stage of action.

The second frequent companion of headache, the cheiro-oral or digitolingual paraesthesia syndrome, involves either the ulnar or the radial digits. It may spread to involve the hand, arm, and shoulder. Often, however, the feelings skip the arm and shoulder and manifest synchronously about the angle of the mouth, one-half of the lips and tongue, and occasionally the cheek (Fig. 8). More rarely, the paraesthesiae manifest in

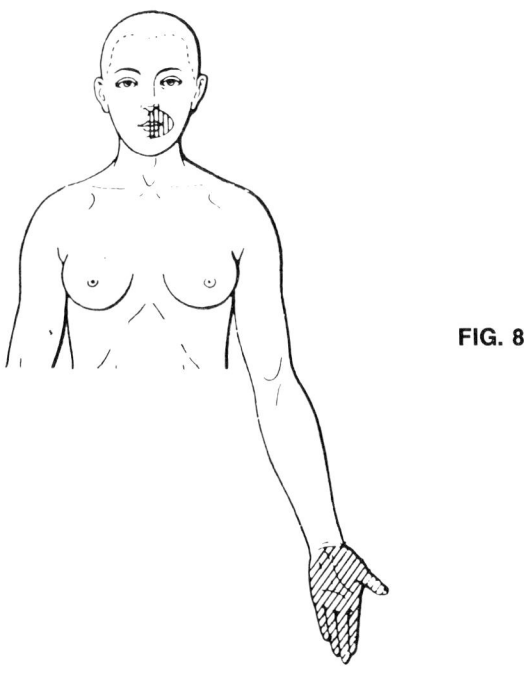

FIG. 8.

the foot, leg, and arm. They are not exceptionally bilateral. Traditional rather than inspired thought attributes this syndrome to involvement of the posterior central convolution as a result of spasm of the paracentral branch of the anterior and the central and parietal branches of the middle cerebral artery. Clinical neurological experience is not compatible with this assumption: (a) manifestation of a sensory cortical lesion prefers the glove-stocking type; (b) there is predominantly lateral facial involvement with sparing of the perioral-nose-eye area; (c) the areas in question are not contiguous (Penfield homunculus); and (d) the absence of reports on unequivocally focal rolandic EEG changes during the cheiro-oral migraine aura makes one raise an eyebrow.

Is posterior central gyrus involvement inference rather than fact? The sensory symptoms can be referred equally well to the ventrobasal thalamic nuclei and *carrefour sensitif* adjacent to the lateral geniculate. Two instances of cheiro-oral paraesthesias followed by hemiparesis were proved at autopsy to be due to a thalamic arteriovenous angioma and a thalamic spongioblastoma. The evidence for thalamic localization was reviewed in 1968 by me. Recent reviews of the clinical syndrome of thalamic sensorimotor infarction have been provided by Mohr et al. (42), Walshe et al. (61), and Donat (16).

The same critical reserve applies to the presumably cortical origin of migrainous dysarthria and aphasia. The speech disturbances, not often present in migraine accompagnée, consist of dysarthria rather than unequivocal expressive aphasia, seldomly amnestic aphasia, rarely receptive aphasia. If speech disturbances result from cortical impairment *(migraine du territoire sylvien),* the absence of a straightforward relationship between the parameter speech disturbance and the parameters handedness, cheiro-oral paraesthesiae, hemianopsia, scotoma, or hemiparesis is neurologically surprising. For (pseudobulbar) dysarthria to occur, bilateral corticobulbar (putaminal) damage must be present, making the cortical hypothesis weaker than it appears *a prima facie.* Unilateral thalamic lesions (6) are as likely to offer an explanation, since abundant evidence of speech disturbance appearing on thalamic lesions has become available (15).

Whether familial hemiplegic migraine, hemiplegic migraine, and classic migraine associated with hemiparesis nosologically belong to one category (a question already negatively answered with respect to familial hemiplegic migraine) is not a point of discussion here. The point is whether these paralyses are of cortical origin. Involvement of the precentral motor cortex is usually considered as the seat of the dysfunction in hemiplegic migraine due to spasm of the rolandic and precentral arteries. On this basis, the clinical neurologist should be suspicious upon encountering a hemiparesis instead of a typical cortical monoparesis; in addition, he should require the paralysis to be flaccid and not spastic. Third, the paralysis, because of the vascular "spasm," should develop gradually and never acutely. Finally, it should be associated with myoclonias because of ischemia-induced excitation. Why do many reports testify to the hyperacute onset and the spasticity of the paralysis, and why is monoparesis scarcely mentioned in the literature? Conversely, why do the transient ischemic attacks excel in monopareses without the companionship of migrainous headache? Cerebral arteriovenous angiomas, impairing cortical blood flow, manifest with epilepsy or subarachnoid hemorrhage, and rarely present with hemiplegic migraine. Only three cases of complicated migraine due to cortical arteriovenous angiomas have been proved in 25 years.

The case history reported by Troost et al. (59) on a 20-year-old woman with a right occipital lobe angioma is stunning. Her daily scintillating scotoma attacks started in the left visual fields but drifted to the right to involve the central and right visual fields and subsequently inferiorly and to the left fields again, all in all lasting 45 min.

To explain the bilateral occipital lobe involvement by assuming callosal transfer (8) obviously is conjecture or worse, as it is known that callosal connections between the Brodmann areas 17 disappear in the late fetal stage (29). The hypertensive migraineur reported on by Cohen and Taylor (11) with left-sided hemiplegic and hemianesthetic attacks associated with dysarthria and tinnitus between ages 20 and 32 had an old left frontal, an old large left cerebellar, and a fresh right parietooccipital infarction, the latter explaining the hemianopsia. In other words, a stereotyped, nonvariant clinical picture of which the substrate ranges from left frontal to cerebellar to right parieto-occipital location.

With respect to facioplegic migraine, the intriguing family described by Barraquer-Bordas et al. (3) showed attacks of peripheral facial palsy and occasionally attacks of peripheral palsy on one side with central paresis on the other. This *par force majeure* indicates pontine involvement (internal auditory branch of the middle cerebellar artery, (14). In Heyck's (25) material of 45 cases of migraine accompagnée, he listed only one with facial paralysis. It is curious that in all cases of complicated migraine with so-called expressive aphasia and hemiplegia, central facial palsy is so conspicuously rare. If one wants to retain the vascular pathogenesis of migraine, the prosoplegic type must be fit into Bickerstaff's concept of basilar artery migraine.

The cerebellar or vestibular type of migraine accompagnée (with vertigo, nystagmus, and ataxia) lacked a sure footing until Bickerstaff outlined the syndrome of basilar migraine. Essentially, Bickerstaff's concept affirms the notion that any if not all events of the pathogenetic mechanisms of migraine should be localized in the brainstem rather than the cortex. The same applies to the century-old concept of dysphrenic migraine (hemicrania dysphrenica), the slightest form of which one scarcely ever misses in common and classic migraine, i.e., dysphoria. Heralding changes of mood in the form of inadequate elation, or euphoria, is not exceptional. The dysphoria may be associated with irritability, incoherence of thoughts, impairment of memory, confusion, apathy, phobia or terror, impulsive behavior, perceptual illusions and hallucinations, depression, or mania, and may grow into a full-blown, if transient, psychosis. The monographic study by Van der Does de Willebois (60) made a convincing case for the referral of all the symptoms to the diencephalon. Today one might include an area phylogenetically as old as the diencephalon, i.e., the hippocampus, and equally supplied by the posterior cerebral arteries.

The ophthalmoplegic type of complicated migraine has, with the exception of a few anecdotal reports on aneurysms in which the ptosis but not the migraine attacks are understandable, remained refractory to attempts at localization (6). Carroll (10) found no cause in 20 cases.

The vegetative, autonomic symptom-complex of mood changes, nausea, loss of appetite, vomiting, diarrhea, fever, retention of water, and polyuria followed by sleep have been suggested to arise in the hypothalamic part of the diencephalon (7,24). The pituitary-hypothalamic unit is a factory of neuropeptides and endorphin-fragments, of which the influence on mood, thought, and autonomic homeostasis are well established. The eliciting or precipitating influences of fasting and of endocrine factors point to the same area. Contrary to general opinion, fasting suppresses sympathetic nervous activity, and overfeeding (oral sucrose-solution) activates it (36). An exhaustive reappraisal of the hypothalamic causation has been presented recently by Johnson (31), with particular reference to a transient noradrenergic (α-adrenergic) activity burst, as proposed by Crisp (12).

The arguments marshaled in this survey serve to emphasize that the alleged cortical origin of dysfunctions in migraine is far from being a closed chapter, and that phylogenetically old areas of the brain, such as the brainstem, are at least as plausible candidates.

We next examine whether data obtained with the aid of auxiliary methods of examination can save the arteriospastic cortical ischemia hypothesis. The EEG has not yet been able to prove the cortical basis of complicated migraine. Granted, about one-third of migraineurs show abnormalities, and marked localized pathological changes have occasionally been recorded in cases of migraine accompagnée. The skeptical reader notices that these localized changes, often consisting of theta and delta waves, often bear a strict relationship to the cortical area presumably involved on the basis of clinical neurological deficit. The pertinent reports repeatedly state that such transient slow wave loci may (a) outlast the attacks, (b) appear again outside the attacks, (c) be bilateral in the presence of unilateral deficit, or (d) indicate impaired function of deep subcortical structures. Since an earlier review (6), the conclusion remains valid that an unequivocal correlation between clinical and EEG signs has not been established.

The state of affairs is scarcely less gloomy concerning cerebral angiographic evidence. The majority of papers report normal vascular visualization both during and outside the attacks. In rare instances, nonfilling (which essentially leaves matters undecided) or obstructions are reported, and very rarely an arteriovenous angioma is found (see refs. 5,34,48,59,62). Skinhøj (55) interpreted partial basilar artery nonfilling in three of four cases during an attack as decreased basilar artery perfusion pressure. Indeed, craniocerebral angiography is of so little value in migraine accompagnée that, in view of its meager yield and its increased risk in these patients, its use is not warranted, except in cases with permanent neurological deficit or with invariably ipsilateral attacks (50).

Radioisotope studies yield data that rather consistently indicate that the prodromal aura stage is characterized by a generalized reduction and the subsequent headache-stage by a diffuse increase of cerebral blood flow (CBF) (17,21,44,52–55). Even if one realizes that the ^{133}Xe inhalation method includes both external and internal carotid trees while the carotid injection method excludes the basilar artery territory and includes (even if the injection is restricted to the internal carotid artery) also the frontal extracranial tissue, there are a number of interpretative pitfalls. Sakai and Meyer (53) adduced evidence that the cerebrovasomotor responsiveness (cerebrovascular autoregulation) was impaired bilaterally during both aura and headache stages, with excessive response to CO_2 inhalation during the headache-free intervals.

Another noninvasive technique is the Doppler-flow-measurement. Kaneko et al. (33), in a series of 10 controls, 19 migraineurs, and seven cases of complicated migraine, found that the external carotid flow increased in none of the controls and in all the migraineurs upon administration of 1.5 mg nitroglycerine; in all seven cases of complicated migraine, the flow in the vertebral arteries was reduced by this drug. I propose that in migraine, CBF reduction starts in the basilar artery distribution and spreads rostrally.

MICROVASCULATURE

The most outstanding feature is the generalized CBF change in the two stages of the attack, a finding that strongly militates against the naive notion of spasm of certain cerebroarterial branches in one hemisphere. The findings indicate impaired cerebrovascular autoregulation, i.e., decreased sensitivity (dilatation) to CO_2, and inability to maintain

CBF on reduction of arterial blood pressure. The complexity of cerebrovascular autoregulation has been lucidly outlined by Purves (49) and Symon et al. (56). Cerebrovascular resistance has two components: (a) the extrinsic neurogenic baroreflex component of the cervical sympathetic innervating the brain base and pial arteries and having tonic control on (b) the intrinsic metabolic cerebral component, maintaining perfusion constancy on the basis of local tissular pH and vascular pCO_2, hypocapnia producing vasoconstriction, and hypercapnia producing vasodilatation. The CO_2-induced changes occur only if the sympathetic component functions. Stellate ganglion stimulation does not change CBF during normocapnia (2) but decreases it during hypercapnia.

The complex interaction of amines, CO_2, and other substances (Fig. 9) is shown by the fact that indomethacin (which blocks prostaglandin synthesis) also abolishes the vasodilatory response to CO_2. The same applies to serotonin (5-HT) and norepinephrine. Under physiological conditions, the arterioles are insensitive to topical or systemic administration of these compounds (in contrast to uridine-5'-triphosphate and angiotensin), whereas during hypercapnia, intraarterial 5-HT will reduce CBF. In addition, the autoregulatory response is not homogeneous. With lowering of systemic blood-pressure, the major extracranial and basocerebral arteries constrict, whereas the small intracranial arteries dilate in order to reduce the increased perfusion pressure. The adrenosympathetic system constitutes a link between psychological factors and cerebral circulation. The findings by Crisp's group (12) on an adrenergic "burst" preceding by some hours the migraine attack are compatible with the role of the sympathetic.

Blau (4), in a critical analysis of the bases for the traditional concept, rejected the cerebroarterial spasm theory, stipulating the central part played by the leptomeningeal microvasculature (i.e., vessels with lumina < 100 μm diameter) and underlining the neurogenic origin of migraine. The gradually accumulating data on α- and β-adrenergic agonists and blockers (e.g., phenoxybenzamine, propranolol, isoproterenol) supplement the earlier findings of the influence of 10% CO_2, amylnitrite, histamine, and ergotamine,

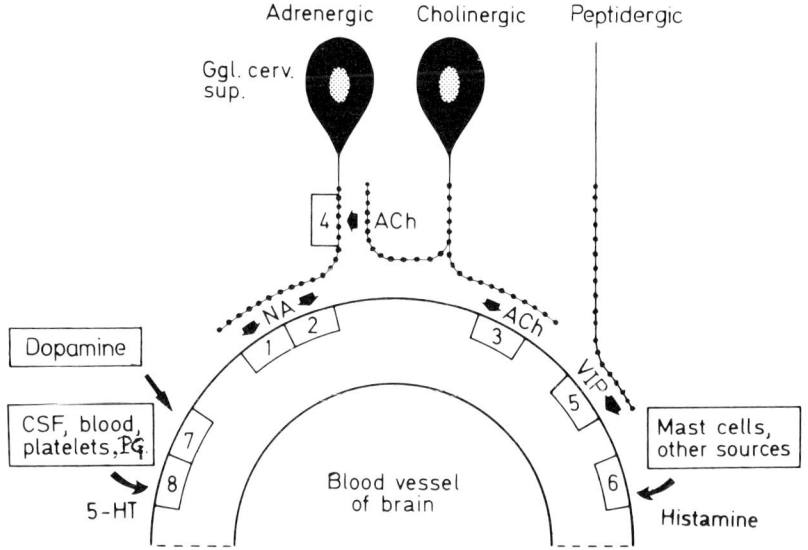

FIG. 9.

as well as Northfield's incisive experiments before World War II showing that histamine injection in the external carotid did not produce headache (18,23,23a,35,45,46). Krabbe and Olesen (34a) recently reviewed the histamine H_1 and H_2 receptor problem, as have Karnushina et al. (33a).

At the microvascular level, adrenergic sympathetic and parasympathetic innervation is rich; histamine is mainly concentrated there (30) (Fig. 10). Presynaptic H_2 receptors inhibit norepinephrine release (40). In addition, there is constrictory serotonergic, dilatatory cholinergic, β-adrenergic, dopaminergic, histaminergic, and peptidergic innervation (Fig. 11) as well as the kinins (Fig. 12). The structural resemblance of the pertinent neurotransmitters makes their effect at multiple receptor sites understandable (Fig. 11A). In this context, it is useful to realize that the blood serotonin changes are an effect rather than a cause, as indicated by the fact that in reserpine- or nitroglycerine-induced attacks, both urinary vanillylmandelic acid (VMA) and 5-hydroxyindoleacetic acid (5-HIAA) excretion increase, whereas urinary VMA remains unchanged when reserpine or nitroglycerine does not succeed in precipitating an attack (9,13). Also, in Anthony's original report, there were two nonmigrainous patients in whom plasma 5-HT fell upon reserpine administration as much as it did in his migraineurs, without a migraine being induced; in one migraineur who had had an attack the previous day, plasma 5-HT was not reduced by reserpine. This observation was confirmed by the experience of Curzon et al. (13), who also pointed out the loose temporal relationship between blood-5-HT and urinary 5-HIAA/VMA and the onset of headache.

Recent studies in this field have shown that (a) brain capillaries receive adrenergic innervation, which opens the possibility of neurogenic control of capillary resistance and of postarteriolar hemodynamics; and (b) in the external carotid bed, β_2-adrenoceptors predominate, whereas vasodilatation of intracranial vessels is subserved by β_1-adrenoceptors, norepinephrine and isoproterenol being much more potent for vasodilatation than epinephrine and the selective β_2-agonist terbutaline; the β_1-mediated vasodilatation is blocked by the selective β_1-agonist practolol (47). The patient reported by Cohen and

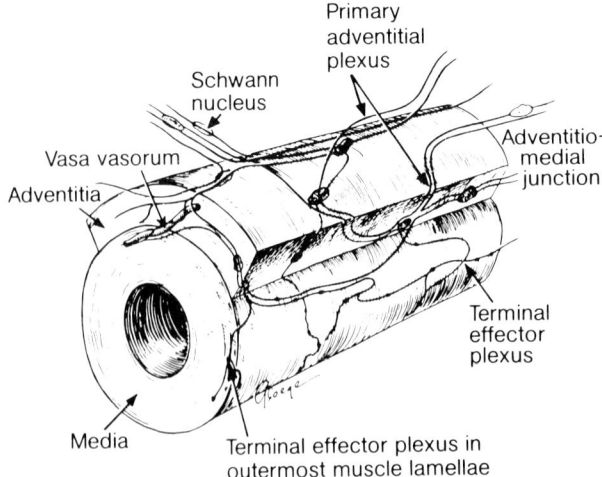

FIG. 10. From: Owman, C. (1979): Neurogenic vasodilatation mediated by the autonomic nervous system. *TRIANGLE* 18/4:89–99.

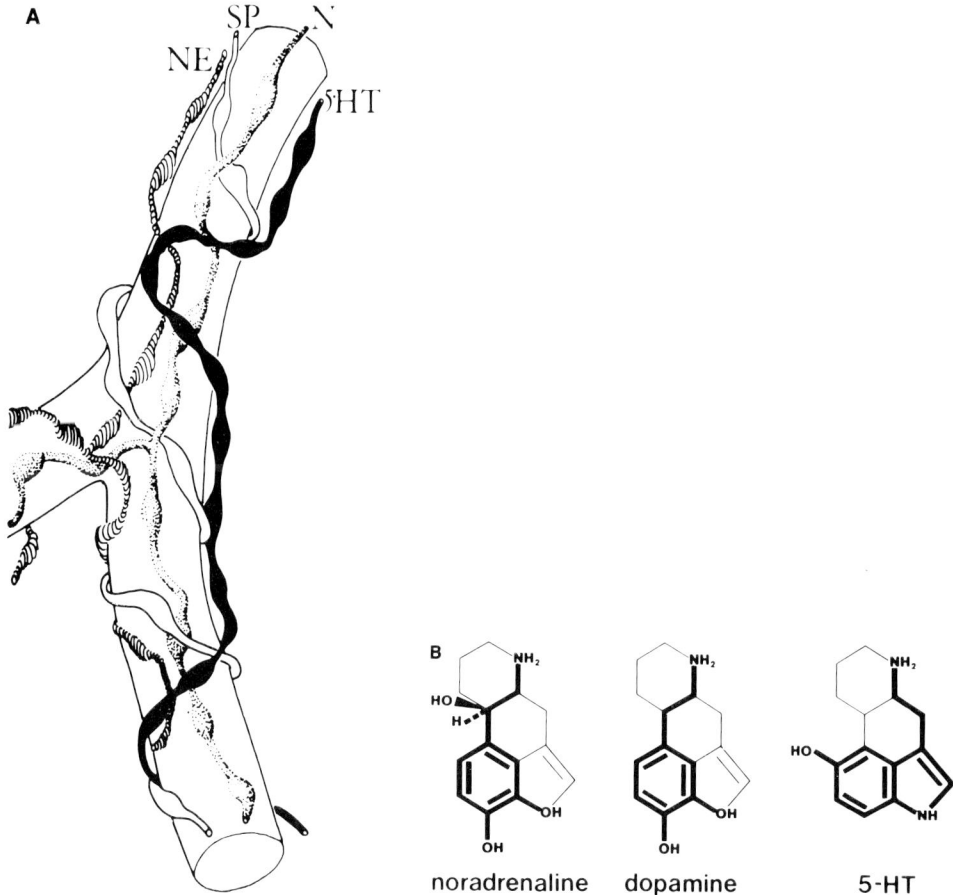

FIG. 11. From: Chan-Palay, V. (1977): *Neurogenic Control of the Brain Circulation,* pp. 39–53. Pergamon Press, New York.

Taylor (11) developed his third attack of basilar migraine deficit after reduction of his propranolol regimen. Beta-blockers with intrinsic sympathicomimetic activity have no beneficial effect in migraine (Tables 1 and 2, Fig. 13). The effects of angiotensin and VIP, one of the important vasodilatory neuropeptides, on the corticopial microcirculation, middle cerebral, and posterior communicating artery await further exploration (38). The neurogenically elicited primary involvement of the microvasculature, together with the reduced blood flow and the tendency to erythrocyte aggregation, may lead to retrograde (upstream) clogging of small caliber arteries with stasis, thus resulting in ischemic infarction in complicated migraine.

If we consider from the epistemological point of view the tenet that craniocerebral arteries with a diameter exceeding 200 μm produce the migrainous symptomatology due to their spasms and dilatations and involve extensive areas of the cerebral cortex, Ockham's venerable razor postulate *(pluralitas non est ponenda sine necessitate ponendi)* contains apotropeic advice. This principle of economy of thought is the main guideline in neurology in any attempt to establish the smallest possible area of the neuroanatomical

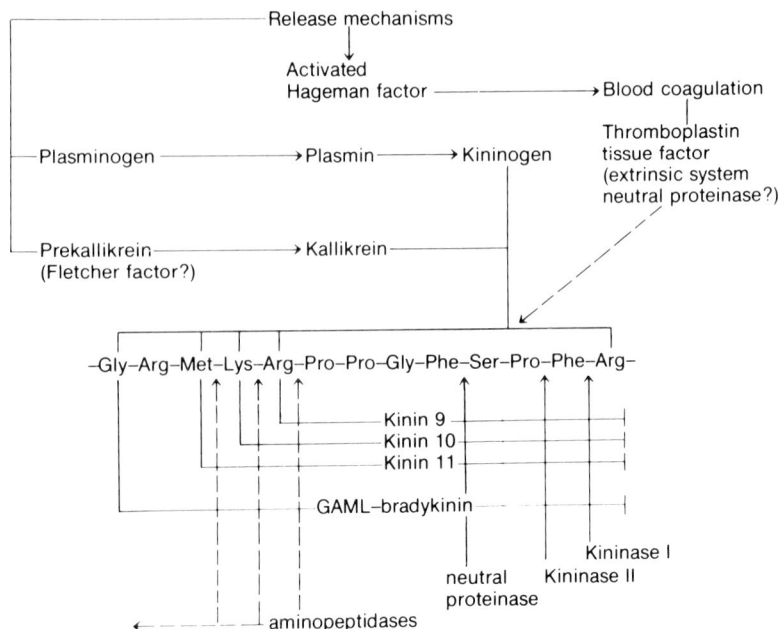

FIG. 12.

TABLE 1. *β-Blockade effect on migraine*

	Intrinsic sympathicomimetic activity	Antimigraine effect
Practolol	++	—
Pindolol	+	—
Butoxamine		—
Alprenolol	?	?
Propranolol	—	+
Timolol	—	+
Metoprolol	±	?
Latetalol	?	?

TABLE 2. *Receptor effects on microvasculature*

Constriction	Dilatation
α-Adrenergic	β_1-Adrenergic
Serotonin	H_2
Cholecystokinin?	Dopamine
Angiotensin?	Neurotensin
	VIP

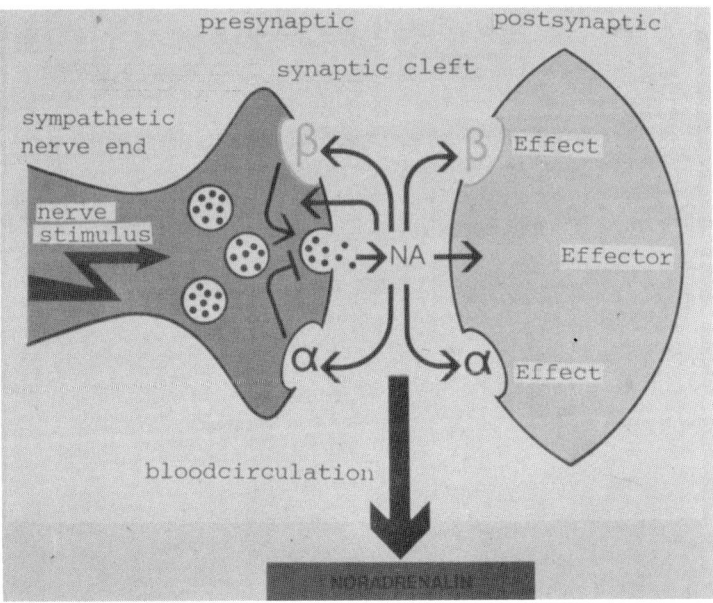

FIG. 13. Presynaptic and postsynaptic differential effects of α- and β-receptors. From: E. Muller-Schweinitzer and G. Engel (1978): α- *und* β-*Rezeptoren. Sandorama* III:9–12.

substrate sufficient to accommodate all the observed neurological symptoms. If applied to the issue *sub iudice,* a region meeting this requisite is the part of the upper brainstem that contains the mesencephalic central gray, the basal thalamus, lateral geniculate body, posterior limb of the internal capsule and hypothalamus and is embraced by the hippocampus. It is the smallest possible region accommodating all dolorous, sensory, visual, motor, speech, autonomic, and mental symptoms in migraine. This area is supplied by the anterior and posterior choroidal arteries and Duret thalamogeniculate artery, all three branches deriving from the (vertebro)basilar artery. If one wants to retain the concept of causative arterial constriction and dilatation, these three branches qualify. Sufficient neuropathological evidence was marshaled a decade ago (6) to justify this area as worthy of serious consideration in any attempt to define more accurately the cerebral structures putatively involved in migraine.

Insufficient data are available on the nature, extent, and quantity of autonomic innervation of these basal branches. Edvinsson et al. (19) pointed out that the ratio of α- and β-adrenergic innervation varies considerably in several brain regions. This sympathetic vascular innervation is heterogeneous in the sense that the phylogenetically oldest part of the brain subserving vitally important functions (pons, mesencephalon, thalamus) is protected against (or refractory to) a $\pm 35\%$ reduction of CBF produced by (nor)epinephrine infusion. Isoprenaline (an α- and B_1-receptor activator) infusion augments CBF in this old part of the brain; the basilar branches apparently have a predominantly α-adrenergic innervation.

We know next to nothing about the balance between carotid (telencephalic) and basilar perfusion, vasoreactivity, and its neurogenic control. One may assume that nature will safeguard the blood supply of the vital brainstem more carefully than that of other parts of the brain. Desequilibration of it may resound throughout the rostral end of the neuraxis with respect to both activity through the activating system of the reticular formation and aminergic activity through the medial forebrain bundle.

The nonspecificity of factors provoking the migraine attack in constitutionally liable people (Fig. 14), the specific stereotyped sequence of function disturbances constituting the attack itself, and the long latency between the impact of the triggering "stressor" event and the manifestation of the attack indicate that the (stressful) information received by the brain is processed and funneled down to the hypothalamus (Fig. 15), where a single factor, a neuropeptide or neurohormone, is released. This sets a preprogrammed set of changes (the attack itself) in motion. The hypothalamus and pituitary, as well as the neuron-specific-enolase-containing platelet (a model for APUD-cell system), are the "interface" between the neural and humoral terms of CNS-language (Fig. 16). I suggest the "serotonin-releasing factor" to be a 130 to 140 amino acid-containing neuro-peptide.

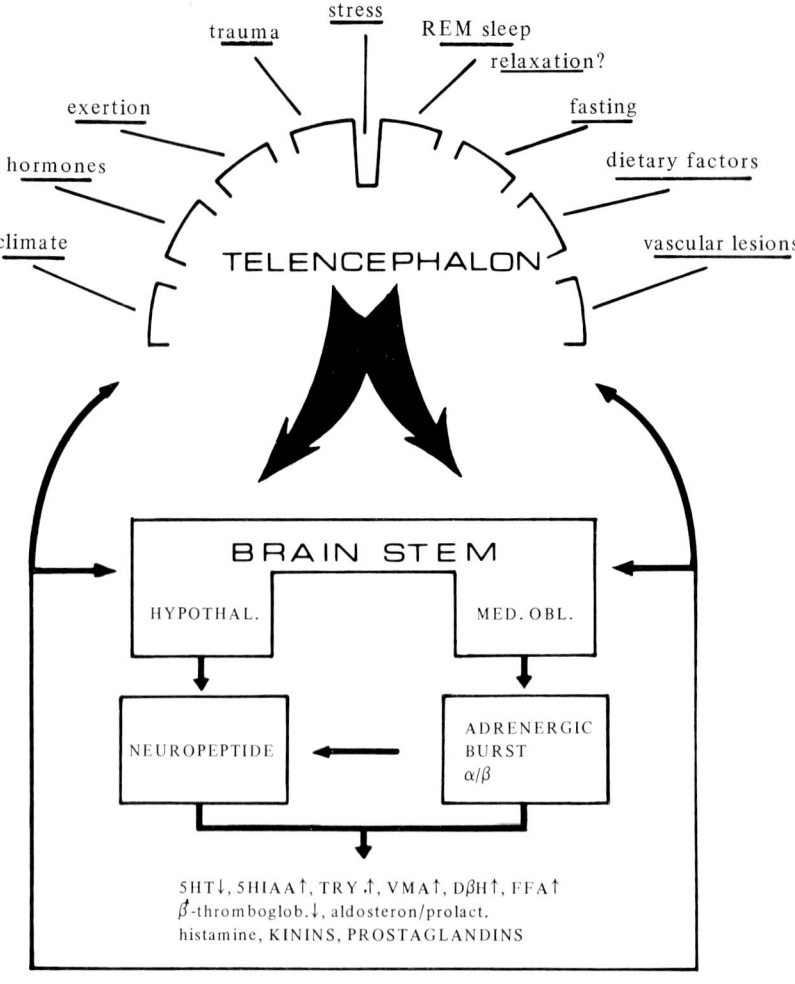

FIG. 14.

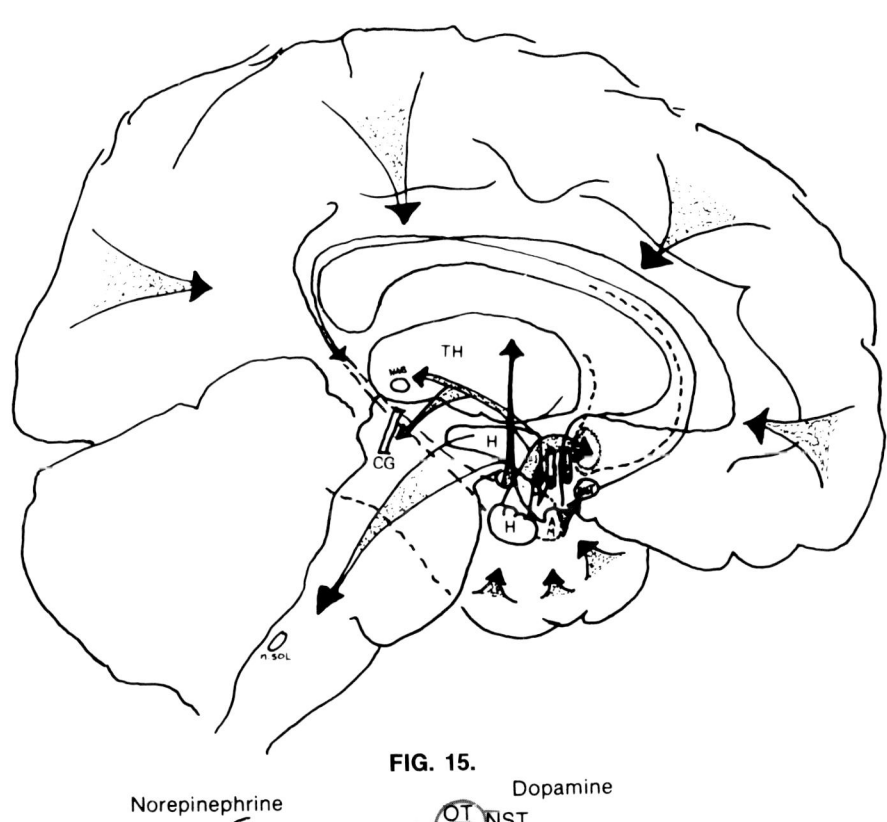

FIG. 15.

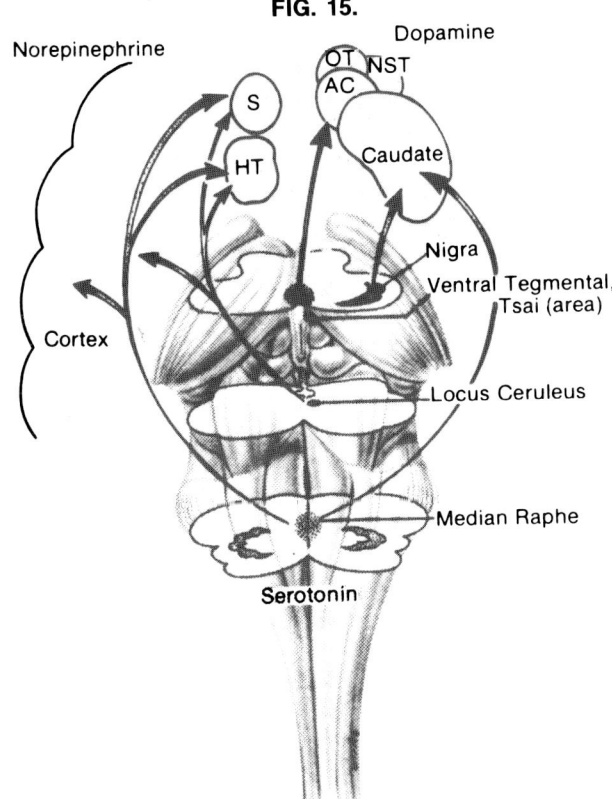

FIG. 16.

This clearly is deductive speculation rather than inductive reasoning based on experiment. The only remedy consists of clinicopharmacological experiments, which has become a nearly closed road in our era. It is also understood that the problem has been concentrated and displaced from many areas to a single one without touching the fundamental process.

REFERENCES

1. Abernethy, J. (1904): Looking back. *Lancet,* Oct. 22:1170.
2. Barker, B. J., Martin, J. S., and Rapela, C. E. (1978): Analysis of bilateral sympathetic stimulation effects on cerebral and cephalic blood flow in the dog. *Stroke,* 9:29–34.
3. Barraquer-Bordas, L., Peres-Serra, J., Grau-Veciana, Sagimon-Rabassa, E. (1970): Migraine prosoplégique familiale. *Acta. Neurol. Belg.,* 70:301–308.
4. Blau, J. N. (1978): Migraine, a vasomotor instability of the meningeal circulation. *Lancet,* 2:1136–1139.
5. Bruyn, G. W., and Gathier, J. C. (1967): Circulation veineuse corticale cérébrale dans le syndrome chéiro-oral. *Rev. Neurol. (Paris),* 114:271–280.
6. Bruyn, G. W. (1968): Complicated migraine. In: *Handbook of Clinical Neurology,* edited by P. J. Vinken and G. W. Bruyn, vol. 5, pp. 59–95. North-Holland, Amsterdam.
7. Bruyn, G. W. (1980): The Biochemistry of migraine. *Headache (in press).*
8. Bücking, H., and Baumgarten, G. (1974): Klinik und Pathophysiologie der initialen neurologischen Symptome bei fokalen Migraine. *Arch. Psychiatr. Nervenkrh.,* 210:37–52.
9. Campus, S., Fabris, F., and Rapelli, A. (1967): Escrezione urinaria di acido-5-idrossindolacetico durante crisi cefalalgici in dotto par hidroglicerina. *Boll. Soc. Biol. Sper.,* 43:1844–1847.
10. Carroll, J. D. (1975): Ophthalmoplegic migraine. Review of 20 cases. In: *Kopfschmerz/Headache 1975,* edited by G. S. Barolin, D. Baumgartner, and W. Hemmer, pp. 303–306. Lehmans, München.
11. Cohen, R. J., and Taylor, J. R. (1979): Persistent neurologic sequelae of migraine. *Neurology,* 29:1175–1177.
12. Crisp, A. H. (1979): Holistic speculations concerning the origin of migraine. *Trends in Neuroscience,* 2:116–118.
13. Curzon, G., Barrie, M., and Wilkinson, M. I. P. (1969): Relationships between headache and amine changes after administration of reserpine. *J. Neurol. Neurosurg. Psychiatry,* 32:555–561.
14. David, M., Angelergues, R., and Hécaen, H. (1956): Un cas de migraine prosoplégique par anévrysme artérielle de la fosse cérébrale postérieure. *Rev. Neurol.,* 94:716–718.
15. Demeurisse, G., Derouck, M., and Crehaerts, M. J. (1979): Study of two cases of aphasia by infarction of the left thalamus without cortical lesion. *Acta Neurol. Belg.,* 79:450–459.
16. Donat, J. R. (1980): Unilateral asterixis due to thalamic hemorrhage. *Neurology,* 30:83–84.
17. Edmeads, J. (1977): Cerebral blood flow in migraine. *Headache,* 17:148–152.
18. Edvinsson, L., Owman, C., and Sjoberg, N. (1976): Autonomic nerves, mast cells and amine receptors in human brain vessels. *Brain Res.,* 115:377–393.
19. Edvinsson, L., Lacombe, P., and Owman, C. (1979): Quantitative changes in regional cerebral blood flow of rats induced by α- and β-adrenergic stimulants. *Acta Physiol. Scand.,* 107:289–296.
20. Engel, G. L., Ferris, E. B., and Romano, J. (1945): Focal EEG changes during the scotoma of migraine. *Am. J. Med. Sci.,* 209:650–657.
21. Hachinski, V. C., Olesen, J., Norris, J. W., Larsen, B., Enevoldsen, E., Lassen, N. A. (1977): Cerebral hemodynamics in migraine. *Can. J. Neurol. Sci.,* 4:245–249.
22. Hardebo, J. E., Hansen, K., and Peters, E. (1940): Syndrome der Arteria Choriodea anterior. *Klin. Monatsbl. Augenheilkd.,* 105:521–542.
23. Hardebo, J. E., Edvinsson, L., and Owman, C. (1978): Potentiation of serotonine receptors in intracranial arteries. *Neurology (Minneap.),* 28:64–70.
23a. Hardebo, J. E., and Owman, C. (1980): Characterization of the in vitro uptake of monoamines into brain microvessels. *Acta Physiol. Scand.,* 108:223–229.
24. Herberg, L. J. (1975): The hypothalamus and migraine. In: *Modern Topics in Migraine,* edited by R. Greene, pp. 85–95. Heinemann, London.
25. Heyck, H. (1973): Varieties of hemiplegic migraine. *Headache,* 12:135–142.
26. Hubel, D. H., and Wiesel, T. N. (1972): Laminar and columnar distribution of geniculocortical fibers in the macaque monkey. *J. Comp. Neurol.,* 146:421–450.
27. Hubel, D. H., Wiesel, T. N., and Stryker, M. P. (1978): Anatomical demonstration of oriental columns in Macaque monkey. *J. Comp. Neurol.,* 177:361–380.
28. Hubel, D. H., and Wiesel, T. N. (1979): Brain mechanisms of vision. *Sci. Am.,* 241:130–144.
29. Innocenti, G. M., Fiore, L., and Caminiti, R. (1977): Exuberant callosal projection from visual cortex in newborn cats. *Neurosci. Lett.,* 4:237–242.
30. Jarrott, B., Hjelle, J. T., and Spector, S. (1979): Association of histamine with cerebral microvessels in bovine brain regions. *Brain Res.,* 168:323–330.

31. Johnson, E. S. (1978): A basis for migraine therapy. The autonomic theory reappraised. *Postgrad. Med. J.,* 54:231–243.
32. Jung, R. (1978): Cerebral correlates of conscious experience. In: *INSERM Symposium No. 6,* edited by P. A. Buser and A. Rougeul-Buser, pp. 24–35. North-Holland, Amsterdam.
33. Kaneko, Z., Shiraiki, J., and Inaoka, H. (1978): Intra- and extracerebral hemodynamics of migrainous headache. In: *Current Concepts in Migraine Research,* edited by R. Greene, Raven Press, New York.
33a. Karnushina, I. L., Palacios, J. M., Barbin, G., Dux, E., Joó, F., and Schwartz, J. C. (1980): Studies on a capillary-rich fraction isolated from brain: Histaminic components and characterization of the histamine receptors linked to adenylate cyclase. *J. Neurochem.,* 34(5):1201–1208.
34. Kattah, J. C., and Luessenhop, A. J. (1980): Resolution of classic migraine after removal of an occipital lobe AVM. *Ann. Neurol.,* 7:93.
34a. Krabbe, A. A., and Olesen, J. (1980): Headache provocation by continuous intravenous infusion of histamine. Clinical results and receptor mechanisms. *Pain,* 8:253–259.
35. Kupersmith, M. J., Hass, W. K., and Chase, N. E. (1979): Isoproteronol treatment of visual symptoms in migraine. *Stroke,* 10:299–305.
36. Landsberg, L., and Young, J. B. (1978): Fasting, feeding and regulation of the sympathetic nervous system. *N. Engl. J. Med.,* 298:1295–1301.
37. Leão, A. A. P. (1944): Pial circulation and spreading depression of activity in the cerebral cortex. *J. Physiol.,* 7:391–396.
38. Larsson, L. I., Edvinsson, L., Fahrenkrug, J., Håkonsong, R., Owman, Chin, Schaffälitzky de Muckadell, O., and Sundler, C. (1976): Immunohistochemical localization of a vasodilatory polypeptide (VIP) in cerebrovascular nerves. *Brain Res.,* 113:400–404.
39. Marshall, W. H. (1969): Spreading cortical depression of Leão. *Physiol. Rev.,* 39:239–279.
40. McGrath, M. A., and Vanhoutte, P. M. (1978): In: *Mechanisms of Vasodilatation,* edited by P. M. Vanhoutte and I. Leusen, p. 248. Karger, Basel.
41. Milner, P. M. (1958): Note on a possible correspondence between the scotomas of migraine and spreading depression of Leão. *EEG Clin. Neurophysiol.,* 10:705.
42. Mohr, J. P., Kase, C. S., Meckler, R. J., and Fisher, C. M. (1977): Sensorimotor stroke due to thalamocapsular ischaemias. *Arch. Neurol.,* 34:739–741.
43. Northfield, D. W. C. (1938): Some observations on headache. *Brain,* 61:133–159.
44. O'Brien, M. D. (1971): Cerebral blood changes in migraine. *Headache,* 10:139–143.
45. Owman, C., Edvinsson, L., and Nielsen, K. C. (1974): Autonomic receptor mechanism in brain vessels. *Blood vessels,* 11:2–31.
46. Wahl, M., and Kuschinsky (1977): Autonomic receptors as studies in pial vessels—microapplication in situ. In: *Neurogenic Control of Brain Circulation,* edited by Owman, C., and Edvinsson, L., pp. 185–195. Pergamon Press, New York.
47. Owman, C. (1979): Neurogenic vasodilatation mediated by the autonomic nervous system. *TRIANGLE,* 18:89–100.
48. Pearce, J. H. S., and Foster, J. B. (1965): An investigation of complicated migraine. *Neurology (Minneap.),* 15:333–340.
49. Purves, M. J. (editor) (1972): *The Physiology of the Cerebral Circulation.* Cambridge University Press, London.
50. Rascol, A., Cambier, J., Guiraud, B., Manelfe, C., David, J., Clanet, M. (1979): Accidents ischémiques cérébraux au cours de crises migraineuses. *Rev. Neurol.,* 135:867–884.
51. Richards, W. (1971): The fortification illusions of migraine. *Sci. Am.,* 224:88–96.
52. Sakai, F., and Meyer, J. S. (1978): Regional cerebral hemodynamics during migraine and cluster headache. *Headache,* 18:122–132.
53. Sakai, F., and Meyer, J. S. (1979): Abnormal reactivity in patients with migraine and cluster headache. *Headache,* 19:257–266.
54. Simard, D., and Paulson, T. B. (1973): Cerebral vasomotor paralysis during migraine attacks. *Arch. Neurol.,* 29:207–209.
55. Skinhøj, E. (1973): Hemodynamic studies within the brain during migraine. *Arch. Neurol.,* 29:95–98.
56. Symon, L., Bull, J. W. D., du Boulay, E. O. G. H., Marshall, J., Ross Russell, R. W. (1973): Reactivity of cerebral vessels. In: *Background to Migraine,* edited by J. N. Cumings, pp. 18–41. Heinemann, London.
57. Szentagothai, J. (1975): The module concept in cerebral cortex architecture. *Brain Res.,* 95:475–496.
58. Szentagothai, J. (1978): The neuron network of the cerebral cortex. *Proc. Soc. Lond. [B.],* 201:219–248.
59. Troost, B. T., Mark, L. E., and Maroon, J. C. (1979): Resolution of classic migraine after removal of an occipital lobe AVM. *Ann. Neurol.,* 5:199–210.
60. Van der Does de Willebois, J. J. M. (1932): Over migraine, in het bijzonder over hemicrania. Doctoral dissertation, Utrecht.
61. Walshe, T. M., Davis, K. R., and Fisher, C. M. (1977): Thalamic hemorrhage. *Neurology,* 27:217–222.
62. Welch, K. M. A., Chabi, E., and Nell, J. H. (1976): Biochemical comparison of migraine and stroke. *Headache,* 16:160–167.

Advances in Neurology, Vol. 33, edited by
M. Critchley et al. Raven Press, New York © 1982

Impairment of Memory Pathways in Adult and Child Headache

G. A. Buscaino

Neurological Clinic, Second School of Medicine, University of Naples, Naples, Italy

The history of a certain forgetfulness among headache patients led Gori-Savellini and co-workers to investigate memory during intercritical periods in both adults and children. As mentioned by these authors, the Rey test is a suitable means in young headache patients to find alterations in the three components of the memory process: (a) recording of data, (b) fixation of the data, and (c) the possibility to voluntarily reproduce the data. These results are of interest because such investigations are rare; Valquist (11) and Bille (1) do not mention it, and in a review of the problem in 1970, Weters (12) did not find any significant differences in adult headache patients regarding intelligence, social class, or predisposition to headache.

The mechanism of memory is so complex and delicate that it can be blocked by a small upset, an emotion, or loss of serenity and tranquility; attention is less acute, and one forgets. Anguish, insecurity, stress, conflicts in affection, and all forms of neurosis cause a clear reduction of memory. Also, loss of sleep or rest disturbed by noise affect memory. American soldiers, who remained awake at night longer than usual, were asked to locate pictures chosen the previous day from a pack of photographs. They chose the wrong pictures with a percentage directly proportional to the lost hours of sleep.

With respect to Rey's test, poor visual perception of the lines could hinder memorization on the basis of imprecise information. Headache in school often is found in relation to underestimated refractory or visual disturbances. Sorge et al. (7,8) carried out an epidemiological investigation on a group of school children with headache (60 were found in a population of 1,800 elementary school children from several working-class areas of Naples). From a questionnaire worked out by these investigators to determine some of the factors underlying headache during development, three groups emerged. The first consisted of those in whom the headache was an abnormal relational incident in a disturbed family context. In the second group were children affected by essential headache but who often used this manifestation as a preferred instrument to strike out at parental figures. The third group consisted of children with essential headache in a family context that was not particularly disturbed.

Although the problem of memory is not the object of specific study, the investigation (8) showed that the children who responded to the questionnaire corresponding to "nonessential headache in a relatively disturbed family context" were those with low scholastic ability who were easily distracted, restless, and timid.

The coexistence of particular character disturbances with essential headaches (4) and psychosomatic headaches (2) leads one to infer that the biological basis of these symptomatologies may be founded on the deficits of particular neurotransmitters, e.g., serotonin and endorphin turnover or phenomena of transport at the level of RNA synthesis (3,5,6). In these cases (i.e., depressive, conversion, or muscular tension headache), memory disturbances are frequent and at times severe. It should be noted from the data of Terenius (10) and those observed in our clinic by Steardo (9) that there is a reduction of cerebrospinal fluid endorphins in essential headache patients during an attack; under the same conditions, patients with psychogenic headaches had normal levels of this peptide (11). Moreover, after the administration of naloxone, there was a lowering of the pain threshold during a headache in the organic patients; there was no alteration in response in the psychogenic headache sufferers.

Regarding the neurobiological mechanisms that may underlie the memory disturbances that occur in headache patients, all conclusions are premature. That neurotransmitters play a role in determining algogenic phenomena and in the mechanisms of consolidation of memory is an attractive hypothesis, but further documentation is required. In fact, even though data indicate that peptides rather than any other substance are responsible for the transfer of memory in laboratory animals, the increase in memorization ability following the administration of RNA or other substrates that increase the RNA content of neurons is less promising in humans than in laboratory animals.

REFERENCES

1. Bille, B. (1962): Migraine in school children. *Acta Paediatr. [Suppl.],* 51:136.
2. Dixon, A. W. (1980): Psychogenic headache. *Headache,* 47–54.
3. Herz, A., and Blasig, I. (1979): *Endorphin in Mental Health Research,* edited by E. Cloding, MacMillan, London.
4. Packard, R. C. (1976): What is psychogenic headache? *Headache,* 16:20–23.
5. Sicuteri, F. et al. (1979): *Psychopharmacology,* 65:205–209.
6. Sicuteri, F. et al. (1979): *Neuroscience,* suppl. 351–S380.
7. Sorge, F., Steardo, L., di Furia, U., Florio, C., di Pietro, G., and Orzalesi, B. (1979): Le cefalee nell'età evolutiva: Inquadramento nosografico mediante schede valutative e tests diagnostici. *Q. Acta Neurol.,* 39:123–134.
8. Sorge, F., Steardo, L., Giani, U., and di Pietro, G. (1980): An epidemiological study of headache in school children of Naples. *Int. Congr. Headache 1980,* Florence, March 17–19.
9. Steardo, L. (1979): Livelli di encefaline nel CSF in pazienti con algie organiche o psicogene. *XXI Congr. Soc. Ital. Neurol.,* Catania, November 8, p. 273.
10. Terenius, L. (1978): *Advances in Psychopharmacology, Vol. 18.* Raven Press, New York.
11. Valquist, B. (1955): Migraine in children. *Int. Arch. Allergy,* 7:348–355.
12. Weters, W. E. (1971): Migraine: Intelligence, social class and familial prevalence. *Br. Med. J.,* 81.

Advances in Neurology, Vol. 33, edited by
M. Critchley et al. Raven Press, New York © 1982

Neuroendocrine Approach to Headache

A. Polleri, *G. Nappi, P. Masturzo, *E. Martignoni,
G. Murialdo, *G. Bono, E. Testa, and *F. Savoldi

*Institute of Internal Medicine, University of Genoa, Genoa; and *Neurological Clinic,
University of Pavia, Pavia, Italy*

Disturbances in neurochemical processes involved in nociceptive mechanisms are reported to occur in essential headache, making this condition a peculiar example of central pain (28). Evidence has been provided by several authors (see ref. 28 for a review) that in essential headache, changes in brain neurotransmitter concentrations and metabolism are present; also, the sensitivity of monoamine postsynaptic receptors is affected. Most data refer to the serotoninergic system, but other monoaminergic neurons also are involved.

The disorder of nociceptive function might be considered to belong to a group of disorders of the central nervous system (CNS) that depend on neurotransmission changes, together with others concerning motility (parkinsonism, Huntington chorea) or mood (depression). In these disorders, the most evident disturbance of neurotransmission regards the neural systems that take part in cerebral function, which is clinically altered; thus pain, motility, and mood symptoms appear. A deeper analysis shows that the neurotransmission disorders are not confined to the neuronal systems more specifically involved in the symptomatology.

Neurotransmitters take part in neuronal function and in the regulation of pituitary function as well; therefore, endocrine counterparts are sought. Several contributions indicate that, besides the main symptomatology typical of each of these disorders, neuroendocrine disorders also are detectable (6,10,14,16,23). These possibilities emerged in an early review of brain-endocrine relationships (1) and were more recently stressed by Barbeau (2).

This chapter shows that also in headache, neuroendocrine disturbances occur and correlate with the painful symptoms, confirming an analogy with endocrine involvement in parkinsonism, Huntington chorea, and depression (for review, see ref. 18). Evidence is presented that changes in the regulation of hormone secretion by the pituitary are present in various forms of headache, even independent of the actual pain attacks. The data obtained indicate that the endocrinological approach may be useful for the clinical evaluation of the headache subject, as demonstrated by the presence of neurotransmission disturbances.

From the methodological standpoint, it must be stressed (21) that we are not dealing with gross changes, comparable to those occurring in typical endocrine diseases: the hormone levels are not pathological. Rather, the disturbances lie with the secretion regulation and are qualitative in nature. The investigation takes advantage of methods that study either spontaneous secretory changes over time using chronobiological techniques or the effects of endocrinological and pharmacological challenges.

MATERIALS AND METHODS

The following types of headache are considered: (a) posttraumatic chronic headache (PTCH), (b) cluster headache (CH), (c) face algic vasomotor syndrome (Charlin-Sluder syndrome) (FAS), and (d) migraine.

Chronobiological studies have been performed determining prolactin (PRL) in sera collected at 2-hr intervals throughout a 24-hr period, according to a method of harmonic analysis by the Fourier's equation, previously described and discussed (18). Stimulation of pituitary hormone secretion has been performed administering 100 μg i.v. luteinizing hormone releasing hormone (LHRH) (Relisorm, Serono, Rome), 200 μg thyrotropin-releasing hormone (TRH) (Relefact, Hoechst Italia, Milan) and regular insulin, 0.1 IU/kg body weight, simultaneously. In these experiments PRL, somatotropin (STH), thyrotropin (TSH), luteotropic hormone (LH), and follicle-stimulating hormone (FSH) were assayed. In pharmacological studies, PRL secretion was challenged with reserpine, sulpiride, fenfluramine, and benserazide, by methods described elsewhere (8,11–13,17,19, 22,25). Hormones were determined by a radioimmunoassay (RIA) method, using reagents obtained from Biodata, Milan. Reference preparations used are the following: PRL WHO 222/71 (1 ng equals 23 μIU); STH WHO 68/38 (1 ng equals 2 μIU); LH and FSH 2nd IRP hMG; TSH WHO 68/38.

RESULTS

PTCH

When the rhythmicity of PRL secretion is studied, no changes are apparent between the patients (16 males) and the age-matched controls, when either the average PRL levels are considered or the harmonic analysis data for each patient are compared by the χ^2 method. However, when the clinical seriousness of each case is evaluated by a score considering skull fracture, duration of unconsciousness, presence of focal neurological signs, and electroencephalographic (EEG) and computerized tomographic (CT) findings, a coincidence is found between the seriousness of the condition and the frequency of the occurrence of harmonic within a period of 24 hr; all patients in the most serious group show only that harmonic (Table 1) (27).

Changes in pituitary function were observed in the same group (9), chiefly concerning a decreased response of TSH to TRH. No differences occurred in baseline levels, whereas the attained peak values are significantly lower ($p < 0.05$) with respect to controls (11.72 $\pm$ 6.48 μIU/ml versus 26.80 $\pm$ 6.42 − mean $\pm$ S.D.). A direct correlation can be drawn ($r = 0.9999$; $p < 0.01$) between the impairment of the response expressed as the mean of the peak values and the clinical severity (Fig. 1). The responses of PRL, STH, and LH are slightly increased, although not significantly. The FSH response is not changed (data not shown).

CH

The mean levels of PRL in 24 hr in nine male patients with CH (8.181 $\pm$ 1.607 ng/ml) were compared to levels in normal, age-matched controls (7.753 $\pm$ 1.560 ng/

TABLE 1. *Common features in males with PTCH*

| Subjects | Mean 24-hr PRL (ng/m) | Periods | | | | | | | | |
| | | 24 hr | | | 12 hr | | | 8 hr | | |
		%	A	ϑ	%	A	ϑ	%	A	ϑ
Controls[a] (6)	7.8 ± 1.4	33.3	1.94	19:40	16.7	1.35	00:20	33.3	1.89	22:20
Patients (16)	12.8 ± 5.2	68.7	4.96	00:54	25.0	3.65	06:42	6.3	2.61	00:47
Clinical score[b]										
0–3 (10)	13.3 ± 6.1	60.0	5.52	02:13	30.0	3.42	06:00	10.0	2.61	16:43
4–7 (3)	13.0 ± 2.6	66.7	7.12	03:20	33.3	4.35	08:59	—	—	—
8–11 (3)	10.7 ± 4.0	100.0	2.40	20:40	—	—	—	—	—	—

A, amplitude; ϑ, phase. Number of subjects in parentheses.

[a] Other harmonics within a period of less than 8 hr are not shown.

[b] Clinical score: Skull fracture, no (point 0); yes (point 2). Duration of loss of consciousness, none (0); <3 days (1); 3 to 6 days (2); 6 to 10 days (3); >10 days (4). CT, negative (0); positive (2). EEG changes (0–1–2). Focal neurological signs, none (0); present (2).

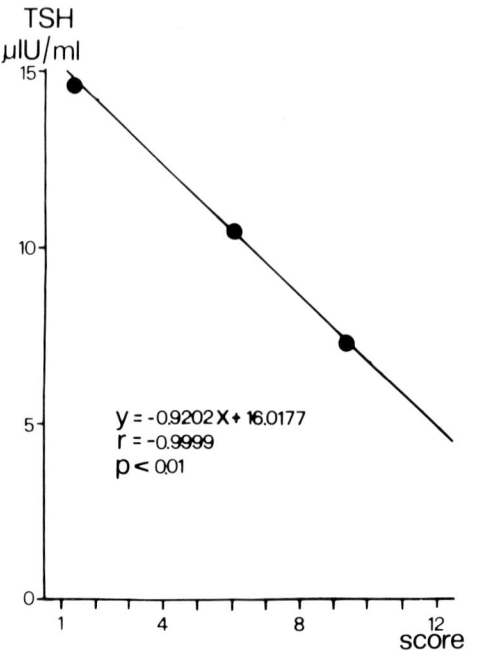

FIG. 1. Correlation between the means of the peak values of TSH upon TRH administration and the clinical score in PTCH.

$y = -0.9202 X + 16.0177$
$r = -0.9999$
$p < 0.01$

ml). The periodicity of hormone secretion is not the same. When the single cases are evaluated by means of harmonic analysis, the number of cases in whom the PRL levels do not show any rhythmicity is larger in normal subjects (one of 13), either in the untreated (four of nine) or lithium-treated CH series (two of nine). The χ^2 value found when the control and the untreated CH series are compared is 4.0903 ($p < 0.05$), which is scarcely significant due to the small number of cases. The trend is better shown when the harmonic analysis is made using the averages of the values obtained in the single cases of each series. With this analytic procedure, no significant rhythmicity is apparent. Lithium treatment has no effect (Table 2).

If pain occurred on the day when PRL secretory periodicity was evaluated, a secretory rhythm could be detected. The mean time of pain occurrence and the detected acrophase of PRL (namely, the time of the day when the peak level of hormone occurs) are similar (11:23 for PRL and 11:35 for pain). In this series, a circadian rhythm is apparent when lithium treatment is performed, even if no pain is occurring during the investigation.

FAS

The occurrence of a PRL secretory rhythmicity in seven men with FAS is not different from that occurring in 10 normal age- and sex-matched controls.

In most of the cases studied, pain was present during observation; when rhythmicity was studied, a rhythm was always present, independent of the occurrence of pain, with a preserved synchronization on sleep. In CH patients, a periodicity was always detectable only in patients with painful accesses (Table 2).

TABLE 2. *PRL rhythmicity in CH and in FAS*

Subjects	Mean 24 hr PRL (ng/ml)	Period (hr)	Amplitude	Phase
Controls (13)	7.75 ± 1.56	24	1.325	23:47
		12	1.302	01:24
Cluster headache				
Untreated (9)	8.18 ± 1.61	NS	—	—
Lithium (9)	8.28 ± 2.26	NS	—	—
Pain (5)	7.95 ± 1.55	12	2.147	11:23
FAS (7)	8.55 ± 2.87	24	2.248	06:26

NS, not significant; $p > 0.05$.
No. of subjects in parentheses.

Migraine

Six adult males with migraine were studied for their PRL secretory periodicity; no differences were found compared to normal controls.

A pharmacological study was performed in migraine patients. Reserpine, a drug that depletes monoamines within and outside the CNS, induces an increase in PRL concentrations in normal men and women, the response in the latter being larger than in the former. No difference in response is present in migrainous women. In men, the obtained increase of serum PRL is similar to that of controls, but the return of the hormone to baseline levels is delayed ($p < 0.001$). The percent increase of PRL concentrations in migrainous men is comparable to that observed in migrainous and healthy women (Fig. 2). A similar although less impressive effect is induced by 60 mg oral fenfluramine, which increases the release and blocks the reuptake of serotonin (5-HT) (Fig. 3).

Benserazide, an inhibitor of the aromatic amino acid decarboxylase, which decreases the concentration of peripheral monoamines and increases it within the blood-brain

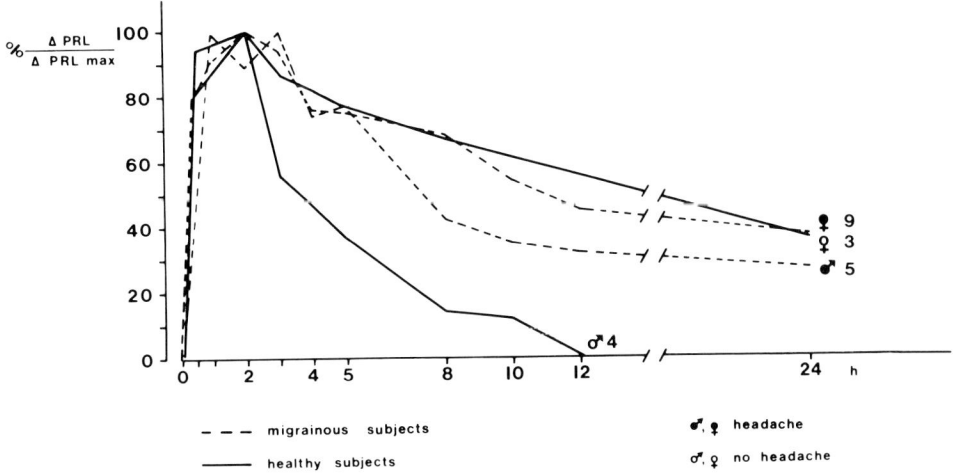

FIG. 2. Percent increase of PRL upon reserpine administration in migraine.

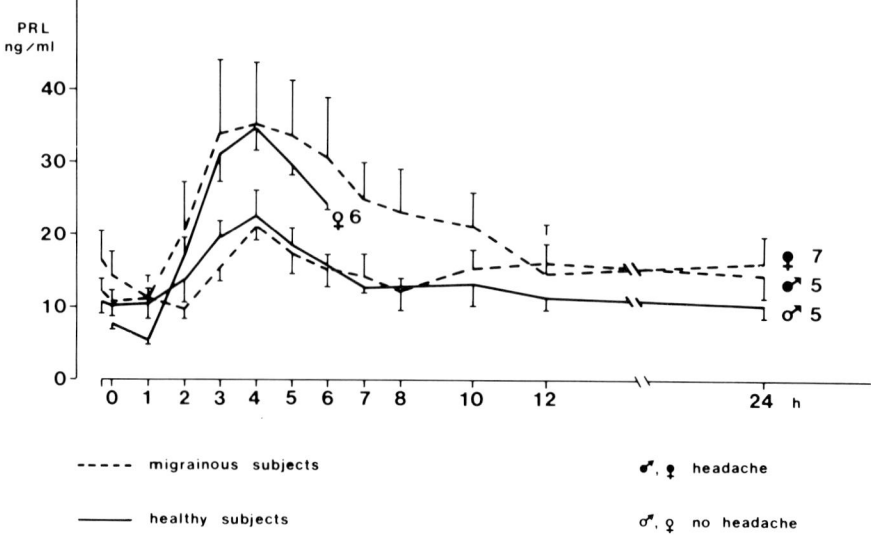

FIG. 3. PRL levels after fenfluramine (60 mg/o.s. at 9 A.M.).

barrier, enhances PRL, with larger peaks in women than in men. Migraine subjects respond to benserazide administration (125 mg orally) in a fashion comparable to normal subjects. However, migrainous women exhibit a slower decrement of the peak in comparison to normal controls ($p < 0.01$) (Fig. 4).

Sulpiride is a blocker of dopamine (DA) receptors at the periphery for doses smaller

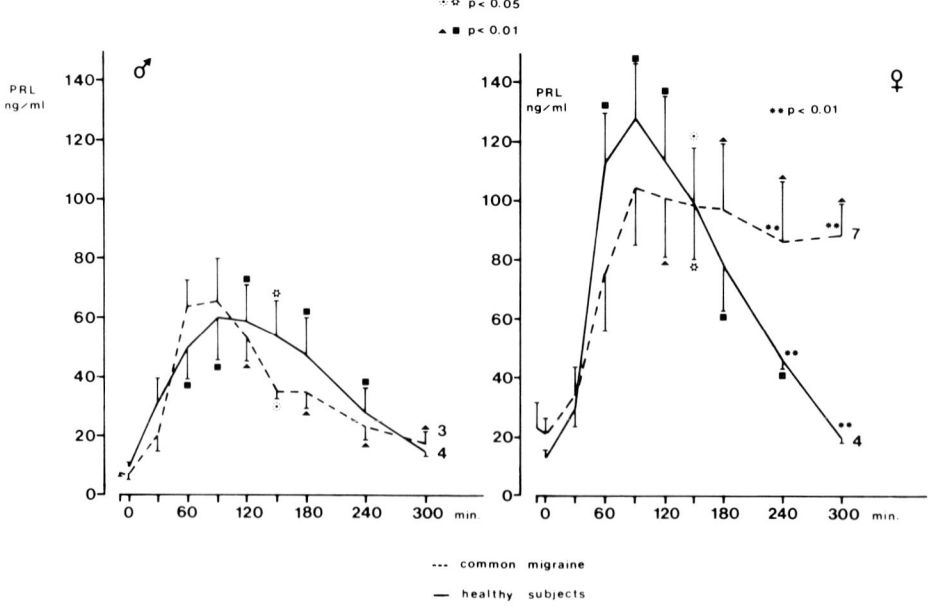

FIG. 4. Increase of PRL in migraine subjects given benserazide (125 mg/o.s. at 9 A.M.).

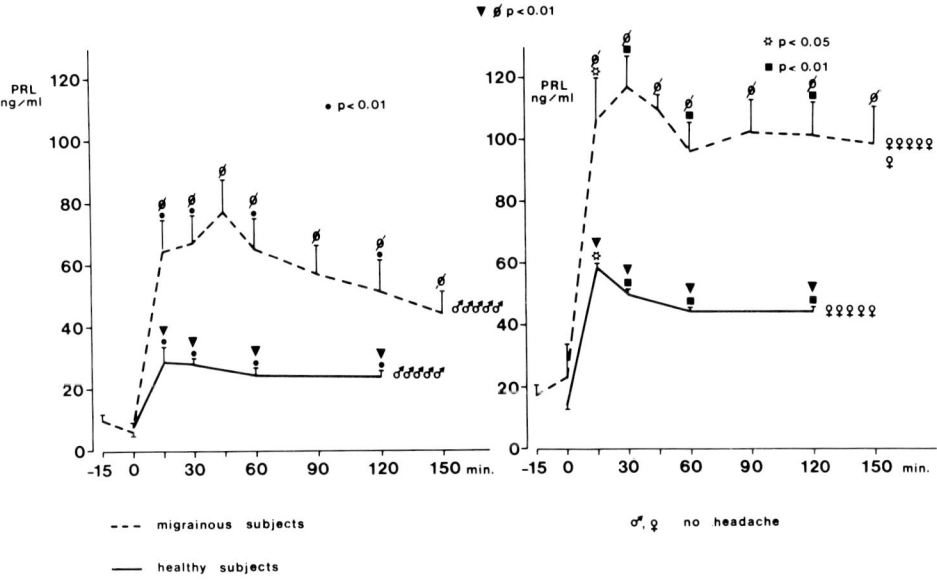

FIG. 5. Effects of sulpiride on PRL in migraine patients (15 mg/m² i.v. at 9 A.M.).

than 100 mg/m² body surface. When a dose of 15 mg/m² is given to men and women, an increase of PRL occurs, which is larger in women than in men in both normal and migraine subjects. In the latter group, however, peak values are larger ($p < 0.01$) than in age- and sex-matched subjects, and the subsequent slope is less steep in both cases (Fig. 5). In a migraine subgroup, consisting of catamenial headache, the peak is larger than in migrainous women ($p < 0.01$) (data not shown).

The occurrence of pain has been sought in these pharmacological studies. Reserpine was able to induce headache in all the 14 migrainous women tested and in 11 of 15 migrainous men. The onset of pain and its maximum were delayed in regard to the hyperprolactinemic response. A similar effect was observed after fenfluramine and benserazide; in these latter instances, however, autonomic symptoms with slight pain were present since the beginning of the PRL rise. Upon benserazide administration, only migrainous women showed pain. No pain was observed in the sulpiride series.

DISCUSSION

Little is known about the mechanisms of the synchronization of hormone secretion, although synchronizing effects of different exogenous events are well known. In the case of PRL and STH, sleep enhances a rhythmicity within a 24-hr period. The cause of secretory PRL episodes with a period shorter than 24 hr, which the harmonic analysis shows to be present in part of the adult male population, remains unknown. It is not possible to explain satisfactorily the presence of a PRL circadian rhythm within a 24-hr period, which has been found in all the most serious patients with PTCH. The strongest rhythm, which occurs earlier in life (20) and is synchronized with sleep, remains, while secretory episodes with a shorter period disappear.

Harmonic analysis gives a more detailed picture of the periodicity of a phenomenon than does the cosinor procedure described by Nelson et al. (15). This may explain why, in the present series, we were unable to find a significant periodicity in PRL levels in CH, in contrast to what we previously observed with a cosinor evaluation (3).

The disturbance is not influenced by lithium, which decreases the occurrence and the intensity of pain (25). Pain, however, has a rhythmicity-entraining effect, since in most subjects with painful bouts, the presence of a rhythm is seen. In some cases, it is not possible to demonstrate a simultaneous occurrence of the pain and of the acrophase of the hormone; when behavior is considered as the average, the effects coincide. PRL is known to increase because of painful stimuli (4).

A difference is present when the behavior of PRL is compared in CH and FAS. In FAS, a rhythmicity is present; regardless of when the pain occurs, the secretory periodicity of PRL is sleep-entrained, as in normal subjects.

No change in rhythmicity occurs in migraine. Challenges to pituitary function demonstrate changes in secretion in PTCH. This involves norepinephrine (NE)-dependent events, such as TSH regulation (7). The pituitary reserve of this hormone seems to be diminished. Whether or not this finding indicates an involvement of the brain NE system must be further investigated.

Regulation of PRL secretion in migraine is grossly impaired. Migrainous subjects show either sustained hyperprolactinemia or higher peaks when agents pharmacologically active on monoaminergic effects are administered. Although in general, the peak sex-linked response is preserved, differences observed indicate that they are most striking when the DA-dependent direct regulation at the pituitary level is challenged, as in the case of benserazide and sulpiride. To assess the relevance of the reported data, it may be useful to recall that neither drug crosses the blood-brain barrier (17,18).

Reserpine and fenfluramine act on monoamine systems at both the brain and peripheral levels. The PRL increase due to the reserpine-induced DA depletion is a central and a peripheral effect as well, whereas the stimulatory effect of 5-HT due to fenfluramine occurs via hypothalamic serotoninergic synapses. At the employed doses, benserazide and sulpiride do not cross the blood-brain barrier in sufficient amounts; they directly affect the DA-dependent regulatory system at the pituitary level. In these conditions, PRL rises. An antagonism between estrogen and DA has been demonstrated at this site (24), which explains the sex-dependent differences in PRL response.

Pain may be elicited by various manipulations of the monoaminergic systems both within and outside the brain. The release and decrease of catecholamines and 5-HT induced both peripherally and centrally by reserpine is a powerful event in pain production. Less effectively, pain may be provoked by fenfluramine. Benserazide, which increases monoamines in the brain and depletes them outside the blood-brain barrier, may also elicit pain. The pharmacological properties of these drugs that have been confirmed by their endocrinological effects suggest that no single monoaminergic system may be implicated in inducing pain; rather, migraine depends on multiple alterations of neurotransmitters.

All the tested drugs induce PRL release. Our sulpiride data rule out the possibility that the hormone acts as a causative agent of pain, as previously suggested (5). The findings suggest that induction of changes in PRL secretion or pain requires different types of modifications in neurotransmitter concentrations and effects. The former responds to individual agents; it gives a direct response. To cause pain, a more complex change in neurotransmitters must be provoked. An equilibrium must be unbalanced at both central and peripheral levels. The neuroendocrinological counterpart of this situation is the alteration of pituitary reserves, which depends on continuous modulation by neurotransmitters. Their signals, stimulating or inhibiting the synthesis and release of the hormone, determine the amount of its storage. The alteration of pituitary response to pharmacological or hormonal challenges is an index of imbalance of a neurotransmitter, which exists in headache subjects as an underlying feature of the condition, even when it is not enough to give rise to pain.

REFERENCES

1. Antognetti, L., and Polleri, A. (1968): L'encefalo endocrino. In: *Trattato di Endocrinologia, Vol. II,* edited by L. Antognetti, pp. 955–1538. CEA, Milan.
2. Barbeau, A. (1977): Brain peptides and neurotransmitters. In: *Proc. 11th World Congress of Neurology, Amsterdam,* pp. 290 (Abstr.).
3. Ferrari, E., Nappi, G., Vailati, A., Martignoni, E., Bossolo, P. A., and Polleri, A. (1979): Circadian periodicity of plasma prolactin in some neurological diseases. *J. Chronobiol.,* 6:231–242.
4. Frantz, A. G. (1973): The regulation of prolactin secretion in humans. In: *Frontiers in Neuroendocrinology,* edited by W. F. Ganong and L. Martini, pp. 337–374. Oxford University Press, New York.
5. Horrobin, D. F. (1973): Prevention of migraine by reducing prolactin levels. *Lancet,* I:777.
6. Müller, E. E., and Agnoli, A. (editors) (1979): *Neuroendocrine Correlates in Neurology and Psychiatry.* Elsevier, Amsterdam.
7. Müller, E. E., Nisticò, G., and Scapagnini, U. (1977): *Neurotransmitters and Anterior Pituitary Function.* Academic Press, New York.
8. Murialdo, G., Masturzo, P., Reforzo, F., and Traldi, S. (1979): Changes in serum titres of prolactin, somatotropin and thyrotropin induced by fenfluramine in humans. *Boll. Soc. Ital. Biol. Sper.,* 55:2135–2141.
9. Murialdo, G., Polleri, A., Testa, E., Martignoni, E., Rossi, M., and Sances, G. (1979): Evaluation of pituitary function in chronic posttraumatic headache. In: *Headache, Pavia 1979,* edited by F. Savoldi and G. Nappi, pp. 45–50. Palladio, Vicenza, Italy.
10. Murri, L., Judice, A., Muratorio, A., Polleri, A., Barreca, T., and Murialdo, G. (1980): Spontaneous nocturnal plasma prolactin secretion and growth hormone in patients with Parkinson's disease and Huntington's Chorea. *Eur. Neurol.,* 19:198–206.
11. Nappi, G., Savoldi, F., Bono, G., Martignoni, E., Rossi, M., and Micieli, G. (1978): PRL response to reserpine test in migraine before and after 2-bromo-α-ergocryptine, DL-5-hydroxytryptophan and methysergide treatment. *The Migraine Trust, 2nd International Symposium,* London, pp. 42–44 (Abstr.).
12. Nappi, G., Savoldi, F., Bono, G., and Martignoni, E. (1979): Reserpine, headache and PRL release in migraine. *Headache,* 19:273–277.
13. Nappi, G., Savoldi, F., Martignoni, E., Murialdo, G., Polleri, A., and Bono, G. (1979): PRL changes in drug induced headache. In: *Headache, Pavia 1979,* edited by F. Savoldi and G. Nappi, pp. 173–183. Palladio, Vicenza, Italy.
14. Nappi, G., Savoldi, F., Martignoni, E., and Polleri, A. (1979): 24-h Prolactin secreting pattern in Huntington's disease. In: *Neuroendocrine Correlates in Neurology and Psychiatry,* edited by E. E. Müller and A. Agnoli, pp. 152–158. Elsevier, Amsterdam.
15. Nelson, W., Liang Tong, Y., Lee, J., and Halberg, F. (1979): Methods for cosinor rhythmometry. *Chronobiologia,* 6:305–323.
16. Polleri, A. (1979): Ruolo della patologia e della farmacologia neuropsichiatrica nella ricerca neuroendocrinologica. *Riv. Neurolo.,* 47:1–20.
17. Polleri, A., Gallamini, G., Barreca, T., Gianrossi, R., Masturzo, P., Murialdo, G., Nizzo, M. C., and Rolandi, E. (1979): Sulpiride effects on prolactin secretion. In: *Sulpiride and Other Benzamides,* edited by P. F. Spano, M. Trabucchi, G. U. Corsini, and G. L. Gessa, pp. 163–173. Raven Press, New York.
18. Polleri, A., Masturzo, P., Murialdo, G., Baldassarre, M., Martucci, N., Nappi, G., Savoldi, F., Muratorio, A., Murri, L., and Gasparetto, B. (1980): Cronobiology of prolactin secretion: A marker in physiology and pathology. In: *Control of Central and Peripheral Regulation of Prolactin Function,* edited by R. M. MacLeod and U. Scapagnini. Raven Press, New York *(in press).*
19. Polleri, A., Masturzo, P., Murialdo, G., and Carolei, A. (1980): Dose and sex related effects of aromatic amino acids decarboxylase inhibitors on serum prolactin in humans. *Acta Endocrinol.,* 43:7–12.
20. Polleri, A., Masturzo, P., Vignola, G., Barreca, T., and Gallamini, A. (1978): Sleep-wake differences in serum prolactin levels in children. *J. Endocrinol. Invest.,* 1:347–350.
21. Polleri, A., and Murialdo, G. (1979): The use of neuroendocrine indices in the study of headache: An introduction. In: *Headache, Pavia 1979,* edited by F. Savoldi and G. Nappi, pp. 143–147. Palladio, Vicenza, Italy.

22. Polleri, A., Murialdo, G., Martignoni, E., Nappi, G., and Savoldi, F. (1979): Benserazide induces migraine attacks, irrelevance of concomitant hyperprolactinemia. *Il Farmaco,* 34:465–468.
23. Polleri, A., Murialdo, G., Masturzo, P., Martucci, N., Palese, N., Agnoli, A., and Gasparetto, B. (1979): Spontaneous prolactin secretory patterns in depressive patients. In: *Neuroendocrine Correlates in Neurology and Psychiatry,* edited by E. E. Müller and A. Agnoli, pp. 255–261. Elsevier, Amsterdam.
24. Raymond, V., Beaubiert, M., Labrie, F., and Boissier, J. (1978): Potent antidopaminergic activity of estradiol at the pituitary level on prolactin release. *Science,* 200:1173–1175.
25. Savoldi, F., Nappi, G., and Bono, G., (1978): Lithium salts in treatment of idiopathic headaches and of facial pain syndromes. *Riv. Patol. Nerv. Ment.,* 99:4–9.
26. Savoldi, F., and Nappi, G. (1979): Contributo all 'indentificazione di sottogruppi di cefalee primarie. XXI Congr. S.I.N., Catania, 8–10 Novembre, pp. 145–181 (Atti).
27. Savoldi, F., Nappi, G., Bono, G., Gasparetto, B., Polleri, A., and Murialdo, G. (1979): Changes of 24-hour pattern of prolactin secretion in chronic post-traumatic headache. In: *Headache, Pavia 1979,* edited by F. Savoldi and G. Nappi, pp. 51–54. Palladio, Vicenza, Italy.
28. Sicuteri, F. (1977): Headaches as methonimy of non organic central pain. In: *Headache, New Vistas,* edited by F. Sicuteri, pp. 19–67. Biomedical Press, Florence.

Advances in Neurology, Vol. 33, edited by
M. Critchley et al. Raven Press, New York © 1982

Headache in Children*

G. S. Barolin

Landes Nervenkrankenhaus Valduna, Neurologische Abteilung, 6830 Rankweil, Austria

Literature on headache in children is scarce and usually treats a particular viewpoint, such as the organic reasons (8,12) or the psychological background (11,14). The present chapter is intended as an aid to clinical practice. It is based on evaluation of patients in a neurological department and an outpatient clinic. We discuss here three questions: (a) Do children in fact have headaches? (b) what kind of headaches do they have? (c) what clinical consequences may be drawn from this knowledge?

Children indeed do suffer from headaches. A young girl recently was hospitalized following a serious suicide attempt. The vomiting and collapsing that accompanied her migraine attacks were seen as an attempt to escape her field work. For many years, she suffered regular beatings for this "laziness."

EPIDEMIOLOGY

Bille (9) studied all school children of a Swedish town and clearly showed that headache is as frequent a difficulty in childhood as in adults. This demands discussion because we know that during adult life, many patients develop new headaches. It can be concluded that about one-half of our young patients tend to lose their headaches (with or without treatment) before becoming adults; thus we find about the same proportion of children and adult headache sufferers. According to our findings, the sex distribution is about the same as in adults, being equally distributed between males and females. Migraine, however, shows a distinct preponderance among females.

DIAGNOSIS

A discussion first is necessary regarding the etiology, pathogenesis, and classification of headache as used in our working group. In contrast to the complicated diagnostic scheme (10) inaugurated by the American Ad Hoc Committee (15 groups and several subgroups of headache), our diagnosis (first step) begins from the simple and purely phenomenological viewpoint that distinguishes migraine (mainly attack featured) from cephalea (mostly permanent or undulating). This differentiation is valid for both theoretical and practical reasons. In genetic studies, different modes of transmission could be found between the two groups (7); in daily practice we use different therapeutic means for the two groups (4). In both children and adults, approximately one-third of the headaches are migraine and two-thirds are of other types.

Our second diagnostic step excludes certain monosymptomatic causes for the headache. Otolaryngological and visual disturbances rank first in this respect. Constant EEG focus must lead to thorough neuroradiological examination. In not more than 10% of headache sufferers (6) can a single causal agent be found and the headache disappears by treating

---

* Abridged version.

Headache Pathogenesis

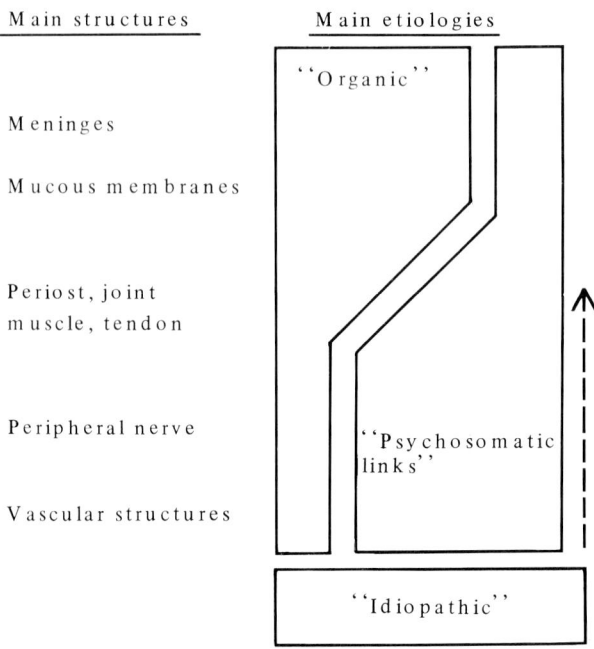

FIG. 1. Structures whose pain receptors are mainly responsible for headaches **(left). Right:** Upper two organic substrates mainly responsible for organic headaches; lower three structures are apt to form "psychosomatic bridges."

this single symptom. Considering pathophysiology, a number of structures are apt to create headaches. We do not believe in a polarity of psychogenic and nonpsychogenic headaches but that given organic structures form psychosomatic bridges between psychological conditions and physical illness, such as headache (2) (Fig. 1). Furthermore, the majority of headache sufferers must be considered of plural etiology (Table 1). Thus our third diagnostic step aims to diagnose these factors and consider them in our therapy. Several specific criteria can be considered for children. Vasolability plays a main role in infantile headache, especially during and after periods of growth. The pale, slim child may raise suspicion of vasolability; he or she should be questioned about dizziness upon awakening and feeling extremely tired. The vertebral column plays a role during childhood by hypermobility, and not by degeneration, which plays the main role in adult life. Depression is less important in children than in adults. Heredity plays a

TABLE 1. *Main etiological factors*

Heredity
Vascular function
Cervical vertebral column
Psychic factors

predominant role in infantile migraine; 50% of children with migraines have migraineurs among their parents. In contrast, in late-onset migraine (after age 45), only 5% of patients have family members with migraine (1).

DISCUSSION

The localization of headache is mostly frontal and connected with the orbits, in accordance with the findings of Bille (9).

The etiology of the headaches is variable (Table 2). True organic findings, whether in clinical neurology, radiology, or the EEG (Table 3), are few and not significant. In cephalea in children, there is a higher incidence of possible organic reasons; in migraine, there is a greater incidence of genetic transmission. (See asterisks in Table 2) Tables 4 and 5 summarize the similarities and differences between adult and infantile headaches.

TABLE 2. *Headache in children*

Possible etiological factors	Cephalea (N = 38)	Migraine (N = 28)	Total (N = 66)
Perinatal lesions	9	3	12
Trauma	6	1	7
Meningitis	2 ⎰23*	— ⎰5	2
ENT/Eyes	5	1	6
Kidney	1	—	1
Heredity	6	16*	22
None	12	8	20

TABLE 3. *Headache in children[a]*

Neurology	Radiology	EEG
Ataxia (slight) (3)	Vertebral column	Focus (8)
Hemisyndrome (slight) (2)	Straight column (few)	Spikes (7)
Occipital pressure point (1)	Hypermobility Pseudospondylolisthesis} (2)	Brain scan (14)[b] Angiography (2)[b]
	Condyls hypoplasia (1)	Pneumoencephalography (1)[b]
	Sinus opacity (few)	

[a] N = 66.
[b] Negative.

TABLE 4. *Commonalities in headaches in adults and children*

Pathophysiology/etiology
Seldom clearly monocausal, including "psychogenic"
Insignificant neurology
General incidence
Proportion cephalea versus migraine
Sex proportion
EEG abnormalities
No connection with epilepsy
Polypragmatic therapy

TABLE 5. *Headache: Adults versus children*

Factors	Children more	Adults more
Localization	Frontal	Other regions
Etiology	Heredity Perinatal defects	Vertebral column depression
Natural history	Spontaneous remission	Chronification
Release factors	Physical stress Television School	Menstruation Weather
Migraine	Combination with fever/ abdominal pains	Combination with vertigo, paresthesias

School athletics should not be excessive but gradually increased to train the underlying vasolability. Other factors in school can be responsible for headache: decompensating ocular factors, poor posture, with bent neck (vertebral column) (13), and hypoglycemia.

PROGNOSIS

A multidimensional therapeutic approach is preferred. We use the same means as in headache treatment of adults (4) but adapted to the special demands of childhood, such as (a) pharmacotherapy in lower doses and for limited periods, (b) psychotherapy, if indicated, including parents and family, (c) physiotherapy mainly coordinated with orthopedic demands and including a great deal of "normal" sport activities in order to make therapy pleasant and acceptable for children.

REFERENCES

1. Barolin, G. S. (1969): *Migräne*. Facultas Verlag, Wien.
2. Barolin, G. S. (1976): Über das Zusammenspiel pyschischer und somatischer Faktoren beim Kopfschmerz. *Fortschr. Neurol. Psychiatr.*, 44:597–614.
3. Barolin, G. S. (editor) (1977): *Kopfschmerz-Headache 1976*. Otto Spatz-Verlag, München.
4. Barolin, G. S. (1977): Medikamentöse Kopfschmerztherapie. In: *Kopfschmerz-Headache 1976*, edited by G. S. Barolin. Otto Spatz-Verlag, München.
5. Barolin, G. S., Saurugg, D., and Hemmer, W. (editors) (1975): *Kopfschmerz-Headache 1975*. Otto Spatz-Verlag, München.
6. Barolin, G. S., Schnaberth, G., Dornauer, U., Gell, G., Samella, A., and Siakos, G. (1972): Zweijahresbericht eines österreichischen Kopfschmerzzentrums. *Wien. Klin. Wochenschr.*, 84:126–130.
7. Barolin, G. S., Schnaberth, G., Dornauer, U., Gell, G., Samella, A., and Siakos, G. (1974): A field study of headache. In: *Archivos De Neurobiologia. Symposium on Headache and Migraine*, Madrid.
8. Berger, H. (1970): Kopfschmerzen beim Kind. In: *Cephalaea*. Bücherreihe der Firma Hommel, Zürich.
9. Bille, B. (1967): Juvenile headache. In: *Headaches in Children*, edited by A. Friedman and E. Harms, Charles C Thomas, Springfield, Illinois.
10. Friedman, A. (1968): Classification of headache. In: *Handbook of Clinical Neurology*, edited by Vinken and Bruyn, North Holland, Amsterdam.
11. Friedman, A., and Harms, E. (editors) (1967): *Headaches in Children*. Charles C Thomas, Springfield, Illinois.
12. Mayr, U. (1975): Über den Kopfschmerz als Leitsymptom chronischer kinderneurologischer Erkrankungen. In: *Kopfschmerz-Headache 1975*, edited by G. S. Barolin, D. Saurugg, and W. Hemmer. Otto Spatz-Verlag, München.
13. Neugebauer, H. (1975): Zum Schulkopfschmerz der Kinder. In: *Kopfschmerz-Headache 1975*, edited by G. S. Barolin, D. Saurugg, and W. Hemmer. Otto Spatz-Verlag, München.
14. Nowak-Vogl, M. (1975): Psychogene Kopfschmerzen bei kindern. In: *Kopfschmerz-Headache 1975*, edited by G. S. Barolin, D. Saurugg, and W. Hemmer. Otto Spatz-Verlag, München.

Advances in Neurology, Vol. 33, edited by
M. Critchley et al. Raven Press, New York © 1982

Multiple Aspects of Headache Risk in Children

Enrico Del Bene

Department of Clinical Pharmacology, Headache Center, University of Florence, Florence, Italy

A child's complaints of headache often are suspect. The truth is, however, that children do suffer from headaches. Epidemiological data confirm the high incidence of headache in children. Valquist (25) reported that 4.5% of 1,236 children ranging in age from 10 to 12 years and 7.4% of 1,375 children aged 16 to 19 suffered from migraine. Bille (3) found 3.9% migraine and 54.8% headache cases in a group of 8,993 children aged 7 to 15.

The study carried out by Oster (15) on 2,178 school children ranging in age from 6 to 19 years showed that 20.6% suffered from headache and 5.5% from migraine. Sillanpää and Peltonen (21) found 21% of recurrent headache and 3.8% of migraine sufferers in a group of 314 Finnish children aged 7 to 15 years. Lanzi (13) studied 246 children aged 6 to 12 years and ascertained 27.6% headache and 9.5% migraine cases. Finally, our recent study on a group of 504 11-year-old school children in Prato (Florence), using standard classification criteria, showed 21.4% headache and 3.6% migraine cases.

The data sometimes are conflicting because both the etiopathogenesis and the classification of headache have not yet been clearly defined.

HEADACHE AS A HANDICAP

At present, headache, one of the most common diseases, is considered to be a dysfunction of the antinociceptive system, having a tendency to get progressively worse. In fact, migraine attacks, rare at the beginning, become more frequent, intense, and disabling as the years go by. Serious and chronic headache usually influences a person's behavior, making him irritable, depressed, aggressive, and hostile. It also alters memory, particularly short-term memory, with harmful consequences to learning ability and self-confidence. Headache affects scholastic performance in students by altering the ability to concentrate; it may even compel the student to interrupt his studies. In adults, headache reduces working capacity and affects the patient's behavior toward his family, work, and society. In this sense, headache is a handicap, however hidden it may be. Hence it is the moral duty of a physician to direct his attention toward the numerous headache sufferers who not only are misunderstood but often fall victim to intolerance and hostility from relatives, schoolmates, or colleagues.

HEADACHE RISK IN CHILDREN

Headache represents a social disease that needs a precocious diagnosis and treatment. Thus it is useful to evaluate those headache risk (HR) factors in children that indicate a predisposition to headache. Analysis of data from observations on migrainous children shows certain clinical symptoms, such as motion sickness, cyclic vomiting, recurrent abdominal pain, limb or growing pains, dizziness, sleeping troubles, and hyperactivity, that accompany and nearly always precede headache.

Kinetosis, or motion sickness, is characterized by pallor, nausea, vomiting, and sometimes headache. Cyclic or periodic vomiting manifests itself with a weakness to vomit, which may occur suddenly as a consequence of an odor or the sight of someone vomiting or even after having heard someone talking about it; it sometimes continues for hours and may last for a few days. Prolonged emesis in children may lead to dehydration and weakness.

Recurrent abdominal pain is a painful, colic-like crisis that occurs suddenly and lasts for a few minutes or hours; it is mainly localized in the appendix or periumbilical region or spread over the entire abdomen. Children with similar painful disorders are occasionally taken to the hospital where they undergo numerous laboratory and X-ray examinations that do not reveal any abnormality; an appendectomy may be performed with no relief.

Limb or growing pains consist of intermittent and sometimes quite disabling pain localized usually in the arms or legs in children and adolescents. This pain is not articular and is occasionally accompanied by restlessness but never by redness or local swelling. It generally arises in the afternoon or evening and disappears in the morning.

Clinical recognition of dizziness is relatively easy when a child says, for example, that his head and body are whirling. Sometimes the dizziness may be accompanied by perspiration, pallor, nausea, and vomiting but not by a loss of consciousness (benign paroxysmal vertigo).

The most common sleeping troubles in young headache sufferers are agitated sleep, talking in sleep, pavor nocturnus, and occasionally, jactatio capitis and somnambulism.

Hyperactivity, an aspect of the much-debated minimal brain dysfunction (MBD), has been considered with particular attention. In 1966, the National Institute of Neurologic Diseases and Stroke Task Force I described the child suffering from MBD as a child of average or above average intelligence, with learning and behavioral disturbances scaled from moderate to serious, associated with an impairment of some of the nervous system functions concerning perception, concept formation, language, control of emotions, impulsiveness, and body motor functions (5). Because this wide and poorly delineated definition includes a vast group of children, it is useful to distinguish a few subgroups in MBD. The diagram of Venn shows three large subgroups and the combinations that may occur (Fig. 1) (22). Clinically, a hyperactive or hyperkinetic child is excessively, often uselessly, active. Hyperactive children often have a poor capacity to concentrate and a short period of attention; therefore, some authors prefer to use the term "syndrome from lack of attention" rather than "hyperactivity." Such children are impulsive, disobedient, sometimes aggressive, and often complain of central symptoms of nocipathy, i.e., headache, growing pains and recurrent abdominal pains.

The above-mentioned clinical symptoms and a family headache history represent the HR factors (Fig. 2). A child who does not complain of headache but exhibits some of the HR factors may be predisposed to headache. A family headache history, particularly when one or both parents are headache sufferers, represents the basic parameter in estimating HR, which may be slight (first degree), medium (second degree), and high (third degree). HR is calculated according to the scheme in Table 1.

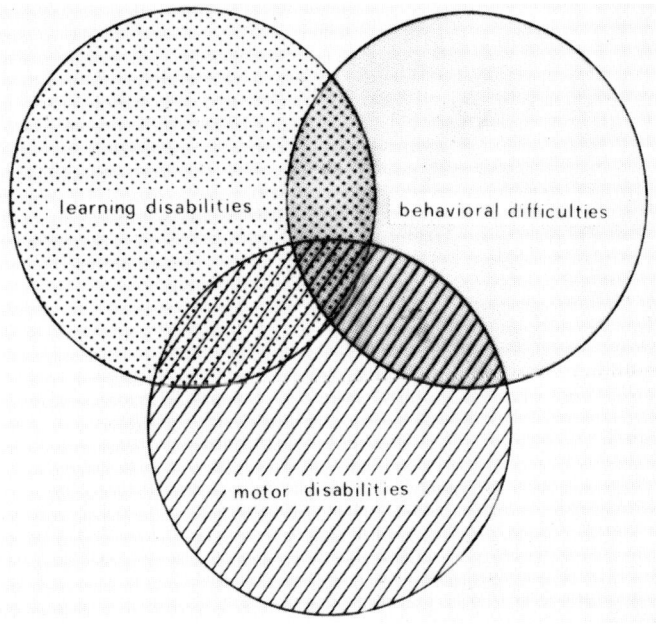

FIG. 1. Venn diagram showing the three subgroups of miminal brain damage (MBD) and their combinations (22).

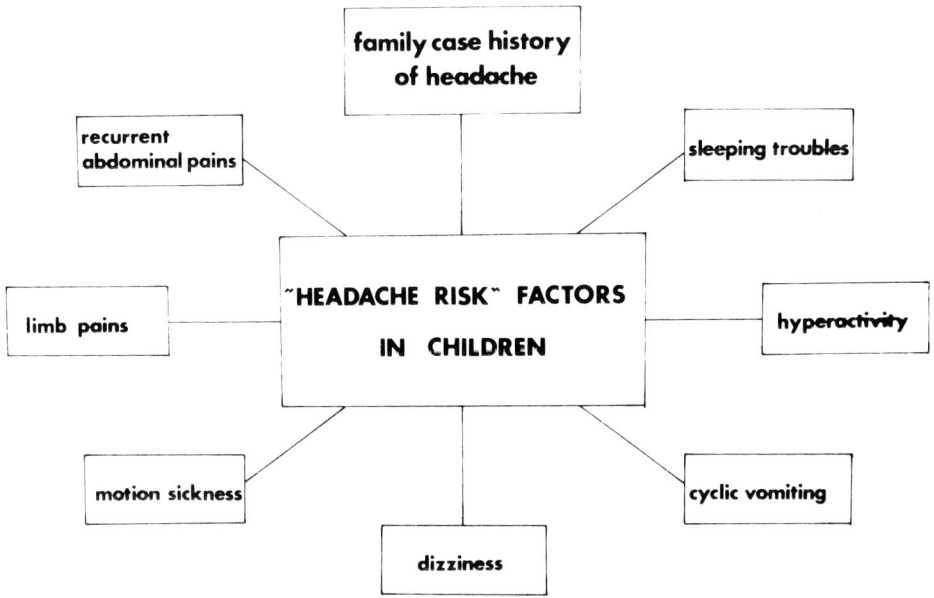

FIG. 2. Headache risk factors.

TABLE 1. *Calculation of headache risk (HR) in children*

Degree	Signs
First (slight HR)	Family headache history; without family headache history, no. of clinical symptoms of HR $\geq$ 3.
Second (medium HR)	Family headache history and no. of clinical symptoms of HR $\leq$ 2.
Third (high HR)	Family headache history and no. of clinical symptoms of HR $\geq$ 3.

EXPERIMENTAL DATA

The problem of child HR was approached from two different directions: (a) clinical and epidemiological investigations in a group of child headache sufferers and in a group of nonselected school children, and (b) pharmacoclinical research using pupillometry tests, which help us study the neuromuscular junction in iris by comparing the response to drugs in children suffering from headache, hyperactivity, and in controls.

Clinical Research

The first was carried out on 562 child headache sufferers (285 males and 277 females), ranging in age from 3 to 16 years, who were visited at the child section of the Headache Center of the University of Florence, Italy. A positive family headache history was present in approximately 80% of cases (mother sufferers, 40%; father sufferers, 20%; both parents, 20%) (Fig. 3).

Clinical symptoms, i.e., the clinical parameters of HR, determined according to data in the literature and to previous personal observations, have a high incidence in child headache sufferers. The following mean values were obtained: motion sickness, 35.3%; cyclic vomiting, 28.5%; dizziness, 19.5%; recurrent abdominal pains, 21.6%; limb pains, 20.6%; sleeping troubles, 20.3%; and hyperactivity, 15.5%. The results, according to sex, indicate a different incidence of certain clinical symptoms between males and females: recurrent abdominal pains are more frequent among girls, whereas hyperactivity or

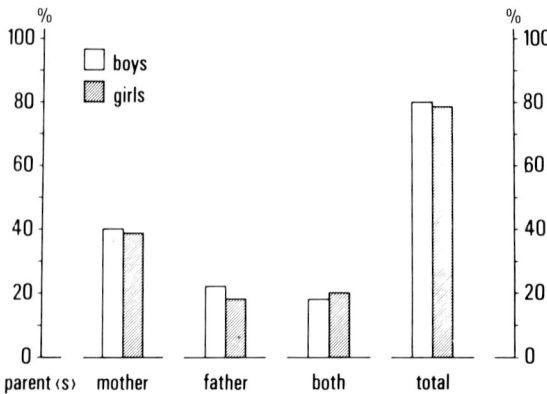

FIG. 3. Incidence of family headache history in 562 headache sufferers.

TABLE 2. *Clinical symptoms of headache risk*[a]

Symptom	Boys (%)	Girls (%)	Total (%)
Motion sickness	33.2	37.4	35.3
Cyclic vomiting	25	32	28.5
Dizziness	18	19	19.5
Sleeping troubles	19	21.6	20.3
Hyperactivity	21	10	15.5
Limb pains	18.4	22.8	20.6
Recurrent abdominal pain	15.4	25.8	21.6

[a] Incidence percentage in 562 headache sufferers (285 males and 277 females) aged 3 to 16 years.

lack of attention has a higher incidence among boys (Table 2). To support the idea that these parameters constitute HR, the percentage incidence of all these clinical symptoms was isolated in another group of children.

This research was performed on 504 11-year-old children who attended the fifth grade in Prato (Florence). They were divided into three groups: (a) headache sufferers, (b) nonheadache sufferers with no family headache history (NH,NF), and (c) nonheadache sufferers with family headache history (NH, F); this gives a clearer picture of HR. In fact, a family headache history is an HR in itself; therefore, it is better to compare the data collected from the examination of headache sufferers (group a) with data collected from nonheadache subjects with no family headache history (group b) rather than simply to compare headache sufferers with nonheadache subjects. Even more informative is the comparison of data obtained from nonheadache sufferers without family headache history (group b) with those of nonheadache sufferers with a family headache history (group c). The incidence of these groups is shown in Table 3.

The comparison between child headache sufferers and normal subjects (NH,NF) shows a statistically significant difference in motion sickness, cyclic vomiting, dizziness, recurrent abdominal pains, limb pains, and sleeping troubles. Comparing the results found in normal subjects (NH,NF) with those in nonheadache sufferers with a positive family headache history (NH,F), the differences are statistically significant with respect to cyclic

TABLE 3. *Clinical symptoms of headache risk*[a]

No.	Symptom	H (%)	NH,NF (%)	NH,F (%)
1	Motion sickness	37.3	22.9	20.3
2	Cyclic vomiting	31.7	16.3	26.4
3	Dizziness	19.8	8.4	15.6
4	Sleeping troubles	24.6	14.5	21.2
5	Hyperactivity	15.5	10.2	15.1
6	Limb pains	24.6	2.4	10.8
7	Recurrent abdominal pains	25.4	12.0	13.2

[a] Incidence percent in 504 children (263 males and 241 females; mean age, 11 years) divided into: headache sufferers (H) ($N = 126$); nonheadache sufferers and no family headache history (NH,NF) ($N = 166$), nonheadache sufferers but with no family headache history (NH,F) ($N = 212$).

H vs NH,NF: $p < 0.05$ (1,4); $p < 0.005$ (2,3,6,7); H vs NH,F: $p < 0.005$ (1,6,7); NH,NF vs NH,F: $p < 0.05$ (2,3); $p < 0.005$ (6).

vomiting, dizziness, and limb pains. Finally, when comparing headache sufferers with nonheadache subjects but with a family headache history (NH,F), statistically significant differences were observed for motion sickness, limb pains, and recurrent abdominal pains.

Clinical Pharmacology

Previous pharmacological studies on headache in adults have shown the existence of a condition of supersensitivity of some structures in the central and peripheral nervous systems. Pharmacological research carried out by using the modified Turner's method of photographic pupillometry (12,24) has shown that the supersensitivity of adrenergic receptors in the iris of adult headache sufferers is probably due to a deficiency of the neurotransmitter (norepinephrine) at that level (9).

A similar study was carried out on children suffering from headache and on hyperactive children in order to ascertain whether a similar alteration in the monoaminic turnover of hyperactivity (a probable HR factor) can be proved at a pupillary level. Thirty children were divided into three groups: (a) 15 migraine sufferers (11 males and four females) ranging in age from 7 to 15 years (mean age, 11.2 years), (b) five hyperactive children (four males and one female) ranging in age from 6 to 11 years (mean age, 7.8 years), and (c) 10 controls (six males and four females) ranging in age from 6 to 12 years (mean age, 10.1 years). One drop of a 1% phenylephrine chloride solution (an α-adrenoceptor agonist) was instilled into the right conjunctival sac. The pupillary diameter was measured before and 30, 60, 90, 120, and 150 min after conjunctival instillation and was expressed as a percentage change over pretest control values. The results of statistical analysis show a significantly greater mydriatic effect in migrainous children with respect to controls 60, 90, 120, and 150 min after phenylephrine (Table 4; Fig. 4).

Even in hyperactive children, mydriasis was significantly greater than that of controls 90, 120, and 150 min after drug installation (Table 5; Fig. 5). Such an increased phenylephrine-induced mydriasis in migrainous and hyperactive children might be due to a modified adrenergic function in the pupil (supersensitivity of sympathetic postsynaptic α-receptors and/or a reduced reuptake of the sympathetic agonist) or to an increased intrinsic cellular energy.

COMMENT

All clinical symptoms of HR, such as motion sickness, cyclic vomiting, dizziness, recurrent abdominal pains, limb or growing pains, sleeping troubles, and hyperactivity, including headache, are important aspects of pediatric pathology. Numerous studies were carried out on these symptoms, but their etiopathogenesis is still unclear.

Only a few conflicting data are available on their incidence. Apley and Naish (2) found abdominal pain in 10.8% of school children; Cullen and MacDonald (6) found that symptom in only 6% of 3,400 children, whereas cyclic vomiting was found in 3%. Lanzi et al. (14) carried out a study on migrainous, epileptic, and healthy (controls) children in whom the incidence of motion sickness, cyclic vomiting, and abdominal pain in the three groups was demonstrated: 35.5% of migrainous children complained of motion sickness, 25.5% of cyclic vomiting, and 17.6% of abdominal pain; 12% of epileptic children suffered from motion sickness, 4.7% of cyclic vomiting, and 4.7% of abdominal pain. In controls, motion sickness was seen in 14.7%, cyclic vomiting in

TABLE 4. *Phenylephrine-induced mydriasis in migrainous children*

Group	Time after instillation of phenylephrine (min)					
	30	60	90	120	150
Migrainous children mydriasis % (mean ± SE)	11.33 ± 3.34	19.73 ± 2.72	19.27 ± 3.23	15.87 ± 2.58	7.57 ± 2.94
Control children mydriasis % (mean ± SE)	4.80 ± 2.19	8.30 ± 3.34	7.30 ± 2.35	5.60 ± 2.14	0.00 ± 0.00
$t =$	1.45	2.65	2.71	2.83	2.08
$p <$	NS	0.05	0.05	0.01	0.05

Statistical analysis between migrainous and control groups ($p <$ values).

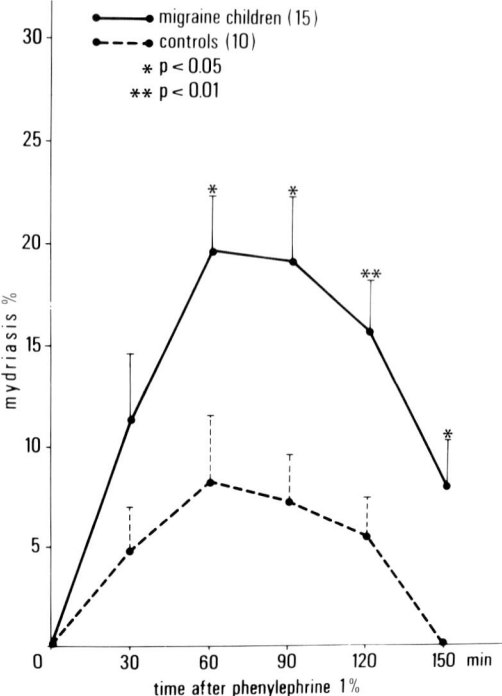

FIG. 4. Pupillary phenylephrine test in migrainous children. Phenylephrine (1%, one drop)-induced mydriasis is greater in migrainous children than in controls (mean ± SE; *p* value between migraine and control groups).

11.8%, and abdominal pain in 3%. The incidence of these symptoms is certainly greater in headache sufferers than in controls, which is in keeping with our observations although our percentages are slightly different. Oster (15) studied 2,178 subjects ranging in age from 6 to 19 years and noticed that 12.3% suffered from recurrent abdominal pains and 15.5% from growing pains; the author also noticed that abdominal pains occurred about 3 years before headache. The connection between headache and some clinical symptoms of HR is already known.

The association of cyclic vomiting, recurrent abdominal pain, and headache was first called "periodic syndrome" (28); fever was also noticed. Later, Apley (1) emphasized the association of recurrent abdominal pains, headache, and limb or growing pains. He suggested that: "these pains may be grouped together as the expression of a reactive pattern which is usually associated with emotional disturbances and is often part of a familial pattern disorder." Many authors found a significant association between cyclic vomiting, motion sickness, and headache in both children and adults (16,26). A correlation between sleeping troubles, behavioral disturbances (hyperactivity), and headache in children (7) was previously detected.

The pathogenetic interpretation of each clinical HR symptom and of its relationship with headache is difficult. These aspects of child pathology are the object of research, study, and considerable doubts, chiefly because of their indefinite etiopathogenesis. Often when a child complains of headache, recurrent abdominal pain, cyclic vomiting, or limb pain, physicians and especially pediatricians and child psychiatrists suspect a psychogenic origin. Headache is the most common clinical expression of a dysfunction in the nociceptive system, correlated to a deficiency of the pain suppressive mechanism (17). Such a disorder is functional and not organic, concerning the turnover of the aminergic

TABLE 5. *Phenylephrine-induced mydriasis in hyperactive children*

Group	Time after phenylephrine instillation (min)				
	30	60	90	120	150
Hyperactive children mydriasis % (mean ± SE)	9.00 ± 3.19	16.20 ± 5.04	26.40 ± 5.37	14.00 ± 2.53	3.40 ± 2.09
Control children mydriasis % (mean ± SE)	4.80 ± 2.19	8.30 ± 3.34	7.30 ± 2.35	5.60 ± 2.14	0.00 ± 0.00
$t =$	1.10	1.34	3.83	2.38	2.40
$p <$	NS	NS	0.01	0.05	0.05

Statistical analysis between hyperactive and control groups (p values).

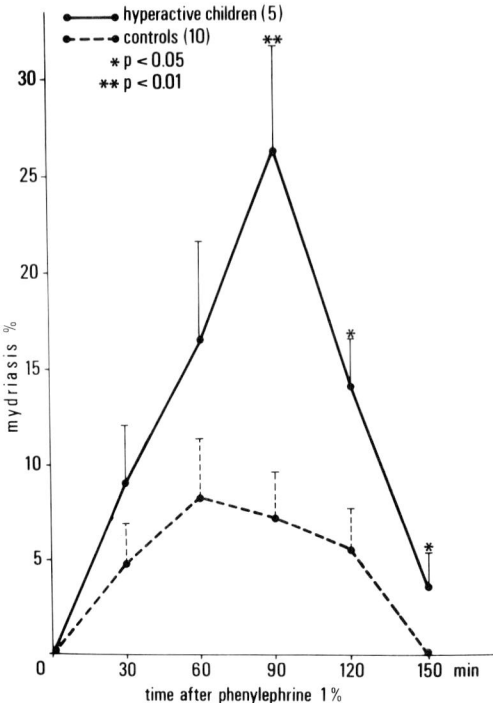

FIG. 5. Pupillary phenylephrine test in hyperactive children. Phenylephrine (1%, one drop) instillation induced a greater mydriasis in hyperactive children than in controls (mean ± SE; *p* value between hyperactive and control groups).

and peptidergic systems involved in the modulation of pain in the central nervous system (CNS). This pathogenetic interpretation of headache is also called central theory or nonorganic central pain (NOCP) (18).

Several pharmacoclinical studies have shown a particular sensitivity at both a central and a peripheral level in headache sufferers. As already known, deficient activity of any neuron results in an increase of postreceptor sensitivity. When supersensitivity is due to surgical, pharmacological, or spontaneous damage of the postganglionic tract, the resulting state of supersensitivity from denervation has high specificity characteristics. When supersensitivity depends on preganglionic damage, it is called "supersensitivity from decentralization" and is characterized by a longer latency and relative lack of specificity (4,23).

The vein supersensitivity to multiple monoamines observed in systemic NOCP patients can be labeled supersensitivity from decentralization rather than denervation (20). The increased sensitivity of α-adrenoceptors of the iris, as seen by an intense and long-lasting mydriasis after conjunctival phenylephrine, supports the supersensitivity hypothesis in adult headache sufferers (9). Such supersensitivity also has been observed in migrainous children (8). The hypermydriatic response from conjunctival phenylephrine instillation in headache and hyperactive children suggests a possible pathogenetic correlation between headache and hyperactivity. In only a few cases (1%) was there a consistent condition of pathogenetic hyperactivity (premature birth, meningeal-encephalitis, or cerebral damage from birth trauma). Instead, there is strong evidence of a functional mechanism, probably genetic in nature, of hyperactivity (27). An impairment of the monoaminergic and peptidergic neuron could be the background for headache and MBD.

Some evidence in headache sufferers shows a particular hypersensitivity of the CNS areas involved in (a) perception of pain, (b) control of arterial blood pressure, (c) vomiting, (d) thermoregulation, and (e) modulation of sexual function, behavior, and sleep (10, 11,18,19).

The headache central theory can be an interpretation for the occurrence of pain in headache and all vegetative and affective phenomena so common in migraineurs. The clinical symptoms of HR, i.e., motion sickness, cyclic vomiting, recurrent abdominal pains, limb or growing pains, dizziness, sleeping troubles, and hyperactivity, may represent a clinical manifestation of supersensitivity of certain areas of the CNS. Thus on one hand we can give a pathogenetic interpretation to many important aspects of child pathology and on the other a correlation between the clinical symptoms of HR and headache. The present clinical study shows a different incidence of HR factors between headache sufferers and controls with no family headache history. Statistical analysis shows that cyclic vomiting, dizziness, and limb pain, as well as family headache history, might be more important when assessing a child's predisposition to headache. The usefulness of HR factors enables us to single out children highly predisposed to headache, to take intensive care of them, and to initiate preventive treatment.

Finally, the pathogenetic interpretation of HR symptoms and their possible correlation with headache suggest further studies on the etiopathogenesis and therapy of different aspects in child pathology.

SUMMARY

Both epidemiological and pharmacoclinical research have been carried out on children suffering from headache. Two epidemiological trials were performed. In the first, 562 migrainous children were questioned about several clinical symptoms that affect child headache sufferers, and the incidence of these symptoms was recorded. In the second, we divided 504 nonselected school children into three groups: headache sufferers and nonheadache sufferers with or without family headache history. The same clinical symptoms were studied. Statistical analysis showed that motion sickness, recurrent abdominal pain, sleeping troubles, hyperactivity, cyclic vomiting, dizziness, and limb pain have different incidences in the three groups. These clinical symptoms and family headache history may be considered HR factors and indicate a predisposition to headache in children. The pharmacoclinical study was carried out on 15 migrainous children, five hyperactive and 10 controls. An increased sensitivity of iris adrenergic receptor in both migrainous and hyperactive children was evidenced by measuring phenylephrine-induced mydriasis.

The possible etiopathogenetic correlations among headache, hyperactivity, and other HR factors are discussed in accordance with the central theory of headache.

ACKNOWLEDGMENTS

This work was supported by a grant from the National Research Council of Rome, Italy.

REFERENCES

1. Apley, J. (1958): A common denominator in the recurrent pains of childhood. *Proc. R. Soc. Med.,* 51:1,023–1,024.
2. Apley, J., and Naish, N. (1958): Recurrent abdominal pains: A field survey of 1000 school children. *Arch. Dis. Child.,* 33:165–170.

3. Bille, B. (1962): Migraine in school children. *Acta Paediatr. Scand.* [*Suppl. 136*], 51:1–151.
4. Cannon, W. B. (1939): A law of denervation. *Am. J. Med. Sci.,* 198:737–750.
5. Clements, S. D. (1966): Minimal brain dysfunction in children: Terminology and identification. PHS Publication 1415, U.S. Department of Health, Education and Welfare, Washington, D.C.
6. Cullen, K. J., and MacDonald, W. B. (1963): The periodic syndrome. Its nature and prevalence. *Med. J. Aust.,* 50:167.
7. Del Bene, E., and Poggioni, M. (1979): Headache risk in children. *Proceedings of the IV Meeting of the Italian Headache Society,* edited by F. Savoldi and G. Nappi, pp. 231–233. Fidia Research Laboratories, Pavia, Italy.
8. Del Bene, E., Poggioni, M., and Fanciullacci, M. (1979): Supersensibilità dei recettori adrenergici pupillari in bambini cefalagici ed in bambini iperattivi. *Abstr. IV Congr. Naz. Soc. Ital. Farmacol. Clin.,* Florence, Italy.
9. Fanciullacci, M. (1979): Iris adrenergic impairment in idiopathic headache. *Headache,* 19:8–13.
10. Fanciullacci, M., Franchi, G., and Sicuteri, F. (1974): Hypersensitivity to lysergic acid diethylamide (LSD-25) and psylocybin in essential headache. *Experientia,* 30:1,441–1,442.
11. Fanciullacci, M., Michelacci, S., Curradi, C., and Sicuteri, F. (1980): Hyperresponsiveness of migraine patients to hypotensive action of bromocriptine. *Headache,* 99:20–24.
12. Galli, P., Fanciullacci, M., Monetti, G., and Assenza, E. (1976): Pupillometria bioculare per studi di farmacologia clinica. *B.S.I.B.S.,* 57:1,948–1,949.
13. Lanzi, G. (1980): *La Cefalea Essenziale nell'eta Evolutiva.* Il Pensiero Scientifico Editore, Rome, Italy.
14. Lanzi, G., Balottin, G., Rosano Burgio, F., and Ottolini, A. (1978): Mal d'auto, vomiti ciclici e dolori addominali ricorrenti come possible espressione della malattia emicrania nel bambino. *Neuropsichiatr. Infant.,* 208:1,153–1,170.
15. Oster, J. (1972): Recurrent abdominal pain, headache and limb pains in children and adolescents. *Pediatrics,* 50:429–436.
16. Selby, G., and Lance, J. W. (1960): Observations on 500 cases of migraine and allied vascular headache. *J. Neurol. Neurosurg. Psychiatry,* 23:23–32.
17. Sicuteri, F. (1976): Headache: disruption of pain modulation. In: *Advances in Pain Research and Therapy, Vol. 1,* edited by J. J. Bonica and D. Albe-Fessard, pp. 871–880. Raven Press, New York.
18. Sicuteri, F. (1977): Headache as metonymy of non-organic central pain. In: *Headache, New Vistas,* edited by F. Sicuteri, pp. 19–67. Biomedical Press, Florence, Italy.
19. Sicuteri, F., Fanciullacci, M., and Del Bene, E. (1977): Dopamine system and idiopathic headache. In: *Headache, New Vistas,* edited by F. Sicuteri, pp. 239–250. Biomedical Press, Florence, Italy.
20. Sicuteri, F., Fanciullacci, M., and Michelacci, S. (1978): Decentralization supersensitivity in headache and central panalgesia. *Research Clin. Stud. Headache, Vol. 6,* edited by A. P. Friedman, M. E. Granger, and M. Critchley, pp. 19–33. Karger, Basel.
21. Sillanpää, M. I., and Peltonen, T. (1977): Occurrence of headache amongst school children in a Northern Finnish Community. In: *Headache, New Vistas,* edited by F. Sicuteri, pp. 5–8. Biomedical Press, Florence, Italy.
22. Swaiman, R., and Wright, M. (1975): *The Practice of Pediatric Neurology.* Saunders, London.
23. Trendelenburg, U. (1966): Mechanism of supersensitivity and subsensitivity to sympathomimetic amines. *Pharmacol. Rev.,* 18:629–640.
24. Turner, P. (1975): The human pupil as a model for clinical pharmacological investigations. *J. R. Coll. Physicians Lond.,* 9:165–172.
25. Valquist, B. (1955): Migraine in children. *Int. Arch. Allergy,* 7:348–355.
26. Waters, W. E. (1972): Migraine and symptoms in childhood: Bilious attacks, travel sickness and eczema. *Headache,* 12:55–61.
27. Wender, P. H. (1972): The minimal brain disfunction in children. *J. Nerv. Ment. Dis.,* 155:55–70.
28. Wyllie, W. G., and Schlesinger, B. (1933): The periodic group of disorders in childhood. *Br. J. Child. Dis.,* 30:1–24.

Advances in Neurology, Vol. 33, edited by
M. Critchley et al. Raven Press, New York © 1982

A New Nonvascular Interpretation of Syncopal Migraine

Federigo Sicuteri, Maria Boccuni, Marcello Fanciullacci, Pietro D'Egidio, and Mara Bonciani

Department of Clinical Pharmacology, Headache Center, University of Florence, Florence, Italy

Migraine attacks may be complicated by loss of consciousness. In some of these patients, electroencephalographic patterns and efficacy of antiepileptic treatment confirm the diagnosis of epilepsy. In others, the mechanism of fainting has not been clarified. Bickerstaff (1,2) has hypothesized that the loss of consciousness is due to ischemia in brainstem provoked by a long-lasting spasm of the basilar artery (basilar artery migraine).

We suggest that the fainting phenomenon might be caused by an acute hypotension which, particularly in standing subjects, may induce a transient brain hypoxia and thus a loss of consciousness. Since headache sufferers exhibit a condition of brain (24) and extrabrain, i.e., smooth muscle of vein and iris (9), supersensitivity, a hyperresponsiveness of dopamine receptors in blood pressure regulating centers can be postulated. In fact, dopamine-dependent cells have a definite inhibiting capacity on the tonic activity of the vasomotor center. Therefore, the stimulation of these cells causes a hypotension central in origin. In general, bromocriptine, a dopamine receptor agonist acting at the central and peripheral levels, is poorly tolerated by headache sufferers (10) because of its hypotensive effect. Paradoxically, ergotamine, a vasoconstrictor agent, when given parenterally during a migraine attack, frequently provokes a collapse (12). This action can be explained in terms of a stimulation of supersensitive dopamine receptors in blood pressure regulating centers. In fact ergot derivatives are considered as powerful dopamine agonists (6).

As a working hypothesis, the loss of consciousness in migraine attacks might be due to an acute hyperresponsiveness of dopamine receptors, which inhibit the vasomotor center. We have evaluated the hypotensive response to bromocriptine and the eventual occurrence of fainting phenomena in syncopal and nonsyncopal migraine.

MATERIALS AND METHODS

Patients

The study included five healthy controls (two males, three females) ranging in age from 24 to 30 years ($\overline{X} \pm SE = 26.5 \pm 0.8$) and two groups of 15 migraine sufferers. Eight patients (two males, six females), ranging in age from 19 to 40 years ($\overline{X} \pm 31.9 \pm 2.2$) previously experienced syncopal episodes during migraine attacks; and seven patients (two males, five females), ranging in age from 17 to 43 years ($\overline{X} \pm SE = 32.4 \pm 4.1$), were free of spontaneous syncopes.

Before the beginning of the experimental procedure, the migraine sufferers (hospitalized in the Department of Clinical Pharmacology at the University of Florence) underwent clinical examinations in order to exclude any organic diseases, with particular attention to cardiovascular disorders.

Syncopal migraine patients did not exhibit neurologic signs, even during their attack periods; flashing lights in the visual fields, postural dizziness, nausea, and vomiting were occasional or frequent but present in migraineurs without syncopes as well.

Drugs

Bromocriptine (CB 154, Parlodel, Sandoz), 2.5 mg, was given in a single oral dose. Domperidone (Motilium, Janssen) was administered in an intramuscular dose of 10 mg.

Experimental Procedure

The subjects assumed a supine position 1 hr before the test and remained recumbent for the entire observation period, except for short periods of orthostasis, during which blood pressure measurements with a mercury sphygmomanometer were performed. After having measured the blood pressure in both supine and standing positions, a single dose (2.5 mg) of bromocriptine was administered orally at 8:30 A.M. During a 7-hr postbromocriptine period, blood pressure recordings were taken in supine and standing positions every hour.

All eight migraine patients with and two without spontaneous syncopes during attacks were kept in an upright position for a period of 10 min for the basal and postbromocriptine blood pressure measurements. Orthostatic blood pressure was registered at 1, 2, 4, 6, 8, and 10 min. The remaining five nonsyncopal migraine sufferers and all the controls were kept in a standing position for a period of 2 min, at the end of which blood pressure was measured before and at each hour after bromocriptine, except for the sixth hour. Clearly, if unable to stand, the patient was replaced recumbent.

When undetectable because of prefainting seizures, the systolic pressure was assigned the value of 50 mmHg, i.e., inferior to the point of critical reduction in cerebral blood flow (60 mmHg). Conventional diastolic pressure values, however, could not be defined in a rational way; therefore, the orthostatic diastolic pressure was not statistically evaluated.

Five days later, the investigation was carried out again on four migraineurs without spontaneous syncopes to study the domperidone-bromocriptine interaction. Domperidone (10 mg) was injected intramuscularly 15 min before bromocriptine in two patients and in the other two 3 hr after bromocriptine, when the hypotensive effect was at its maximum.

Statistical Analysis

The bromocriptine effect was expressed as percent change ($\Delta\%$) of blood pressure with respect to basal values. Mean values $\pm$ SE of systolic (supine and standing) and diastolic (supine only) pressure were calculated for each individual group. Student's *t*-test was employed for intergroup comparison. Student's *t*-test for paired data was used in order to verify intragroup statistical significance of blood pressure changes versus the baseline values. The χ^2 test was used in evaluating the frequency of prefainting seizures.

RESULTS

Clinical Effects of Bromocriptine

Migraine patients in both groups, free of attacks at the beginning of the test, frequently complained of characteristic headache during the period of bromocriptine effect; the pain was usually accompanied by nausea and occasionally by vomiting, postural dizziness, and prefainting seizures. Such subjective disturbances took place only in cases of a severe bromocriptine-induced hypotension; in fact, none of the migraine sufferers without significant falls in blood pressure or the control subjects without hypotensive manifestations complained of any subjective disturbances, except occasional nausea.

Blood Pressure Changes

At the first hour after bromocriptine, none of the migraine patients without previous syncopal experiences exhibited a significant blood pressure fall; the maximum hypotension, lasting usually 1 to 2 hr, was registered from 2 to 4 hr after bromocriptine.

In syncopal migraine patients, the hypotensive effect of bromocriptine was sometimes more precocious, frequently of higher severity and duration (average, 3 to 5 hr); in some, the reaction to bromocriptine was particularly exaggerated (Fig. 1).

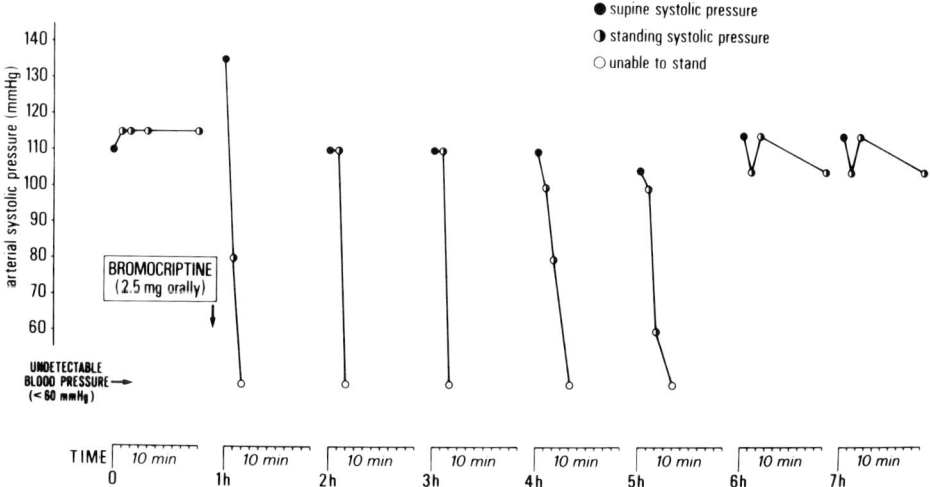

FIG. 1. Dramatic hypotensive reaction to bromocriptine in a 40-year-old woman suffering from syncopal migraine. At 1 hr postbromocriptine, a 60 mmHg fall in systolic blood pressure is observed after 1 min of orthostasis. At 2 min, the systolic pressure becomes undetectable. The patient was unable to maintain an upright position because prefainting disturbances continued to occur in the following hours. At 4 and 5 hr, the ability to stand lasted 4 min. Circulatory adjustments begin to take place 6 hr after bromocriptine administration.

TABLE 1. *Systolic pressure changes induced by bromocriptine in supine subjects*

Subjects	\Delta% Blood pressure after bromocriptine (hr)						
	1	2	3	4	5	6	7
SM[a]							
Mean values	−5.3	−8.6	−14.2	−15.8	−16.0	−12.8	−12.2
SE	4.4	2.3	2.7	4.1	3.4	4.6	4.9
p vs basal values	NS	<0.01	<0.005	<0.01	<0.005	<0.005	<0.05
NSM[b]							
Mean values	−4.9	−11.4	−14.2	−9.4	−8.8	NR[c]	−8.0
SE	2.4	3.7	4.6	3.5	3.0	NR	3.7
p vs basal values	NS	<0.025	<0.025	<0.05	<0.05		NS
Controls							
Mean values	−1.5	−0.9	−3.6	−5.5	−4.2	NR	−1.4
SE	1.4	3.1	3.6	2.9	1.9	NR	2.1
p vs basal values	NS	NS	NS	NS	NS		NS
p (SM-NSM)	NS	NS	NS	NS	NS		NS
p (SM-controls)	NS	NS	<0.05	NS	<0.05		NS
p (NSM-controls)	NS	NS	NS	NS	NS		<0.05

[a] SM, syncopal migraine patients.
[b] NSM, nonsyncopal migraine patients.
[c] NR, not registered.

In the supine position, systolic pressures of syncopal migraine sufferers fell significantly in the period between 2 and 7 hr after bromocriptine, whereas in nonsyncopal migraineurs, systolic pressure changes were not significant at 7 hr. No significant changes of systolic pressure were registered in controls. The differences in values of the two migraine groups (syncopal and nonsyncopal) were not significant; when each migraine group was compared with the control group, the differences became statistically significant (Table 1).

Diastolic pressure changes recorded when the patients were supine were observed to be irregularly significant in the two groups of migraine patients and not significant in control subjects. The differences among the three groups were not significant, except for the comparison between nonsyncopal migraine and control subjects at 7 hr (Table 2). Two minutes after orthostasis, a significant systolic hypotension was registered only in migraine patients of both groups from 2 to 7 hr after bromocriptine. The differences in values between the two groups were not statistically significant, whereas the differences between the migraine and control groups were statistically significant (Table 3).

Domperidone-Bromocriptine Interaction

When administered either 15 min before (Fig. 2) or 3 hr after, domperidone counteracted hypotension, nausea, and postural dizziness induced by bromocriptine in all four tested subjects.

Prefainting Seizures

Prefainting phenomena were constantly correlated with a fall of blood pressure in the standing position. None of the controls, six of the eight (75%) syncopal, and three

TABLE 2. *Diastolic pressure changes induced by bromocriptine in supine subjects*

Subjects	Δ% of blood pressure after bromocriptine (hr)						
	1	2	3	4	5	6	7
SM[a]							
Mean values	0.7	−3.9	−10.3	−0.9	−12.4	−5.7	−6.1
SE	5.4	4.3	6.3	6.7	4.1	6.5	6.2
p vs basal values	NS	NS	NS	NS	<0.02	NS	NS
NSM[b]							
Mean values	−5.4	−9.3	−11.4	−8.3	−6.7	NR[c]	−8.1
SE	2.9	5.2	4.3	4.9	3.5	NR	2.0
p vs basal values	NS	NS	<0.05	NS	NS		<0.05
Controls							
Mean values	4.2	1.5	0.1	−1.7	0.0	NR	1.7
SE	3.9	4.0	3.0	3.5	3.2	NR	4.5
p vs basal values	NS	NS	NS	NS	NS		NS
p (SM-NSM)	NS	NS	NS	NS	NS		NS
p (SM-controls)	NS	NS	NS	NS	NS		NS
p (NSM-controls)	NS	NS	NS	NS	NS		<0.05

[a] SM, syncopal migraine patients.
[b] NSM, nonsyncopal migraine patients.
[c] NR, not registered.

TABLE 3. *Systolic pressure changes induced by bromocriptine after 2 min of orthostasis*

Subjects	Δ% of blood pressure after bromocriptine (hr)						
	1	2	3	4	5	6	7
SM[a]							
Mean values	−10.7	−18.4	−37.7	−33.4	−33.3	−27.9	−27.8
SE	6.8	3.4	6.2	6.4	7.7	8.6	8.7
p vs basal values	NS	<0.001	<0.001	<0.005	<0.005	<0.05	<0.02
NSM[b]							
Mean values	−3.8	−22.7	−33.0	−23.4	−24.0	NR[c]	−13.7
SE	3.9	8.5	6.4	6.8	7.2	NR	2.2
p vs basal values	NS	<0.05	<0.005	<0.02	<0.02		<0.01
Controls							
Mean values	−0.8	−4.9	−3.5	−6.3	−4.6	NR	−1.5
SE	2.2	3.8	2.9	4.5	2.8	NR	2.5
p vs basal values	NS	NS	NS	NS	NS		NS
p (SM-NSM)	NS	NS	NS	NS	NS		NS
p (SM-controls)	NS	<0.025	<0.005	<0.02	NS		<0.05
p (NSM-controls)	NS	NS	<0.005	NS	NS		<0.001

[a] SM, syncopal migraine patients.
[b] NSM, nonsyncopal migraine patients.
[c] NR, not registered.

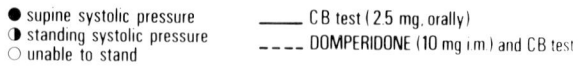

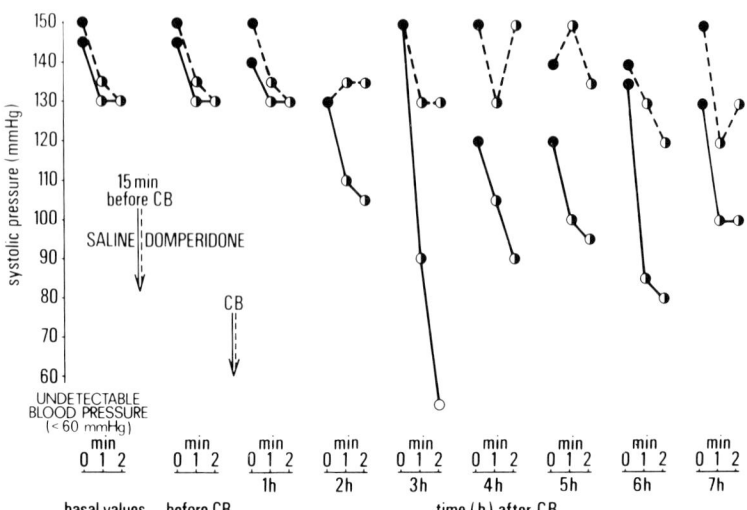

FIG. 2. Domperidone antagonism on bromocriptine (CB)-induced hypotension in a 32-year-old migrainous woman. While saline solution did not abolish the hypotensive reaction to bromocriptine, after domperidone, bromocriptine-induced hypotension did not take place. The small lowering of blood pressure observed during the antagonizing effect of domperidone is comparable to spontaneous blood pressure fluctuations in basal conditions.

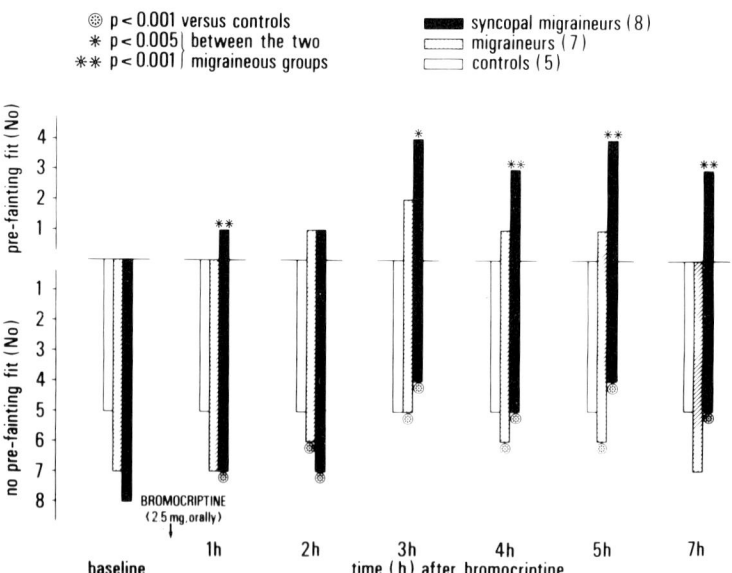

FIG. 3. Prefainting seizures analytically considered at each hour after bromocriptine. In syncopal migraine patients, they are significantly more frequent than in nonsyncopal migraineurs, except at 2 hr. At 7 hr, prefainting episodes occur only in syncopal migraine patients. Both migraine groups are statistically different from controls, who did not experience any prefainting seizures (χ^2 test).

of the seven (43%) nonsyncopal migraine patients experienced prefainting seizures after bromocriptine. The differences between the two migraine groups were statistically significant ($\chi^2 = 21.2$; $p < 0.005$). Both syncopal ($\chi^2 = 120.0$; $p < 0.005$) and nonsyncopal ($\chi^2 = 54.8$; $p < 0.001$) migraine groups showed significant differences when compared to controls.

After bromocriptine, some patients experienced more than one prefainting seizure. Therefore, the relationship between the total number of presyncopal episodes and the number of orthostatic maneuvers was evaluated. The frequency of prefainting phenomena was 33% in the syncopal and 12% in the nonsyncopal migraine groups, a highly significant ($\chi^2 = 12.7$; $p < 0.001$) intergroup difference.

The differences in frequency of prefainting seizures in syncopal ($\chi^2 = 39.5$; $p < 0.001$) and nonsyncopal ($\chi^2 = 12.8$; $p < 0.001$) migraine groups were also highly significant when compared with controls. An analysis of the frequency of prefainting seizures during each hour after bromocriptine showed significant differences between migraineurs and controls. Furthermore, the differences between the two migraine groups were also statistically significant at all hours of the test, except for 2 hr, when the number of prefainting episodes was comparable between the two groups (Fig. 3).

DISCUSSION

Idiopathic headache may be a clinical feature of a dysfunction in pain modulation attributable to a congenital disorder involving the antinociceptive neurotransmitters, endorphin and serotonin in particular (19,20). In cerebrospinal fluid sampled during migraine attacks, reduced amounts of morphine-like factors were detected (21). Therefore, a clinical and biochemical analogy between migraine and morphine abstinence was postulated (20,22). Moreover, an increased responsiveness to endogenous and exogenous monoaminergic agents has been observed in migraine as well as in morphine abstinence (22,24). The mechanism of this hyperresponsiveness is unclear. It might be regarded as an expression of receptor supersensitivity dependent on a preexisting monoamine deficiency at the postsynaptic receptor level or on an adaptive increase of cellular intrinsic energy (cyclic nucleotides) in morphine abstinence (5) and migraine (20).

Dopaminergic neurons are implicated in modulating the nociception, but it remains unclear whether dopamine participates directly or by interfering with serotonin release and turnover (28).

Mating centers are excited by stimulating dopamine receptors in animal (7,13,17); thus the sexual arousal during violent migraine attacks, detected in 10% of sufferers, may be compatible with an acute supersensitivity of central dopamine receptors regulating sexual behavior (8). Nausea and vomiting, the most common extrapain clinical phenomena in attacks, have been attributed to a supersensitivity of dopamine receptors located in the chemoceptor trigger zone. This is supported by the hyperemetic response to low doses of apomorphine, a dopamine receptor agonist, observed in migraine patients (23).

The loss of consciousness during migraine attacks might be a clinical sign of dopamine receptor supersensitivity thought to be particularly pronounced in migraineurs with spontaneous syncopes. This is compatible with the severe hypotension seen in syncopal and nonsyncopal migraineurs, when the dopamine receptors of their blood pressure regulating centers are stimulated by a dopamine agonist (bromocriptine) in doses unable to provoke hypotension in controls.

In the literature, bromocriptine was studied only in patients who used the drug for therapeutic purposes. In patients taking moderate or high doses, a mild hypotension was registered, whereas a blood pressure fall with the loss of standing ability was rarely reported (14,16,18,25–27,31).

In migraine patients, two types of reactions to bromocriptine were observed: moderate, i.e., only with a mild hypotension, and severe, i.e., with a considerable fall of blood pressure constantly associated with prefainting phenomena. This latter response was more frequent among migraine patients with spontaneous syncopes and often reached a long-lasting (hours), complete disability to stand. Since a severe response to bromocriptine was observed in some nonsyncopal migraine sufferers, the positive responses (fainting) to the bromocriptine test cannot be considered specific. Hypotension putatively correlates with the degree of the supersensitivity. Domperidone, a dopamine receptor antagonist unable to cross the blood-brain barrier, abolishes the bromocriptine-induced hypotension. This is not in contrast with the central nature of hypotension, since some blood pressure regulating centers are outside the blood-brain barrier.

The dopamine receptors regulating blood pressure are mainly located on the endings of peripheral and central adrenergic neurons. Their activation provokes a vasodilatation by inhibiting the norepinephrine release from adrenergic neurons (4,18,29,31). The possibility that bromocriptine directly stimulates dopamine receptors in arterial walls (mainly mesenteric and renal arteries) cannot be excluded (3).

Bromocriptine lowers blood pressure in migraine patients apparently without influencing peripheral sympathetic activity; during hypotension, serum dopamine-beta-hydroxylase activity remain unchanged (10). In addition, patients receiving higher doses exhibit decreased levels of norepinephrine in the cerebrospinal fluid, suggesting a central action of bromocriptine (31). Moreover, a hypotensive effect has been obtained in animals after the intracerebroventricular injection of dopamine agonist in low doses (11,15) and after dopamine application into the A_2 region of the nucleus of the tractus solitarius (30).

The peripheral activation of dopamine receptors inhibiting norepinephrine release plays a significant role in the vasodilating and hypotensive action of bromocriptine (4,18,29,31). Therefore, its involvement in provoking an exaggerated hypotensive reaction to bromocriptine in migraine patients can be postulated too.

In conclusion, the chronic supersensitivity of dopamine receptors in blood pressure regulating centers may be acutely enhanced during migraine attacks, with a resulting hypotension and, consequently, brain hypoxia and fainting. This supersensitivity, chronic in nature, spontaneously emerges during attacks and can be unmasked even in attack-free periods by a dopamine agonist (e.g., bromocriptine).

SUMMARY

Migraine sufferers who experience spontaneous syncopes (syncopal migraine) during attacks exhibit a dramatic intolerance to bromocriptine, a dopamine agonist. An oral dose of this drug renders these patients unable to stand, even for some hours, because of precipitously falling of arterial blood pressure. Treatment with domperidone, a specific dopamine receptor antagonist, abolishes the syncopal effect of bromocriptine. This evidence is compatible with a supersensitivity of those dopamine receptors, which exert an inhibiting activity and are located on blood pressure regulating centers as well as on cardiovascular sympathergic neurons.

ACKNOWLEDGMENTS

Our thanks are due to the National Research Council, Rome, Italy, for a grant; to Dr. Savik Shuster for his help in translating the manuscript; and to Mrs. Anna Bassi for typing. We wish to thank also Sandoz Ltd., Milan, Italy, for bromocriptine, and Janssen Pharmaceutica, Beerse, Belgium, for domperidone.

REFERENCES

1. Bickerstaff, E. R. (1961): Basilar artery migraine. *Lancet,* 1:15–17.
2. Bickerstaff, E. R. (1961): Impairment of consciousness in migraine. *Lancet,* 2:1,057–1,059.
3. Clark, B. J. (1977): Dopamine receptor stimulants in hypertension. *Acta Med. Scand.* [*Suppl.*], 606:95–99.
4. Clark, B. J., Scholtysik, G., and Flückiger, E. (1978): Cardiovascular actions of bromocriptine. *Acta Endocrinol.* [*Suppl. 216*], 88:75–81.
5. Collier, H. O. J. (1980): Cellular sites of opiate dependence. *Nature,* 283:625–629.
6. Corrodi, H., Fuxe, K., Hökfelt, T., Lidbrink, P., and Ungarstedt, U. (1973): Effect of ergot drugs on central catecholamine neurons: Evidence for stimulation of central dopamine neurons. *J. Pharm. Pharmacol.,* 25:409–412.
7. Da Prada, M., Bonetti, E. P., and Keller, H. H. (1977): Induction of mounting behaviour in female and male rats by lisuride. *Neurosci. Lett.,* 6:349–353.
8. Del Bene, E., and Sicuteri, F. (1979): Headache and sexual behavior. In: *Headache,* edited by F. Savoldi and G. Nappi, pp. 168–172. Fidia Research Laboratories, Abano Terme, Padova.
9. Fanciullacci, M., Del Bianco, P. L., and Sicuteri, F. (1978): Iris and vein adrenoceptors in migraine and central panalgesia. In: *Recent Advances in the Pharmacology of Adrenoceptors,* edited by E. Szabadi and C. M. Bradshaw, pp. 295–303. Elsevier, Amsterdam.
10. Fanciullacci, M., Michelacci, S., Curradi, C., and Sicuteri, F. (1980): Hyperresponsiveness of migraine patients to the hypotensive action of bromocriptine. *Headache,* 20:99–102.
11. Finch, I., and Hersom, A. (1976): Studies on the centrally mediated cardiovascular effects of apomorphine in the anaesthetized rat. *Br. J. Pharmacol.,* 56:366.
12. Franchi, G. (1979): On the circulatory collapse from ergotamine during migraine attacks: A clinical pharmacological contribution. In: *Headache,* edited by F. Savoldi and G. Nappi, pp. 240–244. Fidia Research Laboratories, Abano Terme, Padova.
13. Gessa, G. L., and Tagliamonte, A. (1974): Role of brain monoamines in male sexual behaviour. *Life Sci.,* 14:425–436.
14. Greenacre, J. K., Teychenne, P. F., Petrie, A., Calne, D. B., Leigh, P. N., and Reid, J. L. (1976): The cardiovascular effects of bromocriptine in parkinsonism. *Br. J. Clin. Pharmacol.,* 3:571–574.
15. Heise, A. (1976): Hypotensive action by central alpha-adrenergic and dopaminergic receptor stimulation. In: *New Antihypertensive Drugs,* edited by A. Scriabine and C. S. Sweet, p. 144. Spectrum, New York.
16. Kaye, S. B., Shaw, K. M., and Ross, E. J. (1976): Bromocriptine and hypertension. *Lancet,* 1:1,176–1,177.
17. Meyerson, B. J. (1964): Central nervous monoamines and hormone induced estrus behavior in the sprayed rat. *Acta Physiol. Scand.* [*Suppl. 241*], 63:1–32.
18. Nilsson, A., and Hökfelt, B. (1978): Effect of the dopamine agonist bromocriptine on blood pressure, catecholamines and renin activity in acromegalics at rest, following exercise and during insulin induced hypoglycemia. *Acta Endocrinol.* [*Suppl. 216*], 88:83–96.
19. Sicuteri, F. (1978): Mini-review, endorphines, opiate receptors and migraine headache. *Headache,* 17:253–257.
20. Sicuteri, F. (1979): Headache as the most common disease of the antinociceptive system: Analogies with morphine abstinence. In: *Advances in Pain Research and Therapy, Vol. 3,* edited by J. J. Bonica, pp. 359–365. Raven Press, New York.
21. Sicuteri, F., Anselmi, B., Curradi, C., Michelacci, S., and Sassi, A. (1978): Morphine-like factors in CSF of headache patients. In: *Advances in Biochemical Psychopharmacology. Vol. 18, Endorphins,* edited by E. Costa and M. Trabucchi, pp. 363–366. Raven Press, New York.
22. Sicuteri, F., Del Bianco, P. L., and Anselmi, B. (1979): Morphine abstinence and serotonin supersensitivity in man: Analogies with migraine mechanism. *Psychopharmacology,* 65:205–209.
23. Sicuteri, F., Fanciullacci, M., and Del Bene, E. (1977): Dopamine system and idiopathic headache. In: *Headache New Vistas,* edited by F. Sicuteri, pp. 239–250. Biomedical Press, Florence.
24. Sicuteri, F., Fanciullacci, M., and Michelacci, S. (1978): Decentralization supersensitivity in headache and central panalgesia. In: *Research in Clinical Study of Headache, Vol. 6,* edited by A. P. Friedman, M. E. Granger, and M. Critchley, pp. 19–33. Karger, Basel.
25. Stumpe, K. O., Kolloch, R., Higuchi, M., Krück, F., and Vetter, H. (1977): Hyperprolactinaemia and antihypertensive effect of bromocriptine in essential hypertension. *Lancet,* 2:211–214.

26. Teychenne, P. F., Calne, D. B., Leigh, P. N., Greenacre, J. K., Reid, J. L., Petrie, A., and Bamji, A. N. (1975): Idiopathic parkinsonism treated with bromocriptine. *Lancet,* 2:473–476.
27. Thorner, M. O., Chait, A., Aitken, M., Benker, G., Bloom, S. R., Mortimer, C. H., Sanders, P., Mason, A. S., and Besser, G. M. (1975): Bromocriptine treatment of acromegaly. *Br. Med. J.,* 1:299–303.
28. Tulunay, F. C., Sparber, S. B., and Takemori, A. E. (1975): The effect of dopaminergic stimulation and blockade on the nociceptive and antinociceptive responses of mice. *Eur. J. Pharmacol.,* 33:65–70.
29. Van Loon, G. R., Sole, M. J., Bain, J., and Ruse, J. L. (1979): Effects of bromocriptine on plasma catecholamines in normal men. *Neuroendocrinology,* 28:425–434.
30. Zandberg, P., De Jong, W., and De Wied, D. (1979): Effect catecholamine-receptor stimulating agents on blood pressure after local application in the nucleus tractus solitarii of the medulla oblongata. *Eur. J. Pharmacol.,* 55:43–56.
31. Ziegler, M. G., Lake, C. R., Williams, A. C., Teychenne, P. F., Shoulson, I., and Steinsland, O. (1979): Bromocriptine inhibits norepinephrine release. *Clin. Pharmacol. Ther.,* 25:137–142.

Advances in Neurology, Vol. 33, edited by
M. Critchley et al. Raven Press, New York © 1982

Sexuality and Headache

Enrico Del Bene, *Carlo Conti, Marco Poggioni, and
Federigo Sicuteri

*Department of Clinical Pharmacology, Headache Center and *Sexuality Section,
University of Florence, Florence, Italy*

In cases of serious headache, there is a hyperreactivity of centers or structures subserving the mechanisms of appetite, vomiting, thermoregulation, hallucinations, diuresis, and blood pressure regulation. It is exhibited by either spontaneous manifestations or direct stimulation with specific drugs (14). Even the mating centers in the central nervous system, which control sexual behavior, show a state of supersensitivity. Some characteristics of sexual arousal in headache sufferers include: (a) lack of spontaneity, (b) accompanied by erotic fantasies, (c) usually experienced at the end of a headache attack (e.g., fever and vomiting), and (d) considered due to a hypersensitivity from poor endorphin modulation of the mating centers.

As demonstrated previously, enkephalin in cerebrospinal fluid decreases critically or disappears completely during migraine attacks (10); naloxone, a morphine antagonist, strongly arouses copulatory behavior in sexually inactive but not in active rats (4,8,9). Endorphins, on the other hand, are strong sexual inhibitors. Parachlorophenylalanine (PCPA), an inhibitor of serotonin synthesis, when given to carcinoid patients and impotent subjects (both groups of nonheadache sufferers), is unable to provoke sexual arousal and the occurrence of pain (1,3,15). In sexually deficient headache sufferers, PCPA elicits an arousal of sexual activity particularly intense if associated with monoamine oxidase (MAO) inhibitors, L-DOPA, or testosterone (2,12,13). These pharmacological manipulations are carried out in order to reduce 5-hydroxytryptamine (5-HT), intended as a mating center inhibitor, and to enhance dopamine, a stimulator, in such a way as to obtain the maximum activity of sexual nervous structures; this has been demonstrated in animals (5–7).

The sexual activity of 16 sexually deficient headache sufferers has been estimated by the number of total penis erections (Fig. 1). During treatment with oral and parenteral placebo for a period of 10 days, only seven erections were registered. In the second 10-day period when oral PCPA was given with intramuscular placebo, 13 erections were counted; when the oral PCPA treatment was associated with intramuscular testosterone, an appreciable increase, 47 erections, was registered. It is noteworthy that all these patients, because of their sexual deficiencies, were previously treated with testosterone without any results. The correlations between sex and pharmacological interactions in sexually deficient headache sufferers are reported in Fig. 2, which presents (a) the basic conditions of headache sufferers, (b) the slight sexual arousal observed when 5-HT levels

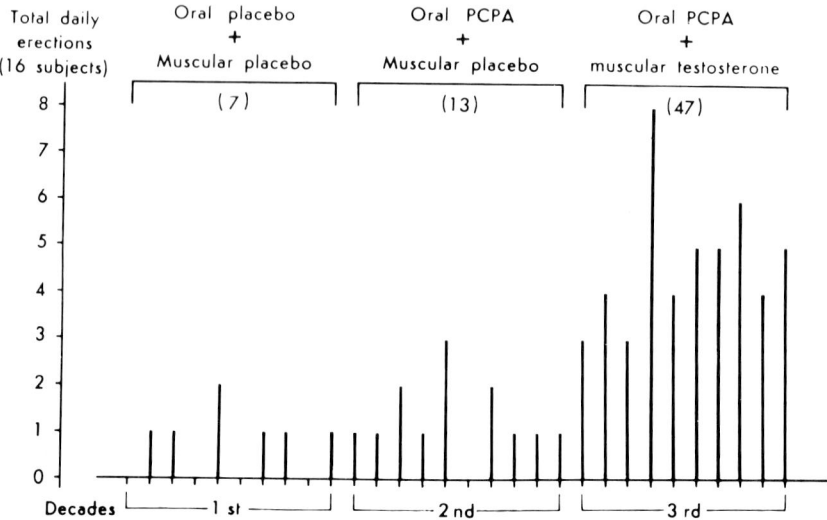

FIG. 1. Sexual activity (experienced by number of erections) by treatment with placebo, parachlorophenylalanine (PCPA), and PCPA plus testosterone, each for a 10-day period (decade) in sexually deficient headache sufferers. Only in the third period (oral PCPA plus muscular testosterone) is the number of erections significantly greater than that of the other two periods.

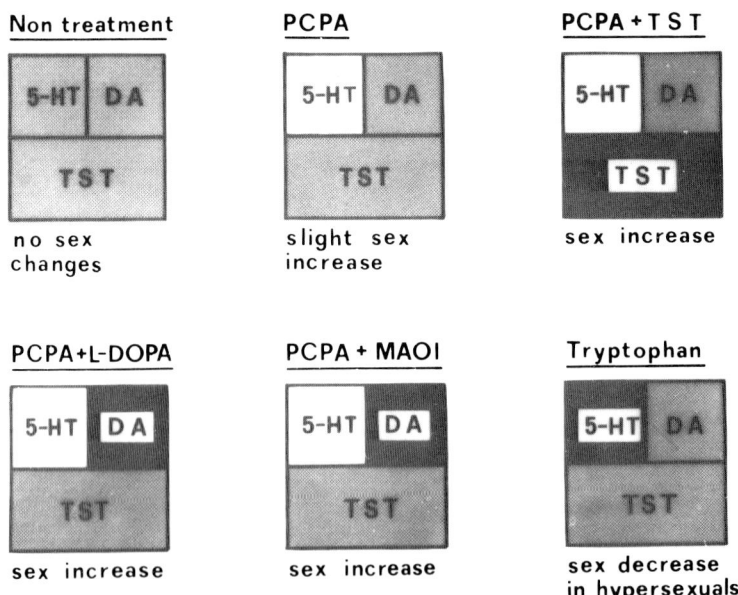

FIG. 2. Pharmacological interactions between plasma testosterone and drugs that affect the monoamine brain concentrations in sexual relationships of headache sufferers.

are lowered by PCPA, and (c) an increase of sexual activity registered when plasma testosterone levels are increased by the addition of testosterone propionate to PCPA. The same sexual stimulating effect is evident in these PCPA-treated subjects when dopamine concentrations are increased by administering L-DOPA or MAO inhibitors. Moreover, in a few cases of sexual hyperactivity in headache sufferers, tryptophan is administered, resulting in an improvement of headache and a normalization of excessive sexual desire.

The disorders of nociception, anhedonia and vegetative imbalance are present only in two syndromes (11): a spontaneous one (headache) and a pharmacologically induced one (morphine abstinence). There are many clinical signs common to both morphine abstinence crisis and migraine attack, such as anxiety, insomnia, lacrimation, rhinorrhea, nausea, and vomiting; another common element is sexual arousal.

CLINICAL ASPECTS

Questioning 362 migraine sufferers revealed sexual arousal in 9% of the females and 14% of the males (Fig. 3). Sexual excitment was more frequent and intense at the end of serious migraine attacks; this desire usually rises also at the end of morphine abstinence crisis. PCPA induces sexual arousal only in headache sufferers and not in impotent, nonheadache subjects. This can be an index of a fragile 5-HT turnover in headache patients. On the other hand, spontaneous sexual arousal during a violent attack might indicate a supersensitivity of the mating centers to dopamine, perhaps secondary to a local endorphin deficiency.

A 38-year-old woman suffering from a typical ophthalmic and hyperpyretic migraine is one of the most significant examples of sexual arousal during headache attack. She was disturbed by an intense sexual arousal, with the desire for intercourse or masturbation during the entire period of the attack. In the attack-free period, the sexual stimulus is slight or absent. One of the most dramatic examples of sexual arousal during violent migraine attack is reported by a 41-year-old male university teacher. The aura of 1 hr characterized by yawning, somnolence, and anxiety is followed by the attack, with typical clinical signs: headache, nausea, vomiting, diarrhea, sensorial hyperesthesia, hot and cold "flashes," gooseflesh, perspiration, oliguria, lacrimation, 3-hr sexual arousal, sometimes spontaneous orgasm, and finally polyuria and sleep. This clinical picture is strikingly identical to the one observed in morphine abstinence.

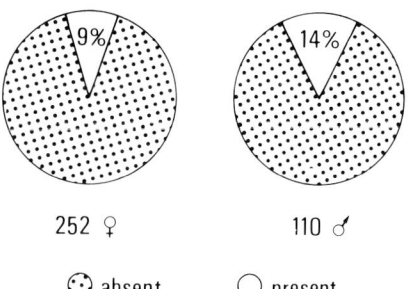

FIG. 3. Percentual incidence of subjects (in 362 migraine headache sufferers) with sexual arousal during attack.

CLINICAL INVESTIGATION BY USING A QUESTIONNAIRE

A statistical empirical research was carried out in order to study the influence headache may have on sexuality in subjects leading a normal life. A questionnaire was given before pharmacological treatment to 16 subjects (eight women) suffering from migraine and to 16 controls (eight women). All patients and controls were similar in age, work, education, and, apparently, type of partner. The questionnaire was designed to cover 1 month and was planned in such a way as to allow the subjects to list each experience (coitus, masturbation, sexual excitement, fantasies, erotic dreams), eventual headache attacks, and sleeping time. The aim was to correlate eventual sexual activity and sleep. The mean age of female headache sufferers was 34 years (range, 20 to 50 years); that of male sufferers was 38 years (range, 23 to 46 years). Because of the small number of subjects, we did not subdivide them according to age. In both groups, six subjects were married, and two had a stable relationship without cohabitation. All subjects were allowed sexual intercourse. The results, taken as a mean number for each subject within 1 month, are reported in Table 1.

When comparing the questionnaires of female headache sufferers with those of healthy controls, one can observe that the number of coiti, either orgasmic or nonorgasmic, was not significantly different between the two groups (14.75 versus 13.37). The number of erotic dreams (3.25 versus 4.87) and the number of sleeping hours (8.7 versus 8.8) for each subject in a month were similar. The number of coiti and the orgasmic response are not influenced by headache. This could be caused either by an insignificant inference of this factor or by a greater importance of sociocultural and relationship factors. Mastur-

TABLE 1. *Clinical investigations on sexuality in 16 headache sufferers and 16 controls*[a]

Mean no. per subject in a 30-day period	Females		
	Headache sufferers (mean age, 34 years)	Healthy controls (mean age, 35 years)	Statistical analysis
Coitus	14.75	13.37	NS
Masturbation	2.12	5.62	$p < 0.05$
Sexual excitement and fantasies	24.37	17.50	$p < 0.05$
Erotic dreams	3.25	4.87	NS
Sleeping hours	8.7	8.8	NS
	Males		
	(mean age, 38 years)	(mean age, 36 years)	
Coitus	10.62	11.00	NS
Masturbation	0.37	3.75	$p < 0.05$
Sexual excitement and fantasies	14.12	22.00	$p < 0.05$
Erotic dreams	4.12	4.50	NS
Sleeping hours	8.0	8.1	NS

bation, however, is significantly less frequent in female headache sufferers than in controls (2.12 versus 5.62). Likewise, the number of coiti is not significantly different between the two male groups (headache sufferers and controls). Masturbation and moments of sexual excitement, evidenced by the number of erections, are significantly less frequent in headache sufferers that in controls (0.37 versus 3.75; $p < 0.05$). These facts point to an evident decrease of sexual desire sometimes present in male headache sufferers.

CONCLUSIONS

Sexual arousal during headache attacks reported in about 10% of patients might be correlated to a supersensitivity of the mating centers, as suggested for all vegetative disorders. Sexual arousal is encountered in cases of morphine abstinence. Numerous clinical analogies, as well as biochemical (lowering of morphine-like factors) and receptoral (peripheral 5-HT supersensitivity) ones, have suggested that the mechanism of headache may be similar to that of morphine abstinence (11).

No definite conclusion can be drawn from the data obtained from clinical investigation on sexuality in headache sufferers because of the limited number of cases examined; also, we have not yet analyzed whether there are significant differences in the sexual experiences of each group over a longer period of time (more than 30 days). An interesting aspect is the relationship between sexual experience and eventual migraine attacks. The number of coiti experienced by migraineurs is the same as that of controls, while the frequency of masturbation is reduced; the headache sufferer may be less inclined to masturbate (perhaps because he fears the consequent onslaught of a headache attack or because of a general state of depression). The number of coiti seems to depend more on sociocultural and relationship factors.

Why erotic fantasies and sexual arousal in women are more frequent among migraineurs, while in men they are more frequent among controls, is unclear. Another aspect is the interruption of a headache attack by sexual intercourse. A strong emotion (sexual in this case) may activate the natural analgesic system; in fact, the analgesic effect of coitus is commonly known.

Some headache sufferers complain of sexual deficiency, which may be due to a marked depression sometimes occurring in cases of chronic headache. In these subjects, drugs acting on the turnover of amines and peptides at the central level could be useful as efficient therapeutic agents.

SUMMARY

Ten percent of 362 headache sufferers reported sexual arousal during migraine attack. Clinical investigations on sexuality in 16 headache sufferers, according to some studies showing correlations between idiopathic headache and sexual behavior, were performed. Patients responding by questionnaire listed each sexual experience, headache attack, and number of sleeping hours every day for 1 month.

In both men and women, the number of coiti, erotic dreams, and sleeping hours were similar in headache sufferers and controls, while the frequency of masturbation was significantly reduced in the former. Sexual excitement and fantasies appeared more often in female headache sufferers than in controls, while the opposite occurred in the male group.

Among the clinical analogies between the crises of migraine and morphine abstinence, sexual arousal may be included.

REFERENCES

1. Benkert, O. (1975): Clinical studies on the effects of neurohormones on sexual behavior. In: *Sexual Behavior: Pharmacology and Biochemistry,* edited by M. Sandler and G. L. Gessa, pp. 297–305. Raven Press, New York.
2. Del Bene, E., and Sicuteri, F. (1979): Headache and sexual behavior. *Proceedings of the IV Meeting of the Italian Headache Society,* edited by F. Savoldi and G. Nappi, pp. 168–172. Fidia Research Laboratories, Pavia, Italy.
3. Engelman, K., Lovenberg, W., and Sjoerdsma, A. (1967): Inhibition of serotonin synthesis by parachlorophenylalanine in patients with the carcinoid syndrome. *N. Engl. J. Med.,* 21:1,103–1,108.
4. Gessa, G. L., Paglietti, E., and Pellegrini-Quarantotti, B. (1979): Induction of copulatory behaviour in sexually inactive rats by naloxone. *Science,* 204:203–205.
5. Gessa, G. L., and Tagliamonte, A. (1974): Role of brain monoamines in male sexual behaviour. *Life Sci.,* 14:425–436.
6. Gessa, G. L., and Tagliamonte, A. (1975): Role of brain serotonin and dopamine in male sexual behaviour. In: *Sexual Behavior: Pharmacology and Biochemistry,* edited by M. Sandler and G. L. Gessa, pp. 117–128. Raven Press, New York.
7. Meyerson, B. J. (1964): Central nervous monoamines and hormone induced estrous behaviour in the spayed rat. *Acta Physiol. Scand. [Suppl. 241],* 63:5–12.
8. Meyerson, B. J., and Terenius, L. (1977): Endorphine and male sexual behaviour. *Eur. J. Pharmacol.,* 42:191–192.
9. Pellegrini-Quarantotti, B., Paglietti, E., Bonanni, M., Petta, M., and Gessa, G. L. (1978): Naloxone shortens ejaculation latency in male rats. *Experientia,* 35:524–525.
10. Sicuteri, F. (1978): Mini-review, endorphins, opiate receptors and migraine-headache. *Headache,* 17:253–257.
11. Sicuteri, F. (1979): Headache as the most common disease of the antinociceptive system: Analogies with morphine abstinence. In: *Advances in Pain Research and Therapy, Vol. 3,* edited by J. J. Bonica, J. C. Liebeskind, and D. G. Albe-Fessard, pp. 359–365. Raven Press, New York.
12. Sicuteri, F., Del Bene, E., and Anselmi, B. (1975): Aphrodisiac effect of testosterone in parachlorophenylalanine-treated sexually deficient men. In: *Sexual Behavior: Pharmacology and Biochemistry,* edited by M. Sandler and G. L. Gessa, pp. 335–339. Raven Press, New York.
13. Sicuteri, F., Del Bene, E., and Fonda, C. (1976): Sex, migraine and serotonin interrelationships. *Monogr. Neural Sci.,* 3:94–101.
14. Sicuteri, F., Fanciullacci, M., and Michelacci, S. (1978): Decentralization supersensitivity in headache and central panalgesia. *Res. Clin. Stud. Headache,* 6:19–33.
15. Sjoerdsma, A., Weissbach, H., Terry, L. L., and Underfriend, S. (1957): Futher observations on patients with malignant carcinoid. *Am. J. Med.,* 23:5–15.

Advances in Neurology, Vol. 33, edited by
M. Critchley et al. Raven Press, New York © 1982

Menstrual Headache

Giovanni Nattero

Headache Center, Institute of Internal Medicine, Turin University, Turin, Italy

About 30% of women suffer from symptoms in the few days preceding each menstrual period. According to many authors (10,11), the association of headache with the sexual rhythm can be found in 60% of female migraine sufferers. Many authors correlate this vasomotor disorder with changes in sex hormone levels (25). Water retention, suggested by oliguria and weight gain, which often herald an attack, and by diuresis and weight loss, which usually accompany recovery, were investigated. Headache is often typical migraine. Nevertheless, some authors (4) expressed doubts about the migrainous nature of the headache; the problem requires reexamination.

STATISTICAL INCIDENCES

A preliminary general investigation was carried out at the Headache Center of the University of Turin (15), in which 1,955 headache sufferers were examined. The major incidence of headache occurred in women (68%); the periods of onset usually are during adolescence (44%) and maturity (37%); accessionality prevails in 60% of the cases. With respect to the hormonal stages in the female absence of premenstrual tension was found in 54%, a chronological connection with menstruation in 55%, no evidence of headache during pregnancy in 78%, a worsening of the headache in 47% of the cases after menopause. All possible correlations existing between the more typical elements of migraine were screened (Fig. 1) by calculating the relative coefficients of correlation at a high significance level. A positive correlation exists between menstrual headache and the absence of headache during pregnancy, and between absence of headache in pregnancy and headache lasting a few days. Recent statistical and mathematical data obtained in a series of 720 women with migraine (21) showed that, in accordance with the parameters elucidated in Table 1, χ^2 analysis within the group revealed two populations: with (a) menstrual and (b) nonmenstrual migraine. In addition, there were statistically significant differences between them with regard to pattern, familial background, history of headache, premenstrual stress, relationship with menstruation and pregnancy, duration of crises, frequency, topography, site, and accompanying symptoms ($p < 0.001$). The presence of such highly significant differences with respect to parameters typical of headache indicates that menstrual headache should be treated as a distinct clinical and/or nosological entity.

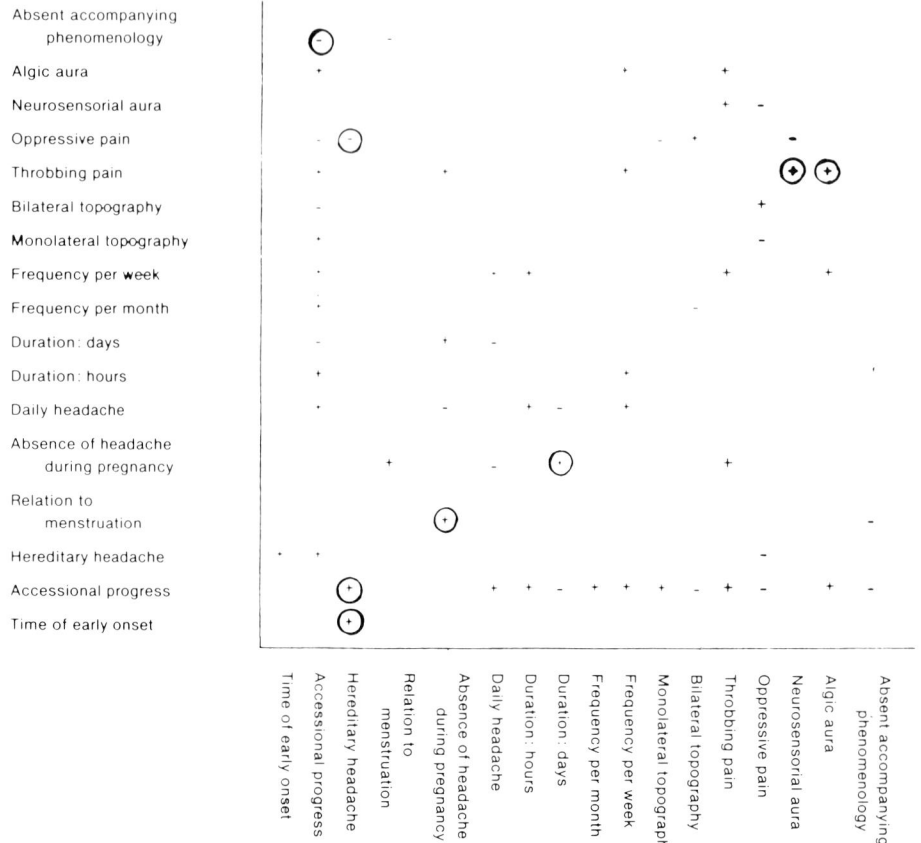

FIG. 1. This screening was done by calculating the relative coefficients of correlations at a high significance level. A positive correlation exists between menstrual headache and the absence of headache in pregnancy and between absence of headache in pregnancy and headache lasting a few days.

BIOCHEMICAL AND CLINICAL ASPECTS

A group of migrainous women, 18 to 42 years of age, with no past or present disease, with regular menses and chronological onset of the premenstrual attack, was studied at our center (18). During this period, patients were kept on a controlled diet.

Hemodynamic Data

By means of the dynamographic method (12), sphygmic waves were recorded during the attack and then compared with those taken during the headache-free period. In eight cases, various hemodynamic changes were recorded during the premenstrual attack in both the affected and pain-free sides.

The constant data observed during a monolateral crisis were the following: a lowering of the systodiastolic ophthalmic pressure on the pain-affected side and, simultaneously,

TABLE 1. *Parameters*

1. Age of onset: prior to puberty, adolescence, senility.
2. Pattern: episodic, continuous, mixed.
3. Familial history of headache: yes, no.
4. Familial history of nervous diseases: yes, no.
5. Psychoneurosis: yes, no, psychic trauma.
6. Premenstrual stress: yes, no.
7. Relationship with menstruation: yes, no.
8. Pregnancy: unchanged, improved, exacerbated, appeared afterward, no pregnancy.
9. Menopause: unchanged, improved, exacerbated, no menopause.
10. Onset: diurnal, nocturnal, varying.
11. Duration of crises: hours, days, until medication.
12. Frequency: monthly, weekly, daily, varying.
13. Site: unilateral, bilateral, spread.
14. Location of pain: generalized, localized.
15. Type of pain: throbbing, dull, various.
16. Associated symptoms: yes, no.
17. Placebo test: positive, negative.
18. Trinitrine test: positive, negative.

an increase of the bilateral diastolic temporal pressure (Fig. 2). These results are in agreement with Pichler's ophthalmodynamographic data (24), observed during spontaneous or pharmacologically induced migraine attacks.

To detect flow changes occurring during the acute pain phase of the premenstrual attack, a biodirectional doppler ultrasound device was applied to a selected group of eight migraineurs, four of whom were suffering from menstrual migraine (22). During a monolateral migraine attack, the rate flow of the temporal artery on the pain-affected side appeared modified in comparison with the contralateral side. Artery flow in 75% of cases was reduced in 50% and increased in 50% of these cases. In all these patients, the flow of the supraorbital artery on the pain-affected side appeared modified but with an inverted relationship with the temporal artery changes. When the temporal flow is increased, the supraorbital flow appears decreased, and vice versa. In the facial artery, a behavior unidirectional with that of the supraorbital artery was noticed in 62% of cases (Fig. 3).

On the basis of these observations, we can conclude that there is a certain vascular and extracranial component in menstrual headache that can be considered as a headache of migraine type.

Biochemical Data

In this connection, the increase of vanillylmandelic acid (VMA) excretion during the menstrual attack lasting 24 hr appears significant (18). This difference is statistically significant (Fig. 4). Our results are in agreement with the data of other authors, including Curran et al. (7) and Curzon et al. (8), who observed an increased VMA excretion during the first stages of spontaneous or pharmacologically induced migraine attacks. 5-Hydroxyindoleacetic acid (5-HIAA) is always lowered during the 24-hr attack periods; this difference, however, is not statistically significant.

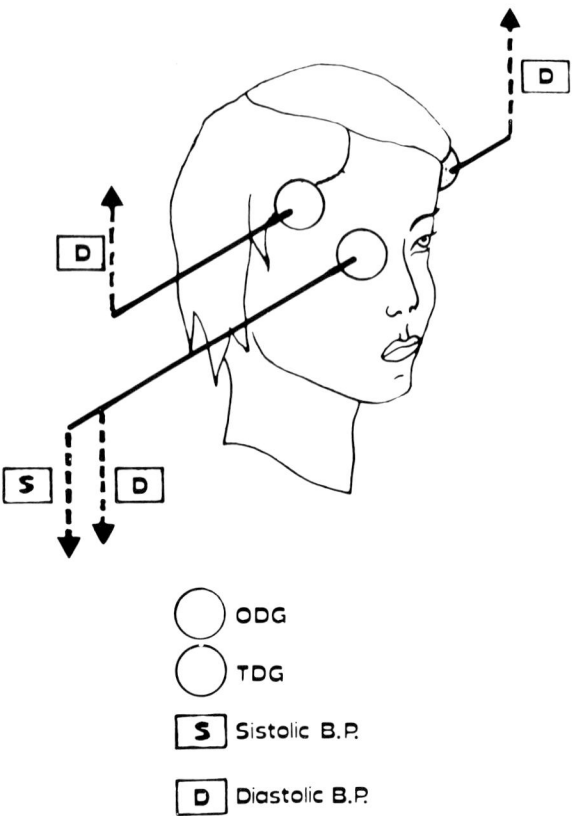

○ ODG

○ TDG

S Sistolic B.P.

D Diastolic B.P.

FIG. 2. Constant data observed during a monolateral crisis; lowering of the systodiastolic ophthalmic pressure on the pain-affected side and, simultaneously, increase of the bilateral diastolic temporal pressure.

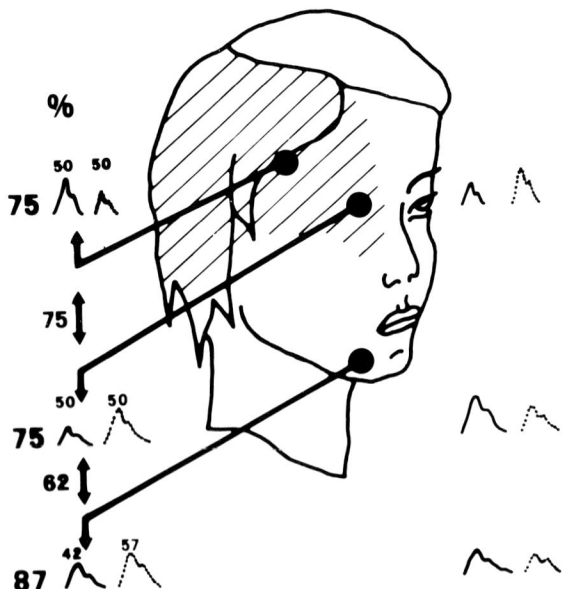

FIG. 3. Doppler measurements of flow signals taken over the terminal branches of the internal and external carotid arteries. When temporal flow is increased, supraorbital flow appears decreased, and vice versa.

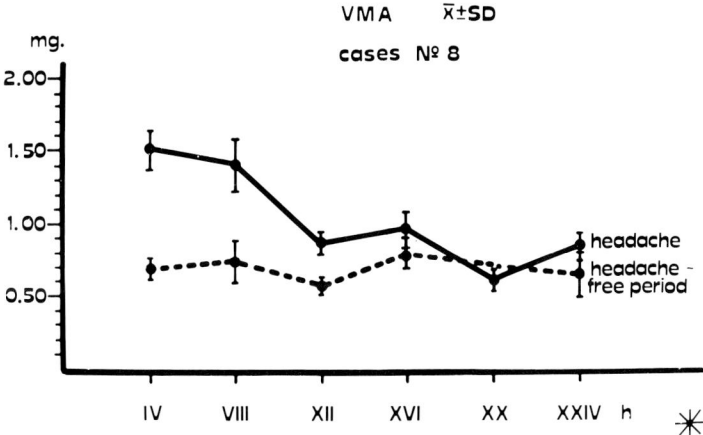

FIG. 4. Average values obtained by means of fractional urinary tests taken at 4-hr intervals of VMA urinary excretion during premenstrual crisis, in comparison with values obtained in headache-free period. Total VMA excretion is always increased during attacks; this difference is statistically significant.

Clinical-Pharmacological Data

Vasoactive substances have long been suspected to be of importance in the genesis of migraine. Sera from premenstrual migraine sufferers were examined in the headache-free periods, in the preattack stages, during the attacks, and immediately afterward. A contracting activity was always present when rat fundus strips were exposed to sera of controls and migraineurs (16). This preparation *in vitro* is particularly sensitive to the presence of serotonin (28).

Remarkably stronger contractions of the rat fundus strip were induced by sera obtained during headache-free periods in 10 patients on the 7th, 14th, and 21st days of the menstrual cycle and on the day preceding the attack. The contractions induced by sera taken on the day of migraine onset, however, were much lower. Approximate quantitation of serotonin-like activity during these intervals showed a maximum of 0.003 ng/ml, minimum (on the day of the migraine attack) 0.0002 ng/ml of serum (Fig. 5).

Extracranial animal arteries (5,9), superficial temporal, were also tested by means of blood samples taken under identical conditions (20,23). No contracting activity from sera taken both in the headache-free period and during the migraine crisis was observed in animal arteries. In contrast, each serum taken after the onset of menstrual migraine showed a synergic effect on the action of norepinephrine, histamine, and serotonin, respectively. This synergic effect increases with the worsening of the attack and decreases as soon as the attack wears off (Fig. 6). Again, it is likely that, on the occasion of a premenstrual attack, vasoactive substances, which enable isolated organs to contract *in vitro*, are released or activated.

Endocrinological Data

Recent literature on menstrual migraine (27) emphasizes that the fall in estrogens during the menstrual cycle is followed by onset of headache. The role of water retention, which often heralds or accompanies an attack of menstrual migraine, in the production of headache is unclear.

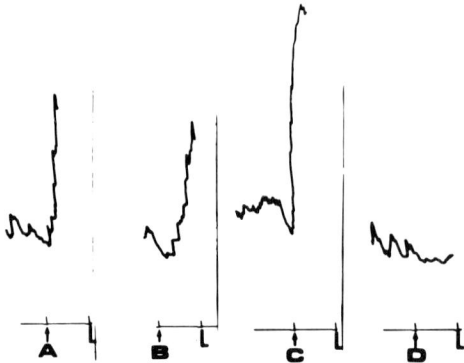

FIG. 5. Rat fundus strip tested by serum samples. On the seventh day, the serum pool is equivalent to 7 ng/ml **(A)**, on the 21st day, 6 ng/ml **(B)**, in the preattack stage, 20 ng/ml **(C)**, and during the attack, 2 ng/ml **(D)**. Mean values.

To evaluate a possible connection between fluid retention and menstrual crisis, sex hormones, prolactin levels, osmolarity, and electrolyte patterns were investigated in a carefully selected group of 10 migrainous women with regular menses and chronological premenstrual attacks (17–19). These investigations included (a) osmolarity, in the span between the two menstrual cycles, (b) estradiol, progesterone, prolactin, and electrolytes in the follicular and luteal stages, and again immediately before the menstrual attack, and (c) aldosterone rhythm in the follicular and luteal stages, and again immediately before and during the migraine crisis. In the migraine group, estradiol and progesterone were higher than in the control group. This difference is statistically significant (Figs. 7 and 8).

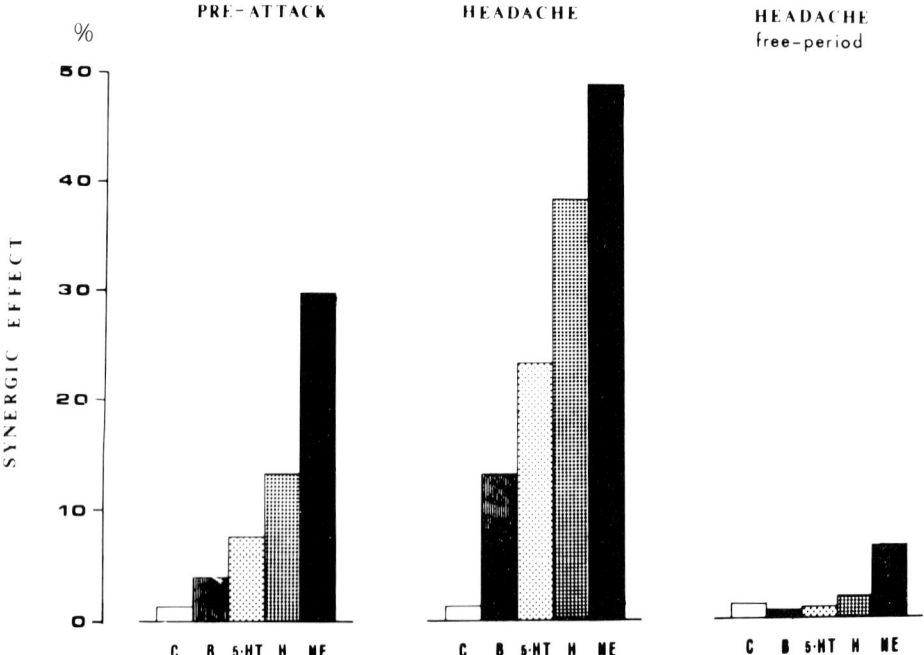

FIG. 6. Each serum taken after the onset of menstrual migraine shows a synergic effect on the action of norepinephrine (NE), histamine (H), and serotonin (5-HT), respectively. C, control; B, bradykinin.

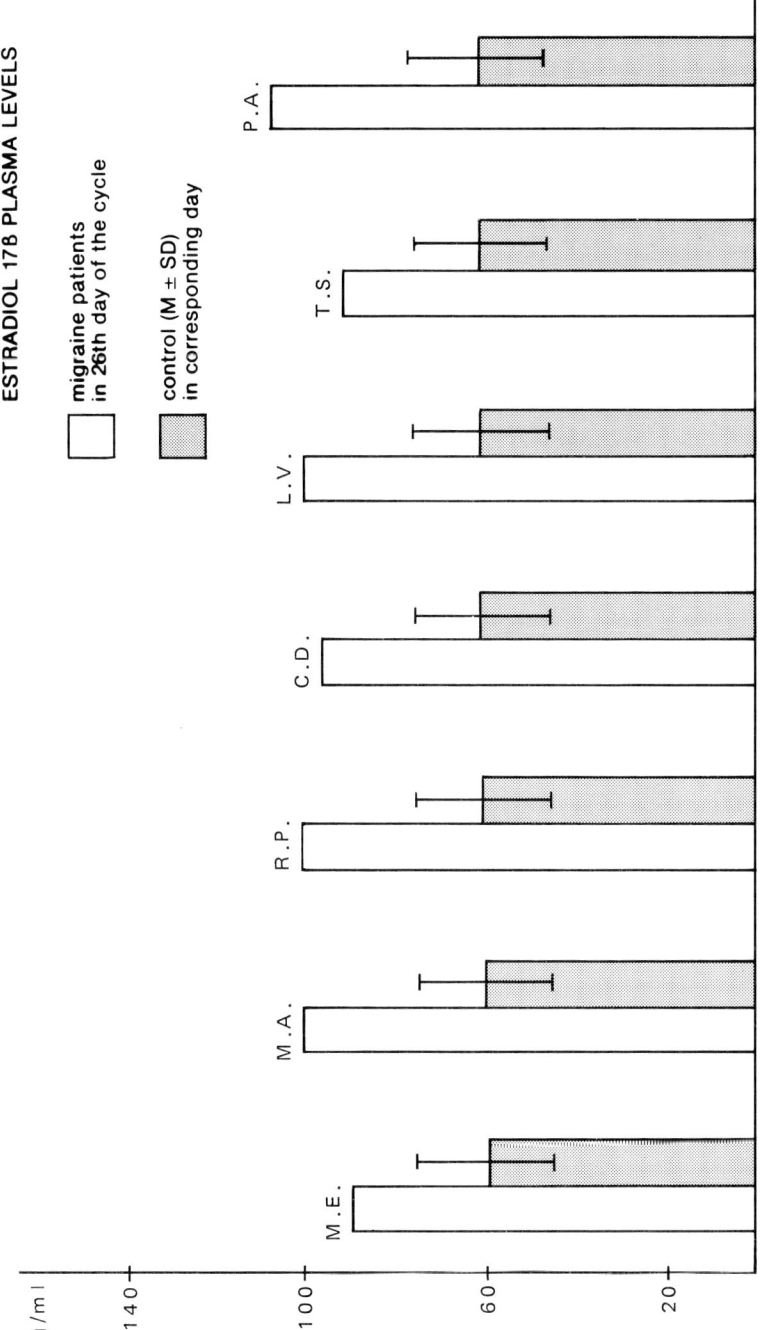

FIG. 7. Estradiol plasma levels in migraineurs on 26th day and in control subjects on the same day.

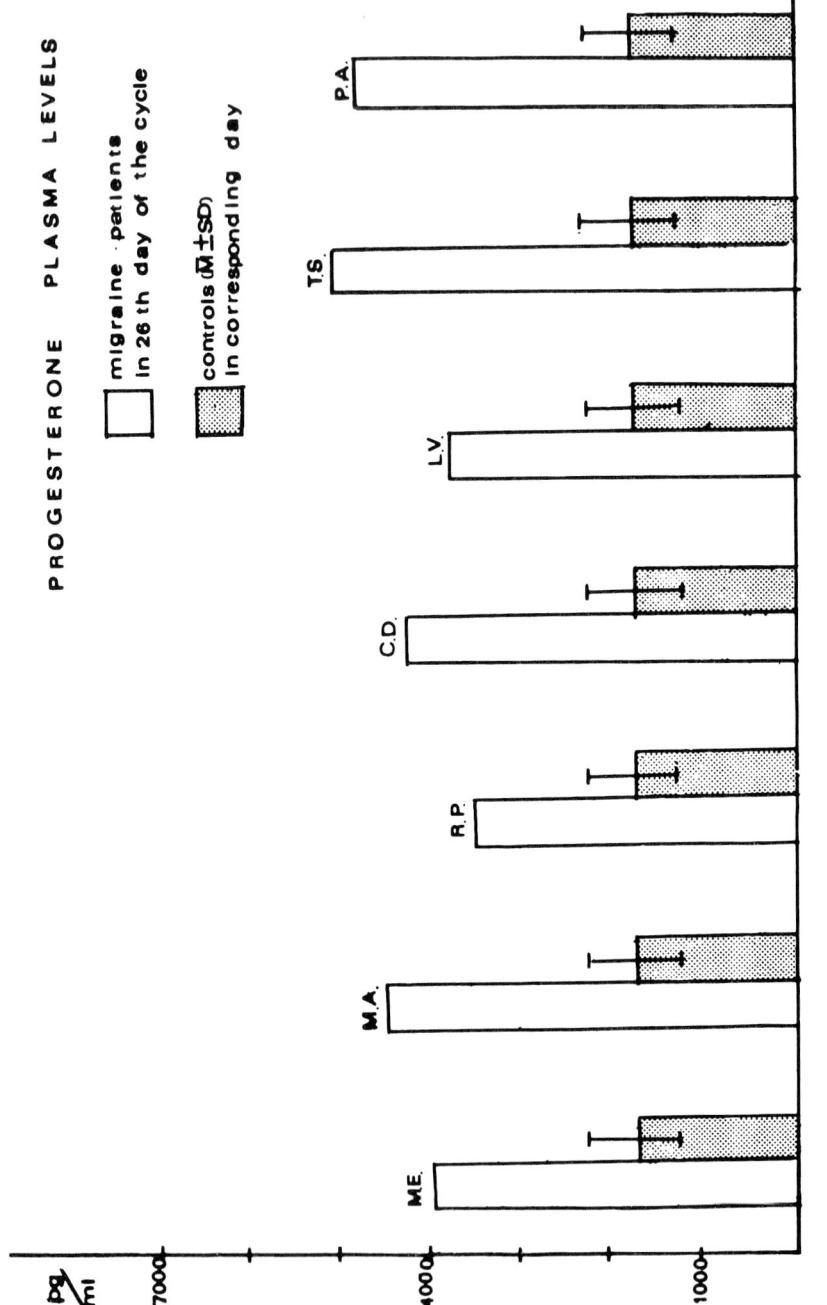

FIG. 8. Progesterone plasma levels in migraineurs on 26th day and in control subjects on the same day.

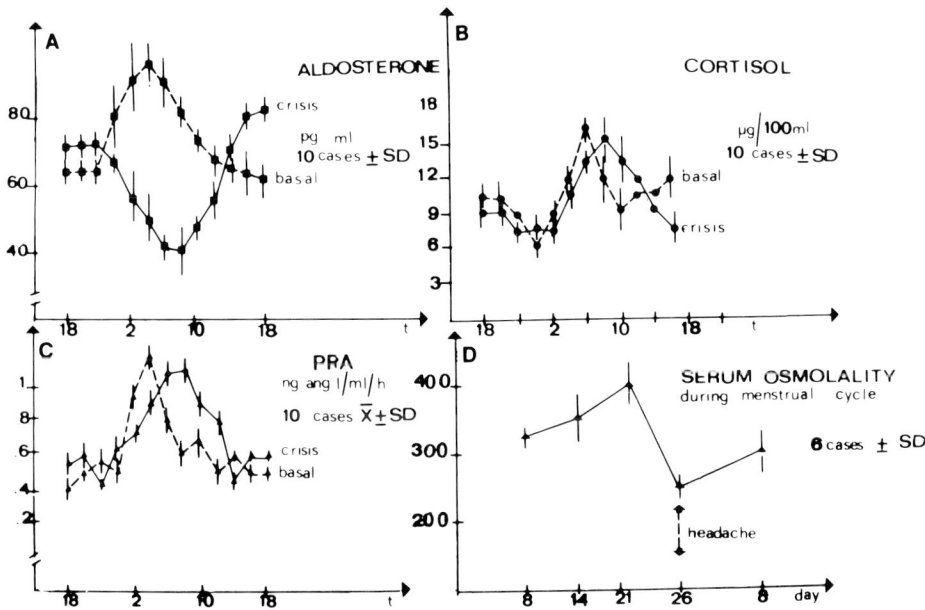

FIG. 9. Curves of aldosterone circadian rhythm **(A)** in headache-free periods and during premenstrual migraine. During the crisis, this rhythm is deeply altered. Cortisol **(B)** and PRA **(C)** do not show any circadian abnormality during the menstrual migraine crisis with respect to control patterns obtained in the follicular phase. Serum osmolarity **(D)** shows higher levels than those of the full crisis.

Prolactin levels were higher in all the migraine patients examined; but this difference is not statistically significant with respect to the control group. Serum osmolarity remained within the normal range; in the immediate preattack stage, however, it showed higher levels than those of the full crisis (Fig. 9D). In the follicular phase, during the headache-free period, plasma aldosterone levels and renin activity (PRA) showed a clear circadian rhythm, their maximum values occurring in the hours following midnight, approximately at 2:00 to 4:00 A.M. (Fig. 9A).

Cortisol and PRA did not show any circadian abnormality during the menstrual migraine attack, with respect to control patterns obtained in the follicular phase (Figs. 9B and C). By contrast, curves of 24-hr plasma aldosterone levels, plotted every 2 hr, were inverted during the headache period when compared with migraine in the headache-free period in all cases (Fig. 9A). The onset of the migraine attack was followed by a drop in plasma aldosterone, which is statistically significant and occurred during the postovulatory phase and at night, a time when aldosterone levels normally rise (Fig. 10). Our data were confirmed by Bana and Graham (3), who observed low aldosterone plasma levels during headache provoked by dialysis. Since PRA, cortisol, sodium, and potassium levels did not change during the menstrual migraine attack, the aldosterone drop is difficult to explain (1). Increased conjugation of aldosterone in the liver, because of increased hepatic blood flow during the attack, might explain decreased plasma levels of this substance. Diuresis decreased with worsening of pain and increased markedly with lessening crisis (Fig. 11).

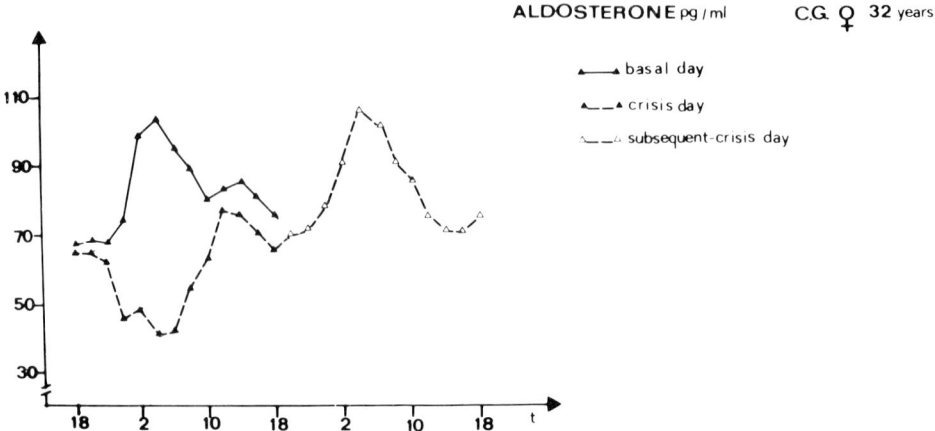

FIG. 10. Curve of 24-hr plasma aldosterone levels inverted during headache period when compared with curves of headache-free period.

A widely held hypothesis claims that estradiol increases the retention of nitrogen and sodium, the latter being considered in its turn as one of the provoking factors of fluid retention. Moreover, progesterone is suspected to interact with estradiol in the postovulatory stage (2,14). Our results show that both estradiol and progesterone levels are significantly higher in premenstrual migraine sufferers than in controls.

Prolactin may cause renal sodium, potassium, and water retention and can also potentiate the renal action of aldosterone and antidiuretic hormone (ADH) (6,13). Our results confirm a general trend toward slightly higher prolactin values in all the migraine patients examined than in the control group, although the mean differences are not statistically significant.

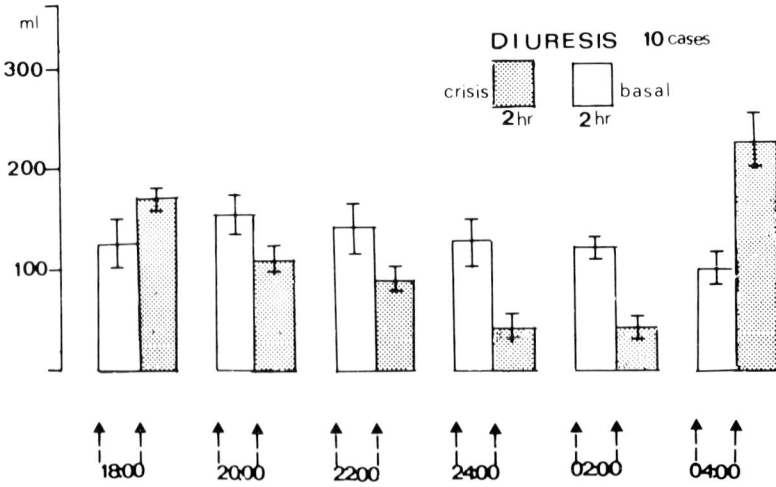

FIG. 11. Changes in the circadian rhythm of diuresis during the crisis and during the control day in migraineurs.

There is evidence of a relationship between osmolarity and ADH. The constant decrease of osmolarity levels in the full crisis, with respect to the immediate precrisis stage, might be related to the oliguria observed by us in this stage.

Progesterone plasma levels appeared to be constantly higher in premenstrual migraine sufferers than in controls. Our results are in agreement with those of Horthe et al. (14). According to Somerville (26), most of the symptoms of the premenstrual syndrome may be attributed to the effects of an insufficiently fast decline of progesterone plasma levels in the last few days of the menstrual cycle. The author postulated that only at the onset of the migraine crisis is there a fast decrease in estradiol values.

CONCLUSION

Our data are far from complete. Further research on menstrual migraine must be carried out. In our view, menstrual headache is but one expression of a more complex picture, described in an oversimple manner as premenstrual syndrome, which includes metabolic, neurological, neuropsychiatric, and vascular features.

ACKNOWLEDGMENTS

I wish to thank for their cooperation: Prof. A. Piazza, Institute of Medical Genetics; Dr. J. Franzone, Institute of Pharmacology; and Dr. D. Bisbocci, 2nd Medical Clinic of the University of Turin.

REFERENCES

1. Ambruster, A., Vetter, W., Beckarhott, R., Bussberger, J., Vetter, H., and Siegenthaler, W. (1975): Diurnal variations of plasma aldosterone in supine man: Relationship to plasma renin activity and plasma cortisol. *Acta Endocrinol.,* 80:95–103.
2. Backstrom, T., and Carstensen, H. (1974): Estrogen and progesterone in plasma in relation to premenstrual tension. *J. Steroid Biochem.,* 5:257–260.
3. Bana, D. S., and Graham, J. R. (1978): Renin-angiotensin-aldosterone system in vascular headache. In: *Current Concepts in Migraine Research,* edited by R. Greene, pp. 111–114. Raven Press, New York.
4. Campbell, D. A., Maj, K. M., and Tonks, E. M. (1951): An investigation of the salt and water balance in migraine. *Br. Med. J.,* 2:1,424–1,429.
5. Cassiano, O. (1969): Azione di farmaci beta stimolanti e beta bloccanti sull'attività contrattile spontanea dei preparati isolati di arteria. *Minerva Anestesiol.,* 3:58–64.
6. Cole, E. N., Evered, D., Horrobin, D. F., Manku, M. S., Mtabayi, Y. J. P., and Nassar, B. A. (1975): Is prolactin a fluid and electrolyte regulating hormone in man? *J. Physiol.,* 252:54–55.
7. Curran, D. A., Hinterberger, H., and Lance, J. W. (1965): Total plasma serotonin 5-hydroxyindoleacetic acid and p-hydroxymethoxymandelic acid excretion in normal and migrainous subjects. *Brain,* 88:997–1,010.
8. Curzon, G., Barrie, M., and Wilkinson, M. I. P. (1969). Relationships between headache and amine changes after administration of reserpine to migrainous patients. *J. Neurol. Neurosurg. Psychiatry,* 32:555–561.
9. Edvinsson, L., and Hardebo, J. E. (1976): Characterization of serotonin receptors in intracranial and extracranial vessels. *Acta Physiol. Scand.,* 97:523–525.
10. Greene, R., and Dalton, K. (1953): The premenstrual syndrome. *Br. Med. J.,* 1:1,007–1,014.
11. Greene, R. (1967): Menstrual headache. In: *Research and Clinical Studies in Headache, Vol. 1,* edited by A. P. Friedman, pp. 62–73. Karger, Basel.
12. Hager, H. (1963): Die ophtalmodynamographie als Methode zur Beurteilung des Gehirnkreislaufes. *Klin. Monatsbl. Augenheilkd.,* 142:827–846.
13. Horrobin, D. F., Lloyd, I. J., Lipton, A., Burstyn, P. G., Durkin, N., and Muiruri, K. L. (1971): Actions of prolactin on the human renal function. *Lancet,* 2:353–354.
14. Horthe, C. E., Wainscott, G., Neylan, C., and Wilkinson, M. I. P. (1975): Progesterone, estradiol and aldosterone levels in plasma during the menstrual cycle of women suffering from migraine. *J. Endocrinol.,* 65:24–29.

15. Nattero, G., Gastaldi, L., Gay, V., Agostoni, A., Cottino, A., and Piazza, A. (1971): Considerations on incidences and statistical correlations obtained through the study of 1500 cases of persistent headache. *Proceedings of the International Headache Symposium, Elsinore, Denmark,* edited by D. J. Dalessio, T. Dalsgaard-Nielson, and S. Diamond, pp. 131–140. Sandoz Ltd., Basil.

16. Nattero, G., Lisino, F., Brandi, G., Bisbocci, D., Bernardi, V., Bottini, A., Griffa, G., Ramella, M. R., and Scalabrino, M. (1976): Rat fundus strip and uterus contracting activity of sera: Relationship to migraine attacks. *Headache,* 16:105–108.

17. Nattero, G., Bisbocci, D., Bottini, A., Brandi, G., Griffa, P. G., Lisino, F., Ansini, A., and Ceresa, F. (1977): Brief report: Humoral and hormonal changes in menstrual migraine. *Headache,* 17:23–24.

18. Nattero, G., Bisbocci, D., Brandi, G., Griffa, P. G., Lisino, F., Franzone, J., Ansini, A., Bottini, A., Ramella, M. R., and Scalabrino, M. (1977): Hemodynamic and humoral aspects in premenstrual headache. In: *Headache New Vistas,* edited by F. Sicuteri, pp. 111–112. Biomedical Press, Florence, Italy.

19. Nattero, G., Bisbocci, D., and Ceresa, F. (1979): Sex hormones, prolactin levels, osmolarity and electrolyte patterns in menstrual migraine: Relationship with fluid retention. *Headache,* 19:25–30.

20. Nattero, G., Franzone, J., Croce, F., Bisbocci, D., and Genazzani, E. (1979): *In vitro* response of animal arteries to serum of migraineurs. *Headache,* 19:209–213.

21. Nattero, G., Borgna, M., Oneglio, G., and Bisbocci, D. (1979): Relationship of migraine with puberty, menstruation, pregnancy and menopause. *Headache, IV Meeting of the Italian Headache Society, Pavia, Italy,* edited by F. Savoldi and G. Nappi, pp. 196–198. Fidia Research Laboratories.

22. Nattero, G., Savi, L., and Pisani, M. (1980): Doppler ultrasound findings during migraine attacks. *International Congress Headache '80, Florence, Italy,* p. 89. Fondazione Internazionale Menarini.

23. Nattero, G., Franzone, J., Croce, F., Bisbocci, D., Cirillo, R., and Genazani, E. (1981): Animal and human arteries *in vitro* response to serum of migraineurs. *Int. J. Clin. Pharmacol. Biopharm.,* 18 *(in press).*

24. Pichler, E., and Strauss, A. (1975): Ophtalmodynamographische Untersuchungen bei experimentellem und Spontankopfschmerz. In: *Kopfschmerz Headache 1975,* edited by G. S. Barolin, D. Saurugg, and W. Hemmer, pp. 191–197. Otto Spatz, Munich.

25. Somerville, B. W. (1971): The influence of hormonal changes upon migraine in women. *Proc. Aust. Assoc. Neurol.,* 84:47–53.

26. Somerville, B. W. (1971): The role of progesterone in menstrual migraine. *Neurology,* 21:853–859.

27. Somerville, B. W. (1972): The role of estradiol withdrawal in the etiology of menstrual migraine. *Neurology,* 22:365–366.

28. Vane, J. R. (1957): A sensitive method for the assay of 5-hydroxytryptamine. *Br. J. Pharmacol. Chem.,* 12:344–349.

Advances in Neurology, Vol. 33, edited by
M. Critchley et al. Raven Press, New York © 1982

Existential Deterrents to Headache Relief Past Midlife

Charles S. Adler and Sheila Morrissey-Adler

955 Eudora Street, Suite 1605, Denver, Colorado 80220

An understanding of the specific developmental tasks and emotional stresses of late middle age is vital for successful treatment of the older headache patient. When headaches have played a dominant role in the patient's life and have caused the patient to alter major life choices and goals, they become part of the patient's identity and acquire existential, psychological, and social, as well as symptomatic, meanings.

Our findings are based on observation and treatment of 56 patients (36 women, 20 men; aged 55 to 70 years; mean age, 60 years) referred to a psychiatrist and a psychologist specializing in headaches. The mean duration of headaches was 36 years; the mean educational level was 3.5 years of college. All but two were or had been married. Although six patients were diagnosed as having cluster headaches, the majority presented with migraine, muscle-contraction, or mixed migraine and muscle-contraction headaches.

The primary developmental task of this period in the life cycle is the resolution of existential questions relating to meaning and identity. Self-appraisal and coming to terms with the finite accomplishments of the central years of one's life are part of the normal and uniquely stressful developmental transition required at this age, and a person's success at doing so has implications for his physical and emotional health. Just as the task of adolescence is to fashion an identity from the experiences of childhood, that of late middle age is to integrate the experiences of adulthood into a more permanent identity. In contrast to the adolescent, however, the older person must derive a satisfactory sense of identity more from what he has been and done than from what he anticipates being or doing. The well-adjusted middle-aged person will audit his losses and accomplishments, mourn what has been missed in life, and take satisfaction in what has not been missed. Success at consolidating an acceptable self-image from the themes and fragments of the central years of life allows the person past age 55 to face his coming years with creativity, purpose, and contentment. His ability to be optimistic about the future depends on his capacity to accept his past as an adequate basis for a satisfactory self-image.

If chronic, disabling headaches and their sequelae have been a major part of his personal history, the patient may find it difficult, if not impossible, to adapt to this transition. Often he is not proud of or satisfied with his life accomplishments and can only justify them by tenuous rationalizations. He may need to cling to these rationalizations because his identity depends on what those earlier years can be fashioned into in his mind. These accrued experiences are seen as more than just a balance sheet of joy and sadness; they provide substantive reasons for a belief that his life up to that point had meaning.

Not only must a lifetime of dealing with headaches be incorporated into this identity, but so must decisions based on the handicap of headaches, the constant dread of their unpredictable onset, and the expectation that they would continue. Examples of such decisions include choosing not to have children, altering career goals, restricting travel, or limiting community and social activities.

Depression in older people often results from being disappointed that they have not realized highly valued goals or dreams in life and that these losses are irretrievable; they may refuse to accept these failings and wish to turn back the clock to redo their past in major ways.

Elaborate systems may have been constructed in the psyche to preserve the self-esteem of a person limited by headaches. When headaches have persisted for 30 or 40 years, they have usually become entwined in a homeostatic equilibrium with the patient's intrapsychic and interpersonal matrix (1). Such an equilibrium may combine both adaptive and maladaptive elements for any given patient. Because of this complexity, the physician who wishes to modify a pattern that seems to be maladaptive for the patient must approach this task with utmost caution. The patient usually has two competing feelings: one is a conscious wish to be rid of the pain and restrictions of the headaches; the second is an unconscious fear that loss of the headaches will devalue his entire past by implying that he spent his life dominated by pain that could have been relieved.

While many patients with a strong and flexible ego structure will be able to relinquish long-standing headaches and successfully compensate for any shifts in their psychosocial equilibrium, others will be so unconsciously defended against reduction of headaches that self-protective mental mechanisms will not allow any treatment to be effective. In some patients, the balance may be so precarious that too rapid amelioration of headaches will precipitate a deep depression. Studies by von Senden (7) appear in the psychological literature of congenitally blind patients whose vision was surgically restored in midlife. When the bandages were removed, instead of the anticipated rejoicing, many patients became unaccountably depressed and some committed suicide. If their sight could have been regained this easily, what, if anything, had been the meaning of their suffering? How could they integrate this past into their concept of their future?

Headache patients, especially migraineurs, are frequently distinguished by personality traits that predispose them to difficulties with the identity consolidation required at middle age. They are often hard-driving, perfectionistic people with exceedingly high expectations of what they should be able to accomplish. They seem to make endless demands of themselves; analysis reveals that their ceaseless attempts are to appease their own harsh and unforgiving conscience (3). Furthermore, the headache problem has been an obstacle to realizing their full potentials and objectives in life. When they reach late middle age and become aware that they have essentially achieved most of what they ever will, this demanding conscience calls them to task unmercifully. The headaches can then provide a vital justification that wards off feelings of self-contempt for having failed to meet these excessive expectations of their conscience.

This knowledge can help us to treat the older headache patient more effectively. First, we can recognize how difficult it is for a patient whose basic identity is connected to headaches to give up those headaches at the time he is striving to stabilize his identity. Since consciously the patient is aware only of his wish to be free of pain, it is the clinician who must be perceptive enough to note cues that reveal conflicting motivation. He should point out these observations with sensitivity and patience. Recognition of these feelings should be facilitated in ways that do not take away from the self-respect so vital to older people. Relinquishing the headaches is expedited if the doctor can help the patient come to terms with his past, either by improving his view of what it was or by reducing his expectation of what it should have been.

The physician can help the patient see that courage was required to struggle on despite continual head pain and thus extract a sense of dignity from his endurance. He can also redirect the patient's self-appraisal by emphasizing that valuable inner strengths, such as increased empathy for others in distress, often accrue from the struggle to come to terms with chronic pain. The patient may then be able to incorporate positive aspects of his experience with headache into his identity and respond to treatment.

However optimistic the physician may feel about the therapeutic prospects of a new treatment, he should leave the expected duration of treatment vague. Thus, if either full or partial remission is medically possible, the patient is given time to make the necessary psychological readjustments without feeling pressured or discouraged. For the same reason, it is best to gradually taper or change the older patient's habitual medications. Even moderate reduction in headache frequency, intensity, or medication requirement can be seen as a significant symbolic victory by the patient over his enemy and have psychological significance of great import.

Similar existential repercussions can occur in the patient's family. They too have lived with and felt victimized by the headaches and may react with feelings of pointless sacrifice or even of having been abused if the patient is relieved of headaches. The patient may intuitively sense this and fear his family's possible resentment. This problem can often be averted by discussing treatment with the spouse in ways that validate the patient's previous attempts to cope with his problem and by indicating how important the family's continuing support is for successful therapy.

A case history will illustrate how these existential impediments can appear in practice. A 60-year-old woman with a history of migraines since childhood was referred to our office for treatment. During her visits, she would repeatedly lament that she had wasted her productive years catering to an irascible husband; she blamed her need for help during migraine attacks for keeping her "trapped" in the marriage. Her bitterness and regret eased when her doctor pointed out that she had provided vital emotional support to help her husband overcome a severely deprived childhood and so had enabled him to become a stable and creative leader in the community and that she could share the credit for his contributions. As she was helped to gain greater empathy for her husband and his struggles, the role of her commitment to him took on greater meaning and she began to recognize that headaches had not caused her life to be "wasted." In addition to bringing into better focus what she had done with her life, she was helped to get a more realistic perspective on what she had not done. For example, she had received a great deal of criticism from her mother for "indulging her migraines" by not flying to a distant city to help care for her chronically ill father, and she had taken these criticisms very much to heart. It was pointed out that her guilt had caused her to misperceive the realities at that time, which were that her proper first priorities were to take care of her own husband and small children, that caring for her father was correctly her mother's responsibility, and that finally, even if she had not had the migraines, her mother's expectations would have been excessive and unreasonable. Having gained these insights, she was able to significantly reduce her problems with migraine through the use of physiological feedback; she experienced a marked decrease in the anger and depression that had plagued her recent years.

In addition to existential problems, age-specific psychosocial difficulties associated with aging can aggravate or initiate head pain. Late middle-age usually is replete with hidden worries. Fears about the future gradually replace a former sense of timeless potential for change. This is the peak period for the occurrence of masked depression, and the proportion of headaches traceable to these is surprisingly large (3). The older patient has been found to have high levels of diffuse anxiety with surprising frequency; increased incidence of alcoholism, medication abuse, and suicide are some of the results (4).

The 55-year-old man is often at the height of his career and probably not experiencing these troubles directly; yet he has the ability to anticipate and fear the future. Losses loom ahead and increase logarithmically with each advancing year. Friends develop infirmities and some die; families disperse; his own fate is portended by the fate of those around him. The anticipation of looking old may come as a profound narcissistic wound to the patient who relied heavily on physical attractiveness for self-esteem. These all can evoke deep concerns about the adequacy of the body's functioning, fear of the helplessness of a "second childhood," and even fear of death, for which our society offers inadequate emotional preparation. The *coup de grace* is often the retirement, a symbolic concretization of the fantasy of being relegated to the unessential. Retirement rates high on the scale of life changes productive of illness. Retirement may force a distant married couple together for the first time and so accentuate all of the marriage's shortcomings. One pertinent example is that the spouse is now face to face with the headaches full time.

Individuals age at different rates physically, intellectually, and emotionally; and age alone cannot predict their inner resources for change. Recent studies have shown that after age 70, most patients have quite adequate intellectual functioning (6), more mature judgment, a greater base of experience to draw upon, and a good ability to be introspective. What appears to be intellectual deficit in the older patient is quite often a manifestation of masked depression and anxiety (2,5).

Many physicians incorrectly consider memory loss, personality change, and social isolation as normal concomitants of aging rather than as failures to adapt to age successfully; they fail to look for specific organic and psychiatric syndromes. The patient is also steeped in this misguided view of his later years and may not reveal his feelings of anxious depression because he sees them as a personal failure to accept the inevitable. Patient and doctor thus can mutually confirm a false and negative stereotype of normal aging.

Many features distinguish treatment of psychological problems of the middle-aged headache patient from that of his younger counterpart. The physician often treats the older patient with approaches designed for younger patients. This results in suboptimal management because it ignores the added dimension that chronicity evokes in any problem (2,4). Just as pediatricians are careful to point out that a child is not simply a small adult, it is important to realize that an aging person is not merely a worn-out adult. The younger physician may need to take a candid look at his own feelings; he may be frightened by the specter of age and wish to categorize and shun the older headache patient in order to gain emotional distance.

If psychopathology is uncovered, an early decision should be made about which facets should be treated supportively and which may be accessible to insight and change. Pointing out certain maladaptive personality traits or unwise decisions will only trigger despair if the time has passed when they could be rectified. Exploring the patient's perceptions of past events, observing the patient's emotional reactions, and use of judicious intuition are the best means for determining which areas may be helped and which should be left alone.

Simple discussion with a trusted physician, not necessarily a psychiatrist, may stimulate the patient to view treatable aspects of his problems in a different light. In these discussions, one of the most powerful tools of the physician is his social authority. Patients often see him as having the power to put the seal of acceptability on their past choices and actions.

Constructive reminiscence involves a reflective consolidation of the past and the individual achievements in it and is an important therapeutic process with which the physician can help his headache patient to start. Finding areas of strength in the patient's history and expressing a curiosity about activities he found most rewarding is one way to help the patient to see his failings and strengths in a more balanced perspective and to restructure his life.

If the existential impediments to headache relief can be overcome, the physician is frequently left with a patient who still feels defeated, hopeless, and passive due to the chronicity of both his disease and the treatment. Here the doctor must tap into the motivations that impelled the patient to seek help once again, as only by the patient's active enlistment of these very motives and of his own inner resources is treatment likely to be rewarding. The physician can help set this in motion by definite expectations of the patient's participation in treatment and by his own active treatment attitude.

Finally, one should be aware of the headache syndromes that actually begin in later life. Even when patients present with a long headache history, the first diagnostic consideration should be that the real reason for this late consultation is the recent onset of a new type of headache superimposed on the chronic one. These headaches can have either psychological or organic origins. Muscle contraction headache triggered by anxiety or depression is the most frequent cause of late onset headaches (5). Cervical arthritis increases with age, but this can be a tricky diagnosis, as many patients with cervical arthritis on X-ray do not experience headaches. Often, a hidden depression concurrent with the arthritis causes the headaches, and both conditions are relieved by antidepressants. Headaches caused by primary or metastatic neoplasia, hypertension, cerebrovascular accidents, chronic hypercapnia from pulmonary disease, temporal arteritis, congestive heart failure, uremia, and arthritis or new dentures affecting the temporomandibular joint are all more prevalent in the older patient. Diuretic use or alcohol abuse may cause headaches due to electrolyte imbalance. Increasing nearsightedness can cause headaches as a result of craning the neck to bring objects into focus. Since true migraine tends to subside with age, one should be extremely cautious about diagnosing a headache of recent origin in an older person as migraine.

In conclusion, the physician who understands the need to integrate the history of headaches into the identity of the middle-aged patient and the complex problems that accompany aging and plans a specific treatment program based on those considerations will find his medical technologies unimpeded by the older person's psychosocial needs and existential imperatives.

REFERENCES

1. Adler, C. S., and Adler, S. M. (1976): Biofeedback psychotherapy for the treatment of headaches: A five year follow-up. *Headache,* 16:189–191.
2. Busse, E. W., and Pfeiffer, E. (1969): *Behavior and Adaptation in Late Life.* Little, Brown, Boston.

3. Dalessio, D. J. (1972): *Wolff's Headache and Other Head Pain,* third edition. Oxford University Press, New York.
4. Howells, J. (1975): *Modern Perspectives in the Psychiatry of Old Age.* Brunner Mazel, New York.
5. Poser, C. (1976): The types of headache that affect the elderly. *Geriatrics,* 31:103–106.
6. Savage, D. R., Britton, P. G., Botton, N., and Hall, E. H. (1973): *Intellectual Functioning in the Aged.* Methune, London.
7. von Senden, M. (1960): *Space and Sight: Perception of Space and Shape in the Congenitally Blind Before and After Operation,* translated by P. Heath. Methune, London.

Advances in Neurology, Vol. 33, edited by
M. Critchley et al. Raven Press, New York © 1982

Blood Platelet 5-Hydroxytryptamine Accumulation and Migraine

J. D. Carroll, *A. Coppen, *C. C. Swade, and *K. M. Wood

*Regional Neurological Unit, Royal Surrey County Hospital, Guildford also University of Surrey, Guildford, Surrey; and *MRC Neuropsychiatry Laboratory, West Park Hospital, Epsom, Surrey, England*

5-Hydroxytryptamine (5-HT) is one of the most potent vasoactive amines that have been implicated in the pathology of migraine. Most of the 5-HT present in whole blood is stored in discrete granules within the blood platelet. The administration of reserpine (4) and tyramine (8), which deplete granular monoamine stores, can precipitate an attack of migraine in susceptible individuals. The aggregation of platelets also releases 5-HT, and an increase in platelet aggregation has been noted in migraine patients (3). These observations, together with the findings of an increase in plasma 5-HT levels and the increased excretion of 5-HT metabolites before and during a migraine attack (1), have led many groups to propose that migraine is associated with abnormally high concentrations of plasma 5-HT. The removal of 5-HT from the plasma is by means of an energy-dependent, saturable process occurring in the plasma membrane of blood platelets (13,14). In a comprehensive review of the literature, Hanington (9) proposed that an abnormality of platelet function is not only a major factor in the pathogenesis of migraine attacks but is their prime cause. In the present study, we have investigated the platelet 5-HT uptake characteristics that may determine the levels of plasma 5-HT in migraine patients.

PATIENTS AND METHODS

Male and female patients with a history of migraine were asked to join an investigation that involved one or two blood samples. Selection for inclusion in this study was made according to criteria laid down by the World Federation of Neurology Research Group on Migraine and Headache (15). Patients with a history of psychiatric disorder were excluded from the study. Ten patients were retested after an interval of 6 months. The patients were asked not to take any medication for 1 week prior to the test and were asked to give the date of their last headache or migraine. The control subjects were normal, healthy volunteers with no history of migraine or physical illness.

Blood was collected by venepuncture after overnight fasting and mixed with one-tenth its volume of a solution containing ethylendiamine tetraacetic acid (EDTA) glucose and sodium chloride. The blood was then centrifuged for 15 min to obtain platelet-rich plasma (PRP). Aliquots of PRP were incubated at 37° and 2°C with C-labeled 5-HT (0.25, 0.5, 2.0, and 4.0 mmoles/ml PRP) for 2 min (7). The uptake of 5-HT was stopped by the addition of 2 ml ice-cold 3% formaldehyde in saline. The platelets were removed from the incubation medium by centrifugation at $2,300 \times g$ for 10 min and dissolved in 1 M KOH. Aliquots were counted for radioactivity in an LKB ultrabeta spectrometer for 30 min.

The values obtained for the passive diffusion of 5-HT into the platelets at 2°C were subtracted from the values for the total uptake at 37°C to yield the values for the active uptake of 5-HT. Lineweaver-Burk analysis (11) was used to obtain the values of K_m (the Michaelis constant) and V_{max} (maximal rate of transport).

RESULTS

There was no significant correlation between age and any of the uptake characteristics and no differences in uptake characteristics between the sexes in either the control subjects or the migraine patients. There were no significant differences in K_m or V_{max} between the control subjects and the migraine patients (Table 1). A significant correlation was found between the length of time since the last migraine attack and V_{max} ($r = 0.50$; $p < 0.05$). Consequently, when the patients were divided into two groups, those who had had a migraine attack within the previous 5 days had significantly lower values of V_{max} than the rest of the patients or the control subjects (Table 2).

Five of the patients who were retested were found to have had a recent headache or migraine on one occasion and no recent attack on the other occasion. Table 2 indicates

TABLE 1. *Characteristics of uptake of 5-HT by platelets from migraine patients and control subjects*

Group	N	Age (years)	K_m (μM)	V_{max} (pmoles/10^8 platelets/min)
Control subjects	18	41.4 ± 3.3	0.51 ± 0.03	32.8 ± 4.3
Migraine patients	25	32.7 ± 2.5	0.50 ± 0.04	24.0 ± 1.8
Migraine patients with headache within previous 5 days	16	31.1 ± 2.8	0.49 ± 0.05	21.7 ± 1.5[a]
Migraine patients without headache within previous 5 days	9	35.7 ± 5.1	0.52 ± 0.08	28.2 ± 4.0

[a] Significantly lower than control subjects, $p < 0.05$.

TABLE 2. *Platelet 5-HT uptake in five patients tested twice, with and without recent migraine*

Occasion	K_m (μM)	V_{max} (pmoles/10^8 platelets/min)
Migraine within previous 5 days	0.51 ± 0.13	22.2 ± 1.7[a]
No migraine within previous 5 days	0.46 ± 0.04	33.7 ± 3.5

[a] Significantly lower than headache-free test, $p < 0.02$.

that the patients tested when they had had a recent headache had a significantly lower V_{max} compared to the occasion when they had had no recent headache.

DISCUSSION

It has been shown that platelet levels of 5-HT fall during a migraine attack. It has been suggested that this is due to the presence in the blood of a releasing factor (6). The uptake of 5-HT is dependent on the Na^+/K^+ distribution across the plasma membrane of the blood platelet. This gradient is generated by the activity of the enzyme Na^+/K^+ adenosine triphosphatase (ATPase).

The release of 5-HT from blood platelets before or during an attack of migraine would increase the concentration of 5-HT in the plasma. The removal of 5-HT from the plasma into the platelet would be hindered by the reduced uptake of 5-HT by the blood platelet. This would lead to elevated plasma levels of 5-HT.

The reduced transport of 5-HT by the platelet reported in this investigation may be due to changes in the activity of ATPase or other disturbances of the Na^+/K^+ gradient across the plasma membrane. There is evidence that adenosine diphosphate (ADP) inhibits the uptake of 5-HT, possibly by changing this Na^+/K^+ gradient (5). It is interesting to note that the ADP content of platelets is significantly higher in migraine patients than in control subjects (12). It is perhaps significant that lithium is used in the treatment and prophylaxis of migraine and headache (7,10) and has the capacity of normalizing the reduced transport of 5-HT into the blood platelets of depressed patients (A. Coppen, *unpublished observations*).

REFERENCES

1. Anthony, M., Hinterberger, H., and Lance, J. W. (1967): Plasma serotonin in migraine and stress. *Arch. Neurol.,* 16:544–552.
2. Coppen, A., Swade, C., and Wood, K. (1978): Platelet 5-hydroxytryptamine accumulation in depressive illness. *Clin. Chem. Acta,* 87:165–168.
3. Couch, J. R., and Hassanein, R. S. (1977): Platelet aggregability in migraine. *Neurology,* 27:843–848.
4. Curzon, G., Barrie, M., and Wilkinson, M. I. P. (1979): Relationship between headache and amine changes after administration of reserpine to migrainous patients. *J. Neurol. Neurosurg. Psychiatry,* 32:555–561.
5. Drummond, A. H., and Gordon, J. L. (1976): Uptake of 5-hydroxytryptamine by rat blood platelet and its inhibition by adenosine 5'-diphosphate. *Br. J. Pharmacol.,* 56:417–421.
6. Dvilansky, A., Rishpon, S., Nathan, I., Zolotow, Z., and Korczn, A. D. (1976): Release of platelet 5-hydroxytryptamine by plasma taken from patients during and between migraine attacks. *Pain,* 2:315–318.
7. Ekbom, K. (1977): Lithium in the treatment of chronic cluster headache. *Headache,* 17:39–40.
8. Ghose, K., Coppen, A., and Carroll, J. D. (1977): Intravenous tyramine response in migraine, before and during treatment with indoramin. *Br. Med. J.,* 1:1,191–1,193.
9. Hanington, E. (1978): Migraine: A blood disorder? *Lancet,* ii:501–502.
10. Kudrow, L. (1977): Lithium prophylaxis for chronic cluster headache. *Headache,* 17:15–18.
11. Lineweaver, H., and Burk, D. (1934): The determination of enzyme dissociation constants. *J. Am. Chem. Soc.,* 56:658–666.
12. Rydzewski, W., and Wachowica, B. (1978): Adenine nucleotides in platelets in and between migraine attacks. In: *Current Concepts in Migraine Research,* edited by R. Greene, pp. 153–158. Raven Press, New York.
13. Sneddon, J. M. (1973): Blood platelets as a model for monoamine containing neurones. *Prog. Neurobiol.,* 1:151–198.
14. Stahl, S. M. (1977): The human platelet: A diagnostic and research tool for the study of biogenic amines in psychiatric and neurologic disorders. *Arch. Gen. Psychiatry,* 34:509–516.
15. World Federation of Neurology (1969): Research group on migraine and headache. *Hemicrania,* 1:3–9.

Advances in Neurology, Vol. 33, edited by
M. Critchley et al. Raven Press, New York © 1982

Platelet Function in Migraineurs

M. J. Gawel and F. Clifford Rose

Department of Neurology, Charing Cross Hospital, London, England

Platelets are involved in thrombus formation. When appropriate stimulus is presented, platelets first undergo the shape change, giving out pseudopods, and then can clump together weakly. If the stimulus is strong enough, they undergo the release reaction and degranulate, liberating 5-hydroxytryptamine (5-HT) and many other products whose function remain uncertain.

Aggregation and/or release can be brought about by catecholamines, ADP, collagen, 5-HT, and other factors, including free fatty acids, especially arachidonic acid. Arachidonic acid is the precursor for postaglandin endoperoxides which, in the platelets, are converted into the potent proaggregating vasoconstricting agent thromboxane A_2 by the action of the enzyme thromboxane synthetase. In the vascular endothelium, the endoperoxides are converted into a strong antiaggregating agent, prostacyclin; the subject is reviewed by Moncada and Vane (20). Free fatty acids, arachidonic acid among them, are released by sympathetic stimulation. Many of the changes that occur during the acute migraine attack are centered around the release of 5-HT by platelets. The lesion in migraine is thought to be a platelet dysfunction (29).

Platelets in circulation are continually undergoing aggregation and disaggregation, and there is a stable proportion of one to the other. This can be assessed directly using a method devised by Wu and Hoak (29). Alternately, the level of a protein released during the release reaction can be measured by radioimmunoassay. This protein is called beta-thromboglobulin (BTG) and is of uncertain biological function but may inhibit prostacyclin activity (16). It is consistently released during the release reaction and can be used to monitor the number of platelets undergoing this reaction *in vivo.* A fairly straightforward immunoassay for BTG recently has become available in kit form from Amersham (1). These two tests measure the steady state in the circulation.

The addition of ADP, collagen, 5-HT, or any other factor that causes platelet aggregation to citrated platelet-rich plasma followed by observation of the transmission of light through the suspension is the principle of aggregometry. The more aggregable the platelets, the more readily will they clump at lower concentrations of aggregating agent (2). The rate of disaggregation also can be measured. Essentially similar information can be obtained using a screen filtration pressure technique (26).

The first two methods concern the state of the platelet-platelet aggregation ratio, whereas the last two supply information about the potential behavior of the platelets in the presence of the appropriate stimulus. Some relationship will exist between results obtained with these methods, since blood containing hyperaggregable platelets will have a slightly higher level of circulating aggregates and BTG. However, it is not until some stimulus threshold is reached that the potential changes may become manifest by measurement found in the first two methods.

STUDIES OF PLATELET FUNCTION

To date, there have been five studies of platelet function in migraine. The first was by Hilton and Cummings (15), who measured the aggregation response of the platelets of migraineurs to 5-HT between attacks and those taken during an attack. These responses were inhibited by ergotamine.

Kalendowsky and Austin (17) studied aggregability to ADP of platelets in migraineurs and controls and plasma coagulation factors. Patients with complicated migraine were more likely to have hyperaggregable platelets and had frequent episodes of focal neurological signs. However, in those patients in whom plasma hypercoagulability also developed, perhaps under the influence of estrogens, serious, more permanent sequelae followed. The authors concluded that the neurological course correlated well with the composition of the blood clots, which might have been postulated on the basis of the abnormalities observed in the coagulation studies. They further suggested that when the migraine occurred, the slowing of the blood flow due to vasoconstriction could have contributed to the development of the signs.

Couch and Hassanein (5) used optical density methods to study aggregation in response to three concentrations of ADP. They found platelet hyperaggregability in the patients as compared to the controls, as manifested by a lower threshold for the platelet release reaction and increased platelet stickiness following aggregation. In contradistinction to the previous two authors, these workers found no correlation of platelet hyperaggregability with the severity of migraine or with occurrences of migraine-associated neurological features.

Deshmukh and Stirling Meyer (7) drew essentially similar conclusions. Using Wu and Hoak's (29) methods, they showed that the migraineurs had more circulating microaggregates between attacks and a higher aggregation response to ADP than non-headache volunteers. Moreover, platelet aggregability and adhesiveness to glass beads measured during the prodrome was high. During the headache phase, adhesiveness increased but aggregation to ADP and epinephrine decreased (exhausted platelets?).

Further reports have implicated the role of platelets in migraine. Dalessio's (6) patient with thrombocytopenic purpura whose migraines improved following splenectomy prompted Hanington (14) to propose that migraine was a disease of platelets. Unfortunately, some gaps have appeared in the argument; not all patients with migraine have aggregation abnormalities (22).

Evidence suggests that in most patients with migraine, there is some increase in platelet activity between attacks. The platelets are more easily triggered to undergo the release reaction and flood the circulation with the products of that reaction, many of which are vasoactive.

STIMULATION OF PLATELET ACTIVATION

The unstable metabolites of arachidonic acid are the most potent agents involved in platelet aggregation. To some extent, they are under the control of circulating free fatty acid levels and perhaps depend on dietary factors; thus people eating, for example, linolenic acid convert it into thromboxane A_3, which is inactive as a platelet-aggregating agent. Free fatty acids can be released by circulating catecholamines and by sympathetic activity. Circulating catecholamines can exert an effect of their own in platelets (22). Allergy, too, can affect platelet function (27), as can infection.

The fifth most recent study of platelet function in migraine (11) involved measurement of BTG, a platelet release reaction-specific product with possible antiprostaglandin activity. In this study, an attempt was made to study the level of stable metabolites of prostaglandin (6-oxoprostaglandin $F_{1\alpha}$) and thromboxane B_2 using a radioimmunoassay method (24). Unfortunately, the method proved not sensitive enough, but the study will be repeated using a more sensitive gas chromatographic technique.

In the study, samples of BTG and the stable products of thromboxane and prostacyclin metabolism were taken from patients during and between migraine attacks, as well as from age- and sex-matched controls. Sex matching is important, as recent evidence suggests that females respond differently to antiplatelet agents with respect to control of transient ischemic attacks and prevention of attacks (3,9). Furthermore, female sex hormones influence the number of 5-HT (23), norepinephrine, and epinephrine receptors on platelets. If this last study is confirmed, it may provide a clue to the female preponderance of migraine.

The study did confirm that platelet release reaction, as shown by the increased level of BTG, does occur during migraine attacks. The level of BTG in migraineurs during the headache-free interval was not significantly higher than that in controls. It must be noted, however, that the level in the clinic controls was higher than in laboratory worker controls (40 ng/ml, possibly indicating an effect of sympathetic stimulation on platelet behavior. O'Neill and Mann (22) suggested that some patients with migraine had normal platelet aggregability and that only those with abnormal aggregability respond to prophylactic aspirin. In the paper by Gawel et al. (11), some patients did not show any change in BTG levels even during a severe attack, although some showed very high levels. This could be explained in three ways: First, if the release of BTG occurs early in the attacks, the level may have fallen to normal by the time the patient presented (the half-life of BTG is 100 min). Second, there may be two populations of migraine sufferers, one with a tendency to platelet activation. Third, the severity of the headache and the stress caused by it may not have been associated with a strong enough stimulus to cause the platelet release reaction in some patients. Further analysis of severity and duration of headache at the time of sampling did not produce any correlation with BTG levels.

These factors raise the question of whether the changes in the platelets are primary or secondary. Platelet aggregation can be caused by many factors, e.g., catecholamines (9) and arachidonic acid. Catecholamine release causes a rise in free fatty acids; thus this could be the mechanism for pathogenesis of migraine whereby the effects of stress, dietary factors, or hunger may precipitate an attack by acting on platelets (14). In this study, it was shown that a generalized platelet release reaction, as measured by BTG levels, occurs during attacks of migraine. It was not shown in these patients whether the change is primary or secondary. Recent work suggests that BTG can inhibit the production of prostacyclin-like activity from bovine endothelia. If this happens in humans, the release of BTG during the migraine attack may prevent the antiaggregating action of the endothelial cells and tend to inhibit vasodilation(15).

Whether primary or secondary, a generalized activation of platelets in these patients increases the probability of thromboembolic events. Patients with migraine have been shown to be more at risk of heart attacks (23) and possibly cerebral infarction, as shown by the computerized tomography scan (18) and biochemical studies (19). The possibility of additive factors affecting platelet aggregation and release reaction, such as the contraceptive pill and nicotine (which causes increased levels of catecholamines), must be considered in this context; there have been reports of increasing migraine attacks leading to focal neurological signs in women taking birth control pills (28). Migraine in certain susceptible individuals may be one of the conditions that increase the likelihood of thromboembolic disease involving either heart or brain; this effect may be mediated through alteration of platelet function. If this susceptible group could be identified, benefit could be derived from antiplatelet therapy not only by preventing thromboembolic consequences (22).

It must also be pointed out that causing platelet activation in normal subjects does not lead to migraine. In the norepinephrine infusion experiment (8), platelet count was also measured and can be seen in Fig. 1. As the norepinephrine level rose, so did the platelet count; but before the norepinephrine level reached its peak, the count began to fall, suggesting that aggregation was taking place. The count continued to fall following the end of the infusion and gradually returned to normal. These changes are precisely the same as those postulated to occur during a migraine. The level of BTG was high during the infusion, as was the ACTH, cyclic AMP, aldosterone, and free fatty acids. None of the healthy volunteers got a headache. This study suggests that there may be peripheral sensitivity to these changes in migraine subjects.

Finally, there is an intriguing link between platelet activation and another aspect of

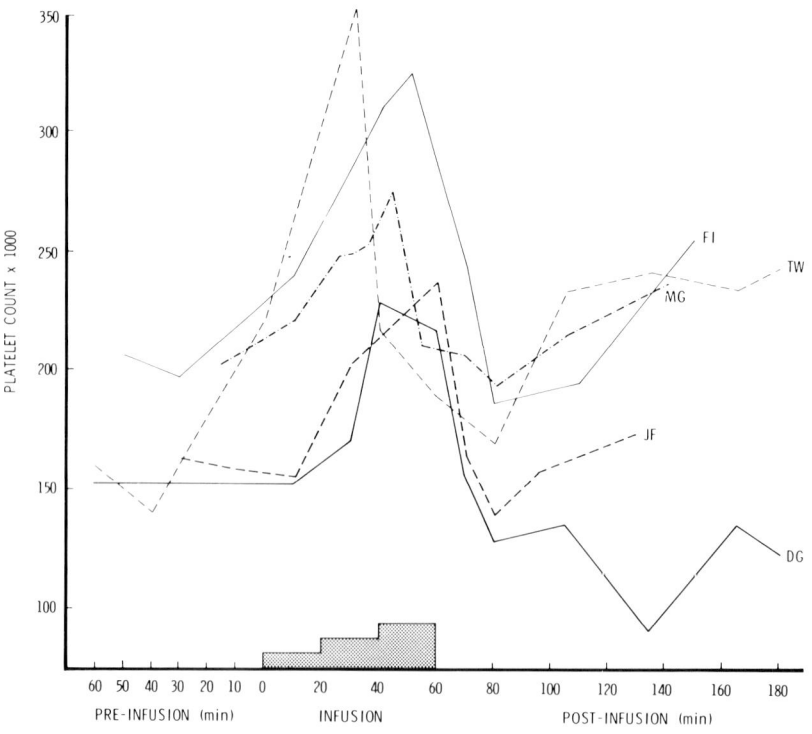

FIG. 1. Platelet count during norepinephrine infusion.

platelet biochemistry, namely, monoamine oxidase (MAO) activity. The levels of MAO are low during migraine attacks (13,25) and in migraine patients free of headache. Experiments in which the platelet count was manipulated either by exercise or by norepinephrine infusion in normal (nonmigrainous) volunteers (M. J. Gawel and F. C. Rose, *unpublished observations*) suggest a strong link between platelet count and MAO activity. Gentil et al. (12) found a similar increase in platelet MAO activity in volunteers given subcutaneous injections of epinephrine. (MAO activity is expressed as activity per unit weight of platelet protein.) This surprising link has two possible explanations: either the catecholamines had some direct effect on platelet MAO (this was not supported by *in vitro* experiments), or freshly released platelets were more active in terms of MAO activity, and changes during migraine attacks are secondary to fluctuation in platelet population following activation, aggregation, and release of fresh platelets. There is evidence for heterogeneity of human platelets with respect to MAO activity (10). At present, we are pursuing this line of investigation.

REFERENCES

1. Bolton, A. E., Ludlam, C. A., Moore, S., Pepper, D. A., and Cash, J. D. (1976): Three approaches to the radioimmunoassay of human B thromboglobulin. *Br. J. Haematol.,* 33:233–238.
2. Born, G. V. R. (1962): Aggregation of blood platelets by adenosine diphosphate and its reversal. *Nature,* 194:927–929.
3. Canadian Cooperative Study (1978): *N. Engl. J. Med.,* 299:53.
4. Carroll, J. D. (1971): Migraine and oral contraception. *Proceedings in Headache Symposium.* Elsinore, Denmark. May 16–18, 1971.
5. Couch, J. R., and Hassanein, F. R. (1977): Platelet aggregability in migraine. *Neurology,* 27:834–848.
6. Dalessio, D. H. (1978): Migraine, thrombocytopenic and serotonin metabolism. *Lancet,* 1:240–241.
7. Deshmukh, S. V., and Stirling Meyer, J. (1977): Cyclic changes in platelet dynamics and the pathogenesis and prophylaxis of migraine. *Headache,* 17:101–108.
8. Few, J., Gawel, M. J., Imms, F., and Jiptaft, E. M. (1978): A delayed effect of noradrenaline infusion on plasma control level in man. *J. Physiol.,* 282:43p.
9. Fields, W. S., Lemak, M. A., Frankowski, R. F., and Hardy, R. J. (1977): A controlled trial of aspirin in cerebral ischemia *Stroke,* 8(3):301–314.
10. Friedhoff, A. J., Miller, C. M., and Karpathin, S. (1978): Heterogeneity of human platelets VII. Platelet monoamine oxidase activity in normals and patients with autoimmune thrombocytopenic purpura. Its relationships to platelet protein density. *Blood,* 51:317–323.
11. Gawel, M. J., Burkitt, M., and Clifford Rose, F. (1979): The platelet release reaction during migraine attacks. *Headache,* 19:323–327.
12. Gentil, V., Greenwood, M. S., and Lader, M. (1975): The effect of adrenaline on human platelet monamine oxidase activity. *Psychopharmalogy (Berlin),* 44:187–190.
13. Glover, V., Sandler, M., Grant, E., Rose, F. C., Orton, D., Wilkinson, M., and Stevens, D. (1977): Transitory decrease in platelet monoamine oxidase activity during migraine attacks. *Lancet,* 1:391–393.
14. Hanington, E. (1978): Migraine—a blood disorder. *Lancet,* 2:501–503.
15. Hilton, B. P., and Cummings, J. N. (1972): 5-Hydroxytryptamine levels and platelet aggregation responses in subjects with acute migraine headaches. *J. Neurol. Neurosurg. Psychiatry,* 35:505–509.
16. Hope, W., Martin, T. J., Chesterman, C. N., and Morgan F. S. Human beta thromboglobulin inhibits PGI₂ production and binds to specific site in bovine aortic endothelial cells.
17. Kalendowsky, Z., and Austin, J. H. (1975): Complicated migraine, its assocation with increased platelet aggregability and abnormal plasma coagulation factors. *Headache,* 15:8–35.
18. Leviton, A., Malvea B., and Graham J. R. (1974): Vascular diseases, mortality and migraine in the parents of migraine patients. *Neurology,* 24:669–672.
19. Matthew, N. T. (1978): Computerized axial tomography in migraine. In: *Current Concepts in Migraine Research,* edited by R. Green, pp. 63–71. Raven Press, New York.
20. Moncada, S., and Vane, J. R. (1978): Unstable metabolites of arachidonic acid and their role in haemostasis and thrombosis. *Br. Med. Bull.* 34(2):129–135.
21. O'Brien, J. R. (1963): Some effects of adrenaline and antiadrenaline compounds on platelets in vitro and in vivo. *Nature,* 200:763.
22. O'Neill, B. P., and Mann, J. D. (1978): Aspirin prophylaxis in migraine. *Lancet,* 2(8101):1,179–1,180.
23. Peters, J. R., Elliott, J. Mu, and Graham-Smith, (1979): Effect of oral contraceptive on platelet noradrenaline and 5 hydroxytryptamine receptors and aggregation. *Lancet,* 1:933–936.

24. Salmon, J. A. (1978): Radioimmunoassay for 6 keto prostaglandins F 1 alpha. *Prostaglandins,* 15(3):383–398.
25. Sicuteri, F., Buffoni, F., Anselmi, B., and Del Bianco, P. L. (1972): *Research and Clinical Studies in Headache,* edited by A. P. Friedman and M. E. Granger. Karger, Basel.
26. Swank, R. L. (1968): The screen filtration pressure method in platelet research, significance and interpretation. *Sem. Haematol.,* 1:146.
27. Weiss, H. J. (1975): Platelet physiology and abnormalities of platelet function. *N. Engl. J. Med.,* 292:531–541.
28. Welch, K. M. A., Chabi, E., Nell, J., Bartosh, K., Meyer, J. S., and Matthew N. T. (1978): Similarities in biochemical effects of cerebral ischemia in patients with cerebrovascular diseases and migraine. In: *Current Concepts in Migraine Research,* edited by R. Green, pp. 1–9. Raven Press, New York.
29. Wu, K. K., and Hoak, J. C. (1976): A new method for the quantitative detection of platelet aggregate in patients with arterial insufficiency. *Lancet,* 2:924–926.

Advances in Neurology, Vol. 33, edited by
M. Critchley et al. Raven Press, New York © 1982

Platelet Activation: Its Possible Role in the Migraine Mechanism

Barbara Wachowicz

Department of Biochemistry, Institute of Biochemistry and Biophysics,
University of Łódź, Łódź, Poland

Platelets, the smallest blood cells, possess well-developed capacities to (a) adhere to biological and foreign surfaces, (b) aggregate, (c) contract or spread, and (d) take up or release substances. The platelet normally circulates as a disk and contains a number of different granules, mainly α-granules and dense bodies. In response to an appropriate stimulus, within seconds platelets may transform their shapes from discs into spherical cells with pseudopods; they can aggregate together and release many different compounds stored in their specific granules.

Numerous stimuli can trigger platelets to various degrees and stages of activity; these agents include thrombin, collagen, serotonin, ADP, epinephrine, prostaglandin (PGEs), and thromboxane A_2 (TxA_2). Platelet response occurs in a graded fashion that depends on the nature, strength, and duration of the stimulus, as well as on platelet physiological and pathological states. Hereditary and acquired disorders, drugs, and certain conditions can limit or modulate platelet responses.

The response of platelets to various stimuli, according to Holmsen (13), can be divided into three phases: (a) induction, (b) transmission, and (c) execution. Induction is an interaction of inducer with the platelet membrane. Transmission phase is an energy-consuming process dependent on the release of a transmitter following the induction stimulus. The transmitter is probably Ca^{2+}, which in some way, possibly by regulation through the cyclic nucleotide system, are mobilized from intracellular storage sites. The execution phase can in turn be divided into four separate reactions normally occurring in series or parallel to each other: (a) shape change, (b) aggregation, (c) dense body release, and (d) α-granule release. The weak inducers (ADP, serotonin) may lead to shape change and aggregation without inducing the release reaction. The strong inducers (thrombin, collagen) normally stimulate the reaction sequence to completion. Thus the platelet membrane plays an important role in the reception of these external stimuli, in the transmission of their message into the cell, and in the execution of the platelet response.

A central role in the initiation of platelet activation is played by the increase of the cytoplasmic Ca concentration and its movement in the cell. Ca^{2+} may be liberated from membranes or from some storage organelles (4). The platelets differ in this respect from other secretory cells in which secretion is induced by Ca^{2+} penetrating the cell from the outside. Since only platelet aggregation *in vitro* can be followed reproducibly in a quantitative manner in the aggregometer (2), aggregation is used as one of the most common parameters of platelet activation.

A new understanding of platelet physiology was gained by the discoveries that platelets can synthesize PGs, converting arachidonic acid via PGEs (PGG$_2$, PGH$_2$) into TxA$_2$ (7–9,23). Most of the platelet arachidonic acid exists in ester linkage of phospholipids. However, because only unesterified or free arachidonic acid is utilized for PG biosynthesis, a phospholipase is required to cleave this fatty acid from phospholipids. Stimulation of platelets by various agents leads to a rapid, Ca-dependent, phospholipase A$_2$-mediated mobilization of arachidonic acid from certain phospholipids and futher transformation to several PGs (6).

Most of the platelet PGEs are transformed to a labile TxA$_2$ (9). Smaller quantities of PGE$_2$, PGF$_{2\alpha}$, and PGD$_2$ are also produced within the platelets. Of these, only PGD$_2$ is sufficiently active to block aggregation or stimulate adenylate cyclase at physiological concentration. TxA$_2$ and PGEs are labile intermediates, which are themselves capable of evoking platelet aggregation and release reaction (18,19). In the presence of active enzymes from vessel walls, PGEs are converted to prostacyclin (16,17).

TxA$_2$ is a potent initiator of the aggregation, inhibiting platelet adenylate cyclase and causing vasoconstriction. The cells of the vessel wall transform the same substrates into prostacyclin (PGI$_2$), which stimulates adenylate cyclase, inhibiting platelet aggregation, and causing vasodilatation (19) (Fig. 1). It should be pointed out that two compounds (TxA$_2$ and PGI$_2$) formed from a common precursor molecule have opposite regulatory activities on cyclic AMP production and platelet aggregation.

When platelets are stimulated, arachidonic acid is liberated and rapidly converted to TxA$_2$, which mobilizes Ca from various storage sites within the platelet. Mobilized Ca then can inhibit the adenylate cyclase and/or initiate platelet secretion (6). A balance between TxA$_2$ and prostacyclin formation regulates platelet cyclic AMP and platelet aggregability. Prostacyclin is a circulating hormone released by the lungs; therefore, platelets may be constantly stimulated by circulating prostacyclin (19).

The involvement of endogenous PGEs and TxA$_2$ in platelet aggregation and the preven-

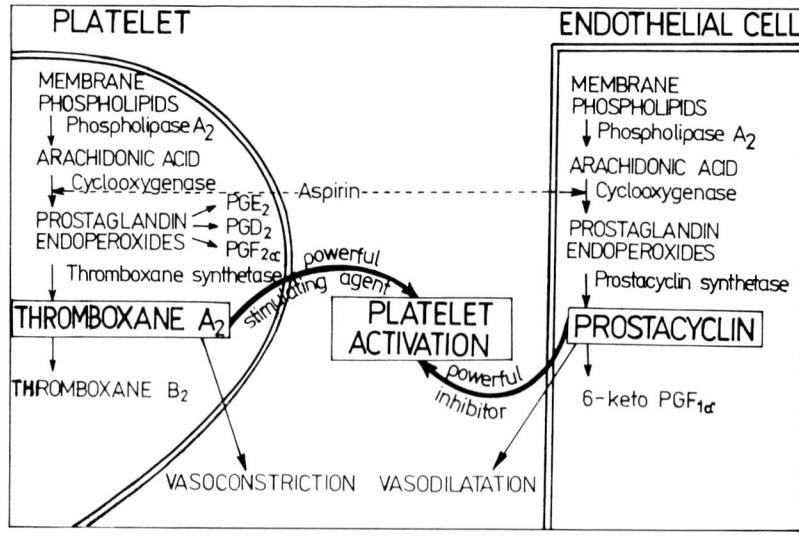

FIG. 1. Simplified scheme of arachidonic acid metabolism in blood platelets.

tion of their formation by inhibition of the cyclooxygenase by aspirin (Fig. 1.) provides a satisfactory explanation of the inhibitory effects of aspirin-like drugs on platelet aggregation and release reaction. Aspirin also inhibits the formation of prostacyclin in the endothelium of the vessel wall; however, it is more effective in blocking the platelet cyclooxygenase than the endothelial enzyme (19).

Different mechanisms are involved in platelet activation, but the role of some compounds and processes is still not understood (15).

Migraine is a disorder associated with an abnormality of platelet function and behavior, particularly manifested by hyperaggregability (3,12,14). Hanington (10,11) hypothesizes that migraine is among the most common disorders of the blood. In migraine, increased platelet adhesiveness, hyperaggregability, release of serotonin, and possibly a decrease in the number of platelets have been observed. Blood platelets as secretory cells release a number of compounds with important biological functions. Of these, serotonin is thought to be significant in the pathogenesis of migraine (1,12). At the onset of a migraine attack, the platelet release reaction, with liberation of serotonin and β-thromboglobulin (5), occurs secondary to earlier stages of platelet activation. Serotonin and other compounds derived from platelets, including PGs, may interact with cranial vessel walls, which in turn may be a target for activated platelets.

Aspirin as an effective treatment of the acute migraine attack (20) is a well-known inhibitor of platelet cyclooxygenase, preventing the formation TxA_2 and PGI_2 from arachidonic acid. This increase of platelet aggregability in migraine may be linked to an alteration of arachidonic acid metabolism in both platelets and vessel wall (Fig. 1). If abnormally sensitive responses of platelets to aggregating agents return toward normal by aspirin, it is likely that the hyperaggregability is a result of enhanced activity or activation of the arachidonate pathway (21). An important role in the pathogenesis of migraine can be played by a balance between TxA_2 and prostacyclin, the two main arachidonic acid metabolites.

Activation of platelets consists of complex cellular responses, which are energy consuming. Our observation that the total adenine nucleotide content in blood platelets of migraine sufferers is significantly higher than that of healthy subjects (22) suggests a biological hyperactivity or an increase of the storage pool of adenine nucleotides in the platelet.

Numerous stimuli, some of which are closely linked with the causes of migraine, can trigger platelets to various degrees of activity. However, certain conditions can limit or modulate platelet responses. The weak stimuli may have a cumulative effect. The common causes of migraine are stress, hormonal factors, and dietary changes. Stress is associated with hyperaggregability of platelets. Hormonal changes influence thrombin level, which is a strong inducer of platelet activation. The amine content of foods can act as a headache precipitant. Moreover, dietary changes result in changes of plasma free fatty acids. These acids are capable of a rapid exchange with membrane fatty acids and release free arachidonic acid. Its availability is a rate-limiting step in platelet activation.

In migraine sufferers, the prodromal symptoms could result from the combined effects of activated (aggregated) platelets and affect cranial blood vessel. PGs, formed during platelet activation, may interact with cranial vessel walls, both intra- and extracerebral, and cause the observed effects. More information is necessary for the complete elucidation of the role of platelets in this disorder.

REFERENCES

1. Anthony, M., Hinterberger, H., and Lance, J. W. (1969): The possible relationship of serotonin to the migraine syndrome. In: *Research and Clinical Studies in Headache,* edited by A. P. Friedman, pp. 29–59. Karger, Basel.
2. Born, G. V. R. (1962): Aggregation of blood platelets by adenosine diphosphate and its reversal. *Nature,* 194:927–929.
3. Cauch, J. R., and Hassanein, F. R. (1977): Platelet aggregability in migraine. *Neurology,* 27:843–848.
4. Detwiler, T. C., Charo, I. F., and Feinman, R. (1978): Evidence that calcium regulates platelet function. *Thromb. Haemost.,* 40:207–211.
5. Gawel, M., Burkitt, M., and Clifford Rose, F. (1979): The platelet release reaction during migraine attacks. *Headache,* 19:323–327.
6. Gorman, R. R., Wierenga, W., and Miller, O. V. (1979): Independence of the cyclic AMP-lowering activity of thromboxane A_2 from the platelet release reaction. *Biochim. Biophys. Acta,* 572:95–104.
7. Hamberg, M., Svensson, J., Wakabayashi, T., and Samuelsson, B. (1974): Isolation and structure of two prostaglandin endoperoxides that cause platelet aggregation. *Proc. Natl. Acad. Sci. USA,* 71:345–349.
8. Hamberg, M., and Samuelsson, B. (1974): Novel transformation products of arachidonic acid in human platelets. *Proc. Natl. Acad. Sci. USA,* 71:3,400–3,404.
9. Hamberg, M., Svensson, J., and Samuelsson, B. (1975): Thromboxanes, a new group of biologically active compounds derived from prostaglandin endoperoxides. *Proc. Natl. Acad. Sci. USA,* 72:2,994–2,998.
10. Hanington, E. (1978): Migraine, a blood disorder. *Lancet,* 2:501–503.
11. Hanington, E. (1979): Migraine, a platelet hypothesis. *Biomedicine,* 30:65–66.
12. Hilton, B. P., and Cumings, J. N. (1972): 5-Hydroxytryptamine levels and platelet aggregation responses in subjects with acute migraine headaches. *J. Neurol. Neurosurg. Psychiatry,* 35:505–509.
13. Holmsen, H. (1976): Classification and possible mechanisms of action of some drugs that inhibit platelet aggregation. *Sem. Haematol.,* 8:51–80.
14. Kalendovsky, Z., and Austin, J. H. (1975): Complicated migraine, its association with increased platelet aggregability and abnormal plasma coagulation factors. *Headache,* 15:18–35.
15. Lüscher, E. F. (1978): Mechanism of platelet function with particular reference to the effects of drugs acting as inhibitors. *Agents Actions,* 282–290.
16. Moncada, S., Gryglewski, R. J., Bunting, S., and Vane, J. R. (1976): An enzyme isolated from arteries transforms prostaglandin endoperoxides to an unstable substance that inhibits platelet aggregation. *Nature,* 263:663–665.
17. Moncada, S., and Vane, J. R. (1977): The discovery of prostacyclin, a fresh insight into arachidonic acid metabolism. In: *Biochemical Aspects of Prostaglandins and Thromboxanes,* edited by N. Kharasch and J. Fried, pp. 155–177. Academic Press, New York.
18. Moncada, S., and Vane, J. R. (1978): Unstable metabolites of arachidonic acid and their role in haemostasis and thrombosis. *Br. Med. Bull.,* 34:129–135.
19. Moncada, S., and Amezcua, J. L. (1979): Prostacyclin, thromboxane A_2 interactions in haemostasis and thrombosis. *Haemostasis,* 8:252–265.
20. O'Neill, B. P., and Mann, J. D. (1978): Aspirin prophylaxis in migraine. *Lancet,* 2:1179–1180.
21. Packham, M. A. (1978): Methods for detection of hypersensitive platelets. *Thromb. Haemost.,* 40:175–195.
22. Rydzewski, W., and Wachowicz, B. (1978): Adenine nucleotides in platelets in and between migraine attacks. In: *Current Concepts in Migraine Research,* edited by R. Greene, pp. 153–159. Raven Press, New York.
23. Samuelsson, B., Hamberg, M., Malmsten, C., and Svensson, J. (1976): The role of prostaglandin endoperoxides and thromboxanes in platelet aggregation. In: *Advances in Prostaglandin and Thromboxane Research, Vol. 2,* edited by B. Samuelsson and R. Paoletti, pp. 737–746. Raven Press, New York.

Advances in Neurology, Vol. 33, edited by
M. Critchley et al. Raven Press, New York © 1982

The Use of Platelet Inhibitors in Migraine

Robert E. Ryan, Sr., and Robert E. Ryan, Jr.

Department of Otolaryngology, St. Louis University School of Medicine; and Ryan Headache Center, St. Louis, Missouri

Platelets, the smallest element found in the blood, usually number between 200,000 and 400,000, depending on a negative feedback mechanism modulated by thrombopoietin. The platelets are removed from the bloodstream by the spleen and liver after they have passed their normal lifespan, which is usually from 8 to 10 days. Platelets contain granules, of which there are two types. One is the amine storage granule, or platelet dense bodies. These granules contain ADP, ATP, serotonin (5-HT), mucopolysaccarides, epinephrine, and calcium. The second type is the alpha granule, which contains lysomal enzymes and possibly fibrinogen.

Abnormalities of platelet aggregation are found in migraine patients, who demonstrate platelet hyperaggregability in the preheadache (prodromal) phase and exhibit an increase in platelet adhesiveness and plasma 5-HT during the headache phase. It seems likely that the changes in platelet aggregation are responsible for the changes in the plasma and 5-HT levels because human platelets contain practically all the total plasma 5-HT. Platelet adhesiveness shows a further increase during the headache phase of the migraine patient; both platelet aggregation and 5-HT levels, however, decrease.

Abnormalities in platelet aggregation are not directly related to the severity of the migraine attack. All the 5-HT contained in the platelets is released during aggregation. Thus the changes that take place in plasma 5-HT may be responsible for the hemodynamic changes that occur in migraine. These are secondary to a change in the platelet aggregation. This suggests that the use of pharmacological agents that change platelet aggregability may be useful in the prophylactic treatment of migraine.

For platelet activation to take place, exposure of the platelet to some form of stimulation must initially take place (13). The platelet then reacts by undergoing a shape change from its natural disk form to that of a rather spiny sphere (1). The platelets then become sticky and form primary aggregates; this is usually referred to as platelet adhesion. Primary aggregation then develops simultaneously. It is a reversible process in which platelets develop an affinity for each other. Primary platelet aggregation is thought to be stimulated by low levels of ADP, a potent aggregating agent. Its escape from platelets undergoing the release reaction causes more and more platelets to become activated (29). The release reaction occurs when the contents of cytoplasmic granules are released extracellularly (25). The released substances are ADP, 5-HT, platelet factor 4, catechols, and factors modifying vascular integrity (18). When a threshold concentration of ADP is obtained, a large number of platelets undergo the release reaction and aggregate irreversibly with each other. This is termed secondary aggregation.

This chapter discusses the possibility that platelet antagonists can prevent migraine attacks. A platelet antagonist consists of a drug that will inhibit a measurable property of platelets, such as adhesion, retention, or aggregation. Although the mechanism involved in platelet aggregation and the release of platelet granule contents is not fully understood, it is known that some drugs, such as dipyridamole and aspirin, do affect these processes.

Dipyridamole and aspirin have been found to increase the inhibitory effects of each other on thrombosis involving small vessels (31). Aspirin also may increase the effect of dipyridamole in increasing platelet survival (9). These two drugs have different mechanisms involving platelet reactions. Dipyridamole probably inhibits platelet aggregation by increasing cyclic AMP levels. On the other hand, aspirin inhibits the cycloxygenase enzyme, which converts the arachidonic acid to prostaglandin G. Aspirin has a marked inhibitory effect on platelet aggregation but does not prolong platelet survival (8,9,22). It inhibits platelets by preventing the synethesis of prostaglandin G_2, the precursor of thromboxane A_2(23,26).

Dipyridamole is a pyrimidopyrimidine compound with vasodilatory properties. It was used initially in the treatment of angina in 1961. The pyrimidopyrimidine compounds inhibit platelet aggregation and the platelet release reactions induced by most aggregating agents (6). Platelet phosphodiesterase is inhibited, which in turn results in an increase of cyclic AMP levels within the platelets (20). Dipyridamole inhibits platelet adhesion to collagen and to the subendothelial structures (3). It has been shown to prolong platelet survival, especially in subjects with a shortened platelet survival (8). It impairs ADP, collagen, epinephrine, and thrombin-induced platelet aggregation (2). It has its most pronounced effect on the first rather than the second phase of aggregation. Platelet function is impaired only while dipyridamole is in the circulation. Its method of action, however, remains unclear.

Aspirin has been shown to acetylate platelet proteins. Because the effect of aspirin cannot be removed by a mere washing of the platelets, it has a long-lasting effect on platelet function (21). Aspirin is an analgesic, antiinflammatory agent with many effects on platelet function. It inhibits the release reaction and aggregation of platelets and adhesion to collagen, which is brought about principally by irreversible acetylation of platelet protein (24). Aspirin also inhibits collagen glucosyltransferase, which has an inhibitory effect on platelet adhesiveness (15), and cyclooxygenase, which is the enzyme involved in the synthesis of prostaglandin G_2. Prostaglandin G_2, along with prostaglandin H_2 and thromboxane A_2, stimulates platelet aggression and platelet release (12).

Dipyridamole has been used as a vasodilator in patients with angina pectoris. It has been reported to be successful in interrupting platelet consumption in patients with atherosclerotic arterial thromboembolic disease (10). It was found to relax the smooth muscles of the cochlear blood vessels and thus increase cochlear blood flow (28). When combined with aspirin, it has been found to reduce the frequency of attacks of idiopathic venous thrombosis (27,30).

One investigation (4) suggests that migraine patients have chronic hyperaggregability of platelets when compared with controls. The authors also found that there was no correlation of platelet hyperaggregability with the severity of the migraine attack or with the occurrence of the neurological symptoms (hemiparesis, dysphasia, loss of consciousness, and hemisensory loss) often associated with an attack of migraine. They concluded that platelet hyperaggregability is a concomitant feature of the migraine attack but is not dependent on the occurrence of the actual headache. Also, since platelet hyperaggregability may be a predisposing factor in the development of intravascular platelet aggregates or mural thrombii, the hyperaggregability found in migraine patients may be the answer to the fact that there is an increase in the incidence of heart attack and in stroke in migraine patients. Another study on platelet hyperaggregability and neurological symptoms (16) postulates that there is a relationship. The initial rate of response of platelets to 5-HT has been found to be higher in migraine patients than in controls in the intermigraine period but lower during the headache phase (11).

It has been demonstrated that the increase in platelet aggregation during the headache phase and during the prodrome of migraine parallel the reported increase in the plasma 5-HT level during these phases. Platelets contain all the 5-HT present in the blood and release it during aggregation. It is possible, therefore, that changes in plasma 5-HT in migraine are secondary to changes in platelet aggregation (5). This study also found that there was hyperaggregability in migraine patients during the headache-free period, which increased during the prodromal phase and decreased during the actual headache attack. Lance et al. (17) observed an increase in 5-HT during the prodromal phase of migraine and a decrease during the actual headache phase.

Release of vasoconstrictor agents resulting from increased platelet aggregability during the prodromal phase of the migraine attack explain the cerebral ischemia, cerebral vasospasm, and reduction of cerebral blood flow that occurs. A significant rise in serum levels of beta-thromboglobulin that occurs during a migraine attack indicates that the platelet release reaction occurs during the headache phase (7).

These recent studies concerning the abnormalities of aggregation of platelets in migraine patients indicate that platelet antagonists might be helpful in the prophylactic phase of the treatment of migraine. These drugs inhibit the agglutination response in several ways. They interfere with the initial phase of platelet aggregation to foreign substances and inhibit the activation of platelet factors 3 and 4 and ADP. Some may also interfere with the transformation of platelet arachidonic acid, which is transformed into several forms of prostagladins. This reaction is critical to the platelet aggregation-release reaction.

Platelet antagonists lengthen the survival time of platelets. Dalessio (14) states that platelet antagonists may prove to be useful in the treatment of migraine. He suggests that vascular permeability related to any type of injury, including neurogenic injury, may be evoked by the release of vasoactive substances from their reservoirs in the circulation, particularly from the platelets. Masel (19) reports that the combination of aspirin and dipyridamole (Persantine®) is effective in preventing migraine attacks and safer than most forms of treatment.

We are testing the hypothesis that platelet antagonists can prevent migraine episodes. The drugs tested were Persantine, which is assumed to prevent the phase of primary aggregation, and aspirin, which is assumed to prevent the secondary phase of aggregation. Each drug was tested alone and in combination with the other. Another group of patients received a placebo. In this double-blind study, the patients were randomly assigned to one of the four treatment groups. We observed 160 patients with either classic or common migraine. The patients were of either sex and varied in age from 21 to 65 years. No pregnant female patients were included. These patients all had at least three migraine attacks per month; the frequency was rather constant for the past 6 months.

Patients were excluded with headache due to trauma, inflammation, uncontrollable hypertension, neurological disturbances, glaucoma, mixed headache, or tumor. Patients with active stomach ulcers were excluded, as were those allergic to aspirin. Also excluded were patients with acute depression and those who would not reliably maintain a daily diary. Patients were not allowed to take aspirin, Persantine, Anturane, beta blockers, steroids, antiinflammatory drugs, or antidepressants throughout the duration of the study.

Before the patients were entered into the study, a complete history was taken. A physical check-up included a chest X-ray, electrocardiogram, SMA-12, CBC, and urinalysis. At the conclusion of the treatment period, the SMA-12, CBC, urinalysis, and physical examination were repeated.

The patients were divided into four groups. One received Persantine (75 mg) and aspirin (325 mg) four times a day. Another received placebo plus aspirin (325 mg) four times a day. A third group received Persantine (75 mg) and placebo four times a day. A fourth group received placebo four times a day. The study medications were used by the patients for a period of 8 weeks, following a period of 4 weeks washout, during which no aspirin or Persantine were used.

Each patient kept an individual diary card noting headache frequency, severity, and duration of attack. Any degree of daily activity limitations was also recorded. Symptomatic medications were also recorded in the diary cards and rated by units (1 unit + analgesics, 2 units = narcotic, and 3 units = ergot preparations). Aspirin and Persantine urine levels were measured after 4, 6, and 8 week periods. Any adverse reactions were recorded on the patients record sheets.

Written uniform consent forms were signed by each patient. Headache frequency was determined for the four groups of patients: 1, dipyridamole plus aspirin; 2, dipyridamole; 3, aspirin; and 4, placebo. The frequency of headaches was determined before treatment and after 4 and 8 weeks of treatment.

In the dipyridamole plus aspirin group, the headache frequency was 9.15 before treatment and 7.15 after 8 weeks of treatment, representing a decrease of 2.00. After 4 weeks of treatment, the headache frequency of this group increased slightly to 9.48, suggesting that more than 4 weeks of treatment are required for benefit from the combination of dipyridamole and aspirin. In the dipyridamole group, the headache frequency was 8.13 prior to treatment and 8.12 following treatment. This shows no change in

TABLE 1. *Headache index*

Treatment	Before treatment	After treatment 4 weeks	After treatment 8 weeks
Dipyridamole + aspirin	13.86	15.18	11.44
Dipyridamole	12.05	15.84	8.02
Aspirin	12.26	10.49	11.33
Placebo	12.03	12.08	11.33

TABLE 2. *Headache frequency*

Treatment	Before treatment	After treatment 4 weeks	After treatment 8 weeks
Dipyridamole + aspirin	9.15	9.48	7.15
Dipyridamole	8.13	9.60	8.12
Aspirin	8.15	7.49	7.13
Placebo	7.79	8.26	7.64

TABLE 3. *Side effects*

Treatment	Nausea	Vomit	Vertigo	Increased headache	Cramps	Skin bruises	Head pressure
Dipyridamole + aspirin	6	2	1	5	2	1	2
Dipyridamole	4	1	2	6			
Aspirin	1						
Placebo				2			

TABLE 4. *Miscellaneous side effects*

Effect	Dipyridamole + aspirin	Dipyridamole	Aspirin	Placebo
Urinary frequency	1			
Sensitive to odors				1
Diarrhea		1		
Chest pain		1		
Chills				1
Rapid heart beat				1
Hot flashes			1	
Tinnitus		1		

this group. The aspirin group showed a decrease from 8.15 prior to treatment to 7.13 following 8 weeks of treatment, a decrease of 1.02. The placebo group prior to treatment was 7.79 and 7.64 after 8 weeks of treatment, showing no change. Thus the greatest change in headache frequency was in the dipyridamole plus aspirin group of patients.

The headache index was also determined for the four groups before treatment and after 4 and 8 weeks of treatment. The dipyridamole plus aspirin group of patients had a headache index of 13.86 prior to treatment and 11.44 following 8 weeks of treatment. This represents a decrease in the index of 2.42. After 4 weeks of treatment, headaches increased to 15.18, again suggesting that more than 4 weeks of treatment are required for improvement. The dipyridamole group prior to treatment was 12.05; after 8 weeks of treatment, the index was 8.02. This group also showed an increase to 15.84 after 4 weeks of treatment. Prior to treatment, the aspirin group had a headache index of 12.26 and 11.33 after 8 weeks of treatment, representing very little change. The placebo group index was 12.03 prior to treatment and 11.33 after treatment, also representing very little change.

Few side effects were reported in this study. Five patients in the dipyridamole plus aspirin group and six in the dipyridamole group reported an increase in headache. Nausea was reported by six patients in the dipyridamole plus aspirin group and by four patients in the dipyridamole group. Only one patient in the aspirin group complained of nausea. The results show that dipyridamole plus aspirin is helpful in reducing both the headache frequency and headache index. Further investigation is indicated; perhaps increasing the drug treatment period to 12 weeks would be advantageous.

REFERENCES

1. Baumgartner, H. P. and Haudenschild, C. (1972): Adhesion of platelets to subendothelium. *Ann. NY Acad Sci.*, 201:22–36.

2. Born, G. V. R., and Mills, D. C. B. (1969): Potentiation of the inhibitory effect of adenosine on platelet aggregation by drugs that prevent its uptake. *J. Physiol. (Lond.),* 202:41P.

3. Cazenave, J-P., Packham, M. A., Davies, J. A., Kinlough-Rathbone, R. L., and Mustard, J. F. (1977): Studies of platelet adherence to collagen and the subendothelium. In: *The Significance of Platelet Function Tests in the Evaluation of Hemostatic and Thrombotic Tendencies. Workshop on Platelets,* edited by H. J. Day, M. B. Zucher, and H. Holmsen.

4. Couch, J. R., and Hassanein, R. S. (1977): Platelet aggregability in migraine. *Neurology,* 27:843–848.

5. Deshmukh, S. V., and Meyer, J. S. (1977): Cyclic changes in platelet dynamics and the pathogenesis and prophylaxis of migraine. *Headache,* 17:101–107.

6. Emmons, P. R., Harrison, M. J. G., Honour, A. J., and Mitchell, J. R. A. (1965): Effect of dipyridamole on human platelet behaviour. *Lancet,* 2:603–606.

7. Gawel, M., Burkitt, M., and Rose, F. C. (1979): The platelet release reaction during migraine attacks. *Headache,* 19:323–327.

8. Harker, L. A., and Slichter, S. J. (1970): Studies of platelet and fibrinogen kinetics in patients with prosthetic heart vales. *N. Engl. J. Med.,* 283:1,302–1,305.

9. Harker, L. A., and Slichter, S. J. (1972): Platelet and fibrinogen consumption in man. *N. Engl. J. Med.,* 287:999–1,005.

10. Harker, L. A., Slichter, S. J., Scott, C. R. et al. (1974): Homocystinemia: Vascular injury and arterial thrombosis. *N. Engl. J. Med.,* 291:537–543.

11. Hilton, B. P., and Cumings, J. N. (1972): 5-Hydroxytryptamine levels and platelet aggregation responses in subjects with acute migraine headache. *J. Neurol. Neurosurg. Psychiatry,* 35:505–509.

12. Holman, R. L. (1977): Atherosclerosis—A paediatric nutrition problem. *Am. J. Clin. Nutr.,* 9:565.

13. Holmsen, H. (1972): The platelet: Its membrane, physiology and biochemistry. *Clin. Haematol.,* 1:235–266.

14. Internal Medicine News (1977): Platelet antagonists seen useful in migraine therapy. *Int. Med. News,* 10:38.

15. Jamieson, G. A., Urban, C. L., and Barber, A. J. (1971): Enzymatic basis for platelet-collagen adhesion as the primary step in haemostasis. *Nature [New Biol.],* 234–235.

16. Kalendovsky, Z., and Austin, J. H. (1975): Complicated migraine. Its association with increased platelet aggregability and abnormal plasma coagulation factors. *Headache,* 15:18–35.

17. Lance, J. W., Anthony, M., and Hinterberger, H. (1967): The control of cranial arteries by humoral mechanisms and its relation to the migraine syndrome. *Headache,* 7:93–102.

18. Marcus, A. I. (1969): Platelet function. *N. Engl. J. Med.,* 280:1,213–1,220.

19. Masel, B. E. (1978): Clinical trial of platelet inhibition, using aspirin and dipyridamole in migraine prophylaxis. *RN,* 41:87.

20. Mills, D. C. B., and Smith, J. B. (1971): The influence on platelet aggregation of drugs that affect the accumulation of adenosine $3':5'$-cyclic monophosphate in platelets. *Biochem. J.,* 121:185–196.

21. Mustard, J., Fraser, P., and Marian, A. (1973): Commentary. Drugs inhibiting platelet function. *Biochem. Pharmacol.,* 22:3,151–3,156.

22. Packham, M. D., and Mustard, J. F. (1977): Clinical pharmacology of platelets. *Blood,* 50:555–573.

23. Rogh, G. J., Stanford, N., and Majerus, P. W. (1971): Acetylation of prostaglandin synthetase by aspirin. *Proc. Natl. Acad. Sci. USA,* 72:3073–3076.

24. Rosenberg, F. J., Gimber-Phillips, P. F., Groblewski, G. E., Davison, C., Phillips, D. K., Goralnick, S. J., and Cahill, R. D. (1971): Acetylsalicylic acid: Inhibition of platelet aggregation in the rabbit. *J. Pharmacol. Exp. Ther.,* 197:410.

25. Salzman, E. W., Kensler, P. C., and Levine, L. (1972): Cyclic $3'5'$-adenosine monophosphate in human blood platelets. IV. Regulatory role of cyclic AMP on platelet function. *Ann. NY Acad. Sci.,* 201:61–71.

26. Smith, J. B., and Willis, A. L. (1971): Aspirin selectively inhibits prostaglandin production in human platelets. *Nature [New Biol.],* 231:235–237.

27. Steele, P. P., Weily, H. S., and Genton, E. (1973): Platelet survival and adhesiveness in recurrent venous thrombosis. *N. Engl. J. Med.,* 288:1,148.

28. Suga, F., and Snow, J. B. (1969): Cochlear blood flow in response to vasodilating drugs and some related agents. *Laryngoscope,* 79:1,956–1,979.

29. Weiss, H. J. (1975): Platelet physiology and abnormalities of platelet function. *N. Engl. J. Med.,* 293:531–541.

30. Wu, K. K., Barnes, R. W., and Hoak, J. C. (1976): Platelet hyperaggregability in idiopathic recurrent deep vein thrombosis. *Circulation,* 53:687.

31. Zacharski, L. R., Walworth, C., and McIntyre, O. R. (1971): Antiplatelet therapy for thrombotic thrombocytopenic purpura. *N. Engl. J. Med.,* 285:408–409.

Advances in Neurology, Vol. 33, edited by
M. Critchley et al. Raven Press, New York © 1982

Migraine as a Blood Disorder: Preliminary Studies

Edda Hanington

City of London Migraine Clinic; Princess Margaret Migraine Clinic, Charing Cross Hospital; and The Wellcome Trust, London, England

My colleagues and I are testing (16,17) the hypothesis that migraine is a blood disorder and due primarily to an abnormality of platelet function. Any hypothesis for migraine must explain its frequently familial nature as well as the fact that it sometimes arises for the first time later in life in people without a family history of migraine. I suggest that migraine is caused by a platelet abnormality which, although most often hereditary, can also be acquired under certain circumstances. The diverse features of migraine attacks can be explained by the great variability in factors affecting even normal platelet function. At the same time, this variability makes it difficult to detect minor abnormalities in platelet behavior. We are investigating patients with classic migraine in whom changes in platelet function would be expected to be most marked. We hope to show that their platelets differ at all times from those of nonmigraine sufferers. If differences in platelet behaviour are detected only during attacks, then it could be argued that these are secondary in nature and dependent on other factors at the time of an attack. To prove any hypothesis for a disorder, a number of clinical, biochemical, pathological, and therapeutic criteria must be fulfilled.

Migraine often is a familial disorder. When 500 patients were questioned routinely about the occurrence of migraine in their families, nearly 70% gave a close family history. Two of three stated that at least one parent, grandparent, or sibling also suffered from migraine. The familial link appears to be stronger on the maternal side, since 38% of these patients had a mother who suffered from migraine, while 14% had a father with a history of migraine.

Platelet behaviour is influenced by genetic factors, which could explain the familial incidence of migraine. Other factors affecting platelet behaviour also influence the incidence of migraine. Sex, age, and hormonal status play a major role in platelet function and in migraine. Migraine is more common in women than in men. The incidence of migraine rises to a peak in women between the ages of 20 and 45 years when hormonal changes, which have a marked effect on platelet function, are most active (26). This could also explain why migraine sometimes arises for the first time in women at the time of menopause and in women using oral contraception (21).

The most common precipitant of migraine is stress. In this context, stress includes such states as anxiety, fatigue, excitement, anger, and exertion. The hormonal changes occurring in the normal menstrual cycle and the use of oral contraceptives both have an influence on the incidence of migraine attacks. A proportion of migraine sufferers report that the eating of certain foods, notably chocolate, cheese, alcohol, and, less frequently, citrus fruits and coffee, is linked with some of their attacks. Fasting is another recognized precipitant of migraine in some sufferers (3,7). The important fact about the precipitants of migraine is that they are cumulative in nature and result in an increase in vasoactive amine metabolism. The catecholamines epinephrine and norepinephrine increase in the plasma under conditions of stress or fasting; and a number of vasoactive amines, including tyramine, octopamine, and betaphenylethylamine, are found in various migraine-precipitating foods (15). The vasoactive amines concerned in migraine are broken down by the monoamine oxidase (MAO) group of enzymes.

Platelet levels of MAO have been shown to be reduced in migraine sufferers (24). This reduction becomes highly significant during migraine attacks (14). Sicuteri and his colleagues first reported changes in 5-hydroxytryptamine (5-HT) metabolism during migraine attacks 20 years ago (25). Platelets contain all the 5-HT present in blood and release this when they aggregate or in response to certain vasoactive amines, such as epinephrine.

Many workers (6,12,19) have observed an increase in platelet aggregation in migraine sufferers since the initial report by Hilton and Cumings in 1971 (18). Platelets aggregate in response to a number of factors including, adenosine diphosphate (ADP), 5-HT, epinephrine, norepinephrine, thrombin, collagen, and arachidonic acid.

Plasma levels of 5-HT rise just before the onset of a migraine attack and fall significantly during an attack (1,8,23). Excretion of the major metabolite of 5-HT, 5-hydroxyindole-acetic acid, is increased during migraine attacks (2,11). A significant rise in serum levels of beta-thromboglobulin occurs during migraine attacks, indicating platelet activation (13). Thus the major biochemical changes reported to occur during migraine attacks are inextricably linked with platelet function.

We briefly consider the sequence of events in an attack of classic migraine. Prodromal symptoms usually are visual; occasionally, however, patients report other symptoms, such as aparaesthesias, weakness in one or more limbs, and, in rare cases, hemiparesis. It is difficult to distinguish these symptoms from those occurring in the transient ischemic attacks arising in older patients with cerebral atherosclerosis. In migraine sufferers, they could result from the combined effect of small platelet aggregates in the affected vessels and vasoconstriction following 5-HT release, or even from the effects of severe vasoconstriction following 5-HT release alone. The occipital cortex is particularly sensitive to the effects of cerebral ischemia (22). In rare cases, cerebral atrophy and areas of cortical infarction have been reported in migraine sufferers.

5-HT constricts the branches of the internal carotid artery but has a variable effect on the branches of the external carotid. When the sympathetic tone is high, as it would be at the onset of a migraine attack, 5-HT causes dilation. Some of the branches of the external carotid artery, notably the middle meningeal, enter the skull. Dilation of these vessels in the meninges could produce the pain characteristic of migraine during the headache phase, which is often localized to the sites supplied by the branches of the middle meningeal artery. Thus abnormal platelet behavior could explain an attack of migraine. We cannot ignore the fact that most drugs that are effective in the prophylactic therapy of migraine have an inhibitory effect on platelet aggregation (4,27). Aspirin, methysergide, amitriptyline, propranolol, dihydroergotamine, heparin, phenylbutazone, and imipramine have all been used in the treatment of migraine; all have an inhibitory effect on platelet aggregation.

It has been shown that the platelets of migraine sufferers release their 5-HT content more readily at all times in response to agents, such as tyramine, than do the platelets of control subjects (9). A defect in platelet 5-HT uptake and accumulation in migraine sufferers has been reported, as well as changes in the platelet membrane (5,20). Thus a permanent difference, first discussed by Hilton and Cumings in 1971 (18), appears to exist in the behaviour of platelets from migrainous subjects.

Platelet function is difficult to investigate not least from the clinical point of view. Evidence should be sought in patients with naturally occurring disorders affecting platelet function. For example, there have been reports of migraine attacks occurring for the first time in patients with thrombocytopenic purpura when a sudden fall in platelet count occurred (10). One patient with severe and frequent attacks of classic migraine reported that these ceased during a 4-week spell when she had repeated blood transfusions. Another patient on cytotoxic therapy stated that one advantage of her periods of therapy was that she was migraine free and could eat chocolate and cheese without getting an attack; these were also times when her platelet count was very low. My colleagues and I have been treating a patient whose headaches greatly increased in severity as she developed thrombocythemia.

Although conclusions cannot be drawn from isolated cases, the gradual accummulation of evidence may slowly lead to the recognition of migraine as a blood disorder.

ACKNOWLEDGMENTS

We thank Miss Heather Cooper, City of London Migraine Clinic, for her assistance with these studies; the Wellcome Trustees for the support of this research; and the British Migraine Association.

REFERENCES

1. Anthony, M., Hinterberger, H., and Lance, J. W. (1967): Plasma serotonin in migraine and stress. *Arch. Neurol.,* 16:544–552.
2. Berstad, J. R. (1976): Total 5-hydroxyindoles in blood related to migraine attacks. *Acta Neurol. Scand.,* 54:293–300.
3. Blau, J. N., and Cumings, J. N. (1966): Method of precipitating and preventing some migraine attacks. *Br. Med. J.,* ii:1,242–2,343.
4. Born, G. V. R., Mills, D. C. B., and Smith, J. B. (1973): Pharmacology of the inhibition of platelet aggregation. *Bull. Schweiz. Akad. Med. Wiss.,* 29:215–222.
5. Coppen, A., Swade, C., Wood, K., and Carroll, J. D. (1979): Platelet 5-hydroxytryptamine accumulation and migraine. *Lancet,* ii:914.
6. Couch, J. R., and Hassanein, R. S. (1977): Platelet aggregability in migraine. *Neurology,* 27:843–848.
7. Critchley, M., and Ferguson, F. R. (1933): Migraine. *Lancet,* i:123.
8. Curran, D. A., Hinterberger, H., and Lance, J. W. (1965): Total plasma serotonin, 5-hydroxyindoleacetic acid and p-hydroxy-m-methoxymandelic acid excretion in normal and migrainous subjects. *Brain,* 88:997–1,010.
9. Dalsgaard-Nielsen, T., and Genefke, I. K. (1974): Serotonin (5HT) release and uptake in platelets from healthy persons and migrainous patients in attack-free intervals. *Headache,* 14:26–32.
10. Damasio, H., and Beck, D. (1978): Migraine, thrombocytopenia and serotonin metabolism. *Lancet,* i:240–242.
11. Deanovic, Z., Iskric, S., and Dupelj, M. (1975): Fluctuation of 5-hydroxy-indole compounds in the urine of migrainous patients. *Biomedicine,* 23:346–349.
12. Deshmukh, S. B., and Meyer, J. S. (1977): Cyclic changes in platelet dynamics and the pathogenesis and prophylaxis of migraine. *Headache,* 17:101–108.
13. Gawel, M. J., Burkett, M., Rose, F. C., Sandler, M., Glover, V., and Moncada, S. (1978): Platelet function during migraine attacks. In: *Absts. of 2nd International Migraine Symposium,* p. 34. London.
14. Glover, V., Sandler, M., Grant, E., Rose, F. C., Orton, D., Wilkinson, M., and Stevens D. (1977): Transitory decrease in platelet monoamine oxidase activity during migraine attacks. *Lancet,* i:391–393.
15. Hanington, E. (1967): Preliminary report on tyramine headache. *Br. Med. J.,* ii:550–551.

16. Hanington, E. (1978): Migraine: A blood disorder. *Lancet,* ii: 501–503.
17. Hanington, E. (1979): Migraine: A platelet hypothesis. *Biomedicine,* 30:2–65.
18. Hilton, B. P., and Cumings, J. N. (1971): An assessment of platelet aggregation induced by 5-hydroxytryptamine. *J. Clin. Pathol.,* 24:250–258.
19. Kalendowsky, Z., and Austin, J. H. (1975): "Complicated migraine". Its association with increased platelet aggregability and abnormal plasma coagulation factors. *Headache,* 15:18–35.
20. Malmgren, R., Olsson, P., Tornling, G., and Unge, G. (1979): Migraine, a platelet disorder. *Lancet,* ii:1198.
21. Poller, L., Priest, C. M., and Thomson, J. M. (1969): Platelet aggregation during oral contraception. *Br. Med. J.,* 4:273–274.
22. Ross Russell, R. W., and Bharucha, N. (1978): The recognition and prevention of border zone cerebral ischaemia during cardiac surgery. *Q. J. Med.,* 187:303.
23. Rydzewski, W. (1976): Serotonin (5HT) in migraine: Levels in whole blood in and between attacks. *Headache,* 16:16–19.
24. Sandler, M., Youdim, M. B. H., and Hanington, E. (1974): A phenylethylamine oxidising defect in migraine. *Nature,* 250:335–337.
25. Sicuteri, F., Testi, A., and Anselmi, B. (1961): Biochemical investigations in headache: Increase in the hydroxyindoleacetic acid excretion during migraine attacks. *Int. Arch. Allgery Appl. Immunol.,* 19:55–58.
26. Somerville, B. W. (1972): The influence of progesterone and estradiol upon migraine. *Headache,* 12:93–102.
27. Weksler, B. B., Gillick, M., and Pink, J. (1977): Effect of propranolol on platelet function. *Blood,* 49:185.

Advances in Neurology, Vol. 33, edited by
M. Critchley et al. Raven Press, New York © 1982

Serotonin-Releasing Factors in Migrainous Patients

Dorotea Mück-Šeler, Živan Deanović, and *Milivoj Dupelj

*Department of Experimental Biology and Medicine, Institute Rudjer Bošković, and *Department
of Neurology, University Hospital, Zagreb, Rebro, Yugoslavia*

Migraine is a complex disorder which includes combined biochemical (8,14,25), vascular (17), and neurological (6) changes. Among the biochemical factors, the role of biogenic amines has been investigated for many years (1,2,4). A sudden and marked fall in serotonin (5-HT) blood levels during the migraine attack could be directly (3) or indirectly (24) related to the pathomechanism of migraine. Moreover, a 5-HT deficiency in the brainstem, associated with a lower pain threshold, was proposed as a central biochemical theory of migraine (22). Therefore, we followed the blood platelet 5-HT level in migraine patients during different clinical phases, along with their urinary excretion rate of 5-HT and its main metabolite, 5-hydroxyindoleacetic acid (5-HIAA).

The decrease in blood platelet 5-HT concentration during the migraine attack was presumed to be provoked by the appearance of a 5-HT-releasing factor in plasma (2,12). Thus we undertook the cross-incubation experiments with plasma and platelets of migraine sufferers in different clinical phases.

MATERIAL AND METHODS

Patients were women, 15 to 54 years of age, hospitalized for either common or classic migraine. During the period of urine collection, the patients were on a diet without any 5-HT-containing food (banana, walnut, pineapple, or tomato juice). Coffee, tea, and cigarette smoking were also restricted. 5-HIAA in the urine was determined by a colorimetric method according to Dalgliesh (9) and 5-HT by a fluorimetric method according to Oates (19).

We tried to provoke a migraine attack with reserpine, 2.5 mg i.m., in seven patients. All but one had a typical headache attack (10).

The blood donors were healthy persons and patients with classic or common migraine. Blood (9 ml) from cubital vein was collected into a plastic tube containing 1 ml anticoagulant (3.8% sodium citrate and 1% ethylenediaminetetraacetic acid in saline; volume ratio, 1:1). Plasma with or without platelets was obtained by two different centrifugation speeds of blood. The cross-incubation experiments were performed in a water bath at 37°C, as previously described (18). 5-HT content in platelets was determined by the spectrofluorimetric method according to Crawford and Rudd (7). For statistical analysis, the conventional Students t-test and the same test as a method of differences were used (13).

RESULTS

A significant increase in 5-HIAA excretion rate was found during the migraine attack as compared with the attack-free period. The postheadache fall of urinary 5-HIAA was also significant (Fig. 1). In six patients, the reserpine provocation test was followed by an intense enhancement of 5-HIAA excretion rate, but the decrease thereafter was less expressed than after a spontaneous attack (Fig. 2).

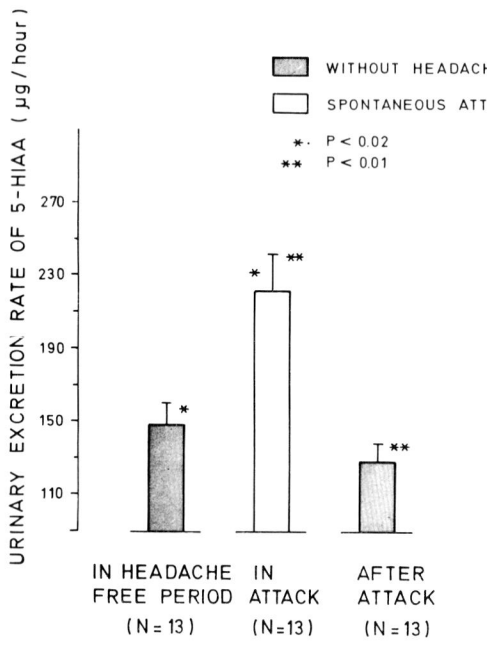

FIG. 1. Urinary excretion rate of 5-HIAA during different clinical phases of migraine. Results are expressed as mean ± SEM. *N*, number of subjects.

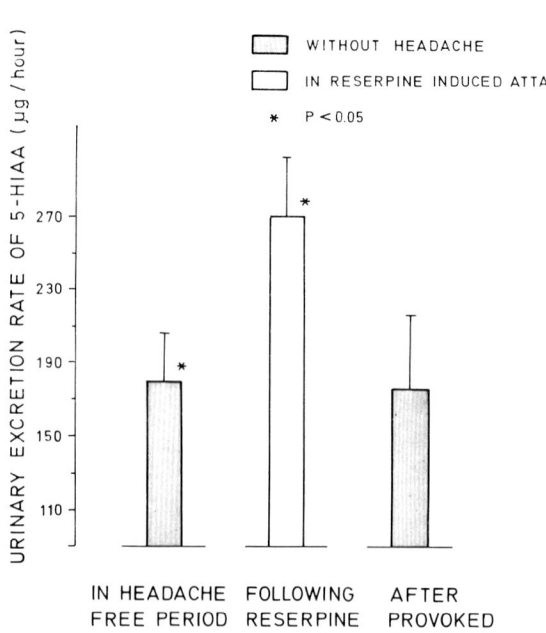

FIG. 2. Urinary excretion rate of 5-HIAA after reserpine provocation test. Results are expressed as mean ± SEM. *N*, number of subjects.

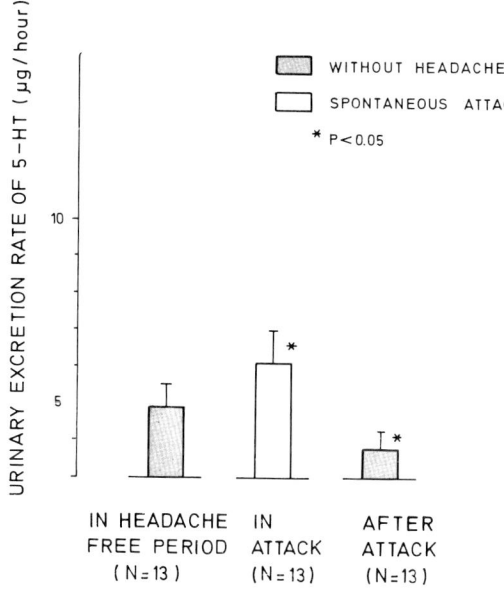

FIG. 3. Urinary excretion rate of 5-HT during different clinical phases of migraine. Results are expressed as mean ± SEM. *N*, number of subjects.

The urinary excretion rate of 5-HT was also followed (Fig. 3). The weak increase in the course of the spontaneous attack was not significant; but after the reserpine test, it was highly significant (Fig. 4). In the period immediately following the attack, the excretion rate of 5-HT was markedly decreased in both the spontaneous and reserpine-provoked headache groups (Figs. 3 and 4).

In six migraine sufferers, it was possible to compare platelet 5-HT levels during head-

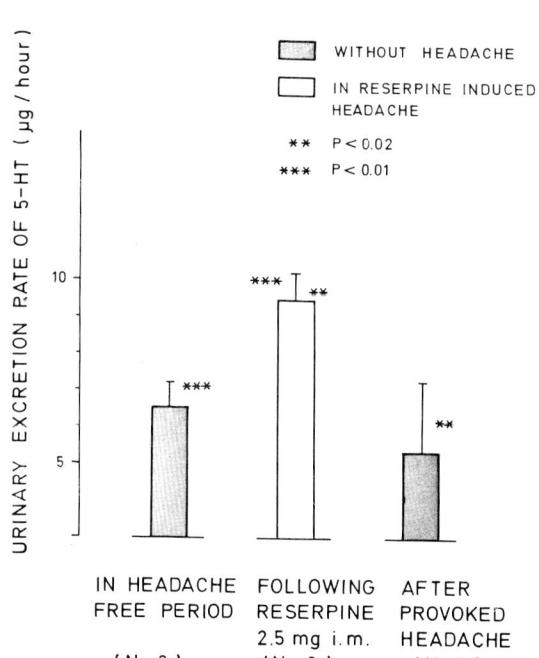

Fig. 4. Urinary excretion rate of 5-HT after reserpine provocation test. Results are expressed as mean ± SEM. *N*, number of subjects.

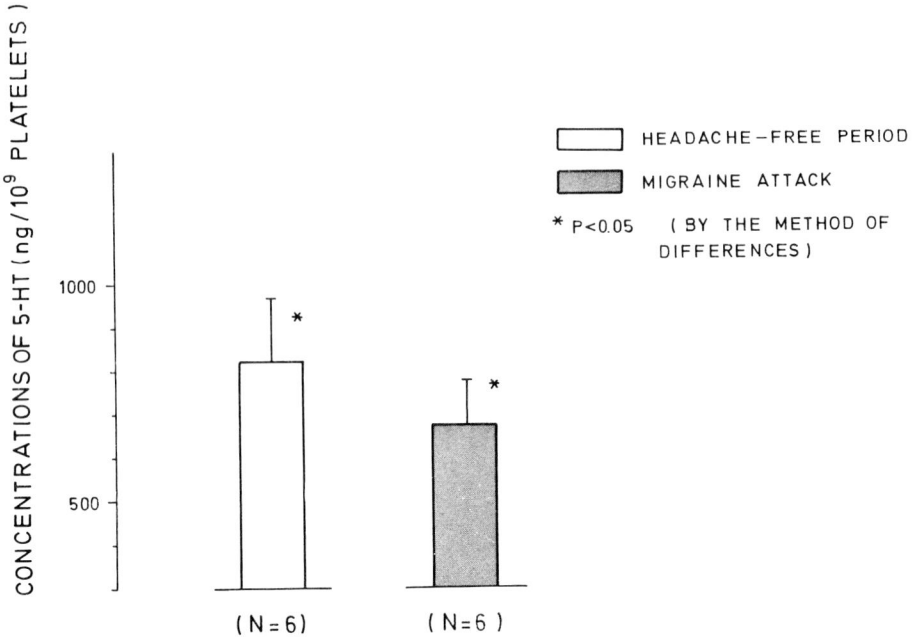

FIG. 5. Difference in platelet 5-HT content in six migraineous patients during headache-free period and during migraine attack. Each column represents the mean ± SEM. *N*, number of subjects.

ache-free periods with the level obtained during the attack (Fig. 5.). The fall of 5-HT concentration during the headache was statistically significant ($p < 0.05$).

The results of cross-incubation experiments are shown in Fig. 6. Platelet-poor plasma (PPP) taken from a migraine sufferer during an attack produced a significant release of 5-HT from blood platelets of other migraineurs isolated during an attack or in the period without headache. The loss of 5-HT was 22% in the first combination and approximately 26% in the second. On the other hand, PPP taken in the headache-free period did not produce any considerable release of 5-HT from migraineous platelets taken during the attack or from the platelets taken in the headache-free period. In cross-incubation experiments with platelets from healthy donors and PPP from migrainous subjects, platelets lost a negligible amount of their 5-HT content in both cases.

DISCUSSION

Among the changes of various humoral factors presumably involved in migraine, a fall of blood 5-HT level appears to be the most consistent (1). No significant difference in platelet 5-HT levels was found between healthy persons and migraine patients during headache-free periods (18). During a migraine attack, however, a significant fall of platelet 5-HT level was established. This decrease of about 15% of the 5-HT content found during the headache-free period is in agreement with the data reported by Anthony et al. (1). The present study reinforces the previous findings that migraine episodes are accompanied by release of 5-HT from platelets into the plasma (2). The free 5-HT undergoes oxidative deamination due to the plasma or vessel wall monoamine oxidase

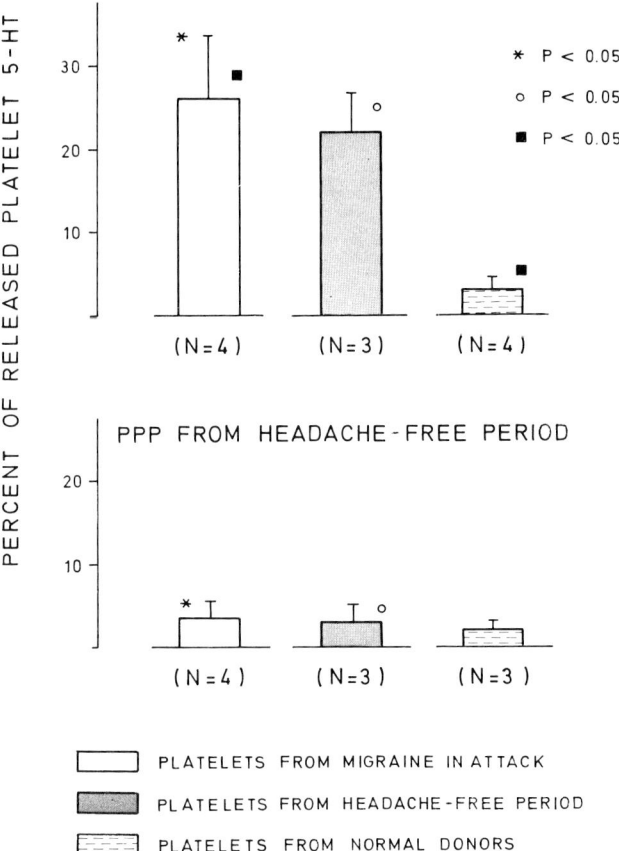

FIG. 6. Percent of released platelet 5-HT in cross-incubation experiments. Results are expressed as mean ± SEM. N, number of cross-incubation experiments. PPP, platelet poor plasma.

(MAO) activity and is finally excreted in the urine mostly as 5-HIAA. The clearance of this acid metabolite is high since its excretion occurs through two different mechanisms: glomerular filtration and tubular secretion (5,11). The small part of the free amine, which has escaped degradation, is eliminated from the bloodstream through tubular secretion only (21,26). Therefore, the oscillation of urinary 5-HT is not so pronounced as in the case of 5-HIAA. On the other hand, the low excretion rate of both 5-hydroxyindoles during the hours after migraine attack could indicate a restitution of the capacity of platelets to take up 5-HT.

Following the application of reserpine, the excretion of both compounds was enhanced; but this phenomenon was not related to headache intensity. The values obtained later (after provoked headache) remained mostly above the control values, which is not surprising because of the well-known protracted effect of reserpine.

The demonstrated fall of 5-HT levels might be involved in the trigger mechanism of migraine episodes owing to a concomitant vasodilatation of scalp arteries (23). However,

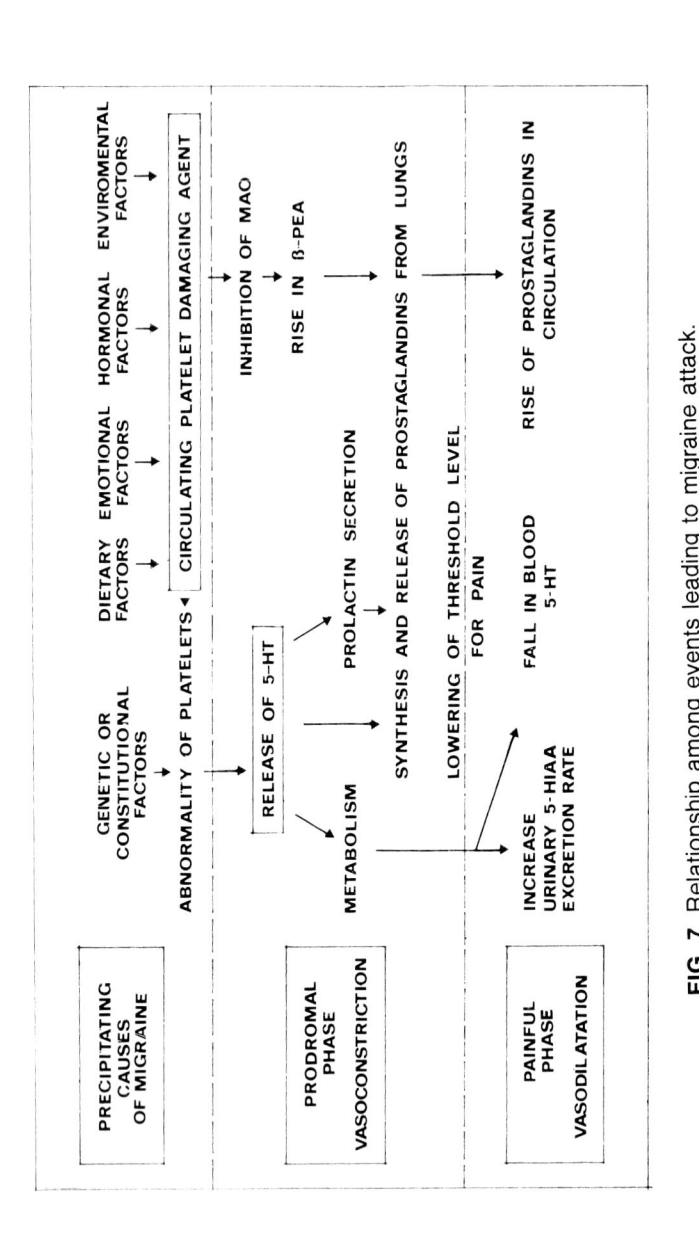

FIG. 7. Relationship among events leading to migraine attack.

the question arises whether this change in platelet 5-HT level is the primary step in the chain of events leading to a migraine attack or is the consequence, i.e. a secondary phenomenon. Our results obtained in the cross-incubation experiments support the hypothesis that 5-HT release and the change in platelet MAO activity are not primary but secondary processes following the appearance of a platelet-damaging agent (20) into the circulation.

In our cross-incubation experiments, only plasma taken from migrainous patients during attacks produced a 5-HT release from platelets of other migraineurs venepunctured in any clinical phase. Moreover, we have shown that the effect of this presumed plasma factor is solely limited to the platelets of migraineurs; it does not affect platelets of healthy subjects. The changes in 5-HT levels during incubation are not to be ascribed to the damage or aggregation of platelets; in this case, the percent of 5-HT release should be greater in other combinations as well.

As considered by Anthony et al. (1), an as yet unidentified 5-HT-releasing factor should appear in plasma provoking the depletion of 5-HT during the migraine attack. We know little about this factor; it is obviously a compound present only in the blood of migraine sufferers in an attack. It is suggested that this compound is not a protein but a low molecular substance; some years ago, Anthony (4) supposed that this compound may be a free fatty acid (for example, linolenic acid).

The relationship between some events leading to a migraine attack is shown in Fig. 7. Commonly observed familial incidence of migraine suggest a genetic origin (17). Dietary, emotional, hormonal, and environmental factors are also known to precipitate migraine. We propose that these factors could influence the appearance of a circulating platelet-damaging agent in the plasma of migraine sufferers. This agent might be able to induce a transitory inhibition of MAO activity (20). Consequently, a rise of beta-phenylethylamine (beta-PEA) concentration may occur; this amine is also known as a vasodilatation-provoking agent (15).

Evidence indicates that a platelet abnormality, e.g., hyperaggregability (16), is present in migraine patients. The platelet-damaging agent might release 5-HT from platelets of these patients early in the prodromal phase. The free 5-HT is rapidly metabolized and excreted as 5-HIAA in the urine. The fall in plasma 5-HT may initiate the dilatation of cranial arteries and hence the pain of migraine. Some findings indicate that substances similar to prostaglandins (PG) play an important role in the pathogenesis of migraine (15). 5-HT, prolactin, and beta-PEA may increase PG synthesis. PG produced a biphasic effect on vascular reactivity; they are vasoconstrictors at low concentrations and dilatators at higher concentrations.

The threshold level for pain probably varies from one sufferer to another, but when biochemical or vascular changes are sufficiently strong, the threshold is exceeded and an attack follows. Many factors could play a role in the pathogenesis of migraine; it is obvious, however, that platelets are closely involved in the mechanism of migraine attack.

ACKNOWLEDGMENTS

These investigations were supported by Fund for Scientific Activities of SR Croatia and NIH PL 480 research agreement 02–015–1. We thank Mrs. Ivanka Fresl for skillful technical assistance. The close collaboration of the staff and patients of the Neurological Clinic, University of Zagreb is also appreciated.

REFERENCES

1. Anthony, M., Hinerberger, H., and Lance, J. W. (1967): Plasma serotonin in migraine and stress. *Arch. Neurol.,* 16:544–552.
2. Anthony, M., Hinerberger, H., and Lance, J. W. (1968): Studies of serotonin metabolism in migraine. *Proc. Aust. Assoc. Neurol.,* 5:109–112.
3. Anthony, M., Hinerberger, H., and Lance, J. W. (1969): The possible relationship of serotonin to the migraine syndrome. *Res. Clin. Stud. Headache,* 2:29–59.
4. Anthony, M. (1975): Some aspects of clinical pharmacology of serotonin. *Agents Actions,* 5:490–491.
5. Barac, G. (1961): Elimination rénale de l'acide 5-hydroxyindoléacétique chez le chien. *C. R. Soc. Biol.,* 155:1732–1738.
6. Blau, J. N. (1978): Migraine: A vasomotor instability of the meningeal circulation. *Lancet,* II:1,136–1,139.
7. Crawford, N., and Rudd, B. T. (1962): A spectrophotofluorimetric method for the determination of serotonin (5-hydroxytryptamine) in plasma. *Clin. Chim. Acta.,* 7:114–121.
8. Curran, D. A., Hinterberger, H., and Lance, J. W. (1965): Total plasma serotonin, 5-hydroxyindoleacetic acid and p-hydroxy-m-methoxy-mandelic acid excretion in normal and migrainous subjects. *Brain,* 88:997–1010.
9. Dalgliesh, C. E. (1958): The 5-hydroxy-indoles. *Adv. Clin. Chem.,* 1:193–199.
10. Deanović, Ž., Iskrić, S., and Dupelj, M. (1975): Fluctuation of 5-hydroxyindole compounds in the urine of migrainous patients. *Biomedicine,* 23:346–349.
11. Despopoulos, A. (1957): Renal metabolism of 5-hydroxy-indole acetic acid. *Am. J. Physiol.,* 189:548–552.
12. Dvilansky, A., Rishpon, S., Nathan, I., Zolotow, Z., and Korczyn, A. D. (1976): Release of platelet 5-hydroxytryptamine by plasma taken from patients during and between migraine attacks. *Pain,* 2:315–318.
13. Fischer, R. A. (1950): *Statistical Methods for Research Workers.* Oliver and Boyd, Edinburgh.
14. Gotoh, F., Kauda, T., Sakai, F., Yamamoto, M., and Takeoka, T. (1976): Serum dopamine-beta-hydroxy-lase activity in migraine. *Arch. Neurol.,* 33:656–657.
15. Horrobin, D. F. (1977): Prostaglandins and migraine. *Headache,* 17:113–117.
16. Kalendovsky, Z., and Austin, J. H. (1975): Complicated migraine—its association with increased platelet aggregability and abnormal plasma coagulation factors. *Headache,* 15:18–35.
17. Lance, J. W. (1972): Clinical features and vascular changes of migraine and cluster headache. *Med. J. Aust.* [*Special Suppl.*], 2:3–6.
18. Mück-Šeler, D., Deanović, Ž., and Dupelj, M. (1979): Platelet serotonin (5-HT) and 5-HT releasing factor in plasma of migrainous patients. *Headache,* 19:14–16.
19. Oates, J. A. (1961): Measurement of urinary tryptamine, tyramine and serotonin. *Methods Med. Res.,* 9:169–178.
20. Sandler, M. (1977): Transitory platelet monoamine oxidase deficit in migraine: Some reflections. *Headache,* 17:153–158.
21. Sanner, E., and Wortman, B. (1962): Tubular excretion of serotonin in chicken. *Acta Physiol. Scand.,* 55:319–925.
22. Sicuteri, F., Anselmi, B., and Del Bianco, P. L. (1973): 5-Hydroxytryptamine supersensitivity as a new theory of headache and central pain; a clinical pharmacological approach with p-chlorophenylalanine. *Psychopharmacologia,* 29:347–356.
23. Sicuteri, F. (1974): Headache biochemistry and pharmacology. *Arch. Neurobiol.,* 37:27–65.
24. Sjaastad, O. (1975): The significance of blood serotonin levels in migraine. *Acta Neurol. Scand.,* 51:200–210.
25. Welch, K. M. A., Chabi, E., Bartosh, K., Achar, V. S., and Meyer, J. S. (1975): Cerebrospinal fluid gama-aminobutyric acid levels in migraine. *Br. Med. J.,* 3:516–517.
26. Williams, W. M., and Huang, K. C. (1970): In vitro and in vivo renal tubular transport of tryptophan derivates. *Am. J. Physiol.,* 219:1,468–1,472.

Advances in Neurology, Vol. 33, edited by
M. Critchley et al. Raven Press, New York © 1982

A Putative 5-HT Central Feedback in Migraine and Cluster Headache Attacks

S. Salmon, M. Bonciani, M. Fanciullacci, *L. Marianelli, S. Michelacci, and F. Sicuteri

*Department of Clinical Pharmacology, and *Department of Pediatrics, University of Florence, Florence, Italy*

The cooperation of analgesic neurotransmitters, serotonin (5-HT) and endorphins, is partly responsible for the control of the pain suppressor system (PSS); thus any impairment of the action of this tandem is expected to disrupt the nociceptive function (1,2), resulting in a lowered pain threshold with an arousal of spontaneous pain. Idiopathic headaches, migraine included, are the most common expressions of a disorder in the PSS (22,24). A deficiency of 5-HT provokes or at least increases pain in animals (11,33) and in man (21). It is not known if in animal or man a deficiency of endorphins induces a similar phenomenon. The evidence supporting the involvement of endorphins in pain control comes from the observation of systemic pain following withdrawal in morphine-tolerant animals (19) and man (25,26,28).

The aim of the present investigation on the 5-HT-headache relationship is twofold: (a) Since our current hypothesis proposes a decreased 5-HT synthesis in the brain during migraine attacks, implying a feedback mechanism, the 5-HT precursor tryptophan (TP) was evaluated in cerebrospinal fluid (CSF) and in plasma of headache sufferers in attack periods. If an urgent request for 5-HT in the brain arises, an elevated availability of free plasma TP, i.e., not bound to albumin and thus disposable for crossing the blood-brain barrier, should be detectable. In such a case, increased concentrations of unbound plasma and CSF TP are expected. (b) Since blood 5-HT, a pain-producing and vasoconstrictor agent, is considered to be responsible for the eruption of a migraine attack by constricting head arteries and stimulating pain receptors, it was necessary to focus the possible correlation between high blood 5-HT levels (carcinoid syndrome and cystic fibrosis patients) with the presence or absence of headache.

Platelet-bound 5-HT, the principal fraction (about 80%) of total blood 5-HT, does not cross the blood-brain barrier. Since no previous reports concern the levels of free plasma 5-HT (4) (which is thought to exert an action on vascular smooth muscle and pain receptors) in carcinoid and cystic fibrosis syndromes, both platelet and plasma free 5-HT were evaluated in subjects suffering from these two pathologies as well as in migraineurs.

RATIONALE

If blood 5-HT was to play a role in the migraine mechanism, severe headaches should constantly be experienced in such diseases such as carcinoid syndrome and cystic fibrosis in which 5-HT concentrations are much higher than in normal conditions. On the other hand, headaches in these patients are just as frequent and intense as in the total population; therefore, the possibility of normal 5-HT levels in plasma of carcinoid and cystic fibrosis patients may not need to be excluded. In fact, platelet-bound 5-HT, being physiologically inactive, does not affect vascular smooth muscle and pain receptors, whereas plasma 5-HT does. Hence we evaluated plasma and platelet 5-HT in the following subjects: (a) normal controls with a negative family history of headache, (b) carcinoid patients who exhibit high levels of total blood 5-HT, (c) cystic fibrosis patients who have elevated blood 5-HT levels (14,15), although less than in cases of carcinoid syndrome, and (d) migraine patients in attack and attack-free periods.

Changes in CSF concentrations of neurotransmitter precursors and/or metabolites reflect their turnover in brain. Therefore, the evaluation of TP in the CSF in pathologic conditions with a putative postulated impairment of brain (brainstem) 5-HT turnover might be informative. Moreover, free and total plasma TP levels, determined after an oral l-tryptophan loading in headache sufferers and normal subjects, appeared to be of great interest in detecting the eventual peripheral modifications of extracerebral 5-HT turnover.

PATIENTS

All the migraine headache patients were hospitalized in the Department of Clinical Pharmacology of Florence. Seven headache sufferers, ranging in age from 22 to 35 years, and five volunteer control subjects, ranging in age from 18 to 28 years, fasting and drug free, were given 8 mg/g i.v. l-tryptophan. Blood samples were taken before and 25 min, 1, 2, and 3 hr after the administration of the drug, as previously suggested (10).

Samples for routine CSF examination and TP evaluation were taken from 36 idiopathic headache sufferers divided into three groups: (a) 10 daily headache sufferers (ranging in age from 22 to 51 years), (b) 26 migraine headache sufferers, 13 in the free period (ranging in age from 22 to 51 years) and 13 during the attack (ranging in age from 24 to 52 years), (c) 13 cluster headache patients, divided in two groups: four in the attack-free period (ranging in age from 32 to 50 years) and nine during the attack (ranging in age from 28 to 48 years), and (d) five neurological patients (ranging in age from 40 to 60 years), who were used as control subjects.

Blood samples for total blood, plasma, and platelet evaluation were collected from (a) 15 migrainous patients (ranging in age from 26 to 47 years) observed during the migraine attack and in the free period, (b) five patients affected by the carcinoid syndrome (ranging in age form 38 to 59 years), hospitalized in the S.M.N. Hospital of Florence, (c) 15 control subjects, nonhospitalized volunteers, with a negative family history of headache (ranging in age from 22 to 56 years), (d) 12 migrainous children observed in the Child Division of the Headache Center in Florence (ranging in age from 6 to 14 years) (9), (e) 11 children affected by cystic fibrosis (11 ranging in age from 2 to 10 years and one 18-year-old), hospitalized in the Division of the Clinic of Pediatrics in Florence (14), and (f) 12 normal children, with a negative family history of headache (ranging in age from 7 to 12 years).

METHODS

TP

Free and total plasma TP, as well as CSF TP levels, were measured using Eccleston's method (6), with an ultrafiltration technique for the free fraction and a spectrophotofluorimetric reaction.

5-HT

Blood, plasma, and platelet 5-HT were evaluated with a spectrophotofluorimetric method (after o-phthaldialdehyde fluorescence), recently modified (16).

RESULTS

Changes in free and total TP levels after intravenous *l*-TP loading are summarized in Fig. 1. Free TP increases four times and total TP three times from baseline levels. The maximum increase is reached 25 min after drug administration. The time course is identical in headache and control subjects.

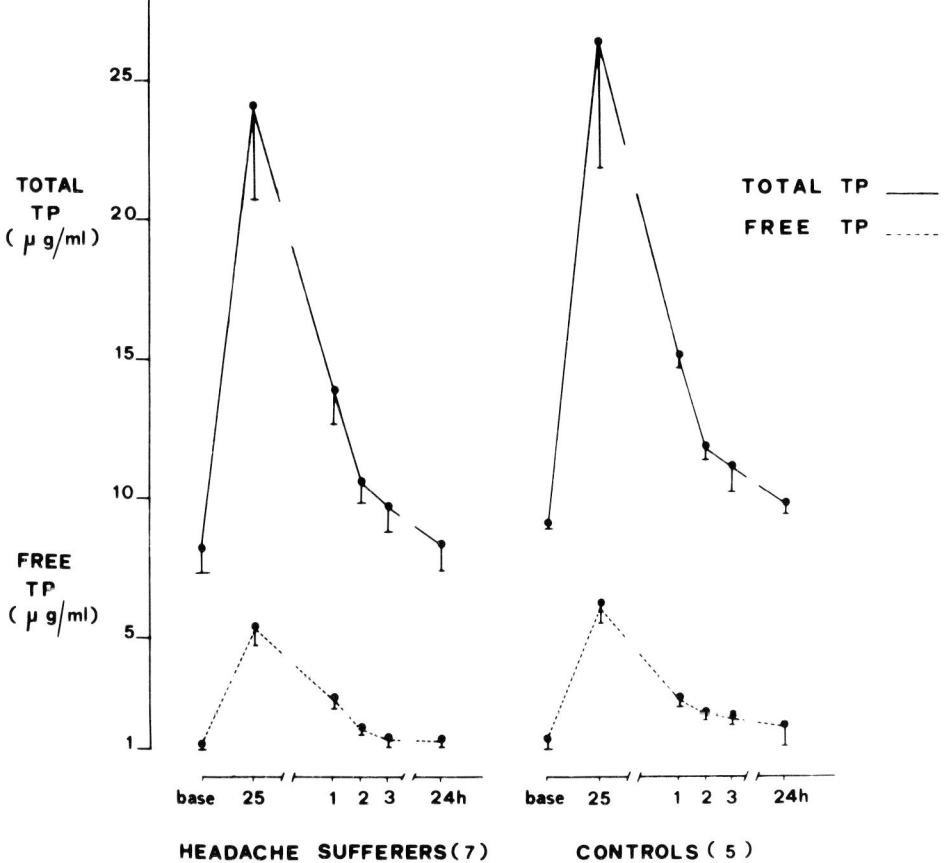

FIG. 1. Plasma free and total TP after *l*-TP loading (8 mg/kg i.v.); no differences between migrainous and nonmigrainous subjects.

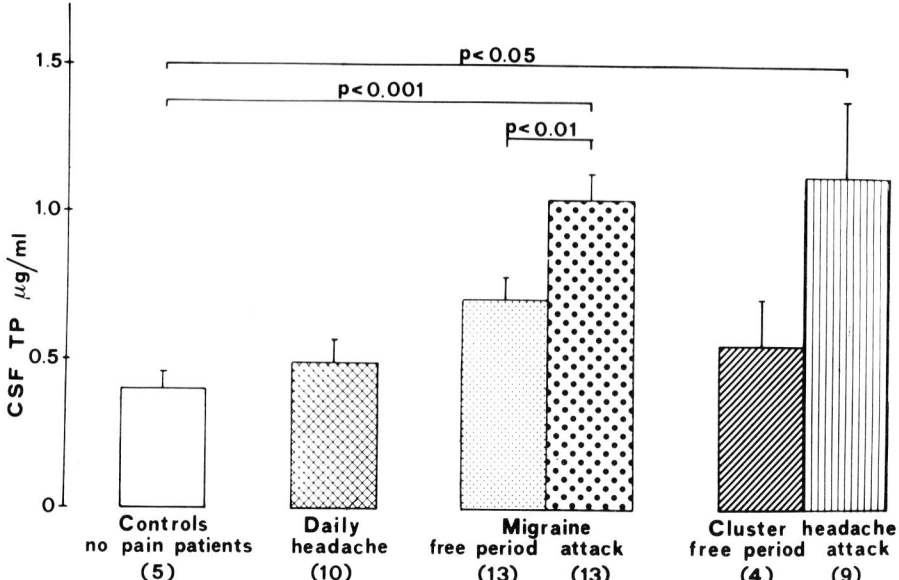

FIG. 2. Significant increase of the 5-HT precursor during migraine and cluster attacks might reflect an increased request for 5-HT (intended as an analgesic neurotransmitter) in the brain to satisfy a putative feedback mechanism.

Mean CSF TP levels are shown in Fig. 2. A highly significant increase is found in migraine patients during the attack (if compared to the free period, $p < 0.01$; if compared to the controls, i.e., neurological patients without pain, $p < 0.001$). A significant increase ($p < 0.05$) is also present in the group of cluster headache patients during the attack period.

Figure 3 shows blood, platelet, and plasma 5-HT levels found in all 35 adult subjects examined. The results are compared to the values previously reported (7). Significant differences between attack and free period were not present in migraine sufferers. Patients affected by the carcinoid syndrome show plasma and, as expected, total blood and platelet 5-HT levels highly increased (about 20 times) when compared with the values in normal subjects (about 20 ng/ml of plasma).

Figure 4 compares blood, platelet, and plasma 5-HT levels of migraine sufferers with those of controls and the five carcinoid patients. When compared with controls, carcinoid patients exhibit higher ($p < 0.001$) plasma levels of 5-HT.

In Fig. 5, blood, platelet, and plasma 5-HT levels of children affected by cystic fibrosis are compared to those found in migrainous children and controls. Platelet 5-HT levels are increased in migrainous as well as in cystic fibrosis patients ($p < 0.05$); plasma 5-HT is increased only in the group affected by cystic fibrosis ($p < 0.001$).

COMMENT

The hypothesis that free plasma 5-HT (the active fraction) is responsible for pain generation in headache by its action on vascular and perivascular pain receptors and/ or on vasomotor (muscular) receptors is hardly acceptable for two reasons: (a) During

5-HT

	blood (ng/ml)	plasma (ng/ml)	platelet (ng/10⁹ plat.)	%	n° platelets
CONTROLS (15)	136.99 ±12.01	25.33 ±2.39	391.62 ±41.23	20.13 ±2.64	289 000 ±17 000
CARCINOIDS (5)	1325.22[**] ±340.92	353.55[**] ±111.96	3104.51[**] ±640.48	27.52 ±6.02	299 000 ±46 000
MIGRAINEOUS (15)	128.47 ±6.99	18.10[*] ±2.26	477.48 ±45.28	14.49 ±1.68	242 000 ±14 000

[*] p < 0.05
[**] p < 0.001

human plasma and platelet 5HT content

| 20 (ng/ml) | 200-600 (ng/10⁹ plat.) |

from Essman W B
Serotonin in Health and Disease
vol 1 Sp Publ Inc 1978

FIG. 3. Blood, plasma, and platelet 5-HT mean levels in migrainous and carcinoid patients and control subjects. Carcinoid patients, who exhibit an usual incidence of headache, have about 20 times higher plasma 5-HT levels (the free active 5-HT) than migraine patients during the attack.

migraine attacks, free plasma 5-HT levels decrease instead of increasing (16,31); and (b) in certain diseases, such as carcinoid syndrome and cystic fibrosis, in which high quantities of 5-HT are not only present in platelet but also are free in plasma, headache complaints are as frequent and intense as in the normal population.

In chronic hyperserotoninemia, however, nociceptors, as well as motoreceptors, are expected to be subsensitive to 5-HT. In fact, when the sensitivity to 5-HT of the smooth muscle of hand dorsal vein is explored by the computerized venotest in carcinoid patients *in vivo,* a five- to 10-fold reduced reactivity is registered (8). Such receptorial subsensitivity might putatively protect vasomotor and pain receptors from the dramatic increase of active 5-HT.

5-HT is able to potentiate the algogenic (20) and vasodilating and permeability-increasing capacities (29,35) of kinins by sensitizing the pain and vascular receptor, respectively. This property of 5-HT has been confirmed and may account for the immediate flushing phenomenon induced by small amounts of intravenous epinephrine, intended as a kinin releaser. Such an influence of 5-HT on kinin activity is additional evidence in contrast to the hypothesis of a peripheral 5-HT role in headache. Brain 5-HT concentrations influence the levels of free plasma TP by a putative feedback mechanism. The oscillations of free plasma TP levels reflect analogous fluctuations of 5-HT concentration in the brain (32); increased levels of TP in CSF of headache sufferers could be compatible with a decrease of 5-HT concentrations in the central nervous system. Increased TP levels are constantly found in CSF during migraine and cluster headache attacks but not in CSF sampled in free periods or in nonheadache sufferers.

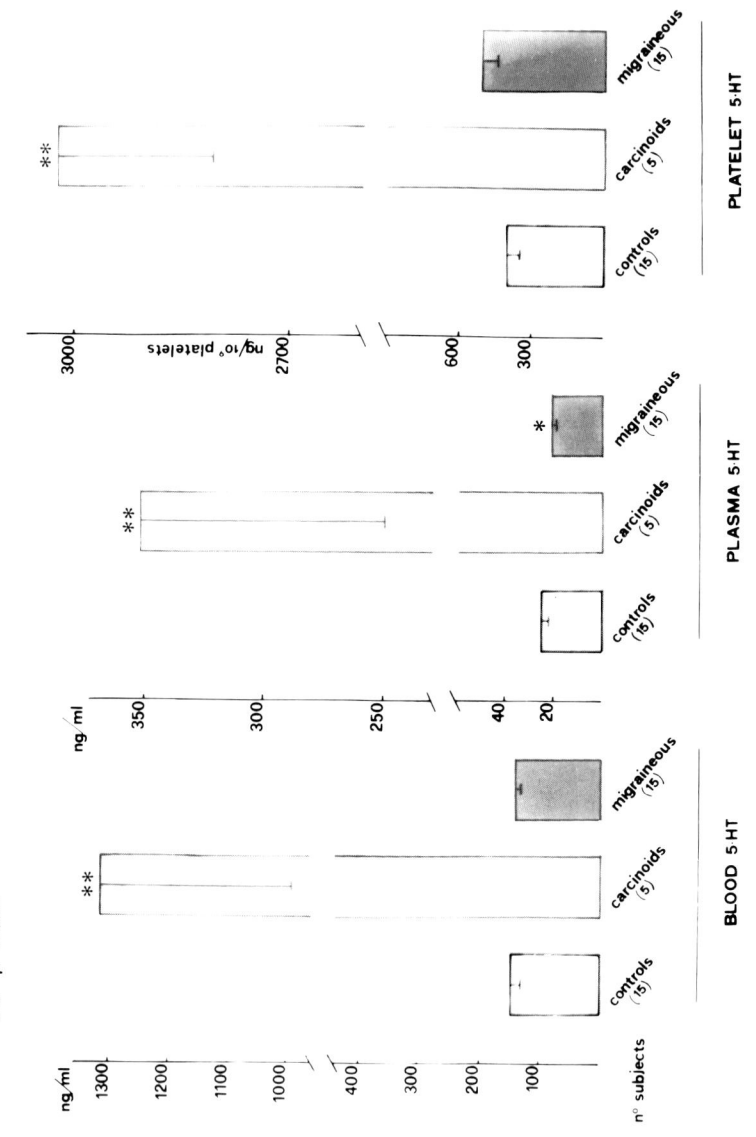

FIG. 4. If spontaneous headache was to depend on the activity of plasma 5-HT (the active part of whole blood 5-HT), carcinoid patients would constantly complain of unbearable headaches.

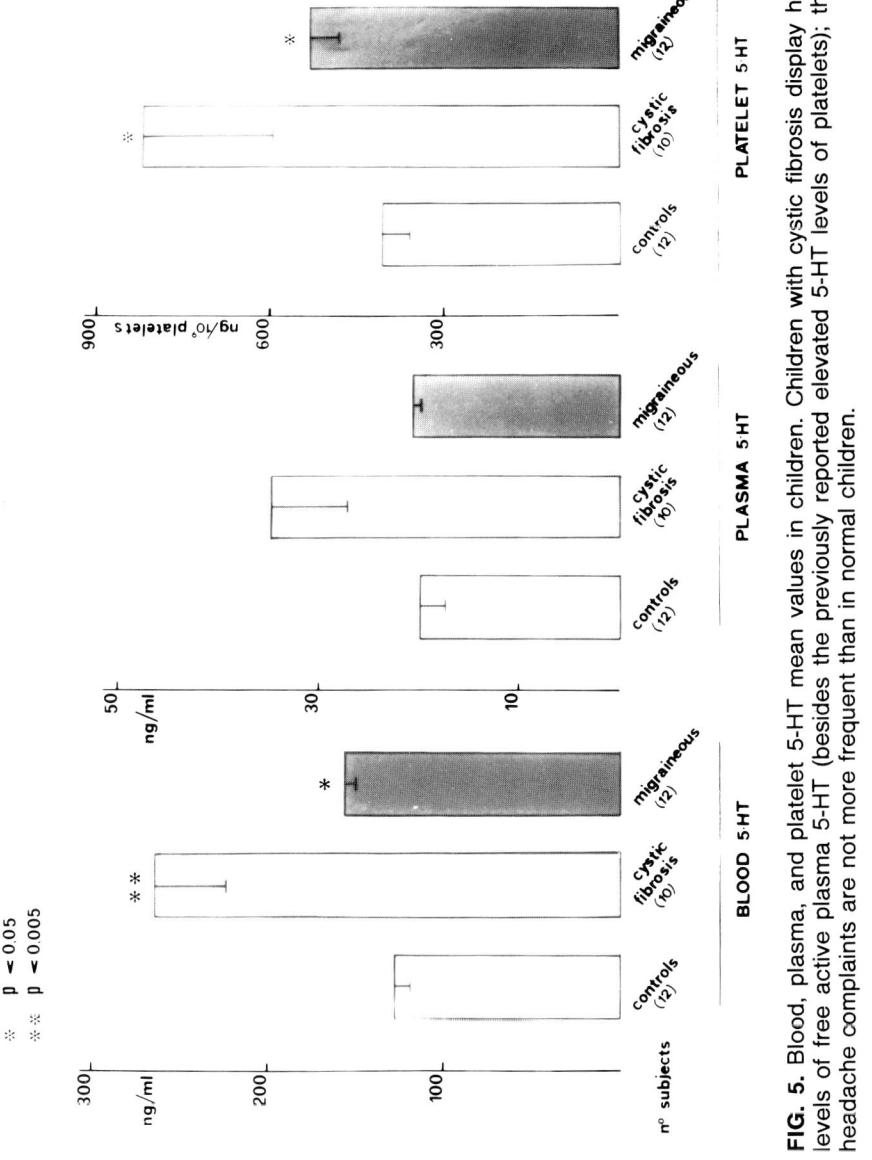

FIG. 5. Blood, plasma, and platelet 5-HT mean values in children. Children with cystic fibrosis display high levels of free active plasma 5-HT (besides the previously reported elevated 5-HT levels of platelets); their headache complaints are not more frequent than in normal children.

Free and total TP increased to the same extent in both headache sufferers and controls after intravenous loading of *l*-TP. This finding disagrees with the hypothesis of an important extracerebral impairment in 5-HT turnover and consequently of the involvement of vascular and pain receptors in headache sufferers. Even if the mechanism underlying the increase of CSF (1) and of free plasma TP (17) during headache attacks is unknown, an interdependence of the analogous phenomena occurring in the two different biological fluids may be postulated. The increased CSF TP concentrations might be due to a greater availability of this amino acid in the free plasma fraction, which is in part able to cross the blood-brain barrier. The pattern of the feedback mechanism which seems to confirm this greater availability of free plasma TP during attack periods may be only hypothesized.

If pain in migraine is assumed to be central in nature, the following sequence of events can be postulated: a putative decrease of 5-HT in the brainstem during migraine attacks triggers a feedback mechanism, the components of which are unknown, with a resulting increased availability of unbound TP in plasma. Obviously, the aim of such a feedback mechanism is to restore the poor amount of neurotransmitter in the brainstem; such a mechanism of increasing synthesis of the analgesic transmitters in PSS remains to be studied. The following serves as indirect evidence of low concentration of 5-HT in the brainstem of headache sufferers: (a) parachlorophenylalanine (PCPA), a 5-HT synthesis inhibitor, induces a panalgesia (systemic pain syndrome, central in nature) only when administered to headache sufferers; such an effect does not take place in normal subjects (21). The same response was observed in parkinsonian patients, in whom 5-HT concentrations in brain were diminished (34); (b) certain drugs able to reduce 5-HT levels in the central nervous system such as reserpine (13) and fenfluramine (5), precipitate migraine attacks; (c) other drugs, such as ergot derivatives, acting as partial 5-HT agonists at either central (12) or vascular (30) levels, exhibit antimigranous activity; (d) the observation that morphine has low or absent analgesic ability in attenuating pain in migraine (23) might agree with the poor morphine analgesia in rats when their 5-HT brain concentrations are lowered (18). Therefore, the absence of morphine analgesia in migraine patients might depend on low 5-HT levels in the brainstem.

In conclusion, the oscillation of TP levels in CSF might occur in parallel with the changes of analgesic neurotransmitter (5-HT and endorphins) quantities (1,27), which in turn are correlated with the fluctuations of pain in headache sufferers. The hypothesis that the migraine attack is an equivalent of depression disagrees with the present findings. In cases of depression, TP levels in CSF were found to be significantly decreased (3), in contrast to the increase occurring during migraine.

SUMMARY

5-HT is considered to play a role in the migraine mechanism; its decrease in the midbrain during migraine attacks has been postulated. CSF TP and plasma and platelet 5-HT levels in migraine and cluster headache sufferers have been evaluated; the values registered were compared to those of neurological and carcinoid patients, respectively.

The following results were obtained: (a) no significant difference in the time course of free and total TP after *l*-TP intravenous loading, (b) increased levels of CSF TP during migraine and cluster headache attacks, and (c) impressively increased levels of plasma 5-HT only in carcinoid patients. These findings suggest the existence of a positive

5-HT central feedback mechanism during attacks of migraine and cluster headache and thus exclude peripheral 5-HT effects in the generation of pain.

ACKNOWLEDGMENTS

Our thanks are due to the National Research Council (C.N.R.), Rome, Italy; to Dr. Savik Shuster for the revision of the English text; and to Mr. Vittorio Vivoli and Mrs. Mara Masi for their technical assistance.

REFERENCES

1. Anselmi, B., Baldi, E., Casacci, F., and Salmon, S. (1981): Endogenous opioids in cerebrospinal fluid and blood in idiopathic headache sufferers. *Headache,* 20:294–299.
2. Basbaum, A. T., and Fields M. L. (1978): Endogenous pain control mechanism: Review and hypothesis. *Ann. Neurol.,* 4:451–462.
3. Coppen, A., Eccleston, E. G., and Peet, M. (1973): Total and free tryptophan concentration in the plasma of depressive patients. *The Lancet,* 2:60–63.
4. Crawford, N. (1963): Plasma free serotonin (5-hydroxytryptamine). *Clin. Chim. Acta,* 8:39–45.
5. Del Bene, E., Anselmi, B., Del Bianco, P. L., Fanciullacci, M., Galli, P., Salmon, S., and Sicuteri, F. (1977): Fenfluramine headache: A biochemical and monoamine receptorial human study. In: *Headache New Vistas,* edited by F. Sicuteri, pp. 101–109. Biomedical Press, Florence.
6. Eccleston, E. G. (1973): A method for the estimation of free and total soluble plasma tryptophan using ultrafiltration technique. *Clin. Chim. Acta,* 48:269–272.
7. Essmann, W. B. (editor) (1978): Serotonin distribution in tissue and fluids. In: Serotonin in Health and Disease, *Vol. 1, Availability, Localisation and Dispositions,* pp. 15–178. Spectrum, New York.
8. Fanciullacci, M., Franchi, G., Curradi, C., Lagi, A., and Sicuteri, F. (1976): Serotonin vascular reactivity and other pharmacological investigations in two intestinal carcinoid patients. In: *Clinical Pharmacology Serotonin, Vol. 3,* edited by F. Sicuteri and E. Schonbaum, pp. 81–87. Karger, Basel.
9. Geppetti, P., Guidotti, R., Baldi, E., Salmon S., and Del Bene, E. (1980): Biochemical aspects of child headache. *Abstr. Int. Congr. Headache,* Florence.
10. Greenwood, M. N., Friedel, J., Bond, A. J., Curzon, G., and Lader, M. M. (1971): The acute effects of intravenous infusion of l-tryptophan in normal subjects. *Clin. Pharmacol. Ther.,* 16(3):435–464.
11. Harvey, J. A., and Lints, C. F. (1971): Lesions in the medial forebrain bundle—relationship between pain sensitivity and telencephalic content of serotonin. *J. Comp. Physiol. Psychol.,* 74:28–35.
12. Higler, H. J., and Aghajanian, G. K. (1977): Serotonin receptors in the brain. *Fed. Proc.,* 36:2,159–2,164.
13. Kimball, R. W., and Friedman, A. P. (1961): Studies on pathogenesis of migraine. *Recent Adv. Biol. Psych.,* 3:220–226.
14. Marianelli, L., Salmon, S., Galluzzi, G., and Repetto, P. (1979): Livelli di serotonina in pazienti con fibrosi cistica. *3° Simposio Italiano sulla Fibrosi Cistica,* Aggiornamento Dieterba Collaborazione Interdisciplinare Patologica Pediatricia 2, S. Remo 30–VI, pp. 449–454.
15. Partington, H. W., and Ferguson, A. L. (1975): Serotonin metabolism in cystic fibrosis. *Arch. Dis. Child.,* 52:386–390.
16. Salmon, S. (1980): Platelet and plasma serotonin, free and bound tryptophan. *Int. Postgrad. Clin. Biomed. Methods Headache,* March 20–22:16–19.
17. Salmon, S., Fanciullacci, M., Bonciani, M., and Sicuteri, F. (1978): Plasma tryptophan in migraine. *Headache,* 17:238–241.
18. Samanin, R., Gumulka, W., and Valzelli, L. (1970): Reduced effect of morphine in midbrain raphe lesioned rats. *Eur. J. Pharmacol.,* 10:339.
19. Schulz, R., and Herz, A. (1977): Naloxone-precipitated withdrawal reveals sensitization to neurotransmitters in morphine tolerant dependent rats. *Naunyn Schmiederbergs Arch. Pharmacol.,* 299:95–99.
20. Sicuteri, F. (1968): Sensitization of nociceptors by 5-hydroxytryptamine in man. *Int. Congr. Pharmacol.,* p. 57. Pergamon Press, New York.
21. Sicuteri, F. (1971): Pain syndrome in man following treatment with p-chlorophenylalanine. *Pharmacol. Rev. Commun.,* 3:401–407.
22. Sicuteri, F. (editor) (1977): Headache as metonomy of nonorganic central pain. *Headache New Vistas,* pp. 19–57. Biochemical Press, Florence.
23. Sicuteri, F. (1978): Mini-review: Endorphins, opiate receptors and migraine headache. *Headache,* 17:253–257.

24. Sicuteri, F. (1979): The nature of pain in headache and central panalgesia. In: *Mechanism of Pain and Analgesic Compounds,* edited by Beers and Bassett, pp. 295–307. Raven Press, New York.

25. Sicuteri, F. (1979): Headache as the most common disease of the antinociceptive system: Analogies with morphine abstinence. In: *Advances in Pain Research and Therapy,* edited by J. Bonica et al., pp. 358–365. Raven Press, New York.

26. Sicuteri, F. (1980): Vascular supersensitivity to serotonin and other monoamines in migraine and in morphine abstinence: A related mechanism? In: *Vascular Neuroeffector Mechanism,* edited by Bevan et al., pp. 357–359. Raven Press, New York.

27. Sicuteri, F., Anselmi, B., Curradi, C., Michelacci, S., and Sassi, A. (1978): Morphine-like factors in CSF of headache patients. In: *Advances in Biochemical Psychopharmacology, Vol. 18, The Endorphins,* edited by E. Costa and M. Trabucchi, pp. 363–366. Raven Press, New York.

28. Sicuteri, F., Anselmi, B., and Del Bianco, P. L. (1980): Dopamine and 5-HT supersensitivity in nonorganic central pain and in morphine abstinence: Fortuitous or real analogy? In: *Neural Peptides and Neuronal Communication,* edited by E. Costa and M. Trabucchi, pp. 523–533. Raven Press, New York.

29. Sicuteri, F., Fanciullacci, M., Franchi, G., and Del Bianco, P. L. (1965): Serotonin-bradykinin potentiation on the pain receptors in man. *Life Sci.,* 4:409.

30. Sicuteri, F., Franchi, G., and Fanciullacci, M. (1974): New perspectives on analgesia from ergotamine and methysergide in migraine. *2nd. Hung. Congr. Pharmacol. Soc.,* Abstr. 1–28.

31. Somerville, B. W. (1976): Platelet bound and free serotonin levels. *Neurology,* 36(1):399–402.

32. Tagliamonte, A., Biggio, G., Vargiu, L., and Gessa, G. L. (1973): Free tryptophan in serum controls brain tryptophan and serotonin synthesis. *Life Sci.,* 12:227–287.

33. Tenen, S. S. (1967): The effects of p-chlorophenylalanine, a serotonin depletor, on avoidance acquisition, pain sensitivity and related behaviour in rats. *Psychopharmacology (Berlin),* 10:204.

34. Van Voert, M. M., Ambent, I. M., and Levine, R. J. (1972): Clinical effects of parachlorophenylalanine in Parkinson's disease. *Dis. Nerv. Syst.,* 33:770–780.

35. Zweifach, B. W. (1966): Microcirculatory effects of polipeptides. In: *Hypotensive Peptides,* edited by E. G. Erdgos, N. Back, F. Sicuteri, and A. F. Wilde, pp. 451–462. Springer Verlag, New York.

Advances in Neurology, Vol. 33, edited by
M. Critchley et al. Raven Press, New York © 1982

Platelet Aggregation in Migraine Patients During the Headache-Free Interval

R. J. Jones, A. M. Forsythe, and J. A. L. Amess

Department of Haematology, St. Bartholomew's Hospital, London, England

It has been proposed that a primary abnormality of platelet function can account for the diverse clinical, biochemical, and pathological findings previously reported in migraine (5). Several aspects of platelet function have been studied, particularly, changes in platelet aggregation. Hilton and Cumings (6) first reported increased platelet aggregation in response to 5-hydroxytryptamine (5-HT) in patients with migraine. Couch and Hassanein (3) documented increased platelet aggregation in migraine patients by showing a lower threshold in response to adenosine diphosphate (ADP) for the platelet release reaction but found no difference in the rate of aggregation. They also demonstrated a slower rate of platelet disaggregation in these patients. The lower threshold for the platelet release reaction was also shown by Deshmukh and Meyer (4). In addition, Kalendovsky and Austin (7), using Swanks screen filtration pressure method, reported increased platelet aggregation in migraine patients in response to ADP, 5-HT, and epinephrine. In this study, platelet aggregation has been studied in the headache-free interval.

SUBJECTS AND METHODS

Patients and Controls

All patients, selected by Hanington (5), had classic migraine. Participants in the study had not taken drugs known to interfere with platelet aggregation for 14 days prior to testing. The female subjects were not taking oral contraceptives. Those studied had fasted overnight and were headache free; all samples were taken between 9 and 11 A.M. The controls had no history of headache and were matched to the migraine patients for sex and age ± 6 years. In addition, some of the patients had a relative control, either a sibling or a parent, neither age nor sex-matched; 17 patient-age/sex-matched control pairs and 13 patient-relative pairs were studied.

Platelet Aggregation

ADP, 5-HT, collagen, norepinephrine, and epinephrine were used to induce aggregation by an optical density method (1). Blood was taken into a plastic syringe with a 19-gauge needle; 27 ml venous blood was mixed with 3 ml of 3.8% trisodium citrate in polycarbonate tubes and centrifuged at 200 × g for 10 min. The platelet-rich plasma (PRP) was harvested using a disposable plastic pipette. The platelets were then counted using a Coulter Thrombocounter C. Platelet-poor plasma (PPP) was obtained by centrifuging the sample for 15 min at 1,800 × g; this was used as a standard for 100% light transmission. The PRP was adjusted by dilution with PPP to give a final platelet count of approximately 200 × 10^9/liter. An ADG aggregometer and Linseis recorder were used for the measurement of platelet aggregation; 200 μl PRP was stirred at 1,000 rpm and brought to 37°C for 2 min prior to adding 20 μl aggregating agent. Aggregation response was shown to five final concentrations of ADP in the range of 0.4 to 10 μm, 20 μm 5-HT, five concentrations of norepinephrine (Sigma reagents) and epinephrine (Antigen Ltd), 1 to 20 μm, and 3.8 μg/ml Collagen (Accu-Tech). The extent of aggrega-

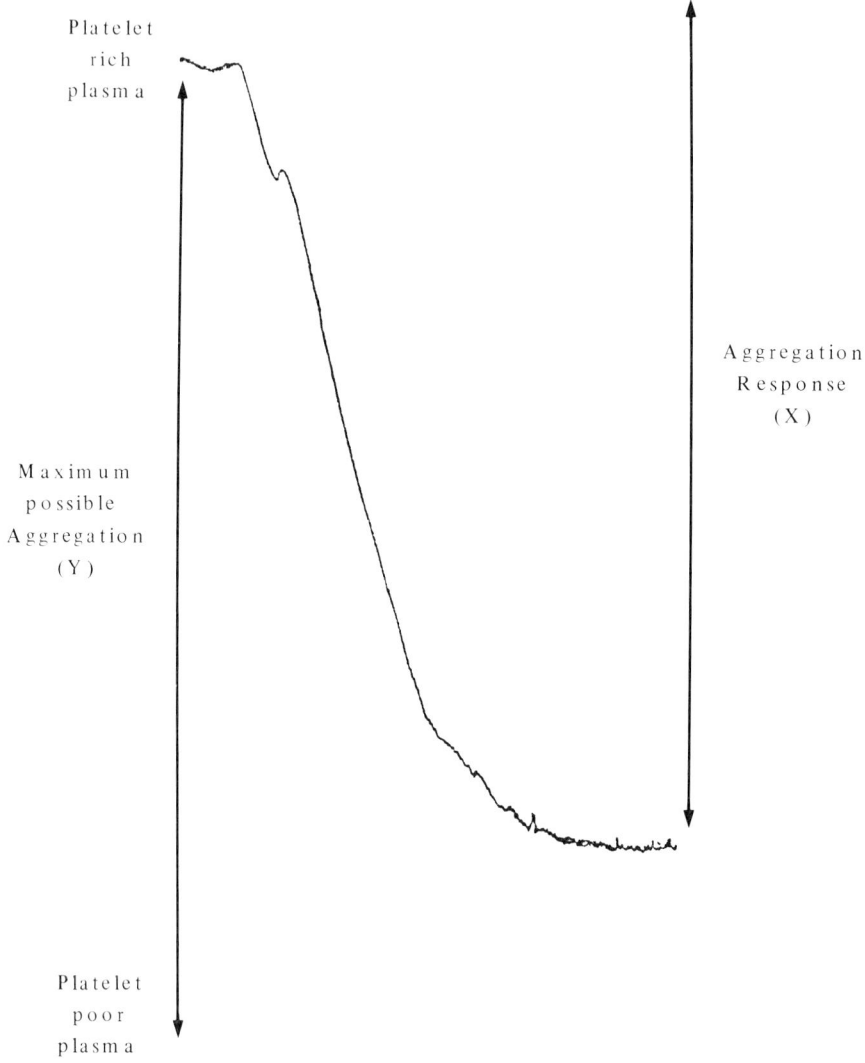

FIG. 1. Extent of aggregation was measured as a percentage: Aggregation response (X)/Maximum possible aggregation (Y) × 100 = percent extent of aggregation. A tangent was drawn to the aggregation curve and rate was calculated in millimeters per minute. This was measured for primary and, where applicable, secondary aggregation.

tion has been presented as a percentage of the maximum possible aggregation (Fig. 1) and the rate of aggregation was measured in millimeters per minute for primary and, where applicable, secondary aggregation.

RESULTS

For each concentration of aggregating agent, we compared the results of both rate and extent of aggregation from the patients with those from age- and sex-matched controls using a paired *t*-test. There was no significant difference in the results. The same finding was obtained when comparing the patients with their relative controls in a similar manner. When comparing six patients with severe prodromal symptoms (selected by Hanington without prior knowledge of the platelet aggregation results) with their age- and sex-matched controls, however, a significant increase ($p < 0.05$) was found in the extent of aggregation induced by 5-HT.

When comparing all aggregation results from each patient with those of their own age- and sex-matched control by Wilcoxon signed ranks test, a significant increase in rate and extent of aggregation ($p < 0.01$) was found in four patients. When individual patients were compared with their relative controls, three showed a significant difference ($p < 0.05$). The patients with these abnormalities were from the small subgroup of six patients with severe prodromal symptoms.

DISCUSSION

The results support the hypothesis that there is an abnormality of platelet function in some patients with classic migraine with severe prodromal symptoms.

The only agent that was found to produce increased extent of aggregation was 5-HT. In addition, some of the patients showed an overall increase in platelet aggregation. Unlike previous workers (3,4,7), no abnormality of aggregation with either ADP or epinephrine was found. Comparison with these studies, however, is difficult. In this work, we have examined only patients with classic migraine and not those with either common migraine or cluster headaches. Because of a difference in methodology, these results cannot be compared with those of Kalendovsky and Austin (7) who used a screen filtration technique. The measurement of the parameters of aggregation has been carried out in many different ways (8). We have measured rate and extent of aggregation; but with the number of agents used, it was not possible to study the platelet release phenomenon or disaggregation (3,4). In addition to the differences in the patients studied and methodology, there are many possible reasons for variation in aggregation results; a recent critical review has been written by Coller (2).

In summary, we have found minor abnormalities of platelet aggregation in patients with severe prodromal symptoms; we intend to study these patients more fully.

ACKNOWLEDGMENTS

This work was supported by grant CFC 2 from the Wellcome Trust.

We thank Nigel Hathaway for statistical analysis of the results; the patients referred by Dr. Edda Hanington from the City of London Migraine Clinic; and Miss Heather Cooper and Mrs. Christine Baker for secretarial assistance.

REFERENCES

1. Born, G. V. R. (1962): Aggregation of blood platelets by adenosine diphosphate and its reversal. *Nature,* 194:927–929
2. Coller, B. S. (1979): Platelet aggregation by ADP, collagen, and ristocetin; A critical review of methodology and analysis. In: *CRC Handbook Series in Clinical Laboratory Science Section I: Haematology,* edited by R. M. Schmidt, pp. 381–397. CRC Press, Florida.
3. Couch, J. R., and Hassanein, R. S. (1977): Platelet aggregability in migraine. *Neurology,* 27:843–848.
4. Deshmukh, S. V., and Meyer, J. S. (1977): Cyclic changes in platelet dynamics and the pathogenesis and prophylaxis of migraine. *Headache,* 17:101–108.
5. Hanington, E. (1978): Migraine: A blood disorder? *Lancet,* 2:501–503.
6. Hilton, B. P., and Cumings, J. N. (1972): 5-Hydroxytryptamine levels and platelet aggregation responses in subjects with acute migraine headache. *J. Neurol. Neurosurg. Pyschiatry,* 35:505–509.
7. Kalendovsky, Z., and Austin, J. H. (1975): "Complicated migraine." Its association with increased platelet aggregability and abnormal plasma coagulation factors. *Headache,* 15:18–35.
8. Yamazaki, H., Takahashi, T., and San, T. (1975): Hyperaggregability of platelets in thromboembolic disorders. *Thromb. Diath. Haemorrh.* 34:94–105.

Advances in Neurology, Vol. 33, edited by
M. Critchley et al. Raven Press, New York © 1982

Platelet Monoamine Oxidase in Migraine

D. V. Thomas

Department of Pharmacology, Institute of Psychiatry, London, England

Involvement of blood platelets in migraine was indicated by significant deficits in platelet monoamine oxidase (MAO) activity in migraineurs both during attacks and in attack-free periods (2,5–7). Consequently, the suggestion was made that migrainous attacks occurred because of inefficient metabolism of circulating amines. Glover et al. (3), however, did not find significant deficits in platelet MAO in attack-free periods in 58 migraineurs and 38 controls. In view of this discrepancy, platelet MAO was measured in subjects participating in the aggregation study.

METHODS

Blood platelets were prepared by the method of Youdim (9), except that potassium EDTA (30 mg/20 ml blood) was used instead of sodium citrate and the number of washes was reduced to two. Prior to assay, platelet samples were disrupted by sonication for 20 sec using a Dawe type 1130A Soniprobe at 2 kHz and then assayed by the ion-exchange method described by Tipton and Youdim (8) using [^{14}C] tyramine or [^{14}C]β-phenethylamine (The Radiochemical Centre, Amersham). Samples were incubated at 37°C instead of 30°C, and the final concentration of β-phenethylamine (specific activity, 1.25 μCi/mmoles) was reduced from 1 to 0.04 mM to eliminate substrate inhibition. Proteins were measured by the method of Lowry et al. (4). Results are presented per milligram protein for 30 females and 15 males, of which 14 and 5, respectively, suffered from classic migraine.

RESULTS

There were no significant differences between controls and migraineurs of either sex in platelet MAO activity using tyramine or β-phenethylamine as substrate. In addition to age-matched controls, the control groups contained migraine-free relatives who, if potential migraineurs, might have biased findings for the control group. Therefore, results were reassessed after regrouping males and females into one group of 10 migraineurs with relatives and another group of 16 migraineurs with age-matched controls; seven migraineurs were common to each group. The results indicated that platelet MAO activity was greater, although not significantly so, in migraineurs and their relatives compared with the age-matched controls of the migraineurs. The subgroup of migraineurs with marked symptoms described by J. Amess and R. J. Jones *(this volume)* also conformed to this pattern. The possibility that significant differences were obscured by the variance introduced by combining results from males and females was tested. In the case of tyramine, the t value increased from 1.79 to 1.9; t would have had to increase to 2.04 to become significant at the 0.5% level. Similarly, no significant differences emerged when migraineurs were subdivided according to sex. Tyramine oxidation (nmoles/hr/mg protein) by platelets from males with classic migraine and their age-matched controls were, respectively 25.5 ± 2.5 and 22.5 ± 8.21 ($N = 4$). The corresponding values for females were 57.37 ± 9.11 and 37.85 ± 3.98 ($N = 12$).

DISCUSSION

The results obtained in the present study are consistent with those of Glover et al. (3) in that there were no significant differences in platelet MAO between controls and migraineurs studied in attack-free periods; although sample size was small, there was no evidence of MAO-related subpopulations. In the present study, values tended to be greater than controls, whereas the reverse was found by Glover et al. (3). It is inappropriate to compare these results with those of Sicuteri et al. (7), who measured platelet MAO activity during both attacks and attack-free periods and presented average values for the duration of the investigation. Nevertheless, there is a discrepancy with those studies (2,5,6) showing significant deficits in platelet MAO in attack-free periods, although large values for 5-hydroxytryptamine oxidation (10 times normal) in two of the studies (5,6) indicate erythrocyte contamination of the platelets.

The conflicting nature of the results from various studies suggests that any conclusion would be premature. Buchsbaum and Rieder (1) attributed discrepant results of platelet MAO activity in schizophrenic patients to the heterogeneity of the disorder. Thus when sample size is small and the particular abnormality occurs in a small proportion of all affected, then significant differences can be expected only in a few studies. The alternative strategy of phenotype subgrouping (1) was also used by Glover, Peakfield, and Sandler *(personal communication.)* Unlike the results of the present study of four males with classic migraine, the authors found a significant deficit in platelet MAO activity in a larger group ($N = 12$) of such males compared to their age-matched controls.

Unfortunately, with so few studies of MAO in migraine, a similar analysis to that of Buchsbaum and Rieder (1) would be unprofitable. The existing results do indicate, however, that a permanent deficit in platelet MAO is not a principal factor in the genesis of migraine. They also support the view that migraine is a heterogeneous disorder, and that a small proportion of migraineurs may have a permanent deficit in platelet MAO activity.

ACKNOWLEDGMENT

The encouragement and advice of Professor E. Marley and the financial support of the Wellcome Trust are gratefully acknowledged.

REFERENCES

1. Buchsbaum, M. S., and Rieder, R. O. (1979): Biologic heterogeneity and psychiatric research. Platelet MAO activity as a case study. *Arch. Gen. Psychiatry,* 36:1,163–1,169.
2. Bussone, G., Giovannini, P., Boiardi, A., and Boeri, R. (1977): A study of the activity of platelet monoamine oxidase in patients with migraine headaches or 'cluster headaches.' *Eur. Neurol.,* 15:157–162.
3. Glover, V., Sandler, M., Grant, E., Rose, E. C., Orton, D., Wilkinson, M., and Stevens, D. (1977): Transitory decrease in platelet monoamine oxidase activity during migraine attacks. *Lancet,* 1:391–393.

4. Lowry, O. H., Rosebrough, N. J., Farr, A. L., and Randall, R. J. (1951): Protein measurement with the folin phenol reagent. *J. Biol. Chem.,* 193:265–275.

5. Sandler, M., Youdim, M. B. H., Southgate, J., and Hanington, E. (1970): The role of tyramine in migraine: Some possible biochemical mechanisms. In: *Background to Migraine, Third Migraine Symposium,* edited by A. L. Cochrane, pp. 103–112. Heinemann, London.

6. Sandler, M., Youdim, M. B. H., and Hanington, E. (1974): A phenethylamine oxidising defect in migraine. *Nature,* 250:335–337.

7. Sicuteri, F., Buffoni, F., Anselmi, B., and Del Bianco, P. L. (1972): An enzyme (MAO) defect on the platelets in migraine. *Res. Clin. Stud. Headache,* 3:245–251.

8. Tipton, K. F., and Youdim, M. B. H. (1976): Assay of monoamine oxidase. In: *Monoamine Oxidase and its Inhibition,* edited by G. E. W. Wolstenholme and J. Knight, pp. 393–403. Elsevier, Amsterdam.

9. Youdim, M.B.H. (1976): Preparation of human platelets. In: *Monoamine Oxidase and its Inhibition,* edited by G. E. W. Wolstenholme, and J. Knight, pp. 405–406. Elsevier, Amsterdam.

Advances in Neurology, Vol. 33, edited by
M. Critchley et al. Raven Press, New York © 1982

Characteristics of Extravascular Serotonin Receptors in the Brain

Henry J. Haigler

Department of Pharmacology, Emory University, Atlanta, Georgia 30322

There are two hypotheses concerning the origin and pathogenesis of migraine headache. The classic one is that a vasoconstriction of cerebral blood vessels is superseded by a vasodilation leading to pain (6); antimigraine drugs are purported to produce a vasoconstriction of the cerebral blood vessels and thus decrease the pain. One basic problem with this hypothesis is that drugs that produce vasodilation generally do not produce headache in normal subjects (23). A more recent hypothesis is that these patients have a biochemical lesion in a serotonergic system of the brain that is associated with modulating nociceptive information. This lesion may lead to hyperalgesia, an increase in the appreciation of pain (21); drugs that are effective in treating migraine headache may act as serotonin (5-HT) agonists rather than antagonists (22).

Both hypotheses may be valid. The vasodilation associated with migraine headache may produce an increase in stimulation of a sensory system that is modulated by 5-HT. Therefore, a biochemical lesion in this system would result in the sensory stimuli arising from the cerebral vasculature being perceived as painful. Furthermore, changes of blood flow in cerebral blood vessels may reflect changes in the availability of 5-HT at both vascular and extravascular neuroeffector junctions in the brain. Because these two hypotheses are not mutually exclusive, migraine headache may be related to both vascular and extravascular 5-HT receptors in the brain.

DIFFERENT 5-HT RECEPTORS

5-HT$_1$ and 5-HT$_2$ Receptors

The 5-HT$_1$ receptors are located on 5-HT-containing cells in the mesencephalic raphe nuclei (dorsal and median raphe nuclei). The 5-HT$_2$ receptors are found on neurons in areas that receive a prominent serotonergic input; neurons in these areas are surrounded by 5-HT terminals (see Fig. 1 in ref. 12).

There is substantial evidence that the 5-HT terminals that surround cells in the forebrain originate in the dorsal and median raphe nuclei (reviewed in ref. 13). Even though 5-HT acting on both of these receptors produces an inhibition of firing, the 5-HT$_1$ and 5-HT$_2$ receptors are not identical, the evidence for which is based on studies with indolethylamines, such as LSD, psilocin, and dimethyltryptamine (Fig. 1; see also ref. 1). In these studies, 5-HT was used as an internal standard; there was no difference in the sensitivity to 5-HT. However, LSD and related compounds have a greater potency in acting on 5-HT_1 receptors than on 5-HT_2 receptors (Fig. 1).

A second characteristic of 5-HT_1 and 5-HT_2 receptors is that the peripheral 5-HT antagonists (methysergide, metergoline, methiothepin, cinanserin, and cyproheptadine), drugs that block the effects of 5-HT on smooth muscle, do not block the inhibitory effects of 5-HT at the 5-HT_1 and 5-HT_2 receptors. Instead, they promote the inhibition of firing produced by 5-HT and act as 5-HT agonists at both the 5-HT_1 and 5-HT_2 receptors. Evidence is now emerging that these drugs, at plasma concentrations achieved clinically, do not block the effects of 5-HT on receptors in blood vessels but instead mimic 5-HT in the human venoconstriction test (3).

A third characteristic of 5-HT_1 and 5-HT_2 receptors is that morphine acts on cells that have these receptors to produce an inhibition of firing. Morphine administered microiontophoretically produces an inhibition of firing in about 33% of neurons that have 5-HT_1 receptors (cells in the dorsal and median raphe nuclei) as well as cells in areas that receive projections from the dorsal and median raphe nuclei (i.e., cells with 5-HT_2 receptors). The areas where 5-HT_2 receptors are located include the subiculum, optic tectum, amygdala, and ventrolateral geniculate (2). Morphine does not act on the forebrain serotonergic system to produce analgesia because it does not have a specific narcotic effect on cells in this system (9). The inhibition of firing produced by morphine was not typically blocked by naloxone; this inhibition was mimicked by dextrorotary isomers of opiate drugs that have no analgesic activity. Therefore, firing in neurons that have 5-HT_1 and 5-HT_2 receptors is inhibited by morphine, but this effect is not a specific narcotic effect. This effect of morphine may be related to changes in body tempera-

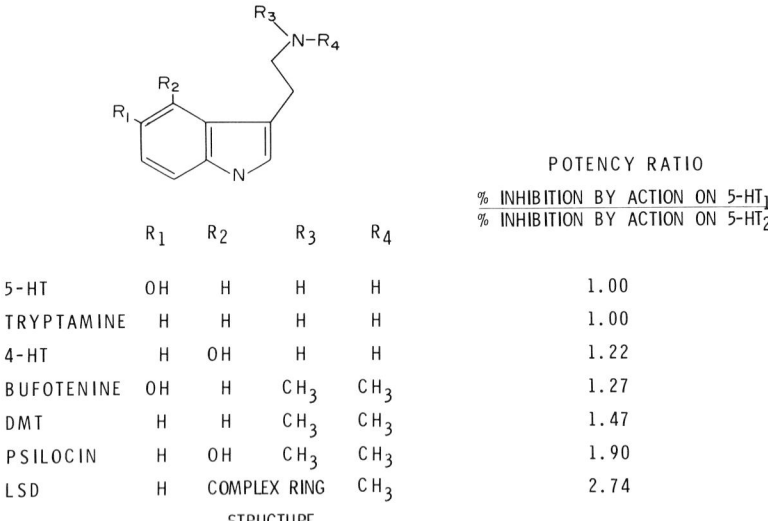

	R_1	R_2	R_3	R_4	POTENCY RATIO $\dfrac{\%\ \text{INHIBITION BY ACTION ON } 5\text{-HT}_1}{\%\ \text{INHIBITION BY ACTION ON } 5\text{-HT}_2}$
5-HT	OH	H	H	H	1.00
TRYPTAMINE	H	H	H	H	1.00
4-HT	H	OH	H	H	1.22
BUFOTENINE	OH	H	CH_3	CH_3	1.27
DMT	H	H	CH_3	CH_3	1.47
PSILOCIN	H	OH	CH_3	CH_3	1.90
LSD	H	COMPLEX RING STRUCTURE	CH_3		2.74

FIG. 1. Comparison of the structures of seven indoleamines with the ratio of their potency on 5-HT_1 and 5-HT_2 receptors. The potency ratio was obtained by dividing the percent inhibition in the raphe by the average percent inhibition on neuronal firing in the two postsynaptic areas; these data are presented elsewhere (see Table 1 in ref. 13). As substituents are added to the terminal amino group and to the fourth position (R_2) of the indoleamine, the potency ratio increases. An ejection current of 5-HT that produced 100% inhibition was always used as a standard in these comparisons. (For further details, see ref. 13.)

ture because both morphine and dextrorphan, a dextrorotary isomer of the narcotic agonist levorphanol, both produce a decrease in body temperature when administered systemically (9).

A fourth characteristic of both the 5-HT$_1$ and 5-HT$_2$ receptors is that morphine can either augment or block the depressant effects of 5-HT. The augmentation of inhibition is apparently a specific narcotic effect because it is antagonized by naloxone (10). This interaction was not studied more extensively because (a) morphine did not consistently alter the response to 5-HT, and (b) the interaction between 5-HT and morphine was not related to the response of the cell to a nociceptive stimulus. Based on the above data, 5-HT$_1$ and 5-HT$_2$ receptors are not associated with an antinociceptive system that is affected by morphine.

5-HT$_3$ Receptors

The 5-HT$_3$ receptors differ from the other two types in that 5-HT acts on these receptors to produce an increase in neuronal firing (see Fig. 3 in ref. 11), which can be blocked by LSD (4) or peripheral 5-HT antagonists (11).

The 5-HT$_3$ receptors are found in areas where 5-HT terminals have a low density; therefore, they may not be related to a 5-HT synapse. Even in the areas where 5-HT terminals are low, 80% of the cells are inhibited by 5-HT when it is administered microiontophoretically (12). Furthermore, electrical stimulation of the raphe nuclei produces an inhibition of neuronal firing in most areas that have been studied, including those where 5-HT terminals have a low density (15; for other references, see ref. 10). Stimulation of the mesencephalic raphe nuclei, however, produces an increase in neuronal firing in some cells in the cerebellum (24), and stimulation of the brainstem raphe nuclei produces an increase in firing of neurons in the reticular formation (5). The increase in firing produced by 5-HT may be related to a modulatory influence of 5-HT on motor neurons (14). Further evidence is needed before it can be concluded that the excitatory action of 5-HT on 5-HT$_3$ receptors is a physiologically relevant response.

MEDULLARY-PONTINE RAPHE NUCLEI

There is now evidence that the medullary-pontine raphe nuclei (MPR; or brainstem raphe nuclei) are an important link in an antinociceptive system. For instance, stimulation of this area produces analgesia in cats because it blocks the behavioral response produced by electrical stimulation of the tooth pulp (16). Furthermore, stimulation of the MPR produces an inhibition of firing in neurons in the spinal cord that are responsive to nociceptive stimuli (7). A third line of evidence supporting this hypothesis is that the intrathecal administration of 5-HT produces an analgesic effect that is comparable to that produced by morphine injected into the periaqueductal gray (25).

Neurons in the MPR differ from those in the dorsal raphe and the forebrain serotonergic system in several respects. For instance, they are not consistently inhibited by LSD, 5-HT, or morphine (Table 1); however, they have action potentials that resemble those recorded in the dorsal raphe (see Fig. 1 in ref. 8); 5-HT-containing neurons in the dorsal raphe contain tryptophan hydroxylase, as indicated by their ability to convert L-tryptophan to 5-hydroxytryptamine (1), and have action potentials with a characteristic waveform and duration (see Fig. 1a in ref. 8).

Because the density of 5-HT-containing cells in the MPR is not as high as in the

TABLE 1. *Effects on spontaneous firing rates in medullary pontine raphe neurons*

Drug	Drugs administered					
	Microiontophoretically[a]			Intravenously		
	+	−	0	+	−	0
Morphine	4	0	39	6	4	5
LSD	0	8	22	0	2	3
5-HT	0	5	12	—	—	—

[a] +, Acceleration; −, slowing or inhibition; 0, no change in spontaneous firing rate.

dorsal raphe, some of the raphe-like action potentials may arise from neurons that do not contain 5-HT. Furthermore, it is possible that only 5-HT-containing neurons in the MPR are inhibited by 5-HT, as are the neurons in the dorsal raphe. If this is so, the electrophysiological characteristics of an action potential that is recorded from a neuron are not an indication of the neurotransmitter content of that neuron. Another possibility is that the electrophysiological characteristics of an action potential accurately reflect the type of neurotransmitter contained by a particular neuron. If so, not all cells that contain 5-HT have the same type of serotonergic receptor (i.e., $5-HT_1$). In fact, some 5-HT-containing neurons in the MPR may not have any 5-HT receptors. It remains to be determined which of the above possibilities is correct.

Morphine does not act directly on neurons in the MPR; when it is applied microiontophoretically, it does not alter the spontaneous firing of these neurons. In contrast, when morphine is administered systemically, there is an increase in firing in some cells in the MPR, which is reversed by the systemic administration of naloxone. These data support the hypothesis that the MPR is an important link in an antinociceptive system that is activated by morphine. However, morphine must act at some site remote to these neurons.

Stimulation of the MPR in cats produces an inhibition of the behavioral response produced by the electrical stimulation of the tooth pulp (16). Stimulation of the dorsal raphe produces a direct inhibition of neuronal firing in the spinal trigeminal nucleus (19). Neurochemically, there are measurable amounts of 5-HT in the trigeminal nucleus (17). These data indicate that both the MPR and dorsal raphe project to the trigeminal nucleus, as indicated in Fig. 2.

If the MPR is an important area with respect to nociception, a biochemical lesion of the MPR could lead to an increase in appreciation in stimuli arising from the cerebral vasculature. This lesion could then be the basis of the pain perceived in a migraine headache. There is also evidence that raphe nuclei in the brain project to blood vessels in the brain (18). Thus the following model may explain the events leading to a migraine attack.

If raphe neurons act to modulate and inhibit sensory input related to nociception, and if there is a biochemical lesion in the serotonergic terminals of these neurons such that the content of 5-HT in these terminals is low, a trigger stimulus (e.g., intense emotion) might result in an increase in the amount of 5-HT released by these terminals.

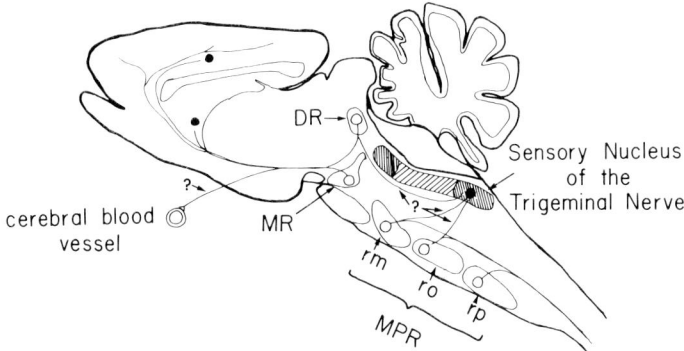

FIG. 2. Diagrammatic representation of projections from the dorsal and median raphe nuclei (DR and MR, respectively) and the MPR in rat brain. 5-HT neurons *(open circles)* in the DR and MR send projections to neurons in the forebrain *(filled circles)* and possibly to cerebral blood vessels. Neurons in the MPR and DR may also send serotonergic projections to the trigeminal nucleus. A decrease in 5-HT levels in the synaptic terminals of axons that project from the MPR and DR to the trigeminal nucleus may be the basis of the pain in migraine headache. rm, raphe magnus; ro, raphe obscurus; rp, raphe pallidus.

This initial phase of release may be correlated with the prodromal stage of the migraine attack and may be reflected in the initial vasospasm of the cerebral blood vessels. As the 5-HT in the synaptic terminals decreases—and the biochemical lesion prevents a rapid replenishment—there would be an escape from tonic inhibition of neurons in the brain that would parallel the vasodilation of the blood vessels. This escape would occur in neurons that receive projections from the dorsal raphe and the MPR. The vasodilation combined with the loss of inhibition in an antinociceptive pathway would lead to the pounding, throbbing pain associated with migraine.

If the 5-HT receptors in the trigeminal nucleus are similar to the 5-HT receptors in the forebrain, drugs that are useful in treating migraine, such as methysergide and ergotamine, might be effective because they act as 5-HT agonists and inhibit neuronal firing in the trigeminal nucleus. These drugs would act to reinstitute the tonic inhibitory effect of 5-HT. Although the above hypothesis may be attractive, it must be tested experimentally. First, the characteristics of 5-HT receptors in the trigeminal nucleus— if there are any—must be determined. Second, a depletion of 5-HT from nerve terminals does not explain all cases of migraine headache; in patients with migraine refractory to other pharmacological treatments, treatment with *p*-chlorophenylalanine, a drug that depletes 5-HT from 5-HT terminals, decreases the frequency and intensity of migraine attacks (20). Finally, drugs that only produce vasoconstriction and do not cross the blood-brain barrier, such as norepinephrine, will reverse a migraine attack (6), although there is disagreement about this point (22). If there is a relationship between 5-HT receptors in the brain and the pain of migraine, it remains to be demonstrated more clearly.

SUMMARY

At least three types of extravascular 5-HT receptors are present in the brain. Peripheral 5-HT antagonists mimic the inhibitory effects but block the excitatory effects of 5-HT in the brain. Although the forebrain serotonergic system is apparently not involved in nociception, the MPR may be an important link in an antinociceptive system; this system may be activated by morphine. A decrease in the amount of 5-HT released by projections from the MPR to the trigeminal nucleus could be partially responsible for the pain experienced in migraine headache. Drugs useful in treating migraine headache may mimic 5-HT at synapses in the trigeminal nucleus that are associated with projections from the MPR. This possibility remains to be tested experimentally.

ACKNOWLEDGMENTS

Preparation of this paper and some of the research were supported in part by NIDA grant 1-RO1-DA-01344-04 and by a grant from the Women's Auxiliary of the Veterans of Foreign Wars.

REFERENCES

1. Aghajanian, G. K., and Haigler, H. J. (1974): L-tryptophan as a selective histochemical marker for serotonergic neurons in single-cell recording studies. *Brain Res.,* 81:364–372.
2. Aghajanian, G. K., Haigler, H. J., and Bennett, J. L. (1975): Amine receptors in CNS. III. 5-Hydroxytryptamine in brain. In: *Handbook of Psychopharmacology, Vol. 6,* edited by L. L. Iverson, S. D. Iverson, and S. H. Snyder, pp. 63–96. Plenum Press, New York.
3. Anselmi, B., Del Bianco, P. L., de Vos, C. J., Galli, P., Lamar, J.-C., Schonbaum, E., Sicuteri, F., and van der Veen, F. (1976): Clinical and animal pharmacology of migraine: New perspectives. *Monogr. Neural Sci.,* 3:45–59.
4. Boakes, R. J., Bradley, P. B., Briggs, I., and Dray, A. (1970): Antagonisms of 5-hydroxytryptamine by LSD-25 in the central nervous system: A possible neuronal basis for the actions of LSD-25. *Br. J. Pharmacol.,* 40:194–201.
5. Briggs, I. (1977): Excitatory responses of neurons in rat bulbar reticular formation to bulbar raphe stimulation and to iontophoretically applied 5-hydroxytryptamine, and their blockade by LSD-25. *J. Physiol.,* 265:327–340.
6. Dalessio, D. J. (editor) (1972): *Wolff's Headache and Other Head Pain.* Oxford University Press, New York.
7. Fields, H. L., Basbaum, A. I., Clanton, C. H., and Anderson, S. D. (1977): Nucleus raphe magnus inhibition of spinal cord dorsal horn neurons. *Brain Res.,* 126:441–453.
8. Haigler, H. J. (1978): Morphine: Effects on brainstem raphe neurons. In: *Iontophoresis and Transmitter Mechanisms in the Mammalian Central Nervous System,* edited by R. W. Ryall and J. S. Kelly, pp. 326–328. Elsevier, Amsterdam.
9. Haigler, H. J. (1978): Morphine: Effects on serotonergic neurons and neurons in areas with a serotonergic input. *Eur. J. Pharmacol.,* 51: 361–376.
10. Haigler, H. J. (1981): Serotonin receptors. In: *Neurotransmitter Receptors,* edited by H. I. Yamamura and S. J. Enna, pp. 1–70. Chapman and Hall, New York.
11. Haigler, H. J., and Aghajanian, G. K. (1974): Peripheral serotonin antagonists: Failure to antagonize serotonin in brain areas receiving a prominent serotonergic input. *J. Neural. Transm.,* 35:257–273.
12. Haigler, H. J., and Aghajanian, G. K. (1974): Lysergic acid diethylamide and serotonin: A comparison of effects on serotonergic neurons and neurons receiving a serotonergic input. *J. Pharmacol Exp. Ther.,* 188:688–699.
13. Haigler, H. J., and Aghajanian, G. K. (1977): Serotonin receptors in the brain. *Fed. Proc.,* 36:2,159–2,164.
14. McCall, R. B., and Aghajanian, G. K. (1979): Denervation supersensitivity to serotonin in the facial nucleus. *Neuroscience,* 4:1,501–1,510.
15. Nakamura, S. (1975): Two types of inhibitory effects upon brain stem reticular formation neurons by low frequency stimulation of raphe nucleus in the rat. *Brain Res.,* 93:140–144.
16. Oliveras, J. L., Redjemi, F., Guibaud, G., and Besson, J. M. (1975): Analgesia induced by electrical stimulation of the inferior centralis nucleus of the raphe in the cat. *Pain,* 1:139–145.
17. Palkovits, M., Brownstein, M., and Saavedra, J. M. (1974): Serotonin content of the brain stem nuclei in the rat. *Brain Res.,* 80:237–249.
18. Reinhard, J. F., Liebmann, J. E., Schosberg, A. J., and Moskowitz, M. A. (1979): Serotonin neurons project to small blood vessels in the brain. *Science,* 206:85–87.

19. Sasa, M., Munekiyo, K., and Takaoria, S. (1975): Dorsal raphe stimulation produces inhibitory effect on trigeminal nucleus neurons. *Brain Res.,* 101:199–207.

20. Sicuteri, F. (1971): Pain syndrome in man following treatment with *p*-chlorophenlalanine. *Pharmacol. Res. Commun.,* 3:401–407.

21. Sicuteri, F. (1972): 5-Hydroxytryphan in the prophylaxis of migraine. *Pharmacol. Res. Commun.,* 4:213–218.

22. Sicuteri, F. (1979): Headache as the most common disease of the antinociceptive system: Analogies with morphine abstinence. In: *Advances in Pain Research and Therapy, Vol. 3,* edited by J. J. Bonica, J. C. Liebeskind and D. G. Albe-Fessard, pp. 359–365. Raven Press, New York.

23. Sicuteri, F., Anselmi, A. and Fanciullacci, M. (1974): The serotonin (5-HT) theory of migraine. *Adv. Neurol.,* 4:383–394.

24. Strahlendorf, J. C., Strahlendorf, H. K., and Barnes, C. D. (1979): Modulation of cerebellar neuronal activity by raphe stimulation. *Brain Res.,* 169:565–569.

25. Yaksh, T. L., and Wilson, P. R. (1978): Spinal serotonin terminal system mediates antinociception. *J. Pharmacol. Exp. Ther.,* 208:446–453.

Advances in Neurology, Vol. 33, edited by
M. Critchley et al. Raven Press, New York © 1982

Pharmacology of Arteriovenous Anastomoses

Egilius L. H. Spierings and Pramod R. Saxena

Department of Pharmacology, Faculty of Medicine, Erasmus University, Rotterdam, The Netherlands

Arteriovenous anastomoses are vascular structures that exist in various parts of the human body. Within a tissue, they are located at a point prior to the capillary bed. They establish a direct communication between the arterial and venous sides of the circulation. Arteriovenous anastomoses have been implicated in the pathophysiology of the migraine headache. Some of the results of this study are presented here; for a more complete review, the reader is referred to recent publications (8,9).

Sucquet (15), in a study published in 1862, was the first to provide indirect evidence for the presence of arteriovenous anastomoses in man. In regard to the head, Sucquet located the arteriovenous anastomoses in the forehead, cheeks, ears, nose, and lips. More than a century later, Rowbotham and Little (7) demonstrated the presence of numerous arteriovenous anastomoses in the human dura mater, an observation subsequently confirmed by Kerber and Newton (6).

The hypothesis on the involvement of arteriovenous anastomoses in the pathophysiology of the migraine headache was formulated in the 1950s by Heyck (3) of Berlin. In his hypothesis, known as the migraine shunt hypothesis, the onset of the migraine headache is ascribed to opening of arteriovenous anastomoses in the cranial (extracerebral) tissues of the head. By a decrease in peripheral resistance, this would lead to an increase in arterial blood flow, widening of the arterial pulse wave pressure, and, by way of a steal mechanism, decreased perfusion of the capillary bed. The latter would in turn give rise to a sterile inflammatory reaction associated with the formation of pain-provoking substances, such as bradykinin and prostaglandins, rendering the increased pulsation and overdistension of the vessels painful. Heyck based his hypothesis on the observation that, while the superficial scalp vessels were distended and excessively filled, the skin at the site of the headache looked hypoperfused and ischemic.

To provide more objective evidence for his hypothesis, Heyck measured the arteriovenous oxygen content difference over the cranial circulation, sampling blood from the external jugular vein. He observed that during the migraine headache, the arteriovenous oxygen content difference was significantly lower ($p < 0.05$) on the side of the headache (0.76 ± 0.44 mmoles/liter) when compared to the other side of the head (1.78 ± 0.76 mmoles/liter). Furthermore, administration of dihydroergotamine, leading to a subsiding of the headache, resulted in a significant increase in the arteriovenous oxygen content difference (from 0.64 ± 0.58 to 2.26 ± 0.74 mmoles/liter; $p < 0.05$). The former observation was confirmed by Graham (1); in experiments in cats, we recently established a dose-response relationship for the effect of dihydroergotamine on the arteriovenous oxygen content difference over the cranial circulation (13) (Fig. 1). However, the question

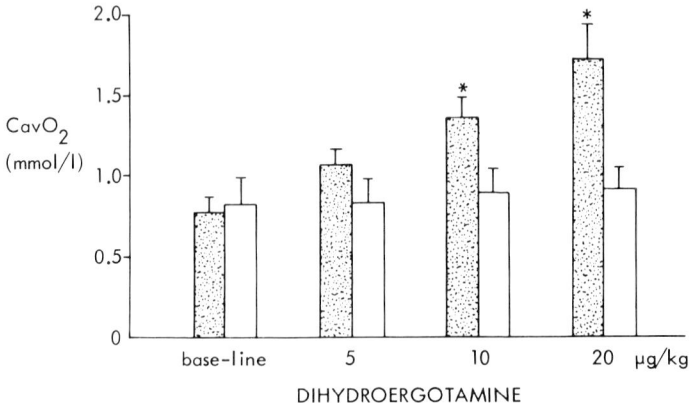

FIG. 1. Effect of dihydroergotamine, 5, 10, and 20 μg/kg i.v., on the arteriovenous oxygen content difference over the cranial circulation of the cat. The venous sample was obtained from the external jugular vein. Both the control group *(open bars)* and the experimental group *(speckled bars)* consist of eight animals. The data are expressed as means $\pm$ SEM. A significant difference ($p < 0.05$) between the means of the control group and of the experimental group is indicated by an asterisk and is calculated according to the two-tailed Wilcoxon rank sum test.

arises: upon what is the assumption based that the arteriovenous oxygen content difference is an index of shunting? The literature does not provide an answer.

In the above-mentioned experiments in cats, apart from the arteriovenous oxygen content difference over the cranial circulation, we also determined the shunting of 15 μm microspheres as an index of arteriovenous anastomotic blood flow (2,4). The microspheres were injected directly into the carotid artery. Using the baseline data of 40 experiments, we found no correlation between the arteriovenous oxygen content difference and the proportional shunting of microspheres (13). When the arteriovenous oxygen content difference was plotted against the carotid blood flow, however, a highly significant correlation was obtained ($r_s = -0.62$, $p < 0.001$) (13). Thus, at least in the cat, the arteriovenous oxygen content difference is an index of arterial blood flow rather than of shunting.

To further investigate Heyck's shunt hypothesis, we studied the effect of antimigraine drugs on arteriovenous shunting in the carotid vascular bed of the cat, using the 15 μm microsphere technique. The results of these experiments are summarized in Fig. 2. The drugs that are effective in the treatment of migraine—ergotamine (5,8,10,13), dihydroergotamine (13), and isometheptene (11)—significantly and dose-dependently altered the distribution of carotid blood flow in favor of perfusion of the capillaries and to the detriment of flow passing through the arteriovenous anastomoses. This mode of action is compatible with a direct constrictor effect of the drugs on the arteriovenous anastomoses, as had been demonstrated for ergotamine in histological studies in the rabbit ear by Stolzenburg (14) in 1937. Methysergide, a drug effective in migraine as a prophylactic agent only, did not significantly change the distribution of carotid blood flow.

In conclusion, the acute antimigraine drugs exert an effect on the distribution of carotid blood flow which is in agreement with, and thus indirectly supports, the notion

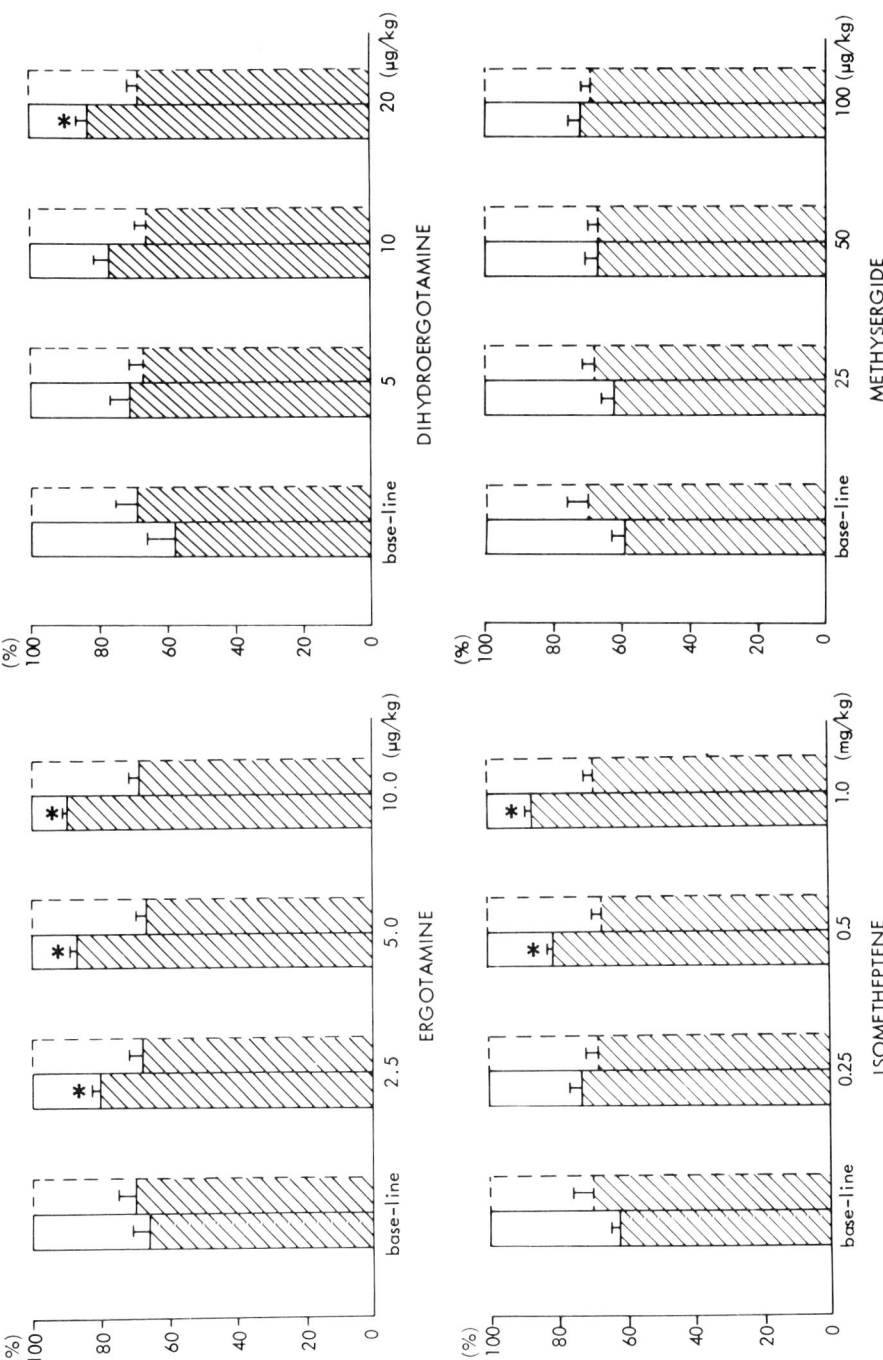

FIG. 2. Effect of the antimigraine drugs ergotamine (2.5, 5, and 10 µg/kg i.v.), dihydroergotamine (5, 10, 20 µg/kg i.v.), isometheptene (250, 500, 1,000 µg/kg i.v.), and methysergide (25, 50, 100 µg/kg i.v.) on the distribution of carotid blood flow over the capillaries *(striped bars)* and the arteriovenous anastomoses *(open bars)* in the cephalic circulation of the cat. The distribution was determined by use of 15 µm isotope-labeled plastic microspheres, which were injected directly into the carotid artery. The data are expressed as means ± SEM; each group consisted of eight animals. A significant difference ($p \leq 0.05$) between the means of the control group *(dashed-lined bars)* and of the experimental group *(solid-lined bars)* is indicated by an asterisk and is calculated according to the two-tailed Wilcoxon rank sum test. (The ergotamine histogram is reproduced from ref. 12.)

that opening of arteriovenous anastomoses constitutes the basic hemodynamic derangement underlying the migraine headache, as Heyck (3) suggested.

ACKNOWLEDGMENT

Dr. M. J. Parnham is acknowledged for reviewing the manuscript.

REFERENCES

1. Graham, J. R. (editor) (1970): The shunting theory of Heyck. In: *Prodromes of Migraine,* pp. 38–40. The Headache Research Foundation, The Faulkner Hospital, Boston.
2. Hales, J. R. S. (1974): Radioactive microsphere techniques for studies of the circulation. *Clin. Exp. Pharmacol. Physiol. [Suppl.],* 1:31–46.
3. Heyck, H. (1969): Pathogenesis of migraine. *Res. Clin. Stud. Headache,* 2:1–28.
4. Heymann, M. A., Payne, B. D., Hoffmann, J. I. E., and Randolph, A. M. (1977): Blood flow measurements with radionuclide-labelled particles. *Progr. Cardiovasc. Dis.,* 20:55–79.
5. Johnston, B. M., and Saxena, P. R. (1978): The effect of ergotamine on tissue blood flow and the arteriovenous shunting of radioactive microspheres in the head. *Br. J. Pharmacol.,* 63:541–549.
6. Kerber, C. W., and Newton, T. H. (1973): The macro and microvasculature of the dura mater. *Neuroradiology,* 6:175–179.
7. Rowbotham, G. F., and Little, E. (1965): New concepts on the aetiology and vacularization of meningiomate; the mechanisms of migraine; the chemical processes of the cerebrospinal fluid; and the formation of collections of blood or fluid in the subdural space. *Br. J. Surg.,* 52:21–24.
8. Saxena, P. R. (1978): Arteriovenous shunting and migraine. *Res. Clin. Stud. Headache,* 6:89–102.
9. Spierings, E. L. H. (1980): *The Pathophysiology of the Migraine Attack.* Stafleu's Wetenschappelijke Uitgeversmaatschappij B. V., Alphen aan den Rijn, The Netherlands.
10. Spierings, E. L. H., and Saxena, P. R. (1979): Effect of ergotamine on cranial arteriovenous shunting in experiments with constant flow perfusion. *Eur. J. Pharmacol.,* 56:31–37.
11. Spierings, E. L. H., and Saxena, P. R. (1980): Effect of isometheptene on the distribution and shunting of 15 μm microspheres throughout the cephalic circulation of the cat. *Headache,* 20:103–106.
12. Spierings, E. L. H., and Saxena, P. R. (1980): The action of ergotamine on the distribution of carotid blood flow—the migraine shunt theory revisited. *Headache,* 20:143–145.
13. Spierings, E. L. H., and Saxena, P. R. (1980): Antimigraine drugs and cranial arteriovenous shunting in the cat. *Neurology,* 30:696–701.
14. Stolzenburg, H. J. (1937): Experimentelle Untersuchungen über das Verhalten der arteriovenösen Anastomosen. *Z. Mikr. Anat. Forsch.,* 41:348–358.
15. Sucquet, J. P. (1862): *D'une Circulation Dérivative dans les Membres et dans la Tête chez l'Homme.* A. Delahaya, Paris.

Advances in Neurology, Vol. 33, edited by
M. Critchley et al. Raven Press, New York © 1982

Basic Mechanisms of Antimigraine Drugs

J. R. Fozard

Centre de Recherche, Merrell International, Strasbourg Cedex, France

Consistently observed biochemical events suggest that 5-hydroxytryptamine (5-HT) is the naturally occurring substance most likely to play a role in the pathophysiology of migraine (10,59). Increased amounts of 5-HT and its metabolite 5-hydroxyindoleacetic acid (5-HIAA) are excreted in the urine during most attacks (see ref. 10 for details). Also, plasma and platelet 5-HT concentrations fall rapidly at the onset of an attack and remain low while the headache persists (1,45,53). Moreover, attacks of migraine have been clearly associated with periods of thrombocytopenia in certain patients (18). The hypothesis receives pharmacological support from the observation that migraine attacks can be triggered by compounds that release 5-HT from tissue stores, such as reserpine (46), fenfluramine (57), or viloxazine (3), and increased in severity during the early stages of treatment with zimelidine (23,66), a specific blocker of 5-HT uptake.

An expected consequence of a role for 5-HT in the etiology of migraine would be that compounds that block its activity at the receptor would be beneficial. In practice, this is so, since methysergide, a potent 5-HT D-receptor antagonist (27), is consistently effective in the prophylaxis of migraine (36); other such antagonists (cyproheptadine, pizotifen) are similarly useful (47,54,64). On the other hand, recognized 5-HT D-receptor antagonists are not the only agents of proven value in the interval treatment of migraine. For instance, propranolol, a nonselective β-adrenoceptor antagonist, amitriptyline, a blocker of monoamine reuptake, and chlorpromazine, whose primary property is nonselective dopamine receptor blockade, have all been used with success in the condition (11,54).

This chapter presents evidence that, along with their other properties, propranolol, amitriptyline, and chlorpromazine share with methysergide the capacity to block 5 HT D-receptors. Moreover, this property cannot be ruled out as an important component in the mechanism of their antimigraine effects. Continuing the theme of 5-HT antagonists being of theoretical benefit in migraine, the mechanism of action of metoclopramide in the treatment of the acute attack is discussed. In particular, the relevance to its clinical mode of action of the recent finding that metoclopramide has potent and selective blocking activity at the receptors for 5-HT present on autonomic and sensory neurons is considered.

5-HT D-RECEPTOR BLOCKADE BY MIGRAINE PROPHYLACTIC DRUGS

Recognized Antagonists at 5-HT D-Receptors

The case for blockade of 5-HT D-receptors being implicated in the mechanism of the antimigraine activity of methysergide, cyproheptadine, and pizotifen has been considered in detail (27) and is not repeated here. Essentially, blockade of 5-HT receptors is the single property these compounds have in common at their lowest active doses. Moreover, judging from animal studies, the doses used clinically would be adequate to supply 5-HT receptor blockade with each of these drugs (27). The precise location and function of these sites remain unknown, although an essential role in some biochemical trigger mechanism for the hypothetical "sterile inflammatory reaction" (17) of the cranial vasculature is consistent with many of the facts (27).

Propranolol

Numerous controlled studies have shown propranolol to be highly effective in the interval treatment of migraine (see, for example, refs. 5,25,70,73). The possibility that blockade of 5-HT D-receptors might be important to the antimigraine effects of propranolol stems from the original work of Weinstock and her colleagues (55,72). Schechter and Weinstock (55) initially demonstrated surmountable blockade of contractile responses to 5-HT on rat stomach and uterus *in vitro*. Weinstock et al. (72) subsequently compared propranolol with methysergide in a number of tests indicative of 5-HT receptor stimulant activity. The data from these experiments and the results from experiments in which propranolol and methysergide were compared as inhibitors of high affinity ^{3}H-5-HT and ^{3}H-lysergic acid diethylamide (^{3}H-LSD) binding to rat brain membranes (12,43) are presented in Table 1.

It is clear that propranolol has activity in each of the tests and that potency resides chiefly in the (−)-isomer, since (+)-propranolol is considerably less active than the racemic mixture. Propranolol varied from being 558 times less potent than methysergide in blocking 5-HT contraction of rat stomach to 1.4 times more potent in blocking the head twitch induced in mice by 5-hydroxytryptophan (5-HTP) (Table 1). As an antagonist of 5-HT-induced sleep in young chicks, propranolol was 33 times less potent than methysergide. The binding of ^{3}H-5-HT and ^{3}H-LSD to rat brain membranes indicates an interaction with two distinct but methysergide-sensitive 5-HT receptors in the brain (63). Propranolol displaced both ^{3}H-5-HT and ^{3}H-LSD from their binding sites, providing direct evidence of an interaction of propranolol with 5-HT receptors (Table 1).

In an attempt to relate the 5-HT receptor-blocking activity of propranolol to the clinical situation, we compare the geometric mean of the potency ratios found in Table 1 with the molar ratio of the daily doses of methysergide and propranolol used clinically in migraine (Table 2). This approach is at best approximate since it takes no account of pharmacokinetic differences between the compounds and therefore ignores the possibil-

TABLE 1. *Comparative effects of propranolol and methysergide on responses mediated by 5-HT receptors*

Drug	Rat stomach[a]	Mouse head twitch[a]	Chick sleep[a]	Displacement of	
				^{3}H-5HT[b,c]	^{3}H-LSD[b,c]
Methysergide	1	1	1	1	1
(±)-Propranolol	558	0.6	33	2.1	78
(+)-Propranolol	6762	>18	>176	43	409

Values are molar dose ratios [methysergide/drug].
From refs. [a]72, [b]43, [c]12.

TABLE 2. *Relationship between potency to block 5-HT responses and clinical dose schedules in migraine for methysergide, (±)-propranolol, amitriptyline, and chlorpromazine*

Drug	Ratio of potency in pharmacological tests[a]	Clinical dose range (mg/day)[b]	Molar ratio
Methysergide	1	2–6	1
(±)-Propranolol	18	80–320	79
Amitriptyline	4.5	30–75	20
Chlorpromazine	5.7	40–150	28

[a] Geometric mean of values presented in Tables 1, 4, and 5.
[b] Data from refs. 33 and 54.

ity that one of the tests is more or less relevant to the antimigraine activity. Nevertheless, in four of five of the pharmacological tests, the potency of propranolol relative to methysergide was less than the clinical molar dose ratio, and the mean ratio of potency was four times less than the ratio between the clinical doses (Table 2). The odds are thus heavily in favor of propranolol being at least as effective as an antagonist of 5-HT D-receptors as methysergide in the doses used clinically in migraine. The important question is whether this property is relevant to the antimigraine effects of propranolol. In any attempt to answer this question, the potential alternative explanations must be considered. To facilitate discussion on this point, the principal pharmacological properties of propranolol are compared with those of the other β-adrenoceptor antagonists that have been used clinically in migraine (Table 3).

Blockade of β_2-adrenoceptor-mediated extracranial vasodilatation is the most likely explanation for the beneficial effects of propranolol in migraine (see, for example, refs. 5,8,29). Yet neither oxprenolol nor alprenolol are of particular value in the condition, despite being potent antagonists at β_2-adrenoceptors (Table 3). Moreover, clinical benefit in migraine has recently been demonstrated following treatment with atenolol, a selective β_1-adrenoceptor antagonist (65). It is clear from Table 3 that a lack of intrinsic sympathomimetic activity may be an important factor. For instance, the basic difference between propranolol and pindolol is the powerful intrinsic sympathomimetic activity of the latter. Furthermore, both timolol and atenolol, which, like propranolol, lack intrinsic sympathomimetic activity, have been shown to have antimigraine activity (Table 3). Precisely how a lack of intrinsic sympathomimetic activity would bestow clinical potency in migraine is unclear. When one considers the case for 5-HT D-receptor blockade as an important factor in the mechanism of action of propranolol, weaknesses are also apparent. Thus alprenolol and oxprenolol have at least some 5-HT receptor blocking activity, yet neither has proved beneficial in migraine (Table 3). Atenolol, which has not been demonstrated to be a 5-HT antagonist, is reported to be clinically effective in migraine (Table 3). No single property of propranolol can explain its undoubted clinical efficacy in migraine. Of the recognized properties of β-adrenoceptor blocking agents, nonselective β-adrenoceptor blockade, lack of intrinsic sympathomimetic activity, and good penetration to the brain are probably the most important. Yet the preeminent position of propranolol as the β-adrenoceptor antagonist with the most consistent effects in migraine must depend on more than this. A unique combination of these properties with significant

TABLE 3. *Effects of β-adrenoceptor blocking agents in migraine and their pharmacological properties*

Drug	Migraine prophylaxis	Selectivity[h]	Intrinsic sympathetic activity[h]	Membrane stabilization	5-HT blockade				Entry to brain[k]
					Fundus[i]	In vitro ³H-5-HT[j]	³H-LSD[j]	In vivo rat hyperactivity[k]	
(±)-Propranolol	Yes[a]	$\beta_1\beta_2$	No	Yes	Yes	Yes	Yes	Yes	Good
Timolol	Yes[b]	$\beta_1\beta_2$	No	Yes/no	NT	NT	NT	Yes	Good
Atenolol	Yes[c]	β_1	No	No	NT	No	No	No	Poor
Pindolol	Yes/no[d]	$\beta_1\beta_2$	Yes	Yes	Yes	Yes	Poor	Yes	Good
Acebutolol	No[e]	β_1	Yes	Yes	NT	NT	NT	No	Poor
Alprenolol	No[f]	$\beta_1\beta_2$	Yes	Yes	NT	Yes	Poor	Yes	Good
Oxprenolol	No[g]	$\beta_1\beta_2$	Yes	Yes	Yes	Yes	Poor	No	Good

[a]See text.
From refs. [b]9, [c]65, [d]60, 20, 2, [e,f]19, [g]20, [h]42, 29, [i]72, [j]12, D. N. Middlemiss, *personal communication*, [k]15.
NT, not tested.

potency as an antagonist at 5-HT D-receptors is likely to be the critical factor determining the clinical response to propranolol.

Amitriptyline

Amitriptyline has been shown to be effective in the prophylactic treatment of migraine (16,32), an effect that occurs apparently independently of its antidepressant activity (16). The principal pharmacological property of amitriptyline is generally considered to be blockade of monoamine uptake with a claimed selectivity toward 5-HT (41); it also has significant blocking activity at cholinergic (50), α-adrenergic (62), and histamine (62) receptors. Recent work has established amitriptyline as a particularly potent antagonist of responses mediated through 5-HT receptors in several pharmacological test systems. For instance, the ED_{50} for blockade of the head twitch induced by 5-HTP in rats was 5.5 mg/kg (38). In the mouse, the equivalent values ranged from 1.3 (38) to 4.6 (30) mg/kg. At even lower doses (0.8 to 1.0 mg/kg), amitriptyline selectively blocked stimulation of the flexor reflex of the hind limb of the spinal rat induced by the 5-HT releasing drug fenfluramine (38). The pooled data from four pharmacological tests where comparisons between amitriptyline and methysergide have been possible are summarized in Table 4. Amitriptyline was 15 times less potent than methysergide in blocking the pressor response to 5-HT in the pithed rat and 11 times less potent against tryptamine-induced seizures in rats. The two drugs were approximately equipotent against head twitches induced in mice by stimulation of 5-HT receptors. Amitriptyline has appreciable affinity for the ^{3}H-LSD binding site in rat brain, being three times less active than methysergide in this respect, but was less active against ^{3}H-5-HT binding (Table 4).

Using the same approach with amitriptyline as was applied above to propranolol, the geometric mean ratio of potency in the pharmacological tests was calculated to be 1:4.5. This can be compared with a value of 1:20 for the molar ratio of the daily clinical doses (Table 2). These data indicate that a degree of 5-HT D-receptor blockade, at least equivalent to that achieved with methysergide, would be established with the doses of amitriptyline used clinically in the treatment of migraine.

The question of whether 5-HT receptor blockade or some other property of amitriptyline is primarily responsible for the positive clinical response in migraine cannot be resolved with certainty. However, anticholinergic, anti-α-adrenergic, and antihistaminic properties are unlikely to be important, since relatively selective agents of these types have not found regular use in migraine (36,54). The capacity to block monoamine uptake may well be relevant to the clinical response. It is important to emphasize, however,

TABLE 4. *Comparative effects of amitriptyline and methysergide on responses mediated by 5-HT receptors*

Drug	Pithed rat blood pressure[b,c]	Mouse head twitch[a,d,e,f,h,]	Rat tryptamine seizures[g]	Displacement of	
				^{3}H-5-HT[e,i]	^{3}H-LSD[e,i]
Methysergide	1	1	1	1	1
Amitriptyline	15	0.8	11	>3.5	3

Values are molar dose ratios $\left[\dfrac{\text{methysergide}}{\text{amitriptyline}}\right]$.

From refs. [a]14, [b]44, [c]26, [d]40, [e]20, [f]72, [g]37, [h]38, [i]12.

that 5-HT D-receptor blockade with amitriptyline occurs at doses below those causing inhibition of monoamine uptake *in vivo* (30,38,52). The above considerations indicate the possibility that blockade of 5-HT D-receptors is an important mechanism contributing to the antimigraine effects of amitriptyline; as with propranolol, however, a multifactorial basis for the clinical response cannot be ruled out.

Chlorpromazine

The phenothiazine tranquilizers, and particularly chlorpromazine, are considered of value in the interval treatment of migraine (11,54,67). As is well known, chlorpromazine has a plethora of pharmacological actions, including blockade of responses mediated through dopaminergic, α-adrenergic, and muscarinic cholinergic receptor sites and the capacity to inhibit monoamine reuptake (33). In addition, it is a powerful antagonist at 5-HT D-receptors, as illustrated by the recent work of Cooper and Wyllie (13). These authors used the perfused hind quarters of the rat *in vivo* and showed the vasoconstrictor response to 5-HT to be markedly reduced by concentrations of chlorpromazine as low as 8×10^{-9} M. Methysergide was similarly effective; it was 43 times more potent than chlorpromazine on a molar basis (Table 5). In four additional tests of 5-HT receptor function, the potency of chlorpromazine ranged from three times more to 31 times less than that of methysergide (Table 5).

The mean molar dose ratio from the pharmacological tests is compared with the clinical molar dose ratio in Table 2. In common with both propranolol and amitriptyline, the doses of chlorpromazine used clinically would be predicted to produce an equal or greater degree of 5-HT D-receptor blockade than that produced by clinical doses of methysergide. With a compound like chlorpromazine, which has multiple pharmacological actions, it would be unrealistic to claim any one of these properties as essential to the production of a clinical response. Nevertheless, chlorpromazine falls into line with the compounds discussed above that provide clinical benefit in migraine and have meaningful 5-HT D-receptor blocking activity.

Final Considerations

The information presented above indicates that propranolol, amitriptyline, and chlorpromazine, drugs with widely different spectra of pharmacological activity but all of benefit in the prophylactic treatment of migraine, are at least as effective as methysergide

TABLE 5. *Comparative effects of chlorpromazine and methysergide on responses mediated by 5-HT receptors*

Drug	Rat limb perfusion[e]	Rat tryptamine seizures[d]	Mouse head twitch[a]	Displacement of	
				^{3}H-5-HT[b,c]	^{3}H-LSD[b,c]
Methysergide	1	1	1	1	1
Chlorpromazine	43	1.6	0.3	31	9.5

Values are molar dose ratios $\left[\dfrac{\text{methysergide}}{\text{chlorpromazine}}\right]$.

From refs. [a]14, [b]6, [c]24, [d]37, [e]13.

as 5-HT antagonists at the doses used clinically. If cyproheptadine and pizotifen are included in the list, the single pharmacological property that the majority of migraine prophylactic drugs have in common is the capacity to block responses to 5-HT mediated through D-receptor. Considering the range of activities displayed by these compounds and the role of serendipity in the introduction into clinical use, it would be remarkable if that single common property were not the important, although not necessarily the exclusive, means through which clinical activity were manifested. Further definition of the site and function of this receptor is a justified priority for future research, since it would inevitably lead to a greater understanding of the disease process itself.

MODE OF ACTION OF METOCLOPRAMIDE

Metoclopramide is used in the treatment of the acute attack ostensibly because of its antiemetic properties (56) but also because, in combination with aspirin, it facilitates the absorption of the latter (69). The compound is a dopamine receptor antagonist (31), which satisfactorily accounts for its antiemetic activity and may also be a factor in its effects on bowel propulsive movement (49,56). Given in an oral dose of 10 mg, metoclopramide relieves the nausea of the attack, but little or no relief of pain is obtained (39,61).

In 1977, Hughes (34), a South Australian general practitioner, reported that he had

> . . . treated four patients who suffered from acute migraine attacks with slow intravenous injection of 10 mg of metoclopramide, which brought immediate relief of symptoms in three cases. The typical response, while nearing the end of the injection, was for the patients to open their eyes, relax their furrowed brow, and say "that feels better, doc!"

The principal difference in this report was that metoclopramide was given by slow intravenous injection rather than orally. At about this time, a novel property of metoclopramide was described, namely, its capacity to inhibit selectively responses to 5-HT mediated through the M-receptors for 5-HT located on the terminal sympathetic fibers of the rabbit heart (28). Figure 1, taken from the work of Fozard and Mobarok Ali (28), shows that blockade of 5-HT is competitive, with the threshold for antagonism being about 6×10^{-8} M or 20 ng/ml. That this concentration would easily be attained in human plasma following a slow intravenous injection of 10 mg metoclopramide is indicated by the data of Bateman et al. (4), reproduced in Fig. 2. The plasma concentration of metoclopramide exceeded the threshold for 5-HT antagonism *in vitro* by four- to fivefold during the first 10 min after injection and remained above 20 ng/ml for more than 1 hr (Fig. 2).

The basic question is whether blockade of 5-HT M-receptors can be rationalized to the immediate relief of clinical symptoms obtained by Hughes (34). It is difficult to envisage a role based on blockade of an autonomic efferent neuronal stimulant effect of 5-HT, the physiological relevance of which is unknown. On the other hand, a role can be conceptualized if these receptors were present on the sensory afferent fibers subserving transmission of pain. 5-HT is a potent pain-producing substance in man (35). Moreover, the receptors involved are known to have the characteristics of the autonomic M-receptor, at least with respect to the relative potency of agonists (35). An animal model of an afferent neuronal stimulant response to 5-HT is the Von Bezold-Jarisch reflex elicited in the anesthetized rat. Intravenous injection of small doses of 5-HT results in transient cardiac slowing, the result of a reflex stimulation of the vagus following activation of sensory afferent fibers located mainly in the right ventricle (48).

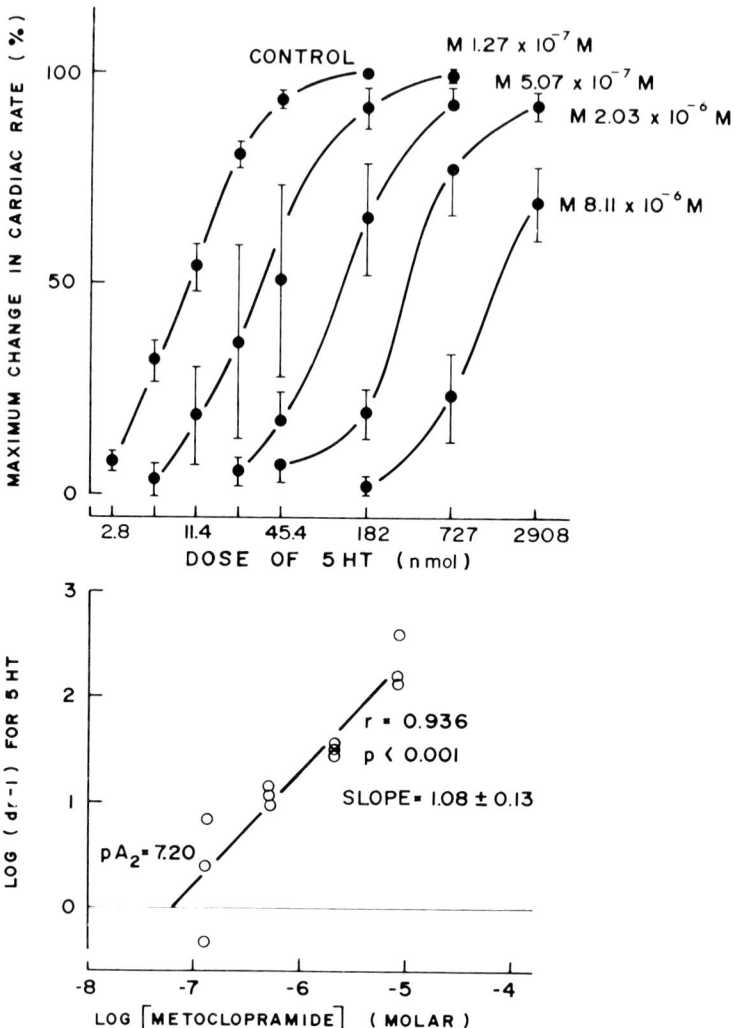

FIG. 1. Effects of metoclopramide (M) on the changes in rate of the isolated rabbit heart evoked by bolus injections of 5-HT. **Upper:** Dose-response curves to 5-HT established (control) and repeated in the presence of metoclopramide at the concentrations shown. Only one concentration was tested per heart; since the control curves did not differ significantly from each other, they were pooled. Points represent the means of three (each concentration of metoclopramide) and 12 (pooled controls) individual determinations with standard errors. Ordinate: maximum change in cardiac rate (%). **Lower:** Plot of log (dr-1) against log [antagonist] (molar) for metoclopramide-5-HT antagonism in isolated rabbit hearts. The points represent results from the experiments shown above, with the 5-HT dose ratios being derived at the ED_{50} level and by individual comparisons with the appropriate control curves. *Ordinate:* log (dr-1) for 5-HT. Response to 5-HT mediated through 5-HT M-receptors is antagonized competitively by metoclopramide. (Data from ref. 28.)

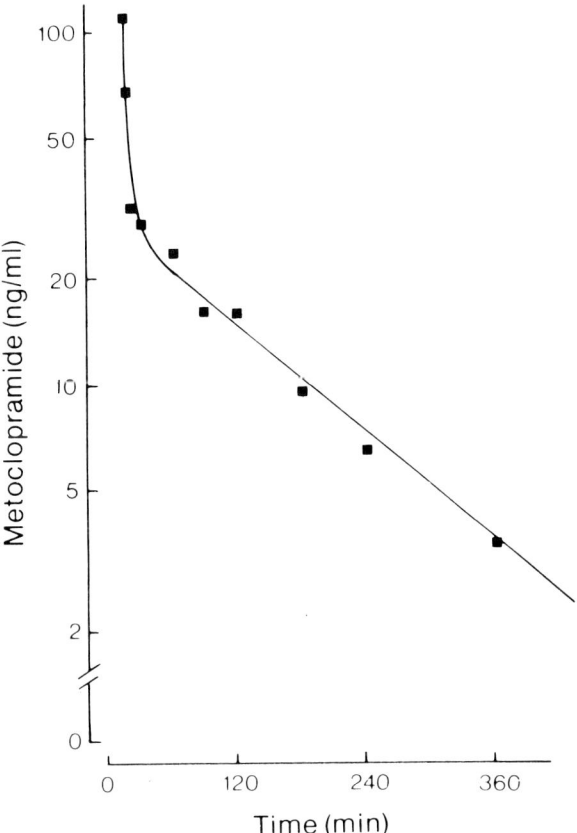

FIG. 2. Plasma concentration profile of metoclopramide following 10 mg metoclopramide hydrochloride given intravenously to a normal human volunteer. (Data from ref. 4.)

The reflex is illustrated in the first part of Fig. 3, which also shows the effect of metoclopramide on the response. At a dose of 1 mg/kg given by slow intravenous injection, metoclopramide markedly inhibited the Von Bezold-Jarisch reflex component of the response to 5-HT. The prolonged depressor response and small increase in heart rate, which arise by different mechanisms (26), were unaffected by metoclopramide (Fig. 3). The threshold dose for blockade of the Von Bezold-Jarisch reflex was 0.23 ± 0.06 mg/kg (mean ± SEM, N = 5); the effect was selective in that the response to afferent vagal nerve stimulation was unaffected even by doses of metoclopramide as high as 5 mg/kg (result not illustrated). It should be noted that blockade of 5-HT-evoked reflex cardiac inhibition is one of the most potent actions of metoclopramide yet described *in vivo*. With the exception of its effects on prolactin secretion (74), the minimum doses of metoclopramide that affect dopamine-mediated function are five to 10 times greater than those affecting 5-HT (22).

The mechanism of the symptomatic relief of migraine afforded by intravenous metoclopramide can be envisaged with the aid of the schematic diagram presented in Fig. 4. According to Blau (7), headache results from activation of afferent sensory nerves in the walls and perivascular areas of the cranial microvasculature, presumably by substances

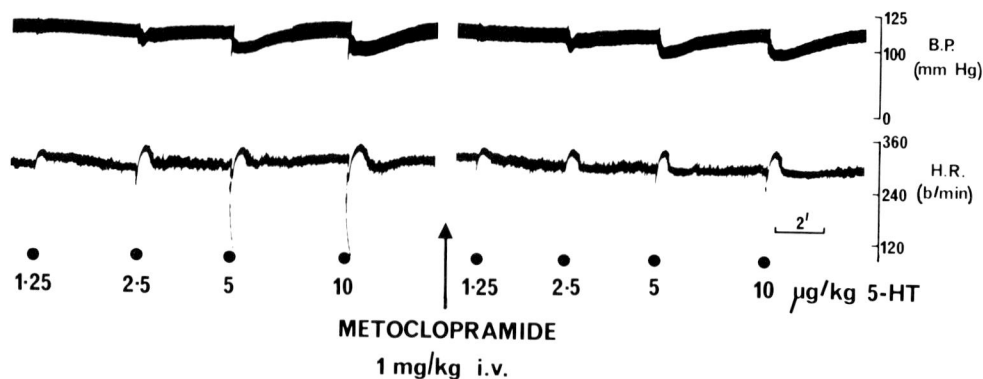

FIG. 3. Effect of metoclopramide, 1 mg/kg i.v., on the Von Bezold-Jarisch component of the cardiovascular response to bolus injections of 5-HT in the rat anesthetized with urethane. **Upper trace,** blood pressure; **lower trace,** heart rate. Initial brief fall in cardiac rate evoked by 5-HT is selectively inhibited by metoclopramide.

released during the hypothetical "sterile inflammatory reaction" (17). 5-HT, which is present in the cerebral microvessels (51), would almost certainly be involved and would, by activating M-receptors on pain-transmitting fibers, generate pain (35). More significantly, perhaps, the presence of 5-HT would sensitize the nerves to other nociceptive stimuli, such as the kinins, inorganic cations, and possibly the mechanical stimulation arising from pulsatile flow (58). Metoclopramide, given intravenously, would exceed the threshold for blockade of the 5-HT M-receptors and by this means block the 5-HT component of the sensory afferent neuronal stimulant response and diminish the pain of migraine.

At present, the only published data showing the beneficial effects of intravenous metoclopramide in migraine are those of Hughes (34); clearly, they must be confirmed by

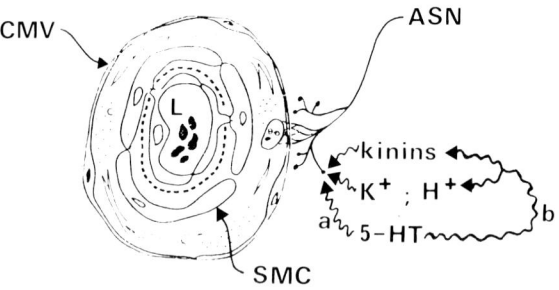

FIG. 4. Diagrammatic representation of the possible involvement of 5-HT in pain production in migraine and the effect of metoclopramide. Afferent sensory neurons (ASN) situated in and around the cranial microvasculature (CMV) are stimulated by substances released during development of a "sterile inflammatory reaction" (17) and are responsible for the pain of migraine (7). 5-HT, which is present in brain microvessels (51), will contribute to the response by (a) stimulating the nerves directly (35) and (b) sensitizing the nerves to other nociceptive stimuli (58). The receptor mediating these effects of 5-HT is the M-receptor; by blocking at these sites, metoclopramide may produce its beneficial effects. L, lumen; SMC, smooth muscle cell. (For further details, see text.)

others under controlled, clinical trial conditions. The general thesis, however, is supported by recent studies carried out with propranolol. Tokola and Hokkanen (68) reported results from a pilot study showing an excellent or good response in 56% of patients whose acute attacks were treated with 40 to 80 mg propranolol. This clinical observation is of relevance since propranolol has been shown to be a potent and selective antagonist at the 5-HT M-receptors of the cat superior cervical ganglion (71).

That intravenous metoclopramide alleviates the symptoms of the acute attack in part by blocking neuronal excitation arising from, or facilitated by, stimulation of 5-HT M-receptors is consistent both with the facts as known and with current concepts of the mechanism of production of headache. It carries the obvious assumption that activation of 5-HT M-receptors is a significant event in the development and maintenance of an attack that points yet again to the importance of 5-HT in the etiology of the condition.

CONCLUSION

That 5-HT is the naturally occurring substance with the strongest claim for a role in the pathophysiology of migraine is reinforced by the facts presented. Collectively, these observations suggest that blockade of 5-HT receptors or function may be the common mechanism by which a number of drugs with widely different pharmacological activities produce their beneficial effects in migraine. Moreover, blockade of the D-receptors for 5-HT would be a key factor in achieving prophylactic protection, whereas blockade of the M-receptor would afford symptomatic relief in the acute attack.

REFERENCES

1. Anthony, M., Hinterberger, H., and Lance, J. W. (1967): Plasma serotonin in migraine and stress. *Arch. Neurol.,* 16:544–552.
2. Anthony, M., Lance, J. W., and Somerville, B. (1972): A comparative study of pindolol, clonidine and carbamazepine in the interval therapy of migraine. *Med. J. Aust.,* i:1,343–1,346.
3. Barnes, T. R. E., Kidger, T., and Greenwood, D. T. (1979): Viloxazine and migraine. *Lancet,* ii:1,368.
4. Bateman, D. N., Kahn, C., Mashiter, K., and Davies, D. S. (1978): Pharmacokinetic and concentration-effect studies with intravenous metoclopramide. *Br. J. Clin. Pharmacol.,* 6:401–407.
5. Behan, P. O., and Reid, M. (1980): Propranolol in the treatment of migraine. *The Practitioner,* 224:201–204.
6. Bennett, J. P., Jr., and Snyder, S. H. (1976): Serotonin and lysergic acid diethylamide binding in rat brain membranes: Relationship to postsynaptic serotonin receptors. *Mol. Pharmacol.,* 12:373–389.
7. Blau, J. N. (1978): Migraine: A vasomotor instability of the meningeal circulation. *Lancet,* ii:1136–1139.
8. Børgesen, S. E. (1977): Propranolol for migraine. *Compr. Ther.,* 3:53–57.
9. Briggs, R. S., and Millac, P. A. (1979): Timolol in migraine prophylaxis. *Headache,* 19:379–381.
10. Bruyn, G. W. (1976): The biochemical basis of migraine: A critique. In: *Clinical Neuropharmacology, Vol. 1,* edited by H. L. Klawans, pp. 185–213. Raven Press, New York.
11. Caviness, V. S., Jr., and O'Brien, P. (1980): Headache. *N. Engl. J. Med.,* 302:446–450.
12. Connell, D. J., Middlemiss, D. N., and Stone, M. A. (1980): Further evidence for an interaction of propranolol with the central 5-hydroxytryptamine (5-HT) receptor. *Br. J. Pharmacol.,* 68:173P–174P.
13. Cooper, M., and Wyllie, J. H. (1979): Some properties of 5-hydroxytryptamine receptors in the hindquarters of the rat. *Br. J. Pharmacol.,* 67:79–85.
14. Corne, S. J., Pickering, R. W., and Warner, B. T. (1963): A method for assessing the effects of drugs on the central actions of 5-hydroxytryptamine. *Br. J. Pharmacol.,* 20:106–120.
15. Costain, D. W., and Green, A. R. (1978): β-Adrenoceptor antagonists inhibit the behavioural responses of rats to increased brain 5-hydroxytryptamine. *Br. J. Pharmacol.,* 64:193–200.
16. Couch, J. R., Ziegler, D. K., and Hassanein, R. (1976): Amitriptyline in the prophylaxis of migraine. Effectiveness and relationship of antimigraine and antidepressant effects. *Neurology (Minneap.),* 26:121–127.

17. Dallessio, D. J. (1978): Mechanisms of headache. *Med. Clin. North Am.,* 62:429–442.
18. Damasio, H., and Beck, D. (1978): Migraine, thrombocytopenia, and serotonin metabolism. *Lancet,* i:240–242.
19. Ekbom, K. (1975): Alprenolol for migraine prophylaxis. *Headache,* 15:129–132.
20. Ekbom, K., and Lundberg, P. O. (1972): Clinical trial of LB-46 (d, 1-4-(2-hydroxy-3-isopropylaminopropoxy)indol) an adrenergic beta-receptor blocking agent in migraine prophylaxis. *Headache,* 12:15–17.
21. Ekbom, K., and Zetterman, M. (1977): Oxprenolol in the treatment of migraine. *Acta Neurol. Scand.,* 56:181–184.
22. Elliott, P. N. C., Jenner, P., Huizing, G., Marsden, C. D., and Miller, R. (1977): Substituted benzamides as cerebral dopamine antagonists in rodents. *Neuropharmacology,* 16:333–342.
23. Evans, L., Best, J., Moore, G., and Cox, J. (1980): Zimelidine—A serotonin uptake blocker in the treatment of phobic anxiety. *Prog. Neuropsychopharmacol.,* 4:75–79.
24. Fillion, G. M. B., Rousselle, J.-C., Fillion, M.-P., Beaudoin, D. M., Goiny, M. R., Deniau, J.-M., and Jacob, J. J. (1978): High affinity binding of [^{3}H]5-hydroxytryptamine to brain synaptosomal membranes: Comparison with [^{3}H] lysergic acid diethylamide binding. *Mol. Pharmacol.,* 14:50–59.
25. Forssman, B., Henriksson, K.-G., Johannsson, V., Lindvall, L., and Lundin, H. (1976): Propranolol for migraine prophylaxis. *Headache,* 16:238–245.
26. Fozard, J. R. (1968): Studies on the cardiovascular actions of 5-HT in the rat. Doctoral dissertation, University of Bradford.
27. Fozard, J. R. (1975): The animal pharmacology of drugs used in the treatment of migraine. *J. Pharm. Pharmacol.,* 27:297–321.
28. Fozard, J. R., and Mobarok Ali, A. T. M. (1978): Blockade of neuronal tryptamine receptors by metoclopramide. *Eur. J. Pharmacol.,* 49:109–112.
29. Frishman, W., and Silverman, R. (1979): Clinical pharmacology of the new beta-blocking drugs. Part 3. Comparative clinical experience and new therapeutic applications. *Am. Heart J.,* 98:119–131.
30. Fuxe, K., Ögren, S.-O., Agnati, L., Gustafsson, J. K., and Jonsson, G. (1977): On the mechanism of action of the antidepressant drugs amitriptyline and nortriptyline. Evidence for 5-hydroxytryptamine receptor blocking activity. *Neurosci. Lett.,* 6:339–344.
31. Goldberg, L. I., Volkman, P. H., and Kohli, J. O. (1978): A comparison of the vascular dopamine receptor with other dopamine receptors. *Ann. Rev. Pharmacol. Toxicol.,* 18:57–79.
32. Gomersall, J. D., and Stuart, A. (1973): Amitriptyline in migraine prophylaxis. Changes in pattern of attacks during a controlled clinical trial. *J. Neurol. Neurosurg. Psychiatry,* 36:684–690.
33. Goodman, L. S., and Gilman, A. (editors) (1975): *The Pharmacological Basis of Therapeutics.* Macmillan, New York.
34. Hughes, J. B. (1977): Metoclopramide in migraine. *Med. J. Aust.,* ii:580.
35. Keele, C. A., and Armstrong, D. (1964): *Substances Producing Pain and Itch.* Williams & Wilkins, Baltimore.
36. Lance, J. W. (1973): *Mechanism and Management of Headache.* Butterworth, London.
37. Leysen, J. E., Niemegeers, C. J. E., Tollenaere, J. P., and Laduron, P. M. (1978): Serotonergic component of neuroleptic receptors. *Nature,* 272:168–171.
38. Maj, J., Lewandowska, A., and Rawtow, A. (1979): Central antiserotonin action of amitriptyline. *Pharmakopsychiatrie,* 12:281–285.
39. Matts, S. G. F. (1974): Metoclopramide in the treatment of migraine. *The Practitioner,* 212:887–890.
40. Mawson, C., and Whittington, H. (1970): Evaluation of the peripheral and central antagonistic activities against 5-hydroxytryptamine of some new agents. *Br. J. Pharmacol.,* 39:223P.
41. Maxwell, R. A., and White, H. L. (1978): Tricyclic and monamine oxidase inhibitor antidepressants: Structure-activity relationships. In: *Handbook of Psychopharmacology, Vol. 14, Affective Disorders: Drug Actions in Animals and Man,* edited by L. L. Iversen, S. D. Iversen, and S. H. Snyder, pp. 83–155. Plenum Press, New York.
42. McDevitt, D. G. (1979): Adrenoceptor blocking drugs: Clinical pharmacology and therapeutic use. *Drugs,* 17:267–288.
43. Middlemiss, D. N., Blakeborough, L., and Leather, S. R. (1977): Direct evidence for an interaction of β-adrenergic blockers with the 5-HT receptor. *Nature,* 267:289–290.
44. Møller Nielsen, I., Nymark, M., Hougs, W., and Pederson, V. (1966): The pharmacological properties of Melitracen (N 7001) and Litracen (N 7049). *Arzneimittelforschung,* 16:135–140.
45. Mück-Seler, D., Deanovic, Z., and Dupely, M. (1979): Platelet serotonin (5-HT) and 5-HT releasing factor in plasma of migrainous patients. *Headache,* 19:14–17.
46. Nappi, G., Savoldi, F., Bono, G., and Martignoni, E. (1979): Reserpine-headache and PRL release in migraine. *Headache,* 19:273–277.
47. Nelson, R. F. (1973): BC-105 A new prophylactic agent for migraine. Four years' experience in 75 patients. *Headache,* 13:96–103.
48. Paintal, A. S. (1973): Vagal sensory receptors and their reflex effects. *Physiol. Rev.,* 53:159–227.
49. Pinder, R. M., Brogden, R. N., Sawyer, P. R., Speight, T. M., and Avery, G. S. (1976): Metoclopramide: A review of its pharmacological properties and clinical use. *Drugs,* 12:81–131.

50. Rathbun, R. C., and Slater, I. H. (1963): Amitriptyline and nortriptyline as antagonists of central and peripheral cholinergic activity. *Psychopharmacologia,* 4:114–125.

51. Reinhard, J. F., Jr., Liebmann, J. E., Schlosberg, A. J., and Moskowitz, M. A. (1979): Serotonin neurons project to small vessels in the brain. *Science,* 206:85–87.

52. Ross, S. B., and Renyi, A. L. (1975): Tricyclic antidepressant agents. II. Effect of oral administration on the uptake of ^{3}H-noradrenaline and ^{14}C-5-hydroxytryptamine in slices of the midbrain-hypothalamus region of the rat. *Acta Pharmacol. Toxicol.,* 36:395–408.

53. Rydzewski, W. (1976): Serotonin (5-HT) in migraine: Levels in whole blood in and between attacks. *Headache,* 16:16–19.

54. Saper, J. R. (1978): Migraine II. Treatment. *JAMA,* 239:2,480–2,484.

55. Schechter, Y., and Weinstock, M. (1974): β-Adrenoceptor blocking agents and responses to adrenaline and 5-hydroxytryptamine in isolated rat stomach and uterus. *Br. J. Pharmacol.,* 52:283–287.

56. Schulze-Delrieu, K., (1979): Metoclopramide. *Gastroenterology,* 77:768–779.

57. Sicuteri, F., Del Bene, E., and Anselmi, B. (1976): Fenfluramine headache. *Headache,* 16:185–188.

58. Sicuteri, F., Fanciullacci, M., Franchi, G., and Del Bianco, P. L. (1965): Serotonin-bradykinin potentiation on the pain receptors in man. *Life Sci.,* 4:309–316.

59. Sjaastad, O. (1975): The significance of blood serotonin levels in migraine. A critical review. *Acta Neurol. Scand.,* 51:200–210.

60. Sjaastad, O., and Stensrud, P. (1972): Clinical trial of a beta-receptor blocking agent (LB 46) in migraine prophylaxis. *Acta Neurol. Scand.,* 48:124–128.

61. Slettnes, O., and Sjaastad, O. (1977): Metoclopramide during attacks of migraine. In: *Headache: New Vistas,* edited by F. Sicuteri, pp. 201–204. Biomedical Press, Florence.

62. Snyder, S. H. (1980): Tricyclic antidepressant drug interactions with histamine and α-adrenergic receptors. *Pharmakopsychiatrie,* 13:62–67.

63. Snyder, S. H., and Goodman, R. R. (1980): Multiple neurotransmitter receptors. *J. Neurochem.,* 35:5–15.

64. Speight, T. M., and Avery, G. S. (1972): Pizotifen (BC-105): A review of its pharmacological properties and its therapeutic efficacy in vascular headaches. *Drugs,* 3:159–203.

65. Stensrud, P., and Sjaastad, O. (1981): Comparative trial of Tenormin (atenolol) and Inderal (propranolol) in migraine. *Ups. J. Med. Sci. (in press).*

66. Syvälahti, E., Kangasniemi, P., and Ross, S. B. (1979): Migraine headache and blood serotonin levels after administration of zimelidine, a selective inhibitor of serotonin uptake. *Curr. Ther. Res.,* 25:299–310.

67. Thrush, D. (1978): Treatment of migraine. *Br. Med. J.,* i:1,004–1,005.

68. Tokola, R., and Hokkanen, E. (1978): Propranolol for acute migraine. *Br. Med. J.,* ii:1089.

69. Volans, G. N. (1975): The effect of metoclopramide on the absorption of effervescent aspirin in migraine. *Br. J. Clin. Pharmacol.,* 2:57–63.

70. Weber, R. B., and Reinmuth, O. M. (1972): The treatment of migraine with propranolol. *Neurology (Minneap.),* 22:366–369.

71. Weinstock, M., and Schechter, Y. (1975): Antagonism by propranolol of the ganglion stimulant action of 5-hydroxytryptamine. *Eur. J. Pharmacol.,* 32:293–301.

72. Weinstock, M., Weiss, C., and Gitter, S. (1977): Blockade of 5-hydroxytryptamine receptors in the central nervous system by β-adrenoceptor antagonists. *Neuropharmacology,* 16:273–276.

73. Wideroe, T.-E., and Vigander, T. (1974): Propranolol in the treatment of migraine. *Br. Med. J.,* ii:699–701.

74. Yamauchi, J., Takahara, J., and Ofuji, T. (1977): Effect of metoclopramide on rat prolactin secretion *in vivo. Life Sci.,* 20:1,581–1,584.

Advances in Neurology, Vol. 33, edited by
M. Critchley et al. Raven Press, New York © 1982

Agonists and Antagonists of Vascular Receptors

Pramod R. Saxena

Department of Pharmacology, Faculty of Medicine, Erasmus University, Rotterdam, The Netherlands

Substances that can either contract or relax the vascular smooth muscle include (a) those arriving with the circulating blood (e.g., angiotensin, vasopressin, epinephrine, or 5-hydroxytryptamine (5-HT), (b) those released from nerve terminals (e.g., norepinephrine or acetylcholine), (c) those liberated mainly from the vessel wall (e.g., prostaglandins, histamine, or adenine nucleotides), and (d) a number of compounds obtained from plant sources or upon chemical synthesis (e.g., ergotamine, reserpine, or prazocin). Some of these substances act on the neurogenic processes by modifying the biosynthesis or release of neurotransmitters from the presynaptic elements. Other agents have a direct action on specialized molecular components located on the plasma membrane of the smooth muscle cells. These are termed postsynaptic receptors.

Based on the agonist and antagonist activity of the neuromuscular junction of vascular smooth muscle, a number of drug binding sites have been characterized as adrenergic, serotonergic, histaminergic, and cholinergic receptors. A number of other substances, such as prostaglandins, vasopressin, and kinins, may also excite specific receptors; but the evidence remains insufficient.

One of the most salient features, the importance of which is not generally appreciated, is the heterogeneity of response to agonists and antagonists not only in different vessels but also within the different segments of the same vascular bed (55). This chapter, therefore, is restricted to a discussion of receptors in the intra- and extracranial vessels which are involved in the pathophysiology of migraine. The evidence from the experiments characterizing the main vascular receptors in this territory is reviewed, and an attempt is made to define the effects of antimigraine drugs on these vascular receptors.

RECEPTORS IN THE CRANIAL VESSELS

A number of specific receptors have been identified on intra- and extracranial vessels. The most important of these receptors, on which the substances implicated in the pathophysiology of migraine (14,42,46) or the antimigraine drugs act are: (a) adrenergic receptors, (b) histamine receptors, and (c) 5-HT receptors.

Adrenergic Receptors

Although there has been considerable debate about the innervation of cerebral vessels, there is now no doubt that both intra- and extracranial blood vessels have a rich sympathetic innervation and, consequently, adrenergic receptors (20,32).

Alpha-Adrenergic Receptors

Exogenously administered norepinephrine and that released by sympathetic nerves or by tyramine (3,8,51) constrict the cranial vessels by an alpha-adrenergic action (10, 14,27,29,42,54). These studies have been performed both *in vivo* and *in vitro;* therefore, alpha-receptors are located on both small (arterioles) and large intra- and extracranial arteries and subserve vasoconstriction. However, differences in the values of dissociation constants obtained from cerebral vessels and other smooth muscle suggest that the alpha-receptors of cerebral vessels may differ from those elsewhere (10).

Beta-Adrenergic Receptors

Stimulation of beta-adrenoceptors causes hyperpolarization of vascular smooth muscle cells and thus leads to vasodilation in most vascular beds, including the intra- and extracranial vasculature (10,27,45,53). However, cerebral blood flow does not always increase following beta-adrenergic stimulation in *in vivo* studies, probably because of autoregulation, as found in conscious renal hypertensive and normotensive rabbits (6).

Histamine Receptors

Interest in histamine was rekindled by the discovery of histamine H_2-receptor blocking drugs (4,5). The effects of this biogenic amine have been extensively studied both *in vitro* and *in vivo* on cranial vessels.

In vitro studies performed by Edvinsson and Owman (11) showed that histamine can elicit both a contraction and a relaxation of intra- (middle cerebral) and extra-cranial (external maxillary or lingual) arteries in cats. The contraction of the extracranial artery was antagonized competitively but that of the intracranial artery noncompetitively by the H_1-receptor blocking agent mepyramine. On the other hand, the H_2-receptor blocker burimamide was able to antagonize the histamine-induced relaxation of both the vessels in a competitive manner, showing that H_2-receptors mediate vasodilation (11). Similarly, the vasodepressor response to histamine in perfused human temporal arteries was also mediated by H_2-receptors (16).

In vivo studies from our laboratory in dogs have shown that vasodilation induced by local administration of histamine in the internal and external carotid artery bed is at least partially antagonized by H_1-receptor blocking drugs (34,36,41,42). Furthermore, although both H_1- and H_2-receptors subserve carotid vasodilation, the affinity of histamine for H_1-receptors is greater than that for H_2-receptors, but the intrinsic activity via both receptors is comparable (36). In the monkey, H_2-receptors may be more important for vasodilation of the external carotid artery (24). In man, indirect evidence is available for the presence of both types of histaminergic receptors in intra- and extracranial vessels. Betahistine, an agent acting on H_1-receptors, induces vasodilation in both scalp and intracerebral vasculature (26,44), while histamine increases blood flow in the internal and external carotid artery of patients pretreated with promethazine, an antagonist of H_1-receptors (52).

The available evidence suggests that in the large cranial arteries, histamine causes a contraction mainly via H_1-receptors and a relaxation via H_2-receptors. In the resistance vessels (arterioles), there are both H_1- and H_2-receptors that lead to vasodilation in the internal and external carotid arterial bed. It must be pointed out that cerebral blood flow may not increase and may even be decreased following histamine administration in the intact organism (21,22). Furthermore, despite incriminating evidence for histamine in the pathophysiology of cluster headache and migraine, treatment with both types of histaminergic blockers, either alone or in combination, is of little therapeutic value in these cases (33).

5-HT Receptors

Depending on the dose, the blood vessel involved, and its basal tone, 5-HT can cause either vasodilation or vasoconstriction. Although the receptors for 5-HT were generally classified as M- and D-types (15), it is now becoming obvious that such a classification is not strictly applicable to several tissues. Investigations in the cranial vessels, initiated because of the possible involvement of 5-HT in migraine (14,46), have tended to support that 5-HT acts on receptors other than M- and D-types.

Studies performed on cats, dogs, and human intra- and extracerebral arteries *in vitro* show that 5-HT is a potent agonist (1,9,28,29,54). Its contractile effect is antagonized by phenoxybenzamine, methysergide, pizotifen, ergotamine, and dihydroergotamine (1,9,28), suggesting that, at least on these large arteries, the amine acts on D-receptors. In the rabbit ear artery and the dog auricular artery, however, there is sufficient evidence that the 5-HT-induced constriction is mediated, respectively, by alpha-adrenoceptors (2) and by another distinct, but as yet not fully characterized, receptor (1). In addition, 5-HT may also elicit vasodilation in previously contracted intra- and extracranial arteries by a beta-adrenergic mechanism (9).

Conflicting results have been reported in studies using *in vivo* techniques. While clear vasoconstrictor response has been noted on the internal carotid artery (18,24,34,41,42, 51,56), the cerebral blood flow may or may not decrease (7,13,31,40), probably due to differential effects on large and small cerebral arteries (19). Similarly, both an increase (24,34,41,42,51) and a decrease (7,18,25,56) was obtained in the blood flow in the external carotid territory. This difference has been shown conclusively to be due to the absence or presence of sympathetic vascular tone (25,56); 5-HT inhibits the release of norepinephrine by a specific presynaptic mechanism (12). Equivocal results have been reported regarding the effects of 5-HT antagonists on the carotid vascular responses to this amine *in vivo*. Our previous investigations repeatedly showed the ineffectiveness of the usual anti-5-HT drugs (34,41,42); others found some weak antagonistic activity in methysergide (56). More recently, Mylecharane et al. (30) reported that while methysergide only slightly antagonized the vasoconstrictor responses to 5-HT on both internal and external carotid arteries of the monkey, pizotifen did not do so at all. Instead, pizotifen potentiated the external carotid responses, as was reported earlier with cyproheptadine and mianserin in the dog (34,41).

VASCULAR RECEPTORS FOR ANTIMIGRAINE DRUGS

Ergotamine-induced vasoconstriction of the scalp vessels is causally related to its antimigraine action (17); it is now recognized that both ergotamine and methysergide have a selective carotid vasoconstrictor action (34,35,37,42). The ergotamine-induced vasoconstriction was only slightly affected by phentolamine pretreatment but was substantially attenuated by previous dibenzyline administration (42). These findings may indicate that ergotamine, apart from some alpha-adrenergic action (39), may also be acting on

D-type of 5-HT receptors. Similarly, it has been suggested that methysergide may be a (partial) agonist for 5-HT receptors in the carotid vasculature (37). Recent studies of Müller-Schweinitzer (28,29) on isolated human and canine cranial arteries have demonstrated that ergotamine, dihydroergotamine, and methysergide can all be regarded as partial agonists of 5-HT receptors (possibly of D-type) that are antagonized by pizotifen. In addition, methysergide, but not cyproheptadine or pizotifen, can excite another 5-HT receptor (unaffected by a number of known antagonists) detected in the auricular artery and in the saphenous vein of dogs (1). Once an antagonist for this 5-HT receptor is discovered, one would be able to characterize the receptors for 5-HT and for the antimigraine drugs in more detail.

Finally, it should be recognized that studies from our laboratory have shown that a number of antimigraine drugs (ergotamine, dihydroergotamine, isometheptene) constrict the arteriovenous anastomoses (AVAs) in the cranial circulation (23,38,43,47–50). It would be most pertinent to work out the receptors involved in the vasoconstriction of AVAs caused by these antimigraine drugs.

REFERENCES

1. Apperley, E., Feniuk, W., Humphrey, P. P. A., and Levy, G. P. (1980): Evidence for two types of excitatory receptor for 5-hydroxytryptamine in dog isolated vasculature. *Br. J. Pharmacol.*, 68:215–224.
2. Apperley, E., Humphrey, P. P. A., and Levy, G. P. (1976): Receptors for 5-hydroxytryptamine and noradrenaline in rabbit isolated ear artery and aorta. *Br. J. Pharmacol.*, 58:211–221.
3. Bevan, J. A., and Bevan, R. D. (1973): Localized neurogenic vasoconstriction of the basilar artery. *Stroke*, 4:760–763.
4. Black, J. W., Duncan, W. A. M., Durant, C. J., Ganellin, C. R., and Parsons, M. E. (1972): Definition and antagonism of histamine H2-receptors. *Nature*, 236:385–390.
5. Black, J. W., Duncan, W. A. M., Emmett, J. C., Ganellin, C. R., Hesselbo, T., Parsons, M. E., and Wyllie, J. H. (1973): Metiamide—an orally active histamine H2-receptors antagonist. *Agent Action*, 3:133–137.
6. Boom, M. van, and Saxena, P. R. (1980): Regional haemodynamic changes evoked by isoprenaline in conscious normotensive and renal hypertensive rabbits. *Br. J. Pharmacol.*, 68:116P–117P.
7. Deshmukh, V. D., and Harper, A. M. (1971): Effect of serotonin on cerebral blood flow and external carotid artery in the baboon. In: *Brain and Blood Flow*, edited by R. W. R. Russell, pp. 136–137. Pitman, London.
8. Edvinsson, L., Aubineau, P., Owman, C., Sercombe, R., and Seylaz, J. (1975): Sympathetic innervation of cerebral arteries. Prejunctional supersensitivity to norepinephrine after sympathectomy or cocaine treatment. *Stroke*, 6:525–530.
9. Edvinsson, L., Hardebo, J. E., and Owman, C. (1978): Pharmacological analysis of 5-hydroxytryptamine receptors in isolated intracranial and extracranial vessels of cat and man. *Circ. Res.*, 42:143–151.
10. Edvinsson, L., and Owman, C. (1974): Pharmacological characterization of adrenergic alpha and beta receptors mediating vasomotor response of cerebral arteries *in vitro. Circ. Res.*, 35:835–849.
11. Edvinsson, L., and Owman, C. (1975): A pharmacologic comparison of histamine receptors in isolated extracranial and intracranial arteries *in vitro. Neurology*, 25:271–276.
12. Feniuk, W., Humphrey, P. P. A., and Watts, A. D. (1979): Presynaptic inhibitory action of 5-hydroxytryptamine in dog isolated saphenous vein. *Br. J. Pharmacol.*, 67:247–254.
13. Forsyth, R. P., and Saxena, P. R. (1978): The influence of methysergide on 5-hydroxytryptamine induced changes in regional distribution of blood flow. *J. Pharm. Pharmacol.*, 30:503–507.
14. Friedman, A. P. (1968): Migraine—pathophysiology and pathogenesis. In: *Handbook of Clinical Neurology, Vol. 5*, edited by P. J. Vinken and G. W. Bruyn, pp. 37–44. North Holland, Amsterdam.
15. Gaddum, J. H., and Picarelli, Z. (1957): Two kinds of tryptamine receptors. *Br. J. Pharmacol.*, 12:323–328.
16. Glower, W. E., Carroll, P. R., and Latt, N. (1973): Histamine-receptors in human temporal and rabbit ear arteries. In: *International Symposium on Histamine H2-receptor Antagonists*, edited by C. J. Wood and M. A. Simkins, pp. 169–174. Dasprint Limited, London.
17. Graham, J. R., and Wolff, H. G. (1938): Mechanism of migraine headache and action of ergotamine tartrate. *Arch. Neurol. Psychiatry*, 39:737–763.
18. Grimson, B. S., Robinson, S. C., Danford, E. I., Tindall, G. T., and Greenfield, J. C., Jr. (1969): Effect

of serotonin on internal and external carotid artery blood flow in the baboon. *Am. J. Physiol.,* 216:50–55.

19. Harper, A. M., and MacKenzie, E. T. (1977): Effects of 5-hydroxytryptamine on pial arteriolar calibre in anaesthetized cats. *J. Physiol. (Lond.),* 271:735–746.

20. Hume, W. R., and Waterson, J. G. (1978): The innervation of the rabbit ear artery, an ultrastructural study. *Blood Vessels,* 15:348–364.

21. Johnston, B. M., and Owen, D. A. A. (1977): Tissue blood flow and distribution of cardiac output in cats: Changes caused by intravenous infusions of histamine and histamine receptor agonists. *Br. J. Pharmacol.,* 60:173–180.

22. Johnston, B. M., and Owen, D. A. A. (1977): Histamine, histamine antagonists and regional blood flow. *Eur. J. Pharmacol.,* 44:355–363.

23. Johnston, B. M., and Saxena, P. R. (1978): The effect of ergotamine on tissue blood flow and the arteriovenous shunting of radioactive microsphere in the head. *Br. J. Pharmacol.,* 63:541–549.

24. Lance, J. W., Spira, P. J., Lord, G. D. A., and Duckworth, J. W. (1978): Evaluation of drugs applicable to treatment of migraine in cranial circulation of the monkey. *Res. Clin. Stud. Headache,* 6:13–18.

25. Mena, M. A., and Vidrio, H. (1979): Reversal of serotonin vasodilatation in the dog external carotid bed by sympathetic denervation. *J. Cardiovasc. Pharmacol.,* 1:149–154.

26. Meyer, J. S., Mathew, N. T., Hartmann, A., and Rivera, V. M. (1974): Orally administered betahistine and regional cerebral blood flow in cerebrovascular disease. *J. Clin. Pharmacol.,* 14:280–289.

27. Mitchell, G., Seriven, D. R. L., and Rosendorff, C. (1975): Adrenoceptors in intracerebral resistance vessels. *Br. J. Pharmacol.,* 54:11–15.

28. Müller-Schweinitzer, E. (1978): Studies on the 5-HT receptor in vascular smooth muscle. *Res. Clin. Stud. Headache,* 6:6–12.

29. Müller-Schweinitzer, E., and Weidman, H. (1978): Basic pharmacological properties. In: *Ergot Alkaloids and Related Compounds. Handbook of Experimental Pharmacology, Vol. 49,* edited by B. Berde and H. O. Schild, pp. 87–232. Springer-Verlag, Berlin.

30. Mylecharane, E. J., Spira, P. J., Misbach, J., Duckworth, J. W., and Lance, J. W. (1978): Effects of methysergide, pizotifen and ergotamine in the monkey cranial circulation. *Eur. J. Pharmacol.,* 48:1–9.

31. Oleson, J., and Skinhoj, E. (1971): The influence of certain vasoactive amines on the regional cerebral blood flow in man. In: *Proceedings of the International Headache Symposium, Elsinore,* edited by D. J. Dalessio, T. Dalsgaard-Nielsen, and S. Diamond, pp. 145–152. Sandoz, Basel.

32. Owman, C., Edvinsson, L., and Hardebo, J. E. (1978): Pharmacological *in vitro* analysis of amine-mediated vasomotor functions in the intracranial and extracranial vascular beds. *Blood Vessels,* 15:128–147.

33. Russell, D. (1979): Cluster headache: Trial of a combined H1 and H2 antagonist treatment. *J. Neurol. Neurosurg. Psychiatry,* 42:668–669.

34. Saxena, P. R. (1972): The effects of antimigraine drugs on the vascular responses by 5-hydroxytryptamine and related biogenic substances on the external carotid bed of dogs: Possible pharmacological implications to their antimigraine action. *Headache,* 12:44–54.

35. Saxena, P. R. (1974): Selective carotid vasoconstriction by ergotamine as a relevant mechanism in its antimigraine action. *Arch. Neurobiol.,* 37:301–315.

36. Saxena, P. R. (1974): The significance of histamine H1 and H2 receptors on the carotid vascular bed in the dog. *Neurology,* 25:681–687.

37. Saxena, P. R. (1974): Selective vasoconstriction in the carotid vascular bed by methysergide: Possible relevance to its anti-migraine effect. *Eur. J. Pharmacol.,* 27:99–105.

38. Saxena, P. R. (1978): Arteriovenous shunting and migraine. *Res. Clin. Stud. Headache,* 6:89–102.

39. Saxena, P. R., and Cairo-Rawlins, W. I. (1979): Presynaptic inhibition by ergotamine of the responses to cardioaccelerator nerve stimulation in the cat. *Eur. J. Pharmacol.,* 58:305–312.

40. Saxena, P. R., Forsyth, R. P., Johnston, B. M., and de Werk, A. (1978): Regional systemic haemodynamic changes evoked by 5-hydroxytryptamine in awake and anaesthetized rabbits. *Eur. J. Pharmacol.,* 50:61–68.

41. Saxena, P. R., van Houwelingen, P., and Bonta, I. L. (1971): The effects of mianserin hydrochloride on the vascular responses evoked by 5-hydroxytryptamine and related vasoactive substances. *Eur. J. Pharmacol.,* 13:295–305.

42. Saxena, P. R., and de Vlaam-Schluter, G. M. (1974): Role of some biogenic substances in migraine and relevant mechanism in antimigraine action of ergotamine—Studies in an experimental model for migraine. *Headache,* 13:142–163.

43. Schamhardt, H. C., Verdouw, P. D., van der Hoek, T. M., and Saxena, P. R. (1979): Regional myocardial perfusion and wall thickness and arteriovenous shunting after ergotamine administration to pigs with a fixed coronary stenosis. *J. Cardiovasc. Pharmacol.,* 1:673–686.

44. Seipel, J. H. (1971): A rheoencephalographic study of the effect of betahistine hydrochloride on the normal human cerebral and scalp circulations. *Fed. Proc.,* 30:274.

45. Sercombe, R., Aubineau, P., Edvinsson, L., Mamo, H., Owman, C., and Seylaz, J. (1977): Pharmacological evidence *in vitro* and *in vivo* for functional beta-1 receptors in the cerebral circulation. *Eur. J. Physiol.,* 368:241–244.

46. Sicuteri, F. (1967): Vasoneuroactive substances and their implication in vascular pain. *Res. Clin. Stud. Headache,* 1:6–45.
47. Spierings, E. L. H. (1980): The pathophysiology of migraine. Doctoral dissertation, Erasmus University, Rotterdam. Stafleu's Wetenschappelijke Uitgeversmaatschappij B.V., Alphen aan den Rijn.
48. Spierings, E. L. H., and Saxena, P. R. (1979): Effect of ergotamine on cranial arteriovenous shunting in experiments with constant flow perfusion. *Eur. J. Pharmacol.,* 56:31–37.
49. Spierings, E. L. H., and Saxena, P. R. (1980): Effect of isometheptene on the distribution and shunting of 15μ microsphere throughout the cephalic circulation of the cat. *Headache,* 20:103–106.
50. Spierings, E. L. H., and Saxena, P. R. (1980): Effect of the antimigraine drugs ergotamine, dihydroergotamine and methysergide, on cranial arteriovenous shunting in the cat. *Neurology,* 30:696–701.
51. Spira, P. J., Mylecharane, E. J., Misbach, J., Duckworth, J. W., and Lance, J. W. (1978): Internal and external carotid vascular responses to vasoactive agents in the monkey. *Neurology,* 28:162–173.
52. Tindall, G. T., and Greenfield, J. C. (1973): The effects of intra-arterial histamine on blood flow in the internal and external carotid artery of man. *Stroke,* 4:46–49.
53. Toda, N. (1976): Regional differences in the response to nicotine in isolated canine arteries. *Eur. J. Pharmacol.,* 35:151–160.
54. Toda, N., and Fujita, Y. (1973): Responsiveness of isolated cerebral and peripheral arteries to serotonin, norepinephrine, and transmural electrical stimulation. *Circ. Res.,* 33:98–104.
55. Vanhoutte, P. M. (1978): Heterogeneity in vascular smooth muscle. In: *Microcirculation, Vol. II,* edited by G. Kaley and B. M. Altura., pp. 181–309. University Park Press, Baltimore.
56. Vidrio, H., and Hong, E. (1976): Vascular tone and reactivity to serotonin in the internal and external carotid vascular beds of the dog. *J. Pharmacol. Exp. Ther.,* 197:49–56.

Advances in Neurology, Vol. 33, edited by
M. Critchley et al. Raven Press, New York © 1982

Duration of the Biological Effect of Ergotamine Tartrate

Peer Tfelt-Hansen,* Jens H. Eickhoff, and Jes Olesen

*Department of Neurology, and *Laboratory of Surgical Circulation Research, Department D,
Rigshospitalet, Copenhagen, Denmark*

A considerable number of migraine patients abuse ergotamine (2,14). Dige-Petersen et al. (4) showed that patients who take ergotamine daily had decreased peripheral systolic blood pressure, i.e., subclinical ergotism. A study in which these patients were asked specifically for symptoms of ergotamine toxicity has shown that 50% experience such symptoms (7). To avoid a chronic vasoconstrictory state and still obtain maximal therapeutic effect, knowledge of the clinical pharmacology of ergotamine is needed. Because of the high specific activity of ergotamine and its chemical instability, it has been impossible until recently to measure ergotamine in blood; therefore, the clinical pharmacology of ergotamine is virtually unknown. The present study uses a biological response (the decrease in peripheral systolic blood pressure) to investigate the duration of action of ergotamine on human arteries.

PATIENTS AND METHODS

Patients

Migraine patients, defined according to the Ad Hoc Committee (1) and to Olesen (13), attending the Copenhagen Acute Headache Clinic (14) were asked to join the study. Five male and 22 females entered after their informed consent. Their average age was 47 years (range, 26 to 61 years). All had tried ergotamine several times before.

Procedure

In the first series, 17 patients were tested as follows. The patients rested for 30 min lightly dressed in a bed covered with a blanket. Blood pressure cuffs were placed around their upper left arms, proximal phalanges of their left first and third fingers, ankles, and big toes. Systolic blood pressures in these positions were measured with the strain gauge technique described by Nielsen et al. (12). Each systolic blood pressure reported in the following was determined as the average of five measurements. Skin temperatures of fingertips and big toes were measured with a thermocouple. Ergotamine tartrate (Gynergen®, Sandoz), 0.5 mg/70 kg, was injected in the right cubital vein in two divided doses with an interval of 5 min. Severe bradycardia was not observed. Systolic blood pressures and temperatures were measured after 15 and 30 min and 1, 2, 3 (and in 12 cases, 4) hr after the injection of ergotamine tartrate. During the total experimental period of 4 to 5 hr, blood cuffs and strain gauges were left untouched. Fifteen of 17 patients were measured again the next day after bed rest for 30 min. Eight patients were measured again from 2 weeks to 2 months later.

In a second series, 10 other migraine patients were measured with the same procedure before and 24, 48, and 72 hr after their normal therapeutic dose of ergotamine as suppositories. All used Gynergen Comp® (Sandoz) suppositories (content, 2 mg ergotamine tartrate, 100 mg caffeine, 100 mg butalbital, and 0.25 mg Bellafoline®). Eight patients took one, and two patients two, suppositories.

Calculation and Statistics

Peripheral systolic blood pressures were expressed as systolic gradients (toe to arm, ankle to arm, finger to arm). Each systolic gradient was calculated as the mean of five peripheral systolic blood pressures minus the mean of five simultaneous systolic arm blood pressures. Wilcoxon's test for paired data was used for statistical evaluation.

RESULTS

Intravenous Injection

Systolic arm blood pressure was significantly increased from 15 min to 2 hr compared with the preinjection value (Fig. 1). The increase was maximal at 15 min ($p < 0.05$).

All peripheral systolic gradients showed sustained decreases. The decrease in toe to arm systolic gradient is shown in Fig. 2. Similar but smaller decreases were found for finger and ankle to arm gradients. For all peripheral systolic gradients, the decreases were significant from 15 min to 22 hr ($p < 0.01$).

Finger and toe temperatures increased significantly after ergotamine. Skin temperatures

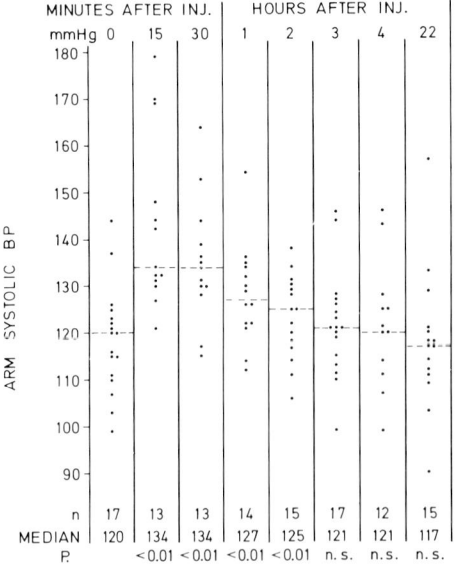

FIG. 1. Effect on arm systolic blood pressure of ergotamine tartrate (0.5 mg/70 kg i.v.) in 17 migraine patients (p given for Wilcoxon's test).

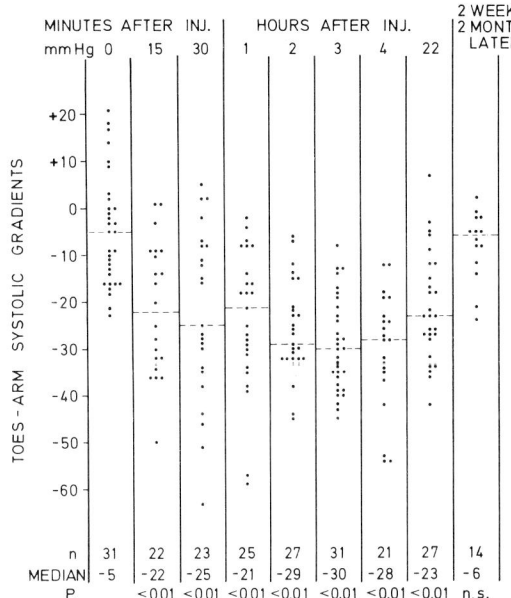

FIG. 2. Toe-arm systolic gradients (big toe minus arm systolic blood pressure) after intravenous injection of ergotamine tartrate (0.5 mg/70 kg) in 17 migraine patients (*p* given for Wilcoxon's test).

from toes are shown in Fig. 3. The increases were significant ($p < 0.05$) from 15 min and further on the same day.

Suppositories

Toe to arm systolic gradients had a median value of -13 mmHg before ergotamine. After 24 hr, the median value showed a significant decrease to -27 mmHg ($p < 0.01$). The values after 48 hr (median -16 mmHg) and 72 hr (-14 mmHg) were not significantly changed. Significant but smaller changes were found for ankles and fingers.

DISCUSSION

Pharmacological Effect of Ergotamine

Animal studies have shown that the direct vasoconstrictory effect of ergotamine on blood vessels is relatively shortlasting and reversible (15). This conclusion was based on the blood pressure elevating effect of ergotamine, presumably an effect on the resistance

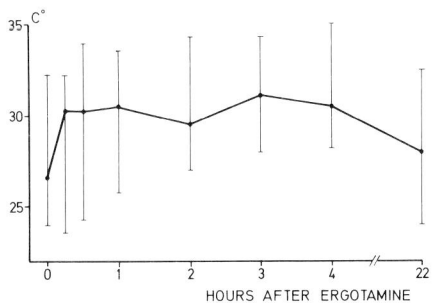

FIG. 3. Reaction of big toe skin temperature after intravenous injection of ergotamine tartrate (0.5 mg/70 kg) (median and range) in 17 migraine patients ($p < 0.05$ from 15 min to 4 hr; Wilcoxon's test).

vessels (arterioles). A relatively short-lasting (1 to 2 hr) increase in blood pressure has been observed in man during spinal anesthesia (5). The present study confirms that the pressor effect of ergotamine (increase of arm systolic blood pressure) is of short duration. In contrast, the effect of ergotamine on peripheral arteries was slow in onset and was well sustained for 24 hr. The discrepancy in the time effect curves for arm and peripheral systolic blood pressure strongly indicates two different mechanisms of action.

The rise in peripheral skin temperature after intravenous ergotamine was an unexpected finding. Fingertips are rich in arteriovenous anastomoses; the increase in finger and big toe skin temperatures must be due to opening of these shunts. Studies of migraine and cluster headache patients during attacks have shown increases of skin temperature (9) and doppler flow (8) in the headache region after ergotamine. In contrast, Spierings and Saxena (18) found a decreased arteriovenous shunt flow in the carotid bed of the cat after ergotamine. At present, we have no explanation for this discrepancy; it should be noted, however, that in all these studies, including this one, ergotamine was given systemically. Thus an effect of ergotamine on central centers for temperature regulation cannot be excluded.

Clinical Implications

The duration of the effect of ergotamine has been considered to be too short for prophylactic use in migraine (10). The present study shows the effect on arteries to be long lasting. Nevertheless, ergotamine should not be used in migraine prophylaxis for several reasons. Migraine patients taking ergotamine daily seem to develop increasing headache frequency and physical dependence with a withdrawal headache (3,16). These patients have subclinical ergotism (decreased peripheral systolic blood pressures) (4); when interviewed specifically, 50% had symptoms of ergotamine toxicity (7). In these studies, the daily dose of ergotamine tartrate was 2 mg or more. Even in patients taking smaller doses (0.9 mg daily) in combination preparations for gastrointestinal dysfunction, fulminant ergotism has been described as due to interaction with antibiotics (11). Thus ergotamine should not be used in migraine prophylaxis, at least until a study proving its efficacy has been conducted.

During the prodromes of classic migraine, cerebral blood flow is considerably decreased (17). In a group of patients with normal cerebral blood flow, intramuscular ergotamine caused no change in regional cerebral blood flow after 15 to 20 min (6). Considering the slow onset of the direct action of ergotamine on arteries demonstrated in the present study after intravenous injections, cerebral blood flow measurements were probably repeated when there was only a small, submaximal effect of ergotamine on arteries. If the arterial constriction observed in arms and legs in the present study are paralleled by the internal carotid artery, ergotamine may well exaggerate the prodromal ischemia. If the prodromes are short lasting, the risk is probably small; but if the prodromes last longer, the risk may be considerable. The problem needs further investigation; we recommend caution in the use of ergotamine on patients with long-lasting migraine prodromes and accompaniments.

ACKNOWLEDGMENT

This study was supported by a grant from the Danish Heart Foundation.

REFERENCES

1. Ad Hoc Committee (1962): Classification of headache of the NIH. *JAMA,* 197:717–718.
2. Ala-Hurula, V., Myllylä, V. V., Arvela, P., Kärki, N. T., and Hokkanen, E. (1979): Systemic availability of ergotamine tartrate after three successive doses and during continuous medication. *Eur. J. Clin. Pharmacol.,* 16:355–360.
3. Andersson, P. G. (1975): Ergotamine headache. *Headache,* 15:118–121.
4. Dige-Petersen, H., Lassen, N. A., Noer, I., Tønnesen, K. H., and Olesen, J. (1977): Subclinical ergotism. *Lancet,* II:65–66.
5. Dunér, H., Granath, A., and Klingenström, P. (1960): The effect of ergotamine on blood pressure and cardiac output during spinal anaesthesia in man. *Acta Anaesth. Scand.,* 4:5–11.
6. Hachinski, V., Norris, J. W., Edmeads, J., and Cooper, P. W. (1978): Ergotamine and cerebral blood flow. *Stroke,* 9:594–596.
7. Hokkanen, E., Waltimo, O., and Kallaranta, T. (1978): Toxic effects of ergotamine used for migraine. *Headache,* 18:95–98.
8. Kudrow, L. (1979). Thermographic and Doppler flow asymmetry in cluster headache. *Headache.* 19:204–208.
9. Lance, J. W., and Anthony, M. (1971): Thermographic studies in vascular headache. *Med. J. Aust.,* 1:240–243.
10. Lance, J. W. (1978): *Mechanism and Management of Headache,* third edition. Butterworths, London.
11. Lorrain, J. M. (1979): Antibiotiques: Interaction avec d'autres médicaments. *Nouv. Presse Med.,* 8:3653–3658.
12. Nielsen, P. E., Bell, G., and Lassen, N. A. (1972): The measurement of digital systolic blood pressure by strain gauge technique. *Scand. J. Clin. Lab. Invest.,* 29:371–379.
13. Olesen, J. (1978): Some clinical features of the acute migraine attack. An analysis of 750 patients. *Headache,* 18:268–271.
14. Olesen, J., Aebelholt, A., and Veilis, B. (1979): The Copenhagen Acute Headache Clinic: Organization, patient material and treatment results. *Headache,* 19:223–227.
15. Rothlin, E., and Cerletti, A. (1949): Untersuchungen über die Kreislaufwirkung des Ergotamins. *Helv. Physiol. Acta,* 7:333–370.
16. Rowsell, A. R., Neylan, C., and Wilkinson, M. (1973): Ergotamine induced headache in migrainous patients. *Headache,* 13:65–67.
17. Skinhøj, E., and Paulson, O. B. (1969): Regional blood flow in internal carotid distribution during migraine attack. *Br. Med. J.,* III:569–570.
18. Spierings, E. L. H., and Saxena, P. R. (1979): Effect of ergotamine on cranial arteriovenous shunting in experiments with constant flow perfusion. *Eur. J. Pharmacol.,* 56:31–37.

Advances in Neurology, Vol. 33, edited by
M. Critchley et al. Raven Press, New York © 1982

Agonists and Antagonists of 5-Hydroxytryptamine on Venomotor Receptors

W. H. Aellig

Experimental Therapeutics Department, Clinical Research Division, Sandoz Ltd., Basle, Switzerland

Since the beginning of scientific investigations on pathogenesis, pathophysiology, and therapy of migraine, 5-hydroxytryptamine (5-HT) and its antagonists have been the subject of many studies; despite the great progress of the last decade, however, much remains unknown. Apart from studies on 5-HT effects in different areas of the brain and on 5-HT receptors in blood platelets, studies on the vascular effects of 5-HT and its antagonists may contribute to an understanding of their actions in migraine. This chapter deals with the effects of 5-HT and 5-HT antagonists on human hand veins. Superficial hand veins are vessels that can be investigated *in vivo* with rather simple clinical pharmacological methods. These allow the study of direct drug actions and drug interactions after local infusion of low doses which do not affect the general circulation.

METHODS FOR STUDIES WITH 5-HT AND 5-HT ANTAGONISTS ON HUMAN HAND VEINS *IN VIVO*

Two main methods are currently used. One is the venoconstriction test described by Sicuteri et al. (13) and its computerized version (7). The general principle is to measure pressure in a dorsal vein of the hand or wrist before and after local infusion of a drug producing venospasm. With the subject in the supine position, a needle is inserted into a superficial hand vein. Pressure in this vein is recorded by means of a pressure transducer. Drugs are administered directly into the vein through the same needle. The effects of agonists leading to an increase in venous pressure are measured by determining the area under the pressure-time curve.

The second method relies on the measurement of venous diameter at a constant pressure. In its original version (12), the diameter of superficial hand veins is determined optically. The subject is resting in the supine position. An arm is placed on a rigid support sloping upward at an angle of 30°, thus allowing complete emptying of superficial hand veins. The summit of a suitable vein is marked with a cross. A stereomicroscope is focused on the mark and refocused 1 to 2 min after inflation to 45 mm Hg of a sphygmomanometer cuff placed on the upper arm. The difference between the two positions of the microscope is a measure of venous diameter under the congestion pressure applied.

A technique has been developed based on the same basic principle to determine compliance of superficial hand veins by measuring venous diameter at a standardized congestion, allowing the direct and continuous recording of venous diameter (3,4). With the aid of a small tripod, a linear variable differential transformer is placed directly on the back of the hand. Its position is adjusted so that a light metal core placed in the central hole of the transformer is situated over the summit of the vein under investigation. The central coil of the transformer is energized by an alternating current. The core placed over the summit of the vein alters the voltage generated in the outer coils; these changes are proportional to its displacement. The device allows a direct registration of venous diameter at a standardized congestion pressure. The main advantages of this technique compared to the optical one are (a) the possibility to record venous diameter directly, and (b) the measuring device is mounted on the back of the hand, thereby reducing the influence of hand swelling and hand movements on the actual measurement.

VENOCONSTRICTOR EFFECTS OF 5-HT

After direct local infusion into superficial hand veins, 5-HT produces a marked and dose-dependent venoconstrictor effect. In the venoconstriction test, this is revealed by an increase in venous pressure (7,13); in the methods measuring venous diameter at a constant pressure, it is shown by a reduction in diameter (4,9). In the venoconstriction test, a dose-dependent venoconstrictor effect of 5-HT is observed with bolus doses of 100 to 500 ng. The activity of 5-HT in this test is greater than that of norepinephrine and epinephrine, of which single doses of 300 to 900 and 500 to 1500 ng, respectively, are required to produce the same effect (7).

In the tests measuring venous compliance at a constant pressure, lower doses of 5-HT are required to establish dose-response curves. The effects of continuous infusion of 2 to 32 ng/min were studied using the optical method (9) as well as the method using a linear variable differential transformer (4). In these experiments, 5-HT was found to be about equipotent with norepinephrine and epinephrine (4,9). Evidence attributes the venoconstrictor effect of 5-HT on human veins to stimulation of 5-HT receptors (5,6).

EFFECTS OF 5-HT ANTAGONISTS

The general cardiovascular actions of 5-HT antagonists after systemic administration usually are very small. Using the venoconstriction test, no direct venoconstrictor effects have been observed after local infusion of antagonists, such as methysergide, pizotifen, and cyproheptadine (7). Two 5-HT antagonists, pizotifen and methysergide, have also been investigated using the optical method for measuring diameters of superficial hand veins at a constant pressure (1,2). Contrary to the results obtained with the venoconstriction test, a dose-dependent reduction of venous diameter was observed after local infusion of both drugs. These results would be in accordance with a partial agonist activity of pizotifen and methysergide of 5-HT receptors on these human veins. That a venoconstrictor effect of pizotifen and methysergide was observed with this method but not with the venoconstriction test can probably be explained by a greater sensitivity for small venoconstrictor effects of the test measuring venous compliance at a constant pressure. In the venoconstriction test, a marked venospasm is required to produce an increase in pressure. This is also apparent from the higher doses of 5-HT required in this test.

INTERACTIONS BETWEEN 5-HT AND 5-HT ANTAGONISTS

Inhibition of the Venoconstrictor Effects of 5-HT

In the venoconstriction test, such drugs as methysergide, pizotifen, cyproheptadine, LSD, and 1-methylergotamine antagonize the strong venoconstrictor effects of 5-HT (e.g., refs. 6,7,13,14). This effect also can be demonstrated with the method in which venous diameter is determined at a constant pressure. Using the linear variable differential transformer, 5-HT dose-response curves were obtained in five healthy volunteers before and after local infusion of 80 ng pizotifen. A parallel displacement of the 5-HT dose-response curves to the right was observed, typical for a competitive antagonism (5). Norepinephrine dose-response curves were not influenced by pizotifen. This specific effect of pizotifen on 5-HT but not on norepinephrine dose-response curves supports the existence of separate 5-HT receptors on human veins, as suggested by Del Bianco et al. (6).

Augmentation of the Venoconstrictor Effect of 5-HT

When low doses of methysergide, ergotamine, and LSD are administered locally, an augmentation of the venoconstrictor effect of 5-HT is observed using the venoconstriction test (10). The type of reaction (i.e., blockade or potentiation of the venoconstrictor effect of 5-HT) depends on the doses used: low doses increase the venoconstrictor effect of 5-HT, whereas higher doses produce a reduction. It was suggested that this augmentation of the effects of 5-HT rather than 5-HT blockade might be responsible for the beneficial effects of these drugs in the treatment of migraine.

Venoconstrictor Effect of Ergotamine

Low doses of ergotamine have been found to increase the venoconstrictor effect of 5-HT (10). Ergotamine also leads to a marked reduction of venous diameter at a constant pressure. This is observed after direct local infusion (1) but also after systemic intravenous administration of the drug (8). Based on experiments on spiral strips of dog's saphenous arteries, Müller-Schweinitzer (11) suggested that the vasoconstrictor effect of ergotamine is at least partly due to a stimulation of 5-HT receptors. This hypothesis was confirmed for the venoconstrictor effect of ergotamine in man (2): 80 ng ergotamine were administered to five healthy volunteers twice on separate occasions, once without pretreatment and once preceded by local infusion of 80 ng of the 5-HT antagonist pizotifen. Ergotamine alone produced a marked reduction (−36%) of venous diameter at a constant congestion pressure. Despite the fact that pizotifen alone also reduced venous diameter (−12%), the cumulative reduction in hand vein diameter when ergotamine was administered after pizotifen was smaller (−17%) than when ergotamine was given alone (−36%).

CONCLUSIONS

Experiments on superficial hand veins obtained with different experimental methods show a dose-dependent venoconstrictor effect of 5-HT. When the venoconstriction test, which relies on pressure increases due to venospasm, is used, this effect is greater than that of the same doses of norepinephrine or epinephrine. When changes in venous compliance are measured at a constant congestion pressure, the venoconstrictor effect of 5-HT is in the same order of magnitude as that of epinephrine and norepinephrine. As with 5-HT, a venoconstrictor effect can be demonstrated with 5-HT antagonists, such as methysergide and pizotifen, when venous pressure is kept constant; this suggests a partial agonist activity of these drugs. 5-HT antagonists inhibit the venoconstrictor effect of 5-HT at higher doses. This is a specific effect; for example, pizotifen shifts 5-HT dose-response curves to the right but does not influence the venoconstrictor effect of norepinephrine. In low doses, some 5-HT antagonists were found to potentiate the venoconstrictor action of 5-HT.

REFERENCES

1. Aellig, W. H. (1976): Influence of ergot compounds on compliance of superficial hand veins in man. *Postgrad. Med. J. [Suppl. 1]*, 52:21–23.
2. Aellig, W. H. (1978): Clinical-pharmacological experiments with pizotifen (Sanomigran®) on superficial hand veins in man. In: *Current Concepts in Migraine Research*, edited by R. Greene, pp. 53–62. Raven Press, New York.
3. Aellig, W. H. (1979): Use of a linear variable differential transformer to measure compliance of human hand veins in situ. *Br. J. Clin. Pharmacol.*, 8:395P (Abstr.).
4. Aellig, W. H. (1981): A new technique for recording compliance of human hand veins. *Br. J. Clin. Pharmacol.*, 11:237–243.
5. Aellig, W. H. (1982): Influence of pizotifen and ergotamine on the venoconstrictor effect of 5-hydroxytryptamine and noradrenaline in man. *Eur. J. Clin. Pharmacol. (in press).*
6. Del Bianco, P. L., Fanciullacci, M., Franchi, G., and Sicuteri, F. (1975): Human 5-hydroxytryptamine venomotor receptors. *Pharmacol. Res. Commun.*, 7:395–408.
7. Del Bianco, P. L., and Sicuteri, F. (1978): Computerized venospasm: A method for exploring the neurovascular junction in man. *J. Pharmacol. Methods*, 1:329–340.
8. Brooke, O. G., and Robinson, B. F. (1970): Effect of ergotamine and ergometrine on forearm venous compliance in man. *Br. Med. J.*, 1:139–142.
9. Collier, J. G., Nachev, C., and Robinson, B. F. (1972): Effect of catecholamines and other vasoactive substances on superficial hand veins in man. *Clin. Sci.*, 43:455–467.
10. Fanciullacci, M., Granchi, G., and Sicuteri, F. (1976): Ergotamine and methysergide as serotonin partial agonists in migraine. *Headache*, 16:226–231.
11. Müller-Schweinitzer, E. (1976): Evidence for stimulation of 5-HT receptors in canine saphenous arteries by ergotamine. *Naunyn Schmiedebergs Arch. Pharmacol.*, 295:41–44.
12. Nachev, C., Collier, J. G., and Robinson, B. F. (1971): Simplified method for measuring compliance of superficial veins. *Cardiovasc. Res.*, 5:147–156.
13. Sicuteri, F., Del Bianco, P. L., Fanciullacci, M., and Franchi, G. (1964): Il test della venocostrizione per la misura della sensibilità alla 5-idrossitriptamina ed alle catecolamine nell' uomo. *Boll. Soc. Ital. Biol. Sperim.*, 40:1148–1150.
14. Sicuteri, F., Fanciullacci, M., Del Bianco, P. L., and Franchi, G. (1964): Inibizione della venocostrizione da 5-idrossitriptamina da parte del metisergide (UML-491) e di·altri antiserotoninici. *Boll. Soc. Ital. Biol. Sperim.*, 40:1151–1152.

Advances in Neurology, Vol. 33, edited by
M. Critchley et al. Raven Press, New York © 1982

Some Aspects of the Dopaminergic Action of Ergot Derivatives and Their Role in the Treatment of Migraine

R. Horowski

Research Laboratories of Schering AG, Berlin (West) and Bergkamen, Federal Republic of Germany

The extensive studies performed since the beginning of this century on the effects of ergot derivatives on smooth muscles of blood vessels and the uterus have been the basis for important new concepts in pharmacology as well as for the development of new therapies. In contrast, the so-called central effects of these compounds have been neglected or disregarded as an expression of toxicity and have been investigated more extensively only during the last decade. In this short time, however, interesting new findings have been obtained, which already resulted in new therapeutic applications as well as in some reevaluation of previous notions in this field. Many different ergot derivatives have a high affinity not only for noradrenergic and serotoninergic but also for dopaminergic receptors within the central nervous system (CNS) and thereby influence profoundly many different physiological systems. In this chapter, we describe pharmacological, biochemical, electrophysiological, and hormonal aspects of the dopaminergic activity of ergot derivatives used in the prophylaxis and treatment of migraine and discuss hypotheses regarding the clinical relevance of these effects. Attention is focused on lisuride (Fig. 1) in view of the pronounced dopaminergic agonist activity of this compound and our involvement in the preclinical and clinical development of this drug.

PHARMACOLOGICAL ASPECTS

Based on neuroendocrine studies concerning the regulation of prolactin secretion, Hökfelt and Fuxe (13) first described a dopaminergic effect of ergot derivatives, such as ergocornine and bromocriptine, in 1972; this was later confirmed by biochemical and pharmacological data (4,22). Other ergot derivatives for which a central dopaminergic effect was claimed include α-ergocryptine, β-ergocryptine, and ergocristine (22), as well as ergometrine (33). In 1975 (19), we reported striking similarities between the effects of apomorphine and lisuride (also called lysenyl at this time), which we interpreted as an expression of dopaminergic activity. These results were extended by our group. For methysergide and d-LSD, two other ergot derivatives with proven activity in the prevention of migraine attacks, a central dopaminergic activity was described (16,20).

This work is dedicated to the memory of Michael Semonský, an eminent scientist in the field of ergot chemistry and pharmacology, who died in 1979.

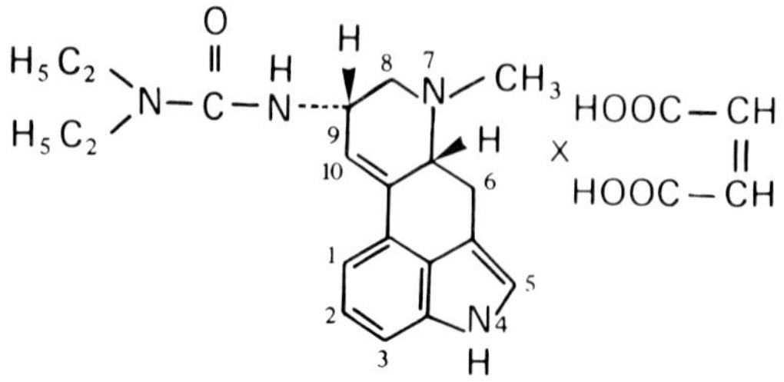

FIG. 1. Structural formula of lisuride.

Pharmacological effects of lisuride in rodents compatible with a high dopaminergic activity include (a) the induction of stereotyped behavior in both naive and reserpinized animals (20), (b) the induction of contralateral turning in rats with lesions of the nigro-neostriatal pathway, (c) a biphasic effect on motor activity, (d) reversal of reserpine-induced immobility, muscular rigidity, and hypothermia, (e) induction of hypothermia in rats maintained in a cold environment, and (f) the induction of hyperreactivity as well as aggressive and mounting behavior in rats maintained in groups (for review, see ref. 21). Other dopaminergic effects of lisuride include a hypotensive action in rats (27), an anorectogenic effect (1), and a potent emetic activity in dogs (20). In many of these tests, lisuride is among the most potent compounds in regard to dosage and total activity, indicating a high affinity for dopaminergic receptors. All these effects can be inhibited or at least impaired by dopamine antagonists, such as haloperidol, spiroperidol, or pimozide. These neuroleptics, however, are less potent antagonists to the effects of lisuride than, e.g., bromocriptine. This observation can be interpreted as an indication of a particularly high affinity of lisuride for dopaminergic receptors (14,15).

In contrast to bromocriptine, and even more to the dopamine-releasing drug D-amphetamine, the effects of lisuride are not inhibited or impaired by depletion of endogenous dopamine levels caused by reserpine and α-methyl-p-tyrosine (AMPT) pretreatment but may even be enhanced in reserpinized animals (1,20). An impressive potentiation of some dopaminergic effects of lisuride can be obtained by repeated treatment: in the case of motor activation in rats, more than a five-fold increase can be observed after 5 weeks of treatment (21). Since in the same animals other effects undergo tolerance development (hypothermic effects) or remain unchanged, and in view of the short plasma half-life of lisuride, this potentiation of activity is not a result of an accumulation of the drug within the body. Rather, changes at the receptor level caused by this drug or a prolonged binding at receptors due to high affinity may be the reason for this increased motor stimulatory effect after repeated administration (21).

BIOCHEMICAL EFFECTS

The high dopaminergic activity of lisuride, as described by us on the basis of pharmacological studies, has led to subsequent biochemical studies from this and other laboratories (24,28). The impairment of the accumulation of L-DOPA caused by pretreatment with the decarboxylase inhibitor NSD 1015, as well as the deceleration of AMPT-induced depletion of brain dopamine, are indirect evidence of stimulation of presynaptic dopaminergic receptors within the brain. In reserpinized rats, evidence for a high dopaminergic activity was obtained using biochemical methods (25). As with other ergot derivatives, unexpected results were found using the dopamine-dependent adenylate cyclase system as a biochemical tool; lisuride, at least at low concentrations *in vitro,* inhibited the effects of dopamine on this system instead of acting as an agonist (23). In contrast, inhibition of ^{3}H-spiroperidol binding showed unusually high competition of lisuride for these receptors, which was higher than that of haloperidol or apomorphine (7). On this basis, it was not surprising that ^{3}H-lisuride itself displays a high specific binding activity within the CNS, which could be displayed best by dopamine antagonists and agonists (8). This high affinity of lisuride for dopamine receptors may explain why lisuride apparently is concentrated four to five times above blood or brain levels within the pituitary (Oshino, *personal communication;* see Table 1).

HORMONAL EFFECTS OF LISURIDE

The concentration of lisuride within the pituitary supports our suggestion that lisuride exerts its prolactin-lowering effects by a direct action on dopaminergic receptors within the pituitary (9,10,16,17). Since lisuride acts on the prolactin cell itself, it can inhibit the secretion of prolactin, irrespective of the physiological situation of this system. Lisuride is highly effective under *in vitro* conditions (26) as well as on pituitaries grafted under the renal capsule of hypophysectomized rats (9,17); also, on parenteral as well as on oral administration, it is a potent inhibitor of both estrogen- and reserpine-induced hyperprolactinemia in rats (10) and inhibits prolactin-secretion in dogs, monkeys, and humans at very low doses (18).

That lisuride lowers prolactin levels at such low doses may reflect a high affinity of ergot derivatives for the dopaminergic system inhibiting prolactin release and correlates with the high concentrations of this compound observed within the pituitary. The high affinity of lisuride for these and other systems has not only resulted in new therapeutic applications for this compound but may become a tool for further investigations of these systems.

As a consequence of its potent prolactin-lowering effect, lisuride also influences prolactin-dependent biological systems. For example, in rats, it inhibits growth of normal breasts as well as of DMBA-induced mammary tumors; it also influences the ovaries (18).

TABLE 1. *Distribution of total radioactivity in rabbit brain 30 min after intravenous injection of 50 μg/kg ^{14}C-lisuride (5 μCi/kg)^a*

Tissue	ng/g, wet tissue
Whole brain	28.2 ± 1.3
Cerebral cortex	26.4 ± 0.8
Putamen	35.3 ± 1.7
Hippocampus	26.5 ± 0.7
Hypothalamus	29.5 ± 0.6
Pituitary	138.2 ± 3.2
Cerebellum	25.5 ± 1.8
Medulla oblongata + pons	21.2 ± 1.8
Plasma	34.9 ± 0.4 ng/ml

$^a N = 3$; x̄ ± SEM.

INFLUENCE OF LISURIDE ON OTHER MONOAMINERGIC SYSTEMS

In addition to its strong dopaminergic activity, lisuride influences other monoaminergic systems. After its synthesis in 1959 by Zikán and M. Semonský (34), lisuride was first developed as a peripheral serotonin antagonist. This similarity to methysergide and *d*-LSD has led to its clinical use as a migraine prophylactic (29). This peripheral antiserotonin effect, observed both *in vitro* and *in vivo,* contrasted with biochemical results from the CNS, where lisuride was described as an agonist of serotonin receptors (24). A central serotonin antagonism, however, was suggested by the observation that single doses of lisuride given to rats elicited stereotyped, long-lasting mounting behavior (Fig. 2), an effect which previously could be obtained only by treatment with an inhibitor of serotonin synthesis, *p*-chlorophenylalanine, combined with dopaminergic agonists (5,20). This apparent contradiction between pharmacological and biochemical results was resolved by the suggestion of Da Prada and his group (5) that lisuride has a preferential affinity for presynaptic serotonin receptors and, by activating these, functionally inhibits serotoninergic neurotransmission.

Electrophysiological studies, using systemic and local microiontophoretic application of lisuride, demonstrated not only a dopaminergic action at the level of the substantia nigra (30,32) but also an inhibition of the spontaneous firing of serotoninergic raphe neurons by very low doses of lisuride (30). With the same (30) and with other biochemical (24) and pharmacological methods, α-adrenolytic effects of high doses of lisuride could be demonstrated. On the basis of *in vitro* results, even a blockade of β-receptors has been reported after rather high concentrations of this compound (3). These data again

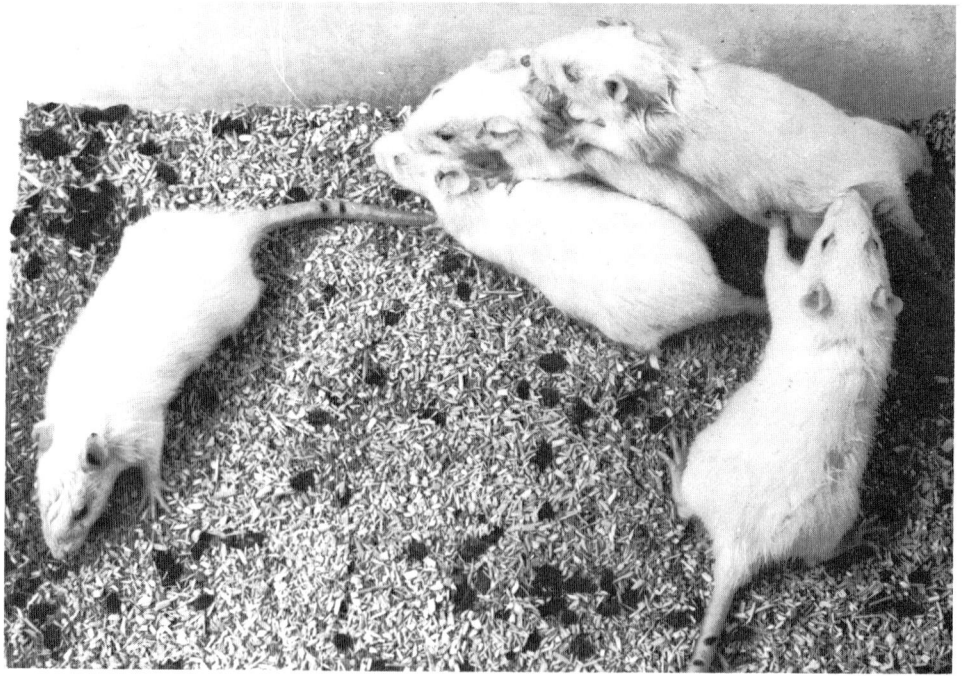

FIG. 2. Typical mounting behavior elicited by a single injection of lisuride (0.5 mg/kg s.c.) in juvenile female rats.

demonstrate that ergot derivatives, such as lisuride, may interact with different monoaminergic systems; only the interaction with dopamine and serotonin receptors, however, is of clinical importance in the case of lisuride.

DOPAMINERGIC EFFECTS OF OTHER ERGOT DERIVATIVES USED IN MIGRAINE

In view of the high sensitivity of the prolactin cells to dopaminergic ergot derivatives, we have found many ergot derivatives that were effective in our test system (see Fig. 3). Young female rats were pretreated with reserpine or primed with estradiol benzoate in order to have elevated prolactin levels, which could easily be lowered by many different dopaminergic compounds (17). Ergotamine is among the ergot derivatives effective under both conditions; this is an expression of dopaminergic activity. In the case of lisuride, methysergide, *d*-LSD, and bromocriptine, we described a prolactin-lowering effect as well as antireserpine activity as early as 1976 and proposed a dopaminergic mechanism for these drug effects (16).

We have extended these studies to include methergoline and bromocriptine, ergoline derivatives for which, as in the case of *d*-LSD, lisuride, and methysergide, a prophylactic effect on recurrent migraine headaches has been reported. We found indications for dopaminergic activity in all cases, even with considerable differences with respect to the intensity of this effect. Lisuride and to a lesser extent *d*-LSD resemble apomorphine, whereas bromocriptine has only slight antireserpine activity, and methergoline has no antireserpine effect. In contrast, a slight hypothermic effect of methergoline can be observed in rats maintained at 4°C; as in the case of bromocriptine (14), this can be reversed by low doses of sulpiride (Fig. 4). A prolactin-lowering effect is common to

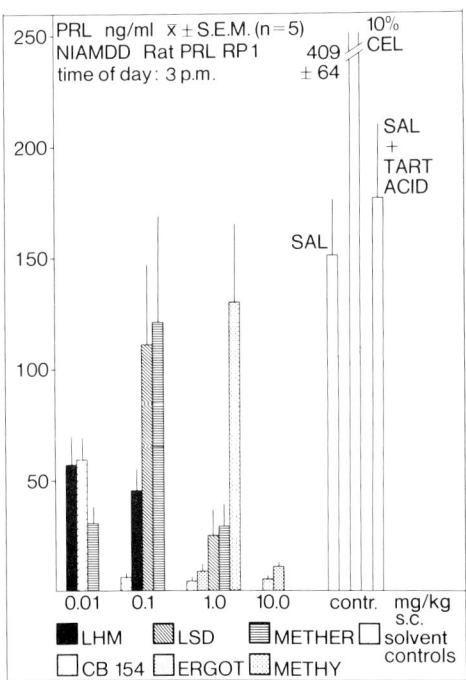

FIG. 3. Serum prolactin levels in rats pretreated with reserpine (2 mg/kg i.p. 30 hr before testing) and various ergot derivatives (6 hr before testing, s.c. injection) as compared with solvent controls. LHM, lisuride; CB 154, bromocriptine; ERGOT, ergotamine; METHER, methergoline; METHY, methysergide.

TABLE 2. *Dopaminergic profiles of ergot derivatives as compared with apomorphine*

Ergot derivative	Prolactin (rats)	Hypothermia at 4°C (rats)	Inhibition of hypothermia by sulpiride (rats)	Reserpine antagonism (mot. act.) (mice)	Stereotyped behavior (mice and rats)
Methergoline	++	(+)	++	−	−
Bromocriptine	++	++	++	(+)	−
d-LSD	++	+	(+)	++	(+)
Lisuride	+++	++	−	++	++
Apomorphine	++	++	−	++	+++

all these compounds, whose central dopaminergic profiles are summarized in Table 2. As can be seen, it is important to define the receptors and their location; the description of an ergot derivative as "dopaminergic" should be given only with a definition of the system tested. This applies also to the effect of ergot derivatives on other (e.g., serotoninergic and noradrenergic) systems and may be illustrated by the observation that several ergoline derivatives, including methysergide, methergoline, *d*-LSD, and lisuride, are all highly effective inhibitors of peripheral serotonin effects both *in vitro* and *in vivo* (29). In the CNS, however, they differ considerably, methergoline being a rather pure antagonist, while the other compounds behave more as agonists on pre- or postsynaptic receptors. We were able to inhibit lisuride-induced mounting behavior using 0.5 mg/kg *d*-LSD s.c., an effect that we interpret to be a reversal of the functional serotonin antagonism of lisuride by a strong direct postsynaptic agonist activity of *d*-LSD. Franchi and his co-authors *(this volume)* have shown that some of these compounds, including lisuride, potentiate serotonin vasoconstriction in a human vein constriction test at very low doses.

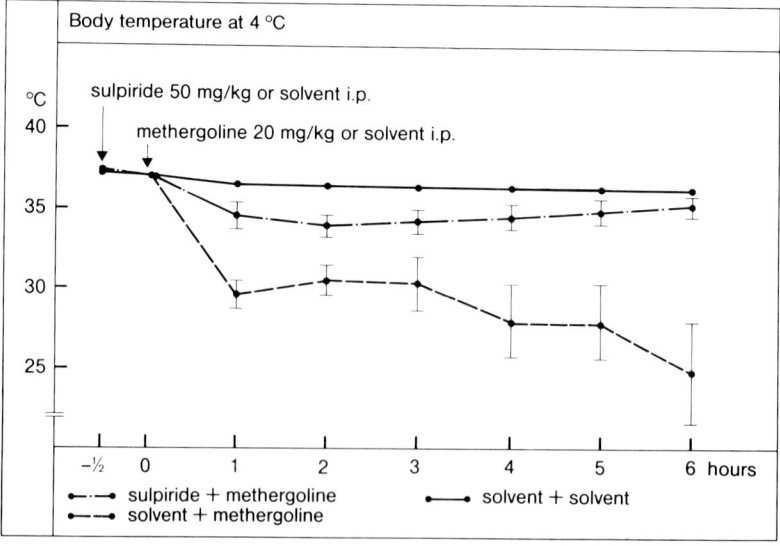

FIG. 4. Hypothermic action of methergoline in rats maintained at an environment of 4°C and influence of pretreatment with sulpiride.

CLINICAL SIGNIFICANCE OF DOPAMINERGIC EFFECTS OF ERGOT DERIVATIVES USED IN MIGRAINE

Compounds derived from ergot structures are still the most powerful drugs used in the prophylaxis and treatment of migraine. Ergotamine is highly effective in the treatment of acute attacks when given at the beginning of an attack; its therapeutic success may even be used as diagnostic evidence for the presence of a true migraine attack. Its use in therapy is limited only by the high incidence of side effects and its poor bioavailability.

Methysergide is still the most potent drug used in long-term preventive treatment of migraine; side effects, however, may be a limiting factor. In a double-blind multicenter study involving 246 patients with severe migraine treated for 3 months, we found no significant difference in efficacy between methysergide (3 × 2 mg/day) and lisuride (3 × 0.025 mg/day), whereas methysergide caused significantly more side effects, even leading to dropouts (11). Despite a surprisingly high placebo success rate, lisuride also proved to be significantly superior to placebo in two other double-blind studies involving 226 patients treated for 6 months, and 66 patients treated for 3 months (12,31). A prophylactic effect on recurrent headache has also been reported for other ergot derivatives, including methergoline, *d*-LSD, and bromocriptine, all of which produced symptoms of dopaminergic activity, including prolactin lowering.

When we first realized that methysergide, bromocriptine, and lisuride had dopaminergic and prolactin-lowering effects, we proposed the hypothesis—in agreement with Horrobin's suggestion of an involvement of prolactin in the pathogenesis of headache—that the migraine prophylactic effect of these compounds might be related to their dopaminergic activity, at least in cases of hormone-dependent migraine (16). Therefore, we compared the influence of pretreatment with low (3 × 0.025 mg/day) or intermediate (3 × 0.1 mg/day) doses of lisuride or placebo on the prolactin-lowering effect of a threshold dose of 0.1 mg lisuride in healthy female volunteers. Since basal prolactin levels cannot be lowered very much, we injected 25 mg sulpiride intramuscularly as a stimulus for prolactin secretion. With this test, maximal values of 160 ng/ml could be achieved 30 min after sulpiride injection in the placebo group. A single oral dose of 0.1 mg lisuride led to a slight reduction in this sulpiride-induced increase in prolactin, which could not be potentiated by a 14-day pretreatment with 3 × 0.025 mg/day lisuride. In contrast, repeated treatment with 3 × 0.1 mg/day lisuride further reduced serum prolactin levels after stimulation with sulpiride (Fig. 4).

From these results, we concluded that the dosage of lisuride used in the preventive treatment of migraine (3 × 0.025 mg/day) had no influence on basal or stimulated prolactin levels. Therefore, another mechanism of action must be involved in the prevention of headache attacks induced by lisuride (6). This interpretation, however, must be confirmed in migraine patients. Sicuteri and co-workers have shown that migraine sufferers may be significantly more sensitive to dopaminergic agonists, including apomorphine and bromocriptine, than normal volunteers (M. Fanciullacci et al., *this volume*). In agreement, low doses of lisuride have been reported to be effective in women with premenstrual breast tension and fertility disorders associated with migraine (O. Pospišil, *personal communication*).

Unfortunately, we know little about the role of the dopaminergic action of ergot derivatives used in headache therapy, and what we do know relates only to side effects and not clinical effectiveness of these drugs. It is well-known that nausea and emesis are associated with dopaminergic agonists and can be prevented by dopamine antagonists

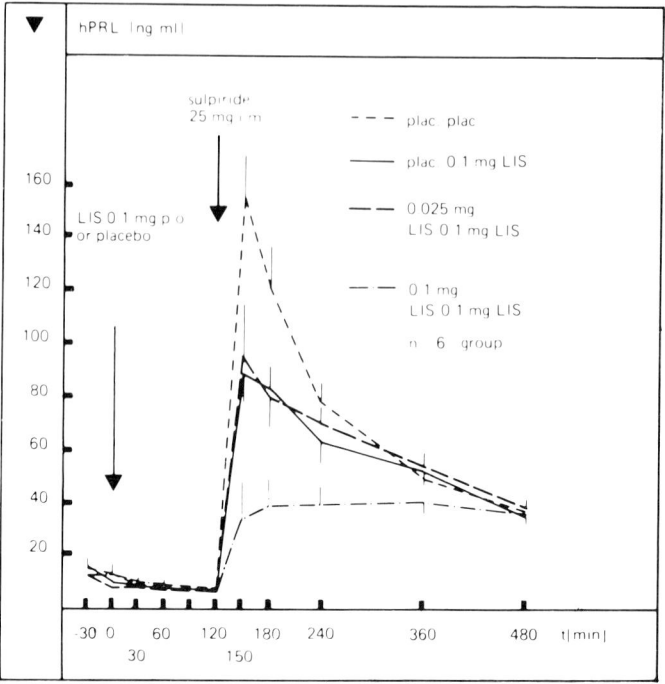

FIG. 5. Influence of treatment for 2 weeks with placebo, 0.025 mg lisuride (LIS) 3 ×/day, or 0.1 mg lisuride 3 ×/day on the acute effect of 0.1 mg lisuride on the sulpiride-induced hyperprolactinemia in healthy female volunteers.

(20). We have observed these effects frequently in patients treated with methysergide but also in some instances after treatment with lisuride (11). Since in healthy volunteers, or even more in women with hyperprolactinemia, higher doses of lisuride are necessary to cause nausea, this observation may be an indication for a higher sensitivity of migraineous subjects to dopaminergic effects.

Orthostatic hypotension and, in rare cases, headache associated with ergot therapy may be expressions of dopaminergic activity of these compounds. Also, symptoms of pituitary adenomas may disappear after treatment with high doses of dopaminergic ergot derivatives, an effect related to the reduction in tumor volume or even an antiproliferative effect caused by these agents (2). This volume reduction may induce important relief in headaches which are often associated with this type of tumor.

Other possibilities exist of how dopaminergic effects of ergot derivatives could influence pathophysiological events associated with a migraine attack. Obviously, the prominent CNS effects of drugs, such as lisuride, may interfere with central events, e.g., caused by a sudden disturbance in brain enkephalins related to pain perception. This may be the initial step in the headache attack where CNS symptoms are known to occur as prodromi. Dopaminergic effects of ergot drugs could also be involved in the vasoconstriction of carotid arteries or, especially, of arteriovenous anastomoses of the face, which have been associated with migraine symptoms by the studies of Heyck. Renal and mesenterial arteries are regulated in part by dopamine receptors, which can be activated by dopaminergic agonists. Finally, it has been proposed that ergot derivatives can inhibit platelet aggregation, an effect that could be mediated by monoaminergic receptors linked with adenylate cyclase on the thrombocytes, and thereby inhibit another phenomenon that seems to be related to migraine attacks.

At present all these possibilities are speculative, and more classification of etiology and pathophysiology of migraine attacks is needed before a conclusion can be drawn. Another more pragmatic approach includes developing and testing new ergot derivatives with more specific pharmacological profiles (e.g., specific dopamine agonist or serotonin antagonist profile versus partial agonists, or compounds that do not penetrate the brain). From these studies, more specific or tolerable therapies for migraine may emerge; thus our knowledge about this important and severe disease may be increased.

REFERENCES

1. Carruba, M. O., Ricciardi, S., Müller, E. E., and Mantegazza, P. (1980): Anorectic effect of lisuride and other ergot derivatives in the rat. *Eur. J. Pharmacol.,* 64:133–141.
2. Chiodini, P. G., Liuzzi, A., Verde, G., Cozzi, R., Silvestrini, F., Marsili, M. T., Horowski, R., Passerini, F., Luccarelli, G., and Borghi, P. G. (1980): Size reduction of a prolactin secreting adenoma during long-term treatment with the dopamine agonist lisuride. *Clin. Endocrinol.,* 12:47–51.
3. Cote, T., Munemura, M., and Kebabian, J. (1979): Lisuride hydrogen meleate: An ergoline with β-adrenergic antagonist activity. *Eur. J. Pharmacol.,* 59:303–306.
4. Corrodi, H., Fuxe, K., Hökfelt, T., Lidbrink, P., and Ungersted, U. (1973): Effect of ergot drugs on central catecholamine neurons: Evidence for a stimulation of central dopamine neurons. *J. Pharm. Pharmacol.,* 25:409.
5. Da Prada, M., Bonetti, E. P., and Keller, H. H. (1977): Induction of mounting behaviour in female and male rats by lisuride. *Neurosci. Lett.,* 6:349–353.
6. Dorow, R., Horowski, R., Lüsse, K. H., and Gräf, K.-J. (1980): Differences between acute and chronic effects of the potent dopaminergic agonist lisuride. *Sixth International Congress of Endocrinology, Melbourne.* Abstr. 873. Union Offset Co., Canberra.
7. Fujita, N., Saito, K., Yonehara, N., and Yoshida, H. (1978): Lisuride inhibits ³H-spiroperidol binding to membranes isolated from striatum. *Neuropharmacology,* 17(22):1,089–1,091.
8. Fujita, N., Saito, K., Yonehara, N., Watanabe, Y., and Yoshida, H. (1979): Binding of ³H-lisuride hydrogen maleate to striatal membranes of rat brain. *Life Sci.,* 25:969–974.
9. Gräf, K. J., Horowski, R., and El Etreby, M. F. (1977): Effect of prolactin inhibitory agents on the ectopic anterior pituitary and the mammary gland in rats. *Acta Endocrinol.,* 85:267–278.
10. Gräf, K. J., Neumann, F., and Horowski, R. (1976): Effect of the ergot derivative lisuride hydrogen maleate on serum prolactin concentrations in female rats. *Endocrinology,* 98:598–605.
11. Herrmann, W. M., Horowski, R., Dannehl, K., Kramer, U., and Lurati, K. (1977): Clinical effectiveness of lisuride hydrogen maleate: A double-blind trial versus methysergide. *Headache,* 17:54–60.
12. Herrmann, W. M., Kriśtof, M., and Sastre y Hernandes, M. (1978): Preventive treatment of migraine headache with a new isoergolenyl derivative. *J. Int. Med. Res.,* 6:476–482.
13. Hökfelt, T., and Fuxe, K. (1972): Effect of prolactin and ergot alkaloids on the tubero-infundibular dopamine (DA) neurons. *Neuroendocrinology,* 9:100–122.
14. Horowski, R. (1978): Differences in the dopaminergic effects of the ergot derivatives bromocriptine, lisuride, and d-LSD as compared with apomorphine. *Eur. J. Pharmacol.,* 51(2):157–166.
15. Horowski, R. (1979): Hypothermic action of lisuride in rats and differences to bromocriptine in the antagonistic effect of neuroleptics. *Naunyn Schmiedebergs Arch. Pharmacol.,* 306:147–151.
16. Horowski, R., von Berswordt-Wallrabe, R., and Gräf, K. J. (1976): Role of serotoninergic mechanisms in the regulation of prolactin secretion and possible mechanism of action of ergot-derivatives. In: *Cellular and Molecular Bases of Neuroendocrine Processes,* edited by E. Endröczi, pp. 183–195. Akadémiai Kiadó, Budapest.
17. Horowski, R., and Gräf, K. J. (1976): Influence of dopaminergic agonists and antagonists on serum prolactin concentration in the rat. *Neuroendocrinology,* 22:273–286.
18. Horowski, R., and Gräf, K. J. (1979): Neuroendocrine effects of neuropsychotropic drugs and their possible influence on toxic reactions in animals and man—The role of the dopamine-prolactin system. *Arch. Toxicol.* [*Suppl.*], 2:93–104.
19. Horowski, R., Neumann, F., and Gräf, K. J. (1975): Influence of apomorphine hydrochloride, dibutyryl-apomorphine, and lysenyl on plasma prolactin concentrations in the rat. *J. Pharm. Pharmacol.,* 27:532.
20. Horowski, R., and Wachtel, H. (1976): Direct dopaminergic action of lisuride hydrogen maleate, an ergot derivative, in mice. *Eur. J. Pharmacol.,* 36:373–383.

21. Horowski, R., and Wachtel, H. (1979): Pharmacological effects of lisuride in rodents mediated by dopaminergic receptors: Mechanism of action and influence of chronic treatment with lisuride. In: *Dopaminergic Ergot Derivatives and Motor Function,* edited by K. Fuxe and D. B. Calne, pp. 237–251. Pergamon Press, Oxford.
22. Johnson, A. M., Vigouret, J. M., and Loew, D. M. (1973): Central dopaminergic actions of ergotoxine alkaloids and some derivatives. *Experientia,* 29:763.
23. Kebabian, J. W., and Kebabian, P. R. (1978): Lergotrile and lisuride: In vivo dopaminergic agonists which do not stimulate the presynaptic dopamine autoreceptor. *Life Sci.,* 23(22):2,199–2,204.
24. Kehr, W. (1976): Effect of lisuride and other ergot derivatives on monoaminergic mechanisms in rat brain. *Eur. J. Pharmacol.,* 41:261–273.
25. Kehr, W., and Speckenbach, W. (1978): Effect of lisuride and LSD on monoamine synthesis after axotomy or reserpine treatment in rat brain. *Naunyn Schmiedebergs Arch. Pharmacol.,* 301:163–169.
26. MacLeod, R. M. (1977): Influence of dopamine, serotonin, and their antagonists on prolactin secretion. *Prog. Reprod. Biol.,* 2:54–68.
27. Mannesmann, G., Haberey, M., Müller, B., and Goedecke, H. (1979): Pharmacological characterization of the cardiovascular activity of lisuridhydrogenmaleate. *Naunyn Schmiedebergs Arch. Pharmacol.* [*Suppl.*] 308:72.
28. Pieri, L., Keller, H. H., Burkhard, W., and da Prada, M. (1978): Effects of lisuride and LSD on cerebral monoamine systems and hallucinosis. *Nature,* 272:278–280.
29. Podvalová, I., and Dlabać, A. (1972): Lysenyl, a new antiserotonin agent. *Res. Clin. Stud. Headache,* 3:325–334.
30. Rogawski, M. A., and Aghajanian, G. K. (1979): Response of central monoaminergic neurons to lisuride: Comparison with LSD. *Life Sci.,* 24:1,289–1,298.
31. Sommerville, B. W., and Herrmann, W. M. (1978): Migraine prophylaxis with lisuride hydrogen maleate— A double blind study of lisuride versus placebo. *Headache,* 18(1):75–79.
32. Walters, J. R., Baring, M. D., and Lakoski, J. M. (1978): Effects of dopamine agonists on dopaminergic unit activity. In: *Catecholamines: Basic and Clinical Frontiers, Vol. 1,* edited by E. Usdin, I. J. Kopin, and J. Barchas, pp. 637–639. Pergamon Press, New York.
33. Woodruff, G. N., Elkhawad, A. O., and Crossmann, A. R. (1974): Further evidence for the stimulation of rat brain dopamine receptors by ergometrine. *J. Pharm. Pharmacol.,* 26:455.
34. Zikán, V., and Semonský, M. (1960): Mutterkornalkaloide XVI. Einige N-/D-6-Methyl-isoergolenyl-8/-,N/D-6-Methylergolenyl-8-/- und N-/D-6-Methylergolin/I/-yl-8/N'-substituierte Harnstoffe. *Collect. Czech. Chem. Commun.,* 25:1,922.

Advances in Neurology, Vol. 33, edited by
M. Critchley et al. Raven Press, New York © 1982

Paradoxical Effects of Frequent
Analgesic Use

Lee Kudrow

California Medical Clinic, Encino, California 91436

One of the major characteristics of chronic pain syndromes is excessive yet ineffective use of analgesic medication. This phenomenon is consistently seen in the condition known as chronic scalp muscle contraction headache, or chronic tension headache. In questioning why a patient with constant pain would persistently use analgesics despite their apparent lack of effect, we examined the natural course of chronic scalp muscle contraction headaches in regard to analgesic use. We found that early in the course of this syndrome, headaches were not constant, as in the "mature" state. They generally began as occasional headaches, ultimately becoming constant. In fact, we were able to discern three stages, which, for descriptive purposes, we categorized as acute, subacute, and chronic.

Acute scalp muscle contraction headache is characterized as a dull, nonthrobbing, generalized headache occurring infrequently, having a duration of 2 to 4 hr; it is not generally associated with nausea, vomiting, photophobia, or sonophobia. Trigger factors include acutely stressful situations, boredom, frustration, "eyestrain," and positional strain. Patients with this type of headache rarely seek medical consultation and successfully self-treat each attack either by discontinuance of the trigger activity, rest, or the use of simple analgesics. This type of headache appears in nonmigraineurs, in contrast to the subacute or chronic conditions (Table 1).

In subacute scalp muscle contraction headache, the frequency of attacks is increased, occurring 2 to 4 times per week, each lasting 6 hr or more. The headache is generally a secondary finding in patients seeking medical consultation for separately occurring migraine headaches. This type often becomes chronic (Table 1).

Chronic scalp muscle contraction headache is the second most common disorder seen at our headache clinic. It generally occurs in migraineurs and may be the major component of posttraumatic headache. It is described as a dull, waxing and waning, constant frontooccipital pain. It is characterized as nonthrobbing and not generally associated with nausea or vomiting. Depression, neuroticism, and analgesic abuse are features commonly associated with this disorder. Amitriptyline, as independently reported by Lance and Curran (9), Diamond and Baltes (2), and Kudrow (7), is the prophylactic drug of choice (Table 1).

In acute scalp muscle contraction headache, analgesic use is limited to the occasional headache episode and is generally effective. In subacute scalp muscle contraction headache, patients often extend analgesic use to headache-free intervals in anticipation of expected headaches. It is at this point (increased frequency of analgesic use) that such

TABLE 1. *Characteristics of scalp muscle contraction headache*

Features	Scalp muscle contraction headache		
	Acute[a]	Subacute[b]	Chronic
Frequency	Occasional	2–4/Wk	Daily
Duration	Hours	1 Day	Constant
Intensity	Dull	Dull	Dull
Location	General	Front-occ	Front-occ
Laterality	Bilateral	Bilateral	Bilateral
Associated symptoms	None	None	None
Migraine status	Negative	Positive	Positive
Analgesic use	Occasional	Often	Excessive
Response to			
Analgesics	Excellent	Fair	Poor
Amitriptyline	—	Excellent	Good

[a] Data obtained from general medical population.
[b] Data obtained from headache clinic population.

treatment becomes less effective. In the chronic type, analgesics are habitually and extensively used, despite the apparent lack of effectiveness (Table 1).

Thus with each successive stage of scalp muscle contraction headaches, increased analgesic use is associated with increased headache frequency. There appears to be an inverse relationship between the frequency of analgesic use and its effectiveness.

The present study addresses itself to several questions: (a) Is analgesic abuse causal or secondary to increased headache frequency? (b) Could analgesic abuse interfere with the expected beneficial effects of tricyclic antidepressants? (c) If causal, what is the mechanism by which persistent analgesic use sustains the headache state? Using chronic scalp muscle contraction headache as the pain model, we evaluated changes in headache frequency with respect to analgesic use and analgesic restriction in amitriptyline-treated and nontreated patients.

PATIENTS AND METHODS

More than 200 patients with chronic scalp muscle contraction headache were admitted to the study. All subjects kept records of headache frequency and analgesic use for a 1-month period prior to the study period. Patients unable to complete the pretrial period were replaced by others to maintain a starting population of 200.

Subjects were randomly divided into two groups and four subgroups. Thus 100 patients in group 1 received amitriptyline medication (25 mg/day for 1 week and 50 mg/day thereafter); 100 patients in group 2 received no amitriptyline medication. In each group, half of the subjects were permitted to continue analgesics without restriction, while the other half was instructed to discontinue analgesic medication. Clinic visits were scheduled weekly during the 4-week study period.

A mean headache index (HI) and a headache index ratio (HIR) were calculated for each group and subgroup. HI is the product of weekly headache frequency and graded pain severity. Dull and moderate intensities were rated as 1 and 2, respectively. The

TABLE 2. *Analgesics used by 200 patients with chronic scalp muscle contraction headache[a]*

Analgesics		Patient distribution	
Class	Generic	N	%
Antipyretics solely (single or combination)	Aspirin, acetaminophen, or phenacetin	56	28.0
Plus sedative, tranquilizer, or muscle relaxant	Barbiturate, meprobamate, orphenadrine, etc.	76	38.0
Plus narcotic	Codeine oxycodone	63	31.5
Plus narcotic-antagonist	Propoxyphene, pentazocine	48	24.0
Others		37	18.5

[a] Based on 1-month prestudy record.

HIR was obtained by dividing the posttreatment by the pretreatment HI. The percent improvement was calculated by subtracting HIR from 1 and multiplying the remainder by 100.

RESULTS

Pretrial Period

One month pretrial records showed that all patients used one or more types of analgesics daily. The greatest number of patients, 76 (38%), used analgesics combined with sedatives, tranquilizers, or muscle relaxants; 63 (31.5%) used analgesic-narcotic combinations; 56 (28%) used mixed or single antipyretic analgesic compounds; and 48 (24%) chronically used narcotic antagonists, such as propoxyphene or pentazocine. The remainder used analgesics combined with agents to reduce side effects, such as buffering agents or anticholinergics (Table 2). Almost two-thirds of the patients used only one type of analgesic, while the rest used two or three types daily. The average daily consumption of analgesics, per patient, was 6.2 pills (Table 3).

TABLE 3. *Distribution of multiple analgesic use*

No. of agents	Patients	
	N	%
One	128	64
Two	64	32
Three	8	4

Mean number of pills per day, per patient, 6.2.

TABLE 4. *Mean age and sex ratios of study patients by group and subgroup*

Groups and subgroups	N	Mean age	F:M ratio
Group 1			
Amitriptyline treated	100	40	5.0:1
+ Analgesics	50	38	5.3:1
− Analgesics	50	43	4.7:1
Group 2			
Amitriptyline withheld	100	36	5.4:1
+ Analgesics	50	37	5.3:1
− Analgesics	50	35	5.5:1
Mean or total	200	38	5.2:1

Trial Period

Two hundred patients were admitted to the study phase. Their mean age was 38 years, and the predominant sex was female (5.2:1). There was no significant difference in mean age or sex ratio between groups or subgroups (Table 4).

Dropouts

In the amitriptyline-treated group, the dropout rate was exceptionally low in those patients permitted to use analgesics (8%). This contrasted dramatically to the analgesic-restricted subgroup, in which 48% of the patients dropped out. The major dropout period occurred by the end of the first week. This distribution was similar in group 2. Thus the dropout rates among analgesic-users and nonusers were 6.0 and 62% respectively. Of the total 200 patients, 62 (29%) could not complete the 4-week study. Dropout or disqualification generally occurred by the first week, the major reason being inability to discontinue analgesics (Table 5). There was little difference in amounts of analgesics used between dropout patients and those who remained in the study.

TABLE 5. *Dropout rates of study patients by groups and subgroups*

Groups	Initial no.	No. patients remaining (wk)			Dropouts	
		1	2	4	N	%
Amitriptyline treated						
+ Analgesics	50	49	48	46	4	8.0
− Analgesics	50	28	27	26	24[a]	48.0
Amitriptyline withheld						
+ Analgesics	50	49	48	47	3	6.0
− Analgesics	50	22	20	19	31[a]	62.0
Total	200	148	143	138	62	29.0

[a] Disqualified, mainly due to inability to stop analgesics.

TABLE 6. *Mean headache index and headache index ratios after 2nd and 4th weeks of study*

Groups and subgroups	Initial Mean HI[a]	2nd Week		4th Week		Improvement %
		Mean		Mean		
		HI	HIR[b]	HI	HIR	
Amitriptyline treated	7.08	4.81	0.69	3.80	0.55	45[c]
+ Analgesics	6.92	5.12	0.74	4.81	0.70	30
− Analgesics	7.24	4.26	0.59	2.02	0.28	72[d]
Amitriptyline withheld	7.04	5.91	0.83	5.30	0.75	25
+ Analgesics	7.12	6.36	0.89	5.83	0.82	18
− Analgesics	6.96	4.82	0.69	3.98	0.57	43[c]

[a] HI, headache index; [b] HIR, headache index ratio.
[c] $p < 0.05$; [d] $p < 0.001$.

Improvement

At the end of 4 weeks, in group 1 (amitriptyline-treated), mean improvement was 30% in the analgesic-using subgroup, in contrast to 72% in the analgesic-restricted subgroup ($p < 0.001$). In subgroup 2 (nonamitriptyline-treated), the corresponding figures were 18 and 43%, the latter barely reaching significance ($p < 0.05$). Overall, group 1 patients scored significantly better than patients in group 2 (45%, $p < 0.05$) (Table 6).

Comparing analgesic-using to analgesic-restricted subgroups of both groups combined, we found significant improvement in only the nonanalgesic-using patients (60%; $p < 0.01$) (Table 7).

DISCUSSION

Analgesic Abuse as a Cause or Result of Increased Headache Frequency

As shown in our pretrial period, daily headaches continued to occur despite or because of frequent analgesic use. Indeed, when patients were asked why they had continued to use analgesics in view of their apparent lack of effect, some replied that when the effects of analgesics wore off, the pain became more intense and required additional medication. Most stated that analgesics offered only temporary reduction of pain, and although relief was incomplete, any reduction was welcome.

TABLE 7. *Improvement by subgroup at the end of 4 weeks*

Subgroup	N	End of 4 weeks		
		HI[a]	HIR[b]	Improvement (%)
+ Analgesics	93	5.33	0.76	24
− Analgesics	45	2.85	0.40	60[c]

[a] HI, headache index; [b] HIR, headache index ratio. [c] $p < 0.01$.

Almost all patients admitted that in earlier years, occasional use of "pain pills" was effective but had gradually become ineffective with increased use or increased headaches.

In this study population, the high dropout rate ($< 50\%$) among analgesic-restricted patients, refractoriness to and increased requirement of analgesics and rebound phenomena represent habituation, tolerance, and possible suppression of antinociceptive function. If frequent analgesic use can suppress antinociceptive function and increase headaches, then discontinuance of the medication should be expected to restore proper antinociceptive mechanisms and result in diminished headache frequency. This appeared to have been the case in our study patients; analgesic-restricted patients scored significantly better than analgesic-users, independent of amitriptyline treatment. Such improvement had not occurred, however, as early as 2 weeks, suggesting that restoration of antinociceptive mechanisms may require an analgesic washout period of 2 weeks or longer.

Analgesic Abuse as an Inhibitor of Effectiveness of Amitriptyline Therapy

In the amitriptyline group (group 1), no improvement occurred in either subgroup by the end of 2 weeks, probably because of the well-recognized response latency period of amitriptyline therapy. By the fourth week, however, analgesic-restricted patients scored significantly improved, in contrast to analgesic users treated with amitriptyline. This suggests that analgesics may have interfered with responsiveness to amitriptyline.

Possible Mechanisms of a Paradoxical Effect of Frequent Analgesic Use in Chronic Pain

As noted earlier, most patients with chronic scalp muscle contraction headaches had migraine attacks, which occurred with varying frequencies from as much as two to three per month to as little as two to three per year. Other data, such as sex distribution and family history of migraine, further suggest an association of chronic scalp muscle contraction headache to migraine. The expression of this type of headache may require several components, of which the genetically determined migraine diathesis is one. This association supports the central unitary concept of idiopathic headache (IH), as proposed by Sicuteri (11). The concept of a central etiology in migraine is strengthened by amine hypersensitivity studies, as reported by this group (3,4,12–14). Peripheral changes, such as cranial vasodilatation and increased cerebral blood flow, have been shown to occur during the migraine attack (10), but a cause-and-effect relationship between these vascular changes and pain remains unlikely. Indeed, profound temporal artery dilatation secondary to internal carotid artery obstruction is generally painless (5). There is also little support for a peripheral pain mechanism in chronic scalp muscle contraction headache (1,6,8). This latter concept was based on earlier reports, which indicated that the pain of chronic scalp muscle contraction headache was caused by sustained muscle contraction (15).

Conceptualization of chronic scalp muscle contraction headache as a central disorder is necessary in order to explain the paradoxical role of analgesic abuse. It is also necessary to recognize that nonnarcotic analgesics have central effects, despite their pharmacological designation as peripherally acting. In fact, direct analgesic and antipyretic effects on the central nervous system have been established for salicylates, acetaminophen, and phenacetin; in toxic doses, the major side effects of analgesics are central.

The results of the present study have demonstrated that excessive use of nonnarcotic analgesics was associated with habituation, tolerance, and rebound pain upon withdrawal.

Furthermore, following a withdrawal or washout period of at least 2 weeks, a significant decrease in headache frequency occurred.

These characteristics are analogous to those of narcotic abuse and withdrawal and strongly suggest shared mechanisms. Thus it is postulated here that nonnarcotic analgesics act on a similar antinociceptive system and may, with persistent use, suppress its function.

Our results suggest that frequent use of nonnarcotic analgesics may paradoxically sustain chronic pain and interfere with the therapeutic effects of tricyclic antidepressants by their suppression of central serotonergic pathways concerned with regulation of dull pain. It may involve a system analogous to, but separate from, the endorphin system—one concerned with lower pain intensities. Our results indicate that in cases of chronic scalp muscle contraction headache, and possibly other chronic pain disorders, analgesics should be discontinued for a period of 2 weeks before instituting other forms of treatment.

REFERENCES

1. Bakai, D. A. (1975): Headache: A biophysiological perspective. *Psychol. Bull.,* 82:369–382.
2. Diamond, S., and Baltes, B. J. (1971): Chronic tension headache treated with amitriptyline—a double blind study. *Headache,* 11:110–116.
3. Fanciullacci, M., Franchi, G., and Sicuteri, F. (1974): Hypersensitivity to lysergic acid diethylamide (LSD-25) and psilocybin in essential headache. *Experimentia,* 30:1,441–1,442.
4. Fanciullacci, M. (1979): Iris adrenergic impairment in idiopathic headache. *Headache,* 19:8–13.
5. Fisher, C. M. (1970): Facial pulses in internal carotid artery occlusion. *Neurology,* 20:476–478.
6. Harper, R. G., and Steger, J. C. (1978): Psychological correlates of frontalis EMG and pain in tension headache. *Headache,* 18:215–218.
7. Kudrow, L. (1976): Tension headache (scalp muscle contraction headache). In: *Pathogenesis and Treatment of Headache,* edited by O. Appenzeller, pp. 81–91. Spectrum, New York.
8. Lader, M. H., and Mathews, A. M. (1971): Electromyographic studies of tension. *J. Psychiatr. Res.,* 15:479–486.
9. Lance, J. W., and Curran, D. A. (1964): Treatment of chronic tension headache. *Lancet,* 1:1,236–1,239.
10. Sakai, F., and Meyer, J. S. (1978): Regional hemodynamics during migraine and cluster headaches measured by the ^{133}Xe inhalation method. *Headache,* 18:122–132.
11. Sicuteri, F. (1972): Headache as possible expression of deficiency of brain 5-hydroxytryptamine (central denervation supersensitivity). *Headache,* 12:69–72.
12. Sicuteri, F., Anselmi, B., and Del Bianco, P. L. (1973): 5-Hydroxytryptamine supersensitivity as a new theory of headache and central pain: A clinical pharmacological approach with *p*-chlorophenylalanine. *Psychopharmacology (Berlin),* 29:347.
13. Sicuteri, F. (1977): Headache as metonymy of non-organic central pain. In: *Headache New Vistas,* edited by F. Sicuteri, pp. 19–67. Biomedical Press, Florence, Italy.
14. Sicuteri, F., Fanciullacci, M., and Del Bene, E. (1977): Dopaminergic system and migraine. In: *Headache New Vistas,* edited by F. Sicuteri, pp. 229–238. Biomedical Press, Florence, Italy.
15. Simons, D. J., Day, E., Goodell, H., and Wolff, H. G. (1943): Experimental studies on headache: Muscles of the scalp and neck as sources of pain. *Assoc. Res. Nerv. Dis. Proc.,* 23:228–244.

Advances in Neurology, Vol. 33, edited by
M. Critchley et al. Raven Press, New York © 1982

Effects on Arterial Receptors of Ergot Derivatives Used in Migraine

E. Müller-Schweinitzer and *A. Fanchamps

*Preclinical Research and *Medical Counsel, Pharmaceutical Division, Sandoz Ltd.,
Basel, Switzerland*

The termination of migraine attacks by ergotamine, a well-established and time-honored therapy, was discovered in 1925 on the basis of the following two assumptions (18): (a) the migraine attack is caused by a vasospasm of sympathicotonic origin; and (b) because of its inhibiting effect on the sympathetic nervous system, ergotamine can prevent or abort such a vasospasm.

In light of further experience, however, both assumptions were found to be incorrect. Migraine is generally not accompanied by a state of hypersympathicotonia and cannot be precipitated by sympathomimetic drugs. The pain phase, with the characteristic nausea and vomiting, has rather vagotonic features. Even the intracranial vasoconstriction of the prodromal phase does not appear to be mediated by sympathetic impulses. In the therapeutic doses used in man, ergotamine is not a potent sympathetic inhibitor. Its antiadrenergic effect on blood vessels is overshadowed by an intrinsic vasoconstrictor action.

As was conclusively demonstrated in the 1930s by Wolff and Graham (5,24), migraine pain is associated with a vasodilation and increased pulsation (indicating passive distension) of an extracranial artery, usually the temporal. Ergotamine terminates the headache by constricting these cranial arteries and thus reducing the amplitude of their pulsations. Norepinephrine (NE) is effective in a similar manner.

When administered to abort a migraine attack, ergotamine acts chiefly by producing a nearly selective vasoconstriction of the hypotonic extracranial arteries. The same is true for dihydroergotamine; however, being a less potent vasoconstrictor, it must be applied in higher doses.

The mechanism of this action remained obscure until the late 1960s, when Salzmann, Weidmann, and Taeschler (19,23) found that, far from consistently antagonizing epinephrine and NE, ergotamine often potentiates the effects of these catecholamines, e.g., the contraction of the cat's nictitating membrane (19,23) or the hypertensive response of the spinal cat (23) (Fig. 1). This suggested that ergotamine acts on the α-adrenoceptors not only as an antagonist but also as a partial agonist, a combination of properties known as "dualism" (17). *In vitro* experiments by Müller-Schweinitzer and Stürmer (8,14,15) on spiral strips of canine veins and trials performed by Aellig (1,2) on superficial hand veins of human volunteers produced further evidence for this assumption. Both ergotamine and dihydroergotamine were found to inhibit competitively the venoconstric-

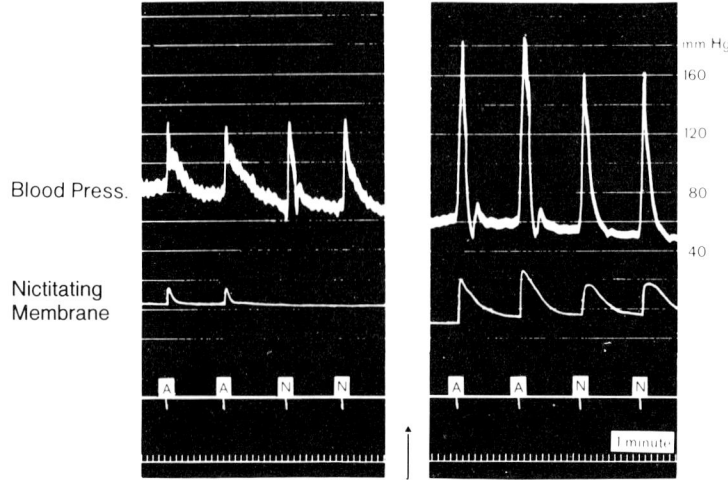

5 µg/kg Ergotamine i.v.
A 2µg/kg Adrenaline N 2µg/kg Noradrenaline i.v.

FIG. 1. Ergotamine potentiates the effects of epinephrine (adrenaline) (A) and noradrenaline (norepinephrine) (N) on blood pressure and contractions of the nictitating membrane in the spinal cat. **Left:** before; **right:** after intravenous ergotamine. (From ref. 23, with permission.)

tor effect of NE while producing a dose-dependent venoconstriction that could be inhibited competitively by an α-blocker, such as phentolamine.

These congruent observations suggested that the vasoconstrictor effect of ergotamine and dihydroergotamine was due to a stimulation of α-adrenoceptors. Arteries, however, do not necessarily react like veins. Furthermore, recent trials on spiral strips from canine, bovine, and human arteries have shown that arteries from the head do not respond to physiologic mediators in the same way as peripheral arteries.

Figure 2 shows dose-response curves for NE, serotonin (5-HT), and ergotamine on canine arteries (16). The limb artery shows a stronger response to NE, whereas the external carotid and especially the basilar, an intracranial artery, exhibit a stronger reaction to 5-HT. Ergotamine is active in much lower concentrations, which points to a high affinity for the receptors, but induces weaker contractions as compared with NE or 5-HT.

In isolated human arteries (Fig. 3), the contractions produced by NE and 5-HT reach the same maximum intensity in both peripheral and intracranial arteries, whereas on the temporal artery, NE produces stronger contractions than does 5-HT. Again, ergotamine is effective in low concentrations but does not produce as strong contractions as the two biogenic amines (16).

The vasoconstrictor effects of 5-HT and NE are additive (Fig. 4). 5-HT alone produces a concentration-dependent constriction, as indicated by the elevated baselines; if NE is applied 30 min later, its constricting action is additive to the 5-HT effect, which suggests that the two substances act on different receptors (16). A differing distribution of these receptors between the various vascular beds might account for the differing sensitivity of the respective vessels to 5-HT and NE.

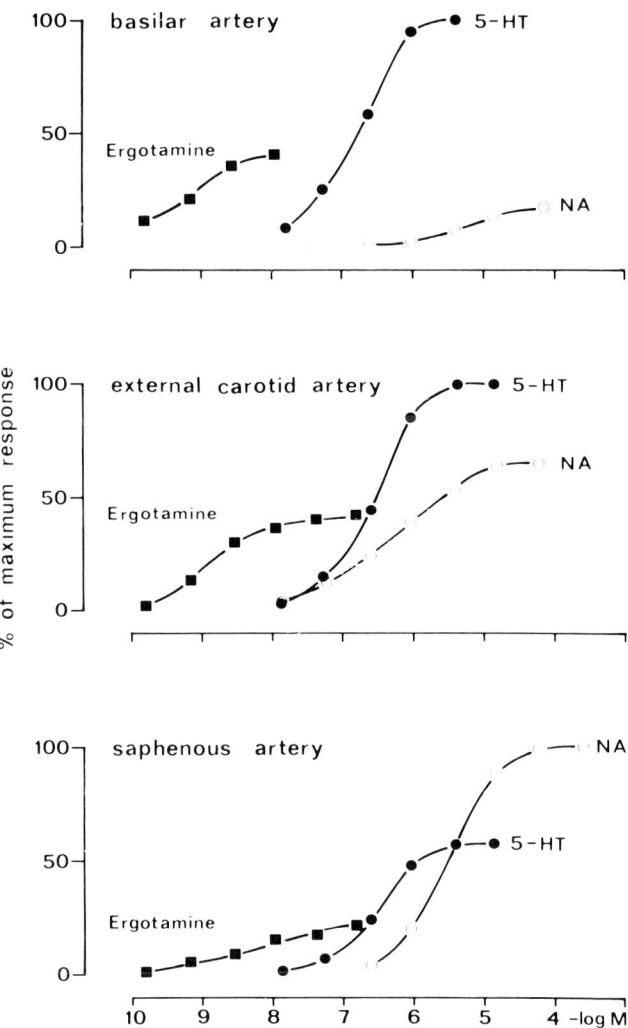

FIG. 2. Dose-response curves for norepinephrine (noradrenaline) (NA), 5-HT, and ergotamine on helical strips from canine arteries. *Ordinate,* intensity of isometric contraction in percent of maximum response; *abscissa,* neg. log of molar concentration (6 means, for example, conc. 10^{-6} or 1:1 million; concentrations thus increase from left to right). Each point represents the mean of six to 10 assays. (From ref. 16, with permission.)

Figure 5 shows the effect of 5-HT on canine arteries, expressed in percent of maximum effect of NE (9). 5-HT produces only 60% of the NE effect on a peripheral artery but 160% on the external carotid and 540% on the basilar artery. The same order of sensitivity is found with ergotamine, although the maximal contractions are weaker: 20, 50, and 210%, respectively, of the NE effect (Fig. 6).

If the effects of ergotamine are expressed in percent of maximum effect of 5-HT (Fig. 7), the curves obtained with the three arteries are nearly interchangeable, suggesting that ergotamine acts on the same receptors as 5-HT (9). Ergotamine, however, has a

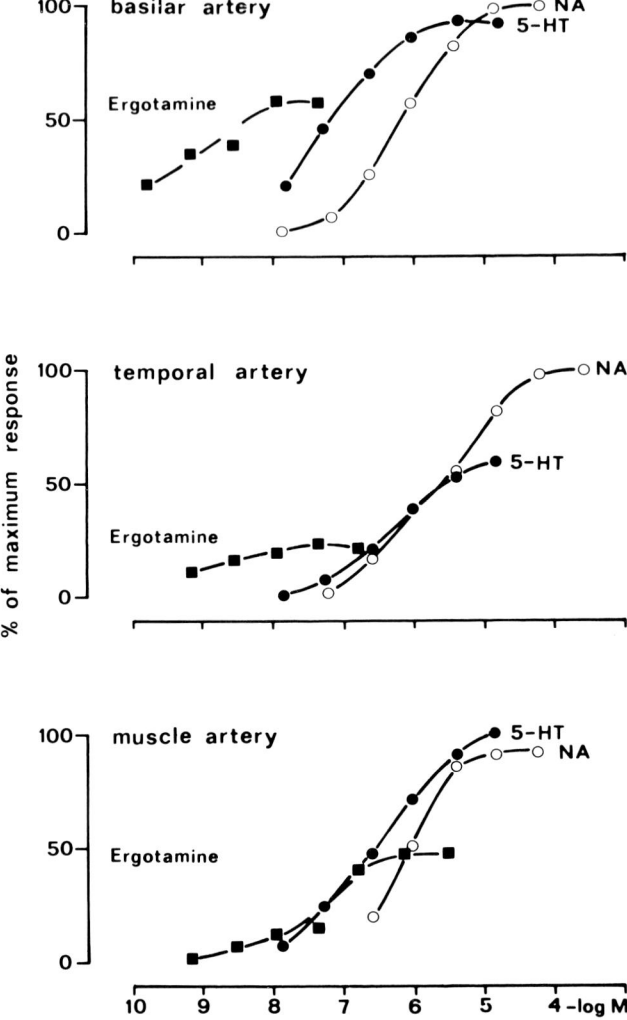

FIG. 3. Dose-response curves on helical strips from human arteries obtained during autopsy within 24 hr after death. Each point represents the mean of 11 to 36 assays for NA and 5-HT and of two to five assays for ergotamine. (From ref. 16, with permission.)

higher affinity than 5-HT itself for the serotoninergic receptor sites in arterial smooth muscle; it is active in about 100 times lower concentrations than 5-HT.

Our assumption that the constrictor effect of ergotamine on arteries is chiefly mediated through serotoninergic rather than through α-adrenergic receptor sites is further supported by experiments carried out with different antagonists on canine limb arteries (Table 1). The concentrations of pizotifen, a specific 5-HT antagonist, required for antagonizing the contractile effect of 5-HT and ergotamine to the same extent are close to each other ($10^{-9.3}$ and $10^{-9.1}$), whereas about 500 times more pizotifen is necessary to inhibit NE. With a specific α-adrenoceptor-blocking agent, phentolamine, higher but again similar concentrations are required to inhibit 5-HT ($10^{-6.2}$) and ergotamine ($10^{-6.5}$),

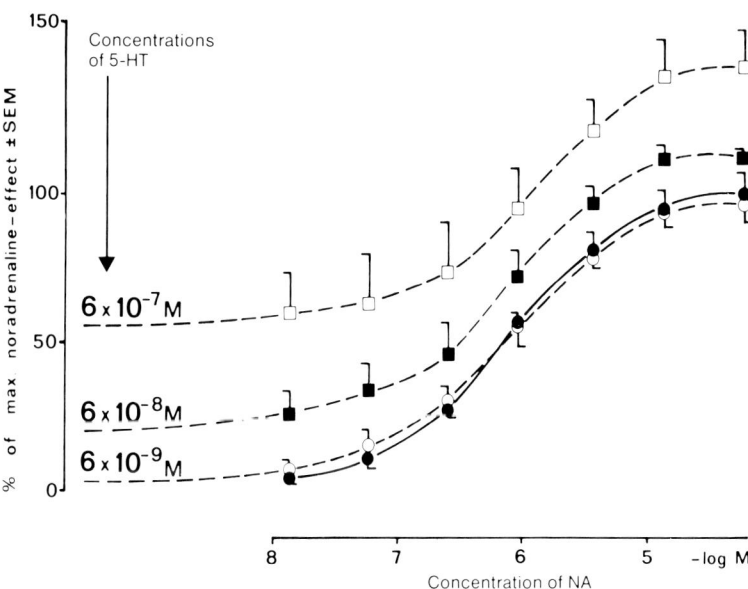

FIG. 4. Cumulative dose-response curves for norepinephrine (noradrenaline) (NA) on spiral strips from canine external carotid arteries. NA alone *(solid line)* or in the presence of 5-HT added to the bath 30 min previously *(dashed line).* For each point, $N = 4$; bars, $\pm$ SEM. (From ref. 16, with permission.)

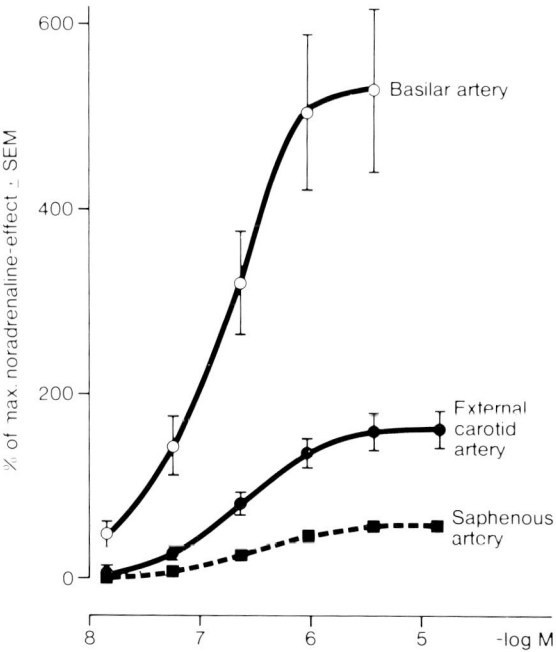

FIG. 5. Cumulative dose-response curves for 5-HT on spiral strips from canine arteries, expressed in percent of maximum response to norepinephrine (noradrenaline). For each point, $N = 6$ to 30. (From ref. 9, with permission.)

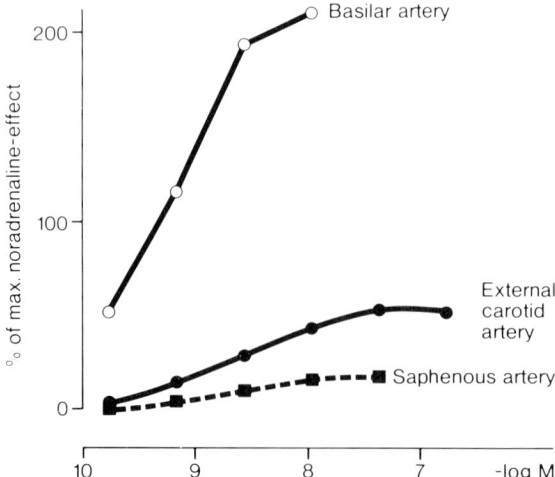

FIG. 6. Dose-response curves for ergotamine on spiral strips from canine arteries, expressed in percent of maximum response to norepinephrine (noradrenaline). For each point, $N = 5$ or 6. (From ref. 9, with permission.)

whereas about 10 times lower concentrations of phentolamine ($10^{-7.4}$) inhibit NE to the same extent (10). Similar results were obtained when pizotifen was tested against 5-HT, ergotamine, and dihydroergotamine on bovine basilar arteries. Pizotifen proved to be nearly equipotent in antagonizing the vasoconstrictor effects of the three agonists (12).

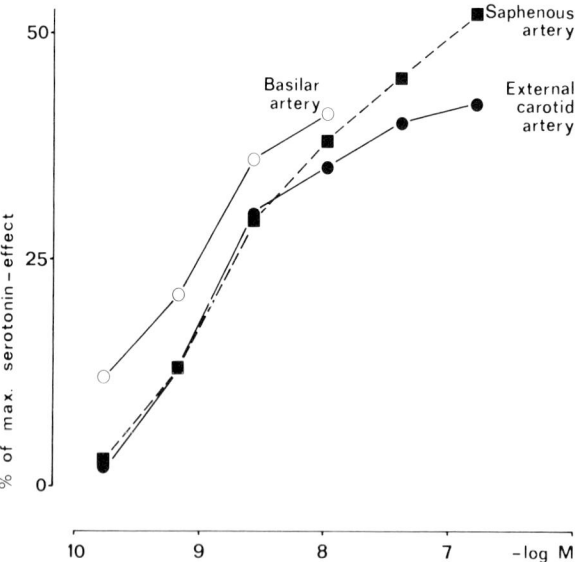

FIG. 7. Dose-response curves for ergotamine on spiral strips from canine arteries expressed in percent of maximum response to 5-HT. For each point, $N = 6$. (From ref. 9, with permission.)

TABLE 1. *Effects of antagonists of 5-HT and NE on spiral strips from canine saphenous arteries[a]*

Antagonists	Agonists		
	NE	5-HT	Ergotamine
Pizotifen (antiserotonin)	$10^{-6.6}$	$10^{-9.3}$	$10^{-9.1}$
Phentolamine (antiadrenergic)	$10^{-7.4}$	$10^{-6.2}$	$10^{-6.5}$

[a]Concentrations of the antagonists making necessary a doubling of the concentration of the agonists in order to obtain a standard response (50% of maximum response).

Ergotamine modifies the vasoconstrictor effects of the two mediators (11,13). According to classic pharmacology, besides its intrinsic vasoconstrictor action, ergotamine inhibits noradrenergic effects in a competitive way. This holds true in peripheral arteries of canine as well as human origin (Fig. 8). The dose-response curves for NE are displaced to the right by previous addition of ergotamine, in a concentration-dependent manner. The intrinsic effect of ergotamine is visible from the higher starting points of the dotted lines in Fig. 8. The parallelism of the shifted curves and the fact that they reach similar maximum levels indicate a competitive antagonism (11).

In cranial arteries, the intrinsic vasoconstrictor effect of ergotamine is again visible. Here, however, the effect of added NE is not antagonized but reinforced when ergotamine is present in the organ bath, as seen in Fig. 9 on canine and human basilar arteries (11) and Fig. 10 in human temporal arteries (16). These additive effects, which resemble those observed with NE and 5-HT, again suggest an action on different receptors.

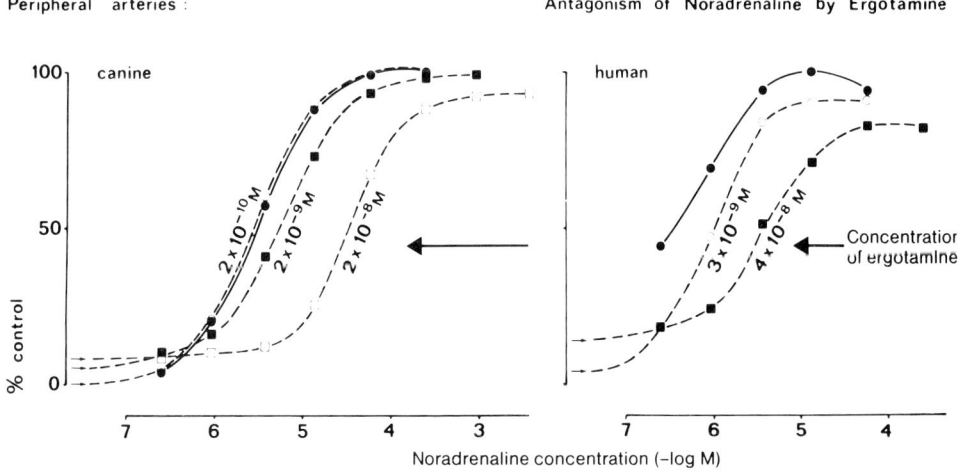

FIG. 8. Cumulative dose-response curves for norepinephrine (noradrenaline) on spiral strips from canine and human limb arteries. Norepinephrine (noradrenaline) alone *(solid line)* or in the presence of ergotamine added to the bath 60 min previously *(dashed line)*. (From ref. 11, with permission.)

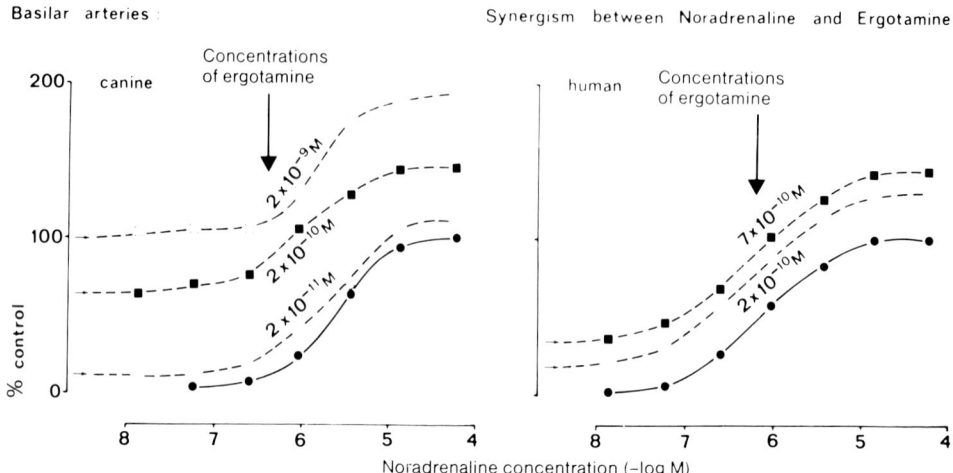

FIG. 9. Cumulative dose-response curves for norepinephrine (noradrenaline) on spiral strips from canine and human basilar arteries. Norepinephrine (noradrenaline) alone *(solid line)* or in the presence of ergotamine added 60 min previously *(dashed line)*. (From ref. 11, with permission.)

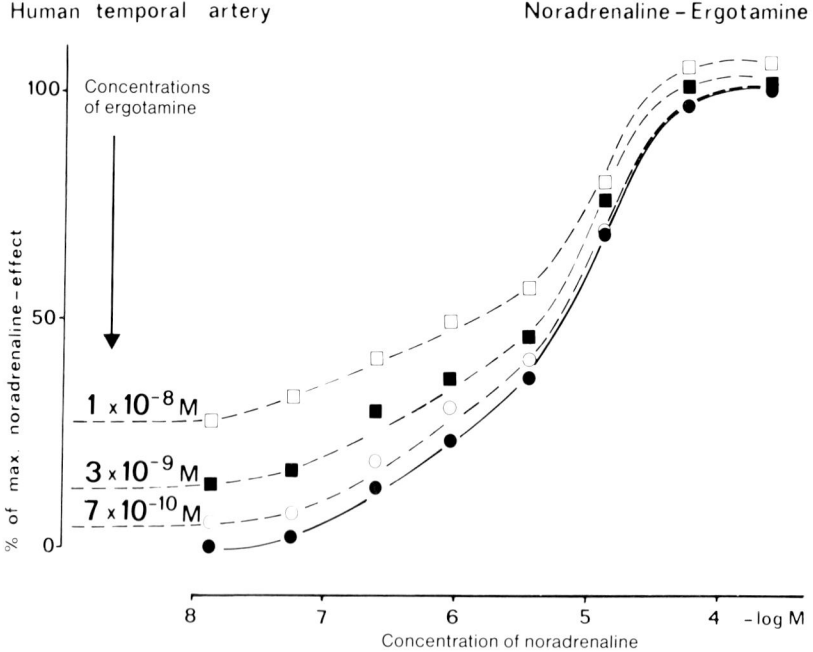

FIG. 10. Cumulative dose-response curves for norepinephrine (noradrenaline) on spiral strips from human temporal artery obtained during autopsy 17 hr after death. Norepinephrine (noradrenaline) alone *(solid line)* or in the presence of ergotamine added 60 min previously *(dashed line)*. (From ref. 16, with permission.)

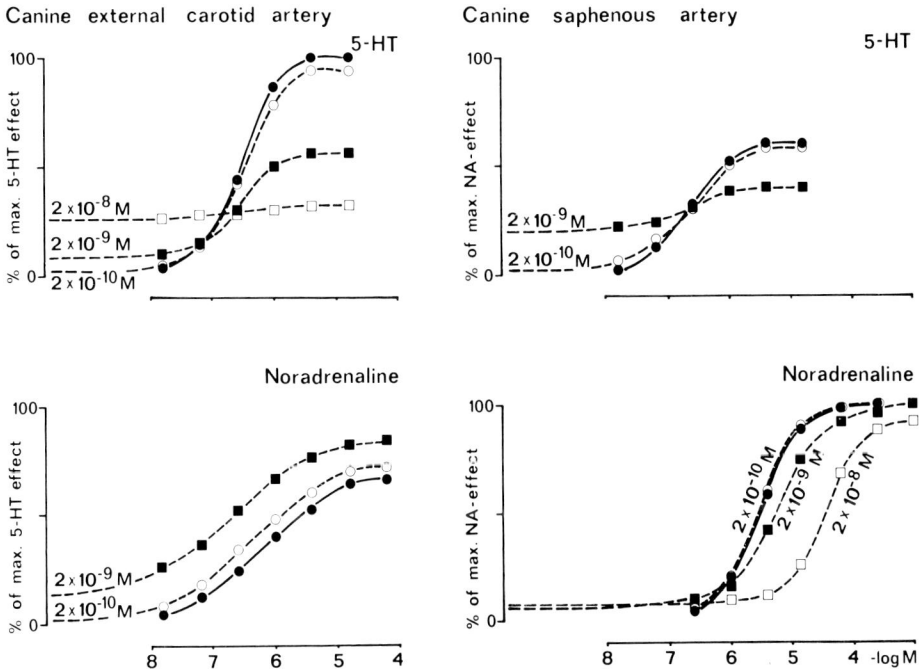

FIG. 11. Dose-response curves for 5-HT **(top)** and norepinephrine (noradrenaline) **(bottom)** on spiral strips from canine arteries. Effects on external carotid **(left)** expressed in percent of maximum 5-HT effect, on saphenous **(right)** in percent of maximum norepinephrine effect. 5-HT or norepinephrine alone *(solid line)* or in the presence of ergotamine in the indicated concentrations *(dashed line)*.

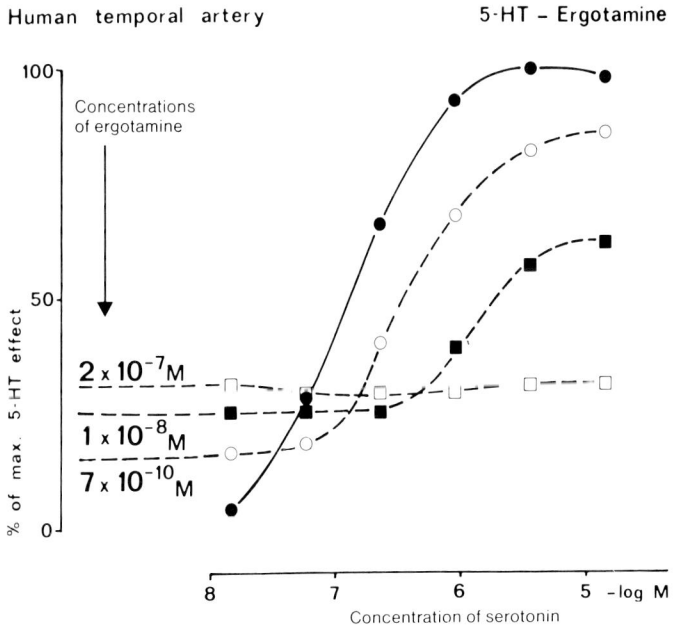

FIG. 12. Dose-response curves for 5-HT on strips from human temporal artery obtained during autopsy 15 hr after death. 5-HT alone *(solid line)* or in the presence of ergotamine added 60 min previously *(dashed line)*. (From ref. 16, with permission.)

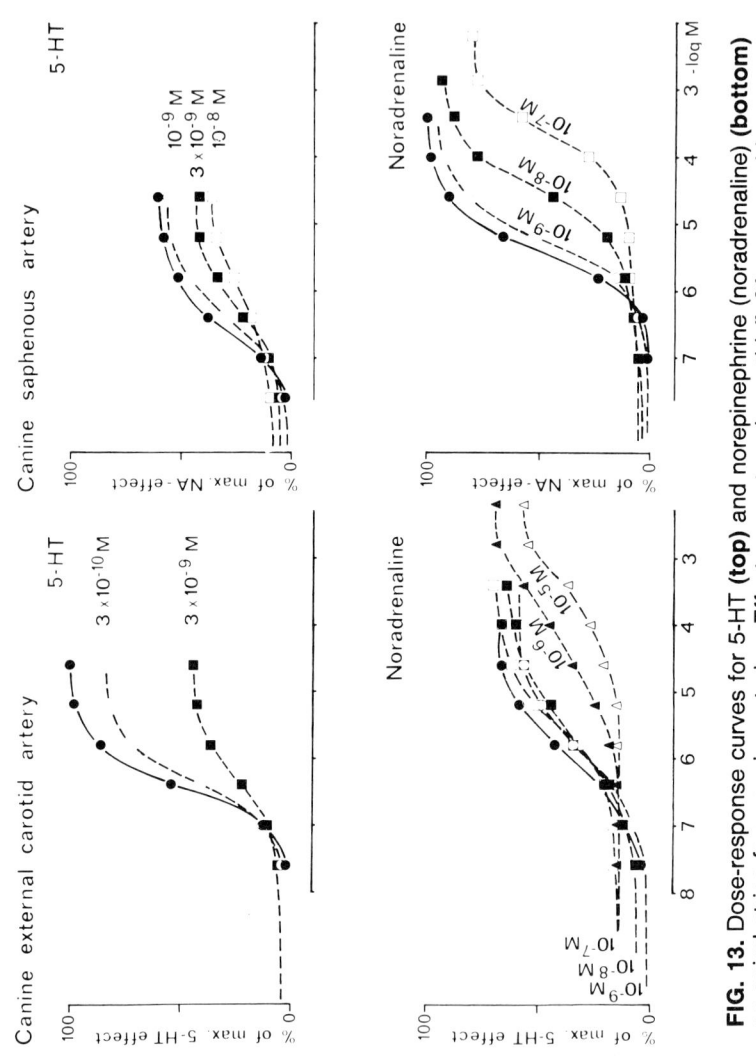

FIG. 13. Dose-response curves for 5-HT **(top)** and norepinephrine (noradrenaline) **(bottom)** on spiral strips from canine arteries. Effects on external carotid **(left)** expressed in percent of maximum 5-HT effect, on saphenous **(right)** in percent of maximum norepinephrine effect. 5-HT or norepinephrine alone *(solid line)* or in the presence of dihydroergotamine in the indicated concentrations *(dashed line)*.

Ergotamine inhibits the effects of 5-HT in all arteries tested. Increasing concentrations of ergotamine produce an increase of the basal tension, but the maximum response to 5-HT added subsequently is progressively depressed, as can be seen in Fig. 11 (external carotid and limb arteries of dog) and Fig. 12 (human temporal artery) (16). This type of interaction suggests that ergotamine acts as a noncompetitive dualist on 5-HT receptors. With dihydroergotamine, the pattern is similar (Fig. 13), except that this drug does not reinforce the vasoconstrictor effect of NE on cranial arteries. Dihydroergotamine is a competitive NE inhibitor on cranial as well as peripheral arteries (13).

These trials on isolated arteries lead to the following conclusions: (a) intra- and extracranial arteries are particularly sensitive to the vasoconstrictor effect of 5-HT, whereas peripheral arteries are more sensitive to NE; (b) ergotamine and, to a lesser extent, dihydroergotamine exert an intrinsic vasoconstrictor action, which results chiefly from the stimulation of 5-HT receptors in cranial arteries and of 5-HT receptors and possibly α-adrenoceptors in peripheral arteries; (c) in cranial arteries, ergotamine reinforces the vasoconstrictor effect of NE while inhibiting its effect competitively in limb arteries; dihydroergotamine inhibits NE in both arteries; (d) in both types of arterial smooth muscle, ergotamine and dihydroergotamine inhibit the vasoconstrictor effect of 5-HT as noncompetitive dualists.

During the migraine attack, 5-HT is first liberated by the blood platelets, then degraded by monoamine oxidase (MAO) and excreted in large quantity as 5-hydroxyindoleacetic

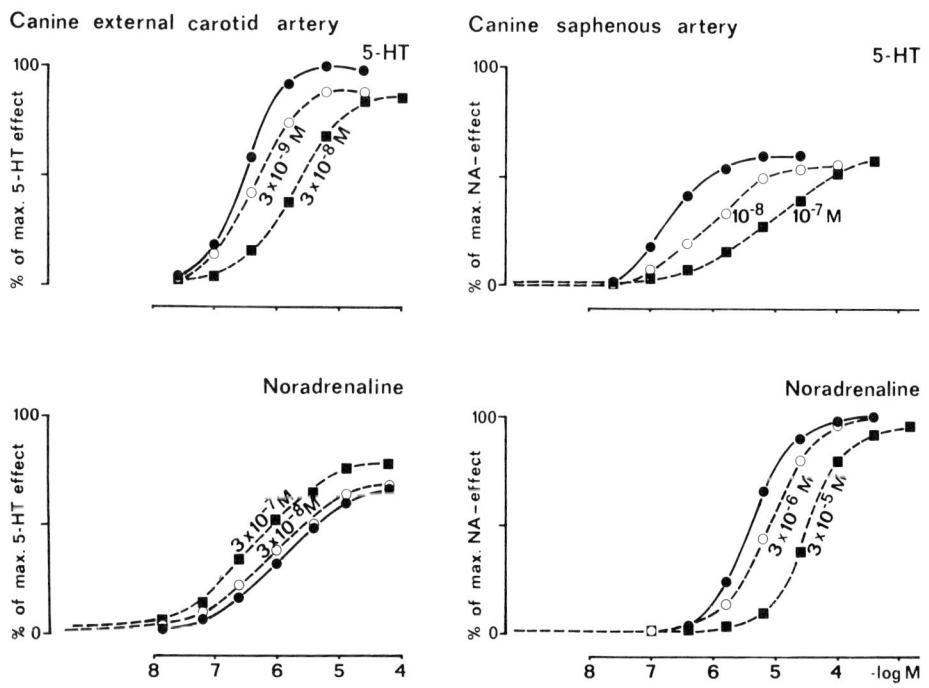

FIG. 14. Dose-response curves for 5-HT **(top)** and norepinephrine (noradrenaline) **(bottom)** on spiral strips from canine arteries. Effects on external carotid **(left)** expressed in percent of maximum 5-HT effect, on saphenous **(right)** in percent of maximum norepinephrine effect. 5-HT or norepinephrine alone *(solid line)* or in the presence of methysergide in the indicated concentrations *(dashed line)*.

acid (5-HIAA) (21). This results in a drop in the 5-HT blood level (3,7), which favors the hypotonicity and passive distension of the cranial vessels. It is against this background that we must consider the effect of ergotamine and dihydroergotamine in migraine: these drugs act by compensating for the deficiency of 5-HT at the receptors, thus counter-acting the loss of tonus of extracranial arteries. The vasoconstrictor effect of ergotamine on these vessels is further fostered by the fact that in this vascular bed, ergotamine does not inhibit but reinforces the action of circulating NE. Dihydroergotamine, besides having weaker intrinsic vasoconstrictor properties, lacks this NE-reinforcing effect on cranial arteries; thus higher doses are needed to abort a migraine attack.

Other ergot drugs, such as methysergide and lisuride, are effective for prophylactic treatment of migraine (4,6,20,22) but are not able to abort an attack; they have negligible intrinsic vasoconstrictor activity.

On isolated canine arteries (Fig. 14), methysergide inhibits competitively the vasoconstrictor effect of 5-HT on the external carotid as well as on the saphenous artery; with respect to NE, it behaves qualitatively like ergotamine, inhibiting NE in a competitive way on limb arteries but enhancing the NE-induced vasoconstriction on the external carotid (13). There is, however, a quantitative difference: with methysergide, the enhancement of NE effects requires 10 times higher concentrations than the inhibition of 5-HT effects, whereas the reverse is true with ergotamine. Lisuride is a noncompetitive 5-HT inhibitor and a competitive NE inhibitor in both canine arteries (Fig. 15). Thus

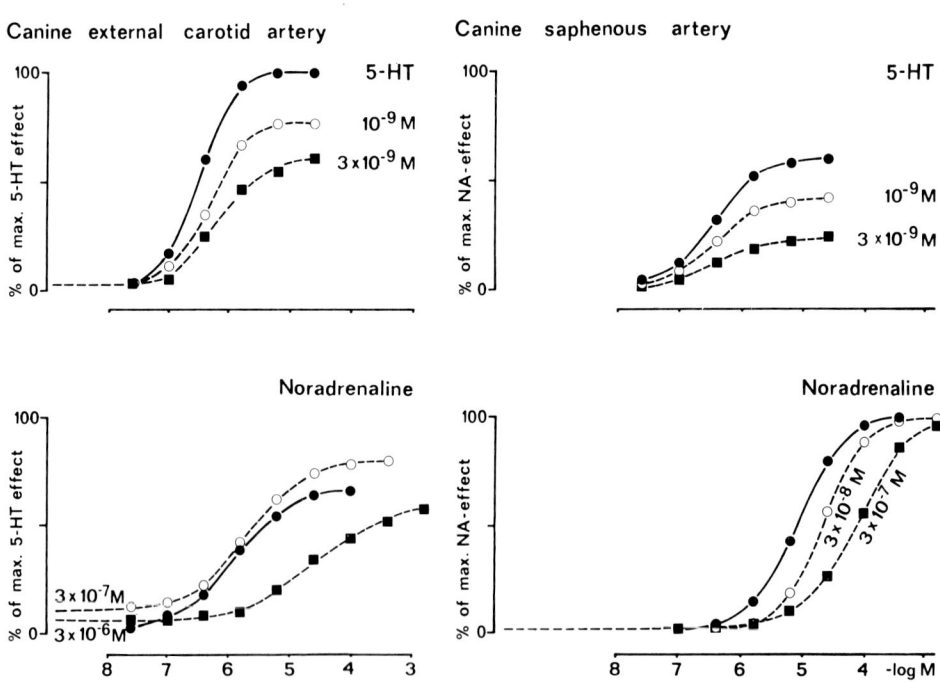

FIG. 15. Dose-response curves for 5-HT **(top)** and norepinephrine (noradrenaline) **(bottom)** on spiral strips from canine arteries. Effects on external carotid **(left)** expressed in percent of maximum 5-HT effect, on saphenous **(right)** in percent of maximum norepinephrine effect. 5-HT or norepinephrine alone *(solid line)* or in the presence of lisuride in the indicated concentrations *(dashed line)*.

methysergide as well as lisuride interfere, each in its own way, with the vasoconstrictor actions of NE and 5-HT. The possible implications of these vascular effects for the prophylactic antimigrainous activity of these two drugs are still unclear.

SUMMARY

When ergot derivatives were tried in the treatment of migraine more than 50 years ago, their use was based on their adrenergic-blocking properties. It was soon recognized, however, that their effectiveness was linked with their constricting effect on dilated extracranial arteries.

Studies on isolated veins from animals and man and on human veins *in situ* subsequently revealed that ergotamine and dihydroergotamine act on α-adrenoceptors not only as competitive antagonists but also as partial agonists (a combination of effects known as dualism). The vasoconstriction brought about by these drugs was thus ascribed to α-stimulation.

Recent experiments on canine, bovine, and human arteries, however, have demonstrated marked regional differences in their pharmacological properties. Cranial arteries are particularly sensitive to the vasoconstrictor effect of 5-HT, whereas limb arteries are more sensitive to NE. Ergotamine and dihydroergotamine inhibit the vasoconstrictor effect of 5-HT in a noncompetitive manner in all arteries. At the same time, both compounds themselves exert a vasoconstrictor action; in cranial arteries, this is due chiefly to the stimulation of 5-HT receptors and in peripheral arteries to the stimulation of 5-HT receptors and α-adrenoceptors. In addition, ergotamine but not dihydroergotamine reinforces the vasoconstrictor effect of NE on cranial arteries while inhibiting its effect on limb arteries. Dihydroergotamine inhibits the action of NE in all arteries. Thus it may be assumed that in the migraine attack, ergotamine and dihydroergotamine act by compensating for the deficiency of 5-HT at the receptors in the extracranial arteries, and that the vasoconstrictor effect of ergotamine on these vessels is further enhanced by reinforcement of the action of endogenous NE.

Methysergide and lisuride possess only a negligible intrinsic vasoconstrictor activity and are therefore unable to abort a migraine attack. Both inhibit the vasoconstrictor effect of 5-HT on cranial and peripheral arteries, the former by a competitive and the latter by a noncompetitive mechanism. Lisuride is a competitive NE inhibitor in all arteries, while methysergide behaves like ergotamine, inhibiting NE competitively in limb arteries but enhancing NE-induced constriction of the external carotid. The possible implications of these vascular effects of methysergide and lisuride for their use in the prophylaxis of migraine are still unclear.

REFERENCES

1. Aellig, W. H. (1974): Venoconstrictor effect of dihydroergotamine in superficial hand veins. *Eur. J. Clin. Pharmacol.*, 7:137–139.
2. Aellig, W. H. (1975): Studies on the venoconstrictor effect of ergot compounds in man. *Triangle*, 14:39–46.
3. Anthony, M., Hinterberger, H., and Lance, J. W. (1967): Plasma serotonin in migraine and stress. *Arch. Neurol.*, 16:544–552.
4. Curran, D. A., Hinterberger, H., and Lance, J. W. (1967): Methysergide. *Res. Clin. Stud. Headache*, 1:74–122.
5. Graham, J. R., and Wolff, H. G. (1937): Mechanism of migraine headache and action of ergotamine tartrate. *Proc. Assoc. Res. Nerv. Ment. Dis.*, 18:638–669.

6. Herrmann, W. M., Horowski, R., Dannehl, K., Kramer, U., and Lurati, K. (1977): Clinical effectiveness of lisuride hydrogen maleate: A double-blind trial versus methysergide. *Headache,* 17:54–60.
7. Lance, J. W. (1973): *The Mechanism and Management of Headache.* Butterworths, London.
8. Müller-Schweinitzer, E. (1974): Studies on the peripheral mode of action of dihydroergotamine in human and canine veins. *Eur. J. Pharmacol.,* 27:231–237.
9. Müller-Schweinitzer, E. (1976): Responsiveness of isolated canine cerebral and peripheral arteries to ergotamine. *Naunyn Schmiedebergs Arch. Pharmacol.,* 292:113–118.
10. Müller-Schweinitzer, E. (1976): Evidence for stimulation of 5-HT receptors in canine saphenous arteries by ergotamine. *Naunyn Schmiedebergs Arch. Pharmacol.,* 295:41–44.
11. Müller-Schweinitzer, E. (1977): Comparative studies on the mode of action of ergotamine in canine and human arteries. In: *Headache New Vistas,* edited by F. Sicuteri, pp. 75–82. Biomedical Press, Florence.
12. Müller-Schweinitzer, E. (1978): Studies on the 5-HT receptors in vascular smooth muscle. *Res. Clin. Stud. Headache,* 6:6–12.
13. Müller--Schweinitzer, E. (1980): Antimigraine drugs: Interaction with 5-hydroxytryptamine and noradrenaline on isolated canine arteries. In: *Vascular Neuroeffector Mechanisms,* edited by J. A. Bevan, Th. Godfraind, R. A. Maxwell, and P. M. Vanhoutte, p. 349–352. Raven Press, New York.
14. Müller-Schweinitzer, E., and Stürmer, E. (1974): Investigations on the mode of action of ergotamine in the isolated femoral vein of the dog. *Br. J. Pharmacol.,* 51:441–446.
15. Müller-Schweinitzer, E., and Stürmer, E. (1974): Studies on the mechanism of the venoconstrictor activity of ergotamine on isolated canine saphenous veins. *Blood Vessels,* 11:183–190.
16. Müller-Schweinitzer, E., and Weidmann, H. (1977): Regional differences in the responsiveness of isolated arteries from cattle, dog and man. *Agents Actions,* 7:383–389.
17. van Rossum, J. M. (1963): Cumulative dose-response curves (II. Techniques for the making of dose-response curves in isolated organs and the evaluation of drug parameters). *Arch. Int. Pharmacodyn. Ther.,* 143:299–330.
18. Rothlin, E. (1925): Ueber die pharmakologische und therapeutische Wirkung des Ergotamins auf den Sympathicus. *Klin. Wochenschr.,* 4:1,437–1,443.
19. Salzmann, R., and Weidmann, H. (1966): Die Wirkung von Ergotamin auf humorale und neuronale Effekte an der Nickhaut der Katze. *Helv. Physiol. Acta,* 24:C117.
20. Sicuteri, F. (1959): Prophylactic and therapeutic properties of l-methyl-lysergic acid butanolamide in migraine. *Int. Arch. Allergy Appl. Immunol.,* 15:300–307.
21. Sicuteri, F., Testi, A., and Anselmi, B. (1961): Biochemical investigations in headache: Increase in the hydroxyindoleacetic acid excretion during migraine attacks. *Int. Arch. Allergy Appl. Immunol.,* 19:55–58.
22. Sommerville, B. W., and Herrmann, W. M. (1978): Migraine prophylaxis with lisuride hydrogen maleate—a double-blind study of lisuride versus placebo. *Headache,* 18:75–79.
23. Weidmann, H., and Taeschler, M. (1967): Influence des substances antimigraineuses sur les effets des catécholamines, de la sérotonine et de la stimulation des nerfs sympathiques. In: *Symposium International sur les Céphalées Vasculaires,* pp. 33–40. L'Expansion Scientifique Française, Paris.
24. Wolff, H. G. (1963): *Headache and Other Head Pain.* Oxford University Press, New York.

Advances in Neurology, Vol. 33, edited by
M. Critchley et al. Raven Press, New York © 1982

Serotonin Precursors in Migraine Prophylaxis

G. Bono, *M. Criscuoli, E. Martignoni, **S. Salmon,
and G. Nappi

*Headache Center, University of Pavia, Pavia; *Instituto Farmochimico Falorni, Florence; and
**Department of Clinical Pharmacology, Headache Center, University of Florence, Florence, Italy*

A possible role of monoaminergic systems in primary headaches is suggested by the observation that some drugs known to interfere with monoamines also may induce or prevent headache attacks. Drugs such as reserpine, parachlorophenylalanine, fenfluramine, and benserazide are known to induce headache attacks in migraine subjects (12, 15,17). These patients also show a particular sensitivity to a series of physiological events involving neurotransmitter turnover, such as stress, sleep deprivation, fasting, and menstruation. Furthermore, the various studies performed to date have not yet completely defined which level (central or peripheral) or which specific aminergic system is involved in the pathogenesis of this disorder.

Migraine attacks are probably caused by a multiple neurotransmitter disturbance. This is suggested by the different sites of action of antimigraine drugs, such as methysergide or pizotifen, or by tricyclic antidepressants (amitriptiline), clonidine, dopaminergic agonists (lisuride), and serotonin (5-HT) precursors. Particularly with respect to experiments with 5-HT precursors, the clinical results are often contradictory.

In 1972, Sicuteri (18), using L-5-hydroxytryptophan (L-5-HTP), 200 mg/day/p.o. for 2 months in 20 cases, obtained therapeutic effects similar to those of methysergide. An analogous response was found by the same author (19) using L-TP, 4 g/day, and by Nappi et al. (11); the latter used doses of 9 g L-TP/day/p.o. for 10 days and found a positive clinical response together with a significant increase of cerebrospinal fluid (CSF) 5-hydroxyindoleacetic acid (5-HIAA) levels. Mathew (10) did not report significant results in a 2-month clinical trial of placebo versus 5-HTP, 300 mg/day/p.o., in 12 cases.

Kangasniemi et al. (8) reported a good clinical response in four of eight cases after a 3-month treatment period with L-TP, 2 g/day/p.o. Besides a significant increase of free TP plasma levels after administration of a single 500 mg L-TP dose, the authors also demonstrated a delayed peak of L-TP absorption in migrainous patients (two responders), who showed particular changes in visual evoked potentials under treatment.

Moreover, most of the studies with acute loading of 5-HT precursors performed in humans and animals have demonstrated the ability of these substances to cross the blood-brain barrier and to produce central effects, such as prolactin and growth hormone release and changes in mood, behavior, and thermoregulation (13).

Despite these positive observations, the transport mechanisms throughout the blood-brain barrier and the correlations between free and bound TP with respect to cerebral 5-HT levels have not yet been completely defined (4). Our data on 5-HT precursors are limited to the therapeutic use of DL-5-HTP, whose pharmacokinetic data are also available.

PHARMACOKINETICS OF DL-5-HTP

The results of orally administered single doses of DL-5-HTP in Winstar rats have been reported by Criscuoli and Savoia (3). The 5-hydroxindole levels were measured by the authors in whole brain by a modified Curzon and Green method before and after oral administration of DL-5-HTP, 25 and 200 mg/kg, respectively. The 25 mg oral dose provokes a striking increase in 5-HTP plasma levels, 100 times higher than basal levels after the first hour, while the cerebral levels nearly doubled within the second hour. Regarding the duration of the phenomenon, the plasma levels still remain elevated after 18 hr, while the cerebral levels return to baseline 3 hr after treatment. After 200 mg, neither the plasma nor the cerebral 5-HTP levels show increases proportional to the dose (increasing only about 600 and 15 times, respectively).

The half-life (t½) values of the 200 mg dose are plasma 3 hr, 22 min for plasma and 3 hr, 15 min for brain, suggesting that cerebral and plasma levels are constantly in balance in a ratio of 0.06. By comparing these plasma and cerebral 5-HTP levels with cerebral 5-HT levels, 5-HTP brain levels higher than 1 μg/kg brain are necessary to support an increase of 5-HT stores. This occurs only with the 200 mg/kg dose. Moreover, as a result of a subsequent series of experiments using a 25 mg/kg dose, 5-HIAA levels rise significantly, simultaneously with 5-HTP. This indicates an increase of 5-HT turnover, even with this low oral dose of DL-5-HTP. On the other hand, most of the pharmacologic effects of the amino acid can be readily observed at doses lower than 25 mg/kg; these doses are clearly independent from changes in brain 5-HT. These effects, which can be defined as thymoleptic and, in part, dopaminergic, may be attributed to an increase of 5-HT turnover or to the involvement of possible dopaminergic mechanisms. However, it cannot be excluded that the 25 mg/kg dose may produce increases in the 5-HT stores of specific brain areas, not detectable by assays in whole brain.

The intravenous administration of the amino acid in the dog has furnished more precise data about the t½ of the substance, which is about 3.5 hr for a single 50 mg i.v. dose (1). When the same dose is administered orally, the highest 5-HTP levels are found within the second hour. By comparing the 5-HTP curves following intravenous and parenteral administration, it appears that the oral dose is absorbed at about 85%. The absorption patterns in the dog were further investigated after 10 days of oral treatment with DL-5-HTP, 25 mg three times per day. As demonstrated by comparing the curves of plasma 5-HTP after two consecutive doses on the 10th day of treatment, even these doses (up to 25 mg) do not alter the basic kinetic parameters nor change absorption, distribution, or elimination mechanisms of the drug.

The plasma levels of hydroxindoles in humans after a single oral 200 mg dose have been reported (14). The curves were obtained from seven migraine subjects. No changes in 5-HT levels can be found, whereas 5-HIAA levels sharply increase even before the 5-HTP peak can be reached. The peak time of absorption falls at the second hour. The t½ is calculated to be 2 hr, 40 min and can exclude any overload phenomenon when the administered dose is equal to or less than 200 mg. With respect to urinary excretion, 5-HTP and 5-HT levels were measured by spectrofluorimetric assays and 5-HIAA by colorimetric methods. In the same patients, 5-HTP was detectable after 48 hr in five of seven cases; at the 24 hr control, 5-HT was detectable in three of seven cases. 5-HIAA levels were particularly elevated only during the 12 hr following treatment.

DL-5-H-TP VERSUS PIZOTIFEN: A DOUBLE-BLIND CONTROLLED CLINICAL TRIAL

The ability of DL-5HTP to functionally interfere with 5-HT pathways and to possibly influence migraine attacks, as well other parameters (e.g., mood, sleep, appetite) has been investigated by means of a double-blind clinical trial.

Methods

The aim of the research plan (Fig. 1) was to evaluate the intrinsic activity of DL-5-HTP as well as to compare it with a common antimigraine drug (pizotifen). After a series of preliminary investigations, the subjects admitted to the study were pretreated with placebo per 30 days and then randomized into two groups: (a) those treated for 60 days with DL-5-HTP (400 mg/day) and (b) those treated with pizotifen (1.40 mg/day).

Eighty subjects were involved in the experiment; all had been suffering from headache (common or classic migraine) for 3 years or more and had been treatment-free for 3 months or more or were never treated. Subjects over 58 and under 18 years of age were excluded, as were those with a headache index less than 6 or with depressive symptoms with a total score exceeding 30 points for the 21 items of the Hamilton rating scale for depression (6).

A self-monitoring system, the "headache time table" of Sicuteri, could furnish for each month, day by day, hour by hour, a complete control of the headache phenomenon as follows:

Frequency (number of attacks per month)
Time of onset and duration
Pain severity, in a 4-degree scale
    4: Total disability, even with medication
    3: Partial disability with medication
    2: No disability after medication
    1: No medication required

RESEARCH PLAN

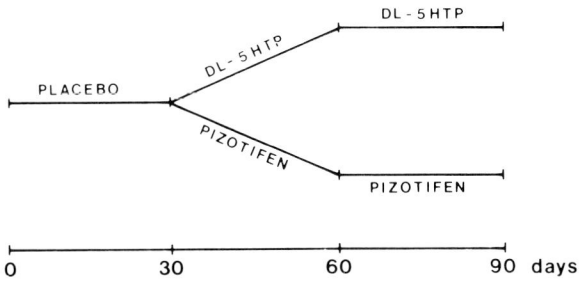

FIG. 1. DL-5-HTP versus pizotifen. A double-blind controlled clinical trial. Research plan.

Analgesic consumption (a suitable index of pain tolerance)
Correlations of headache attacks and the effects of treatments with some physiologic events (sleep-wake rhythm, weight changes, and menstruation).

Moreover, the Hamilton scale permitted the detection of eventual effects caused by DL-5-HTP treatment on the items related to sleep, mood, and ideomotor activity, which may be altered in migraine patients.

During the first clinical control, the patients were given information about the aim of treatment and the necessary instructions for the self-monitoring system. Further controls were planned after the first, second, and third months of treatment for clinical observation and Hamilton scale administration. During treatment, the consumption of normal analgesics was not modified, the only requirement being the accuracy in recording amounts and hours of drug consumption.

All patients, even though free of dietary restrictions, were asked to avoid abuse of food and drinks containing large amounts of amines and amino acids known to compete with TP transport mechanisms through the blood-brain barrier (5).

Results

Of the 80 subjects, 13 were eliminated because of side effects, incomplete self-monitoring, absence at controls, or therapy discontinuation. Thus the analysis of the results were limited to two groups each of 33 patients: seven males and 26 females in the DL-5-HTP group, five males and 29 females in the pizotifen group; the average ages were 37.7 and 36.5 years, respectively.

From the data of each patient's "headache time table," pain total index (PTI) (2), Headache Index (HI) (8), and monthly analgesic consumption were calculated, as were the scores of the Hamilton rating scale for depression at the planned controls.

The aims of the statistical analysis of the results were as follows: (a) comparison between DL-5-HTP and placebo periods of treatment; (b) comparison of DL-5-HTP activity versus pizotifen, preceded by a statistical assessment of the homogeneity between the two groups (age, $p > 0.50$; sex, $p > 0.30$; PTI, $p > 0.80$; HI, $p > 0.40$; analgesic consumption, $p > 0.45$); (c) analysis of the antimigraine activity of DL-5-HTP as a function of the different degrees of headache severity; (d) comparison of DL-5-HTP activity versus pizotifen as a function of the different degrees of headache severity, after statistical assessment of homogeneity between the headache severity subgroup (degree 4, $p > 0.25$; degree 3, $p > 0.20$; degree 2, $p > 0.95$; degree 1 (nonhomogeneous groups), $p < 0.02$); and (e) analysis of the Hamilton scores of the DL-5-HTP group at the various controls.

In the statistical analysis of the antimigraine activity of the drugs, Student's t-test was employed. Cochran t was calculated if Snedecor test was significant. The results of the Hamilton scale were evaluated with Wilcoxon test for series of paired data.

Comparison with placebo (Fig. 2) indicates that DL-5-HTP is capable of reducing analgesic consumption within the first month ($p < 0.02$); PTI and HI showed significant decreases only during the second month of treatment ($p < 0.01$ and $p < 0.02$). These effects are delayed in comparison to pizotifen, with a significant difference after the first month. After the second month, however, no difference can be found between the two for both PTI and analgesic consumption index.

From the analysis of the different activities of the two drugs evaluated as a function

RESULTS

	DL - 5HTP ∕ Placebo		DL - 5HTP ∕ Pizotifen	
PTI	N. S.	p < 0.01	p < 0.05	N.S.
HI	N. S.	p < 0.02	p < 0.01	p < 0.02
analgesic - use index	p < 0.02	p < 0.0001	p < 0.001	N. S.
	60 days	90 days	60 days	90 days

FIG. 2. Results of statistical evaluation of DL-5-HTP activity on PTI, HI, and analgesic-use index, calculated monthly, versus placebo and pizotifen treatments. NS, nonsignificant (Student's *t*-test); *p:* statistical significance (Student's *t*-test).

of the different degrees of headache severity (Fig. 3): (a) with respect to placebo, the effects of DL-5-HTP are selectively distributed in headache severity subgroups 4 and 3, i.e., the more severe headaches. Their duration in hours significantly decreases during both the first and second months of treatment; (b) no significant difference can be found between DL-5-HTP and pizotifen within headache severity subgroups 4 and 3; and (c) within the groups of less severe headaches (headache severity subgroups 1 and 2), the therapeutic response is quite similar for all three kinds of treatment (including placebo).

By the analysis of Hamilton scores in the DL-5-HTP group, significant improvements can be found after the first and second month for items 1 ($p < 0.05$), 2 and 3

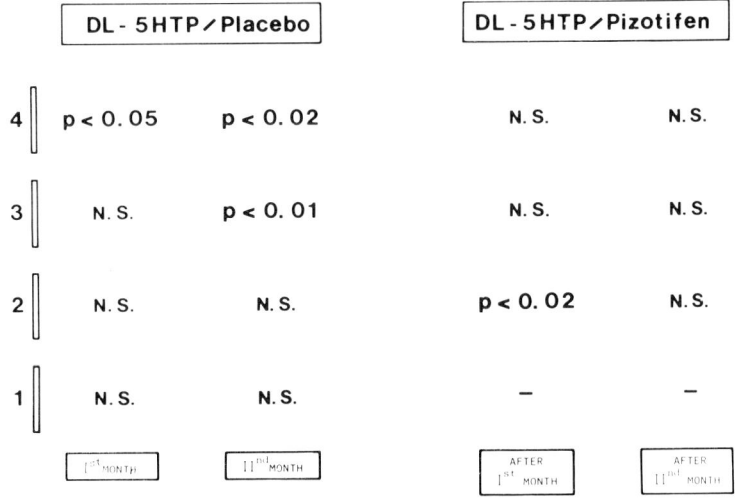

FIG. 3. DL-5-HTP activity versus placebo and versus pizotifen treatment. Evaluation as function of four different degrees of headache severity. NS, nonsignificant (Student's *t*-test); *p*, statistical significance (Student's *t*-test).

($p < 0.07$), 7 ($p < 0.01$), and 8 ($p < 0.01$), and after the second month for items 4, 5, and 6 ($p < 0.05$).

Side Effects

Of 13 subjects, five stopped treatment within the first week because of side effects. All belonged to the DL-5-HTP group and complained of nausea, diarrhea, pyrosis, and drowsiness. Weight gain in the pizotifen group was analogous to previous reports (7), ranging between 1 and 2 kg in four cases and between 2 and 3 kg in 18 cases. In the DL-5-HTP group, only nine of 33 showed weight increase, not exceeding 2 kg.

CONCLUSIONS

The results of our clinical trial demonstrate that DL-5-HTP is capable of influencing migraine symptoms, distinguishing itself from the control treatment by means of its selective activity on pain severity, duration, and tolerance, without significant changes in attack frequency. The administration of this 5-HT precursor has positively influenced parameters related to mood, ideomotor activity, and wake-sleep rhythm. The amount of improvement is such that it cannot be completely and simply attributed to the relief of the migraine symptoms.

The antidepressive activity of TP is well known (13,20). However, the utilization of these results in the formulation of simplistic theories, as well as extrapolations regarding migraine pathogenesis, or other neurotransmitter disturbances (depression), must be avoided.

The hypothesis that acute or short-term administration of 5-HT precursors may determine "functional increases" of cerebral 5-HT turnover has been suggested by a number of studies (13). The effects of these substances on the migraine syndrome, however, cannot be explained simply by investigating individual steps of the central or peripheral turnover of a single neurotransmitter.

The frequent discrepancies in previous clinical reports dealing with 5-HT precursors in migraine prophylaxis underline the necessity to biologically subdivide groups of patients apparently affected by the same disorder. Analysis of our cases shows an unresponsive group within each treatment group. For example, within the less severe headache groups (pain severity degrees 1 and 2), the therapeutic response is similar for pizotifen, DL-5-HTP, and placebo. These data indicate the importance of those psychophysiologic factors that trigger the onset of the attacks.

Thus in these patients, the use of such drugs as beta-blockers or minor tranquilizers may be preferred. Within the groups with milder headaches, we found the highest scores for anxiety and its somatic symptoms on the Hamilton rating scale for depression.

Looking ahead to a specific treatment and better interpretation and planning of clinical trials, new methods must be considered (9,16), capable of identifying the specific biologic disturbance in each subject.

REFERENCES

1. Clement Sarret, M., Meazzini, L., and Ballotti, P. (1979): Neuropharmacological profile of DL-5HTP in animals. *Neurosci. Lett.,* [Suppl. 3]: S241.
2. Couch, J. R., Ziegler, D. K., and Hassnein, R. (1976): Amitriptyline in the prophylaxis of migraine. Effectiveness and relationship of antimigraine and antidepressant effects. *Neurology,* 26:121–127.

3. Criscuoli, M., and Savoia, C. (1979): Effects of oral DL-5-hydroxytryptophan loading on brain 5-hydroxy-tryptophan and 5-hydroxytryptamine levels in the rat. *Neurosci. Lett.,* [Suppl. 3]: S237.
4. Curzon, G. (1979): Relationships between plasma, CSF and brain tryptophan. *J. Neural Transm. [Suppl.]*, 15:81–92.
5. Fernstrom, J. D., and Wurtman, E. J. (1972): Brain serotonin content: Physiological regulating by plasma neutral aminoacids. *Science,* 178:414–416.
6. Hamilton, M. (1960): A rating scale for depression. *J. Neurosurg. Psychiatry,* 23:56–62.
7. Kangasniemi, P., and Rinne, U. K. (1977): Clonidine and pizotiphene in the interval treatment of migraine patients. In: *Headache New Vistas,* edited by F. Sicuteri, pp. 205–212. Biomedical Press, Florence, Italy.
8. Kangasniemi, P., Falck, B., Lånvik, V. A., and Hyyppä, M. T. (1978): Levotryptophan treatment in migraine. *Headache,* 18:161–166.
9. Lechin, F., and van der Dijs, B. (1980): Physiological, clinical and therapeutic basis of a new hypothesis for headache. *Headache,* 20:77–84.
10. Mathew, N. T. (1978): 5-Hydroxytryptophan in the prophylaxis of migraine: A double blind study. *Headache,* 18:111.
11. Nappi, G., Poloni, M., Bono, G., and Savoldi, F. (1974): Livelli liquorali di acido 5-idrossindolacetico in pazienti emicranici prima e dopo trattamento con L-triptofano. *Boll. Soc. Ital. Biol. Sper.,* 50:1,037–1,041.
12. Nappi, G., Savoldi, F., Bono, G., and Martignoni, E. (1979): Reserpine-headache and PRL release in migraine. *Headache,* 19:272–277.
13. Pühringer, W., Wizz-Justice, A., Graw, P., Lacoste, V., and Gastpar, M. (1976): Intravenous L-5-hydroxy-tryptophan in normal subjects: An interdisciplinary precursor loading study. *Pharmakopsychiatrie,* 9:259–354.
14. Savoia, C. (1979): *Personal communication.*
15. Savoldi, F., and Nappi, G. (editors) (1979): *Headache Pavia 1979.* Tipo-litografica Palladio, Vicenza.
16. Savoldi, F., and Nappi, G. (1979): Contributo alla identificazione di sottogruppi di cefalee primarie. Atti XXI Congresso S.I.N., Catania, 8–10 Novembre 1979, pp. 145–181.
17. Sicuteri, F. (1971): Pain syndrome in man following treatment with p-clorophenylalanine. *Pharmacol. Res. Commun.,* 3:401–407.
18. Sicuteri, F. (1972): 5-Hydroxytryptophan in the prophylaxis of migraine. *Pharmacol. Res. Commun.,* 4:213–218.
19. Sicuteri, F. (1973): The ingestion of serotonin precursors (L-5-hydroxytryptophan and L-tryptophan) improves migraine headache. *Headache,* 13:19–22.
20. Van Hiele, L. J. (1980): L-5-Hydroxytryptophan in depression: The first substitution therapy in psychiatry? The treatment of 99 out-patients with "therapy-resistant" depression. *Neuropsychobiology,* 6:230–240.

Advances in Neurology, Vol. 33, edited by
M. Critchley et al. Raven Press, New York © 1982

Disruption of Iris Adrenergic Transmission as an Index of Poor Endorphin Modulation in Headache

Marcello Fanciullacci, Umberto Pietrini, and Maria Boccuni

Department of Clinical Pharmacology, Headache Center, University of Florence, Florence, Italy

The neuroeffector junction is an apparatus probably implicated in a wide variety of human pathological conditions, particularly in so-called functional diseases. The monitoring of this function directly *in vivo,* in order to establish the neuron and/or receptor dysfunction, is difficult in man because of a scarcity of methods. Using pupil size as an indicator, the iris neuromuscular junction is ideal for such purposes, being supplied by adrenergic and cholinergic neuronal transmission. In addition, pupil diameter is measured by noninvasive and acceptable techniques. Moreover, the responses of the iris muscle to autonomically acting drugs are reproducible when repeated under standard conditions (25).

This chapter summarizes our past and recent efforts to pharmacologically explore the pupillary neuromuscular junction, in particular in a disease such as headache which is considered typically functional in nature. Among the different theories of headache, that of an impairment of the neuroeffector junction is apparently verifiable by using the pupillometry technique.

METHODS

Photographic Pupillometry

A modified Sneddon and Turner's (23) photographic technique was used to measure pupil diameter. An ophthalmic headrest mounted on a small table provided a constant and reproducible position of the subject's head. Pupils were photographed with two Nikkormat FT2 single lens reflex cameras, using one camera for each eye. Lenses were provided with bellows and autoteleconverters $2 \times$ positioned between the body and the bellow-lens system. A macrophoto of the pupils in the ratio of 1:1 was obtained; thus the transverse diameter of the pupil was measured directly on the negatives. A manual device permitted a simultaneous click of the two cameras. Standard light conditions were provided by a 150-W lamp fixed at a distance of 40 cm from the eyes. While being photographed, subjects were requested to focus on a red disk situated between the two cameras. The photographic equipment was placed in a small dark room (3 × 1.5 m).

Electronic Pupillometry

A prototype of a microprocessor-controlled device, designed to dynamically track the pupil diameter, was used; the apparatus was developed in the System and Information Section of the Electrical Engineering Department of the University of Genoa, Italy (7,8). The set-up consisted of a television (TV) camera (with infrared tube) equipped with a special optical apparatus that allowed proper magnification of the subject's eye, a digital interface between the TV camera and microprocessor, and a TV monitor that gave visual control during examination of the pupil. Because the pupil is the darkest part of the human eye, the voltage level of a particular TV raster line, crossing the pupil, drops in correspondence to the pupil itself. This line was counted by a microcomputer. To facilitate its normal setting, the patient's eye was visualized on the TV monitor with a superimposed white line on the part of the image to be measured. The display of a white line along the tract, which measures the length of the pupil diameter, has an important role from the point of view of the operator: the visual feedback allows the operator to check the correspondence between the diagram plotted by the microcomputer and the quantity analyzed. The TV camera was mounted on a sliding rule, which rapidly permitted eye focus. A mobile headrest allowed easy and rapid switching from eye to eye during measurement. A white plexiglass sheet of hemispheric shape was placed between the face and TV camera and uniformly illuminated by a 25-W lamp (Fig. 1). Pupil diameter can be expressed as such or as a percentage change over pretest control values.

CLINICAL MATERIAL

Migraine, daily headache, and cluster headache sufferers, both in- and out-patients of the Department of Clinical Pharmacology of Florence, were studied. Migraine and cluster patients were tested during headache-free intervals. Normal subjects included physicians, technicians, and students. Patients were drug-free for almost 2 weeks. All were informed as to the nature and scope of the investigation. Statistical comparisons were done by using Student's *t*-test.

RESULTS

Evidence for Adrenergic Intraneuronal Defect

Fenfluramine exhibits indirect sympathomimetic properties (15,16) and induces mydriasis (9,12). Its mydriatic response is predicted by intact stores of norepinephrine (NE) in adrenergic nerve terminals of the iris. A single oral dose (40 mg) of fenfluramine presented a less evident mydriasis of a shorter duration in migraine patients as compared to controls within 4 to 8 hr after drug administration (Fig. 2).

Conjunctival application of guanethidine provokes a depletion of NE in iris adrenergic synapses and consequently a miosis due to a prevalence of the cholinergic neuronal control (18). Two drops (0.1 ml) of guanethidine 5% instilled into the right conjunctival sac induced a miosis greater and longer lasting in migraineurs than in controls. Recovery of pupillary size was complete at 72 hr in the latter and at 96 hr after instillation in the former (Fig. 3). Guanethidine, when instilled in both eyes in unilateral migraine, induced miosis in the eye ipsilateral to the attack which was not different from that of the unaffected side (Fig. 4).

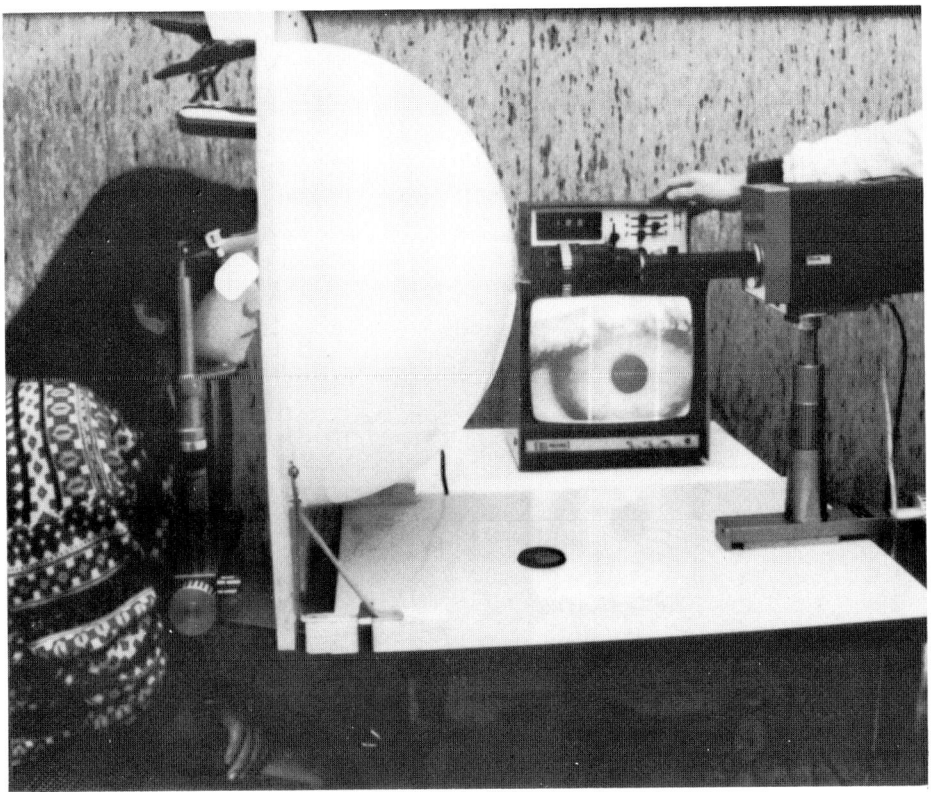

FIG. 1. Apparatus for electronic pupillometry.

One drop of tyramine (2%), a NE releaser, was instilled in both eyes of patients with cluster headache. Pupillary tyramine-induced dilatation of the pain side was less than that of the pain-free side at 45 and 60 min after instillation (Fig. 5). One drop of cocaine 4% was instilled in both eyes and provoked a greater mydriasis in the pain-free side than in the pain side. Reduced mydriatic response to tyramine and cocaine

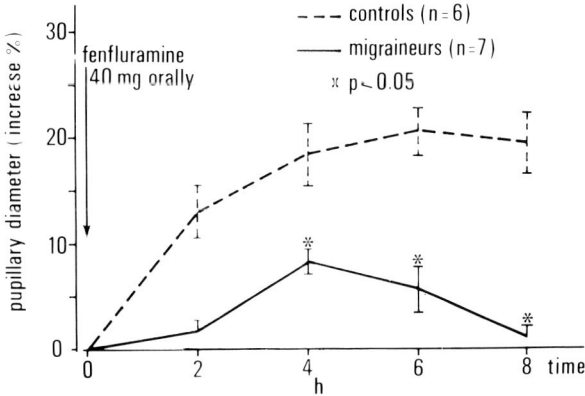

FIG. 2. Mydriatic response to fenfluramine is reduced in headache sufferers. Mean ± SE; *p* between migraine and control groups.

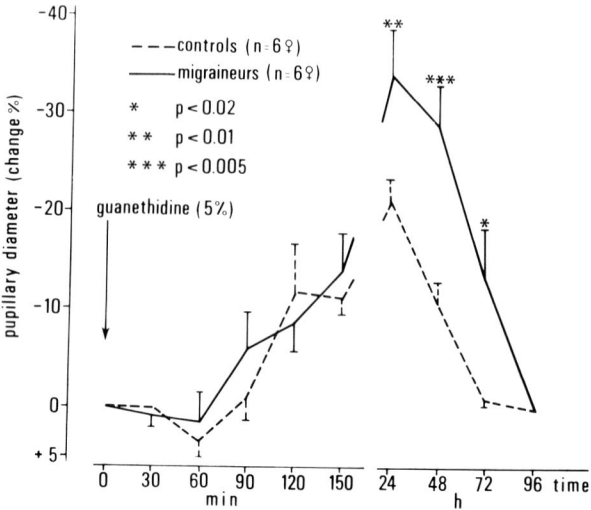

FIG. 3. Guanethidine, one drop instilled into the right eye, induces an intense and prolonged miosis in migraineurs. Mean ± SE; *p* between migraine and control groups.

was more evident during cluster period than in the cluster-free stage. A complete absence of tyramine mydriatic response was observed in the pain side pupil of chronic cluster headache. Therefore, the iris hyporeactivity to NE releasers, such as fenfluramine, tyramine, and cocaine, and the marked NE depletive action of guanethidine demonstrate an intraneural defect of NE content and synthesis that might result in a reduced sympathetic input. Because this last condition causes a hypersensitivity to a direct-acting sympathetic agent (see below), the hyperreactivity to NE depletor stresses a lack of transmitter even more pronounced than that resulting from the tests with NE releasers.

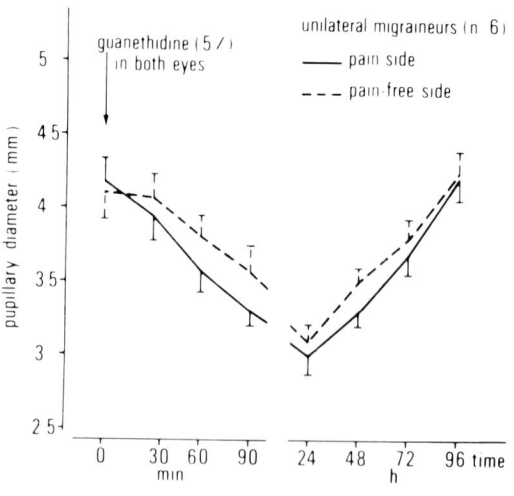

FIG. 4. Topical guanethidine-induced miosis in unilateral migraine patients. The responses of the two pupils are not statistically different. Mean ± SE.

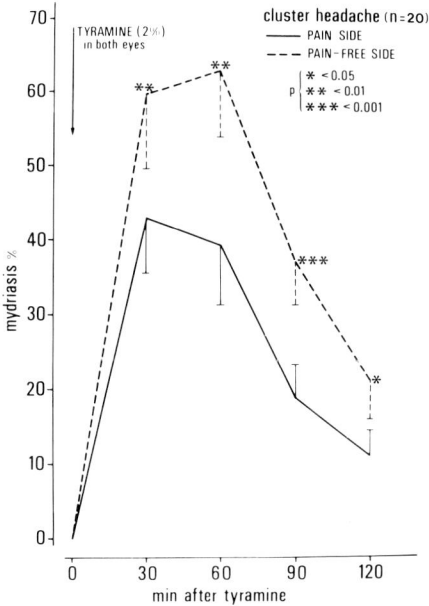

FIG. 5. Mydriasis from conjunctival tyramine is greater in the pupil contralateral to the headache attack than in the ipsilateral one. Mean ± SE; *p* between pain side and pain-free side.

Hyperresponsiveness to Adrenoceptor Stimulation

One drop of phenylephrine 1% provoked only a slight pupillary dilatation in controls, whereas it caused a definite mydriasis in migraineurs (Fig. 6). Hypersensitivity to phenylephrine also occurred in the iris of migraineous children. Conjunctival phenylephrine (1%) instilled in these children caused a mydriasis that was statistically greater than that of controls 60, 120, and 150 min after instillation. Increased mydriatic response to phenylephrine was also observed in both eyes of cluster headache sufferers.

Hyperresponsiveness to Cholinoceptor Stimulation

Aceclidine, a specific cholinergic agonist, has demonstrated a greater miotic activity in migraine patients than in controls. One drop of aceclidine (0.05%) instilled in the right eye provoked an intense and prolonged miosis in headache sufferers. Miotic response to aceclidine was always evident 4 hr after drug instillation in headache sufferers but not controls (Fig. 7).

Morphine Receptors in the Human Iris

Two drops of morphine 4% instilled in the right conjunctival sac induced miosis of the treated eye only. Topical naloxone (0.16%, two drops) reversed the local morphine-induced miosis, thus suggesting a possible existence of opiate receptors in the pupillary neuromuscular junction of man (3). Conjunctival morphine provoked a more prolonged miotic reaction in headache patients when compared to controls. In fact, the complete restoration of baseline pupil diameter was obtained 210 min after morphine in these patients and 240 min in healthy volunteers (Fig. 8).

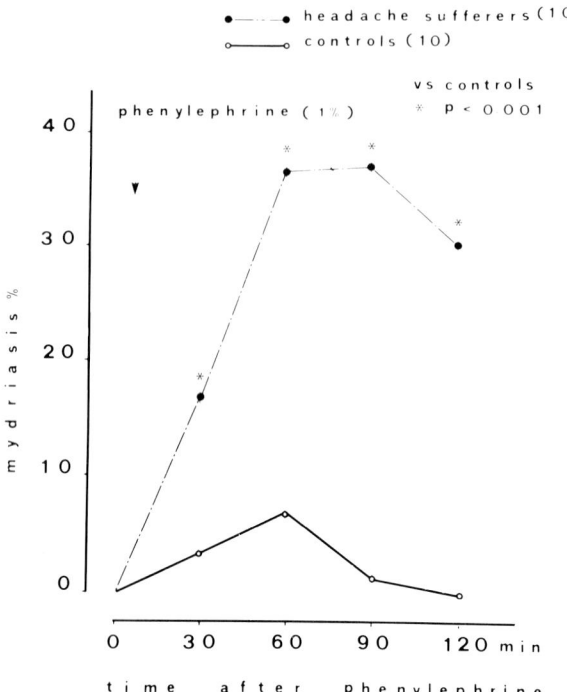

FIG. 6. Hyperresponsiveness to phenylephrine in iris of headache sufferers. Headache patients exhibit an enhanced mydriatic response to phenylephrine instillation (one drop into one eye). Mean ± SE; *p* between headache and control groups.

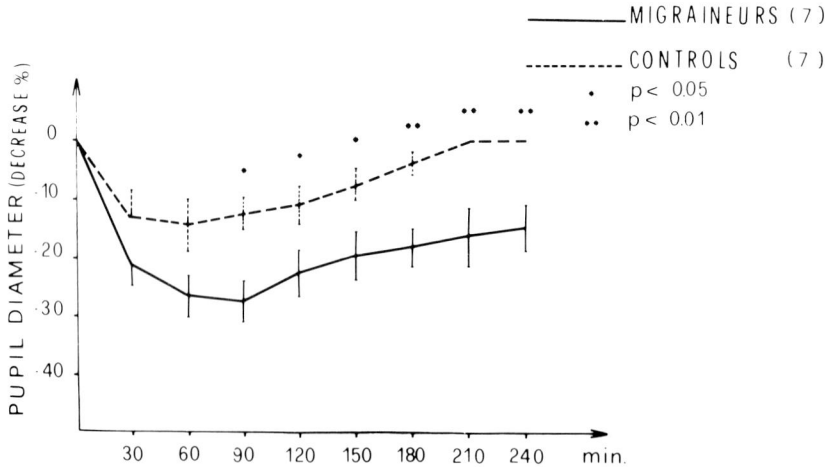

FIG. 7. The miotic response to aceclidine is increased in headache sufferers. One drop of aceclidine (0.05%) was instilled into one eye at time 0. Mean ± SE; *p* between migraine and control groups.

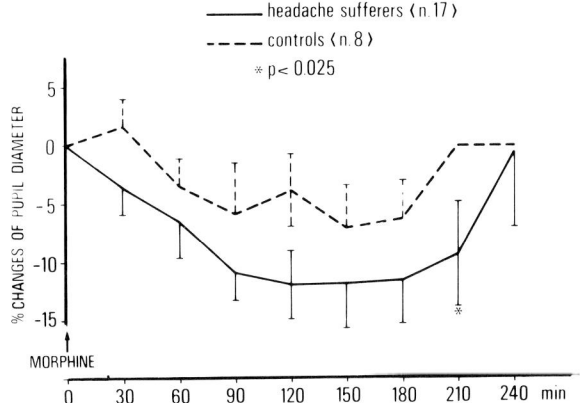

FIG. 8. Topical morphine provokes a prolonged miosis in headache sufferers. Two drops of morphine 4% were instilled into one eye. Mean ± SE; *p* between headache and control groups.

Headache Reduces Pupil Size

It is well known that acute pain induces pupil dilation by activating the sympathetic system. On the contrary, headache reduces the pupil as seen by a smaller pupil size in these sufferers when compared to controls. This reduction was observed in headache patients subsequently divided into daily headache, migraine, and cluster headache (Table 1). No significant difference in pupil size was found among these groups nor in cluster patients between pain-free and pain side.

DISCUSSION

Past (2,5,6) and present results are compatible with a reduced adrenergic transmission in the iris of headache patients. This dysfunction, clinically silent, can be unmasked by pharmacological tests that show that these sufferers have a reduced mydriatic response to NE releaser drugs, such as fenfluramine, tyramine, and cocaine, and a hyperresponsive-

TABLE 1. *Pupil size in headache patients*

Subject	No.	Pupil size (mm) (mean ± SE)	
Controls			
x̄ of both eyes	12	6.00 ± 0.34	
Daily headache			
x̄ of both eyes	15	4.43 ± 0.20[a]	
Migraine (headache free)			
x̄ of both eyes	21	4.74 ± 0.16[a]	
Cluster headache (headache free)			
During bouts	14	4.24 ± 0.18[a,b]	4.32 ± 0.20[a,c]
Out of bouts	15	4.21 ± 0.19[a,b]	4.13 ± 0.20[a,c]

[a] $p < 0.001$ (versus controls).
[b] Pain-free side; [c] pain side.

ness to the direct adreneceptor agent phenylephrine. The process of intraneuronal NE resynthesis is defective in headache patients since guanethidine, a powerful NE depletor, induces a miosis that disappears more slowly than in controls. Therefore, a chronic deficiency of sympathetic input to the iris dilatator muscle might induce the hypersensitivity of alpha-adrenoceptors of this muscle to phenylephrine. Because the action of phenylephrine finishes and tyramine is taken up into the neuron by the amine uptake mechanism (24), a deficiency in this process could determine the abnormal pupillary response to these drugs in headache sufferers. The increased miotic activity of aceclidine, a cholinoceptor agonist, might be considered further indirect evidence of reduced adrenergic transmission. This implies a diminution of the tone of the iris dilatator muscle and thus a defect in counteracting the aceclidine-induced constriction of the iris sphincter. Also, the smaller pupil size of headache sufferers could reflect a predominance of parasympathetic activity because of the insufficient sympathetic input in the iris.

This mechanism considers the hyperresponsiveness to phenylephrine as a phenomenon of "denervation supersensitivity," which implies a shift to the left of the dose-response curve, rather difficult to verify *in situ* in man. If adrenergic nerve transmission is altered, what will be the most likely nature of this abnormality? A disorder of central sympathetic activity regulation and/or a peripheral sympathetic affection may be postulated. A peripheral lesion of sympathetic innervation of the iris has been suggested in cluster headache with clinical signs of oculosympathetic paresis (13,17). The pupillary abnormalities have been attributed to an injury of the internal carotid sympathetic plexus, which results from dilatation of the intraosseous portion of the internal carotid artery during headache attack. However, since pupillary alterations are pharmacologically demonstrated out of a single attack as well as out of a cluster phase, their relationship with vasodilatating episodes is improbable. In addition, guanethidine tests in both eyes of unilateral migraine have demonstrated that the adrenergic impairment is not limited in the affected area but is systemic.

Miosis from topical morphine, reversible with conjunctival naloxone, represents suggestive evidence for the presence of opiate receptors in the iris of humans. Since morphine inhibits some peripheral adrenergic neuroeffector transmissions (10,11), morphine receptors in the human iris, presumably located on the adrenergic neurons, might inhibit NE release. This mechanism could explain mydriatic response to conjunctival naloxone observed in morphine addiction (4). Therefore, adrenergic transmission in the human iris could represent an example of morphine-sensitive neuroeffector junction. Taking into account the long-lasting miotic action of local morphine in headache patients, this might be considered an increased inhibitory effect on NE release due to the poor intraneuronal availability of this neurotransmitter. In addition, a hypersensitivity of the iris morphine receptors due to a deficiency of endogenous opioid substances could also be considered.

Opiate drugs cause inhibition of adrenergic transmission not only in the peripheral but also in the central nervous system; rats, chronically tested with opioid agents, developed a marked disease supersensitivity to NE in cortex (14).

Although the physiological role of endorphins is still an open question, the same link between opioid endogenous agents and adrenergic transmission could be taken into account in order to prospect an inhibitory physiological modulation on some adrenergic systems from these substances. If this inhibitory action is reduced because of a deficiency of endorphins, an unrestricted adrenergic transmission in the endorphin-dependent neurons is expected at both central and peripheral levels. This NE neuronal incontinence can lead to a neuron which is poor in, or completely deprived of, this neurotransmitter (i.e., in chronic cluster headache). The disruption of noradrenergic input might induce homeostatic compensatory mechanisms resulting in postsynaptic receptor supersensitivity which has been found in migraineous children (1). Also, the observed supersensitivity of the smooth muscle of the vein to serotonin and NE, transient during migraine attack (22) or permanent in some chronic headache with panalgesia (21), may be due to a similar mechanism. Therefore, iris adrenergic nerve terminals of headache patients could represent an example of "latent empty endorphin-dependent adrenergic neuron," connectable with the postulated impairment of the endorphinergic system in headache (19,20).

Moreover, the lack of valid endorphin modulation on the central and/or peripheral autonomic nervous system, might explain the autonomic dysfunctions in headache syndrome; in particular vasomotor changes, together with pain, represent the most frequent clinical symptoms in these patients.

This present theory must be confirmed by future research. However, abnormal responses of the iris to autonomically active drugs could acquire the significance of diagnostic pupillary tests in a sine materia disease, such as headache syndrome, where conventional examinations are normal and where the diagnosis is often misunderstood and contested.

SUMMARY

Pupillometry was used to evaluate the effect of oral or topically applied adrenomimetic drugs and of local morphine on pupillary size in headache patients and controls. In headache sufferers, a disruption of adrenergic transmission is suggested since the iris adrenergic nerve terminal is apparently poor in NE; this neuron also exhibits a reduced capacity of neurotransmitter synthesis and an adrenoceptor hypersensitivity. The spontaneous reduction of pupillary size detected in headache sufferers also suggests a decreased sympathetic input. The miosis, registered after conjunctival instillation of morphine, demonstrates that iris is a possible example of an opioid-dependent adrenergic neuron in man. A poor modulation of the iris adrenergic transmission induces, in headache sufferers, a neuronal incontinence and therefore a chronic intrasynaptic leakage of NE, resulting in an exhausted empty neuron on the one hand and a compensatory hyperactivity of the effector muscular cell on the other. Since indirect evidence suggests a morphine modulation of the iris adrenergic neuron, a deficiency of endorphin modulation could be the mechanism of disruption of iris adrenergic transmission. Apart from the theoretical aspects, the exploration of iris neuroeffector junction represents a noninvasive and simple diagnostic tool in headache.

ACKNOWLEDGMENTS

The authors wish to thank Dr. E. Tendi of the Pharmacy of St. Maria Nuova Hospital, Florence, for the preparation of the eye drop solutions. This work was supported by a grant from the Ministry of Public Education.

REFERENCES

1. Del Bene, E., Poggioni, M., and Fanciullacci, M. (1979): Supersensibilità dei recettori adrenergici pupillari in bambini cefalalgici e in bambini iperattivi. *IV Congr. Soc. It. Farmacol. Clin.*, Florence *(Abstr.)*.

2. Fanciullacci, M. (1979): Iris adrenergic impairment in idiopathic headache. *Headache,* 19:8–13.
3. Fanciullacci, M., Boccuni, M., and Ermini, P. (1979): Recettori morfinici nell'iride umana. *IV Congr. Soc. Ital. Farmacol. Clin.,* Florence, *(Abstr.).*
4. Fanciullacci, M., Boccuni, M., Pietrini, U., and Sicuteri, F. (1980): The naloxone conjunctival test in morphine addiction. *Eur. J. Pharmacol.,* 61:319–320.
5. Fanciullacci, M., Del Bianco, P. L., and Sicuteri, F. (1978): Iris and vein adrenoceptors in migraine and central panalgesia. In: *Recent Advances in the Pharmacology of Adrenoceptors,* edited by E. Szabadi, C. M. Bradshaw, and P. Bevan, pp. 295–303. Elsevier, Amsterdam.
6. Fanciullacci, M., Galli, P., Pietrini, U., and Sicuteri, F. (1977): Adrenergic supersensitivity of the pupil in idiopathic headache. *Experientia,* 33:1,082–1,083.
7. Gaglio, S., Marino, G., Morasso, P., and Tagliasco, V. (1978): Systems concepts in the on line control and processing of multiple ophthalmological tests. *Proc. Digital Equipment Computer Users Soc.,* 401–404.
8. Giordano, A., Sandini, G., and Marino, G. (1977): A microprocessor controlled device for dynamic measure of pupillary diameter. *4th Conference and Exhibition on Bioengineering,* pp. 151–153 Budapest.
9. Guidicelli, J. F., Richer, C., and Berdeaux, A. (1976): Preliminary assessment of flutiorex, a new anorectic drug in man. *Br. J. Clin. Pharmacol.,* 3:113–121.
10. Henderson, G., Hughes, J., and Kosterlitz, H. W. (1975): The effect of morphine on the release of noradrenaline from the cat isolated nictitating membrane and the guinea-pig ileum myenteric plexus-longitudinal muscle preparation. *Br. J. Pharmacol.,* 53:505–512.
11. Hughes, J., Kosterlitz, H. W., and Leslie, F. M. (1975): Effect of morphine on adrenergic transmission in the mouse vas deferens. Assessment of agonist and antagonist potiencies of narcotic analgesics. *Br. J. Pharmacol.,* 53:371–381.
12. Kramer, R., Rubick, M., and Turner, P. (1973): The role of fenfluramine in fenfluramine-induced mydriasis. *J. Pharm. Pharmacol.,* 25:575–576.
13. Kunkle, E. C., and Anderson, W. B. (1961): Significance of minor eye signs in headache of migraine type. *Arch. Ophthalmol.,* 65:504–508.
14. Llorens, C., Martres, M. P., Baudry, M., and Schwartz, J. C. (1978): Hypersensitivity to noradrenaline in cortex after chronic morphine: Relevance to tolerance and dependence. *Nature,* 274:603–605.
15. Mitchell, G. E. D., and Mottram, D. R. (1976): Peripheral effects of fenfluramine. *Br. J. Pharmacol.,* 57:185–189.
16. Mottram, D. R., and Washwam, D. (1977): The sympathomimetic activity of fenfluramine hydrochloride on rat vas deferens. *Br. J. Pharmacol.,* 59:615–620.
17. Nieman, E., and Hurwitz, L. J. (1961): Ocular sympathetic palsy in periodic migrainous neuralgia. *J. Neurol. Neurosurg. Psychiatry,* 24:369–373.
18. Riley, F. C., and Moyer, N. J. (1970): Experimental Horner's syndrome: A pupillographic evaluation of guanethidine-induced adrenergic blockage in humans. *Am. J. Ophthalmol.,* 69:442–447.
19. Sicuteri, F. (1978): Endorphines, opiate receptors and migraine. *Headache,* 17:253–257.
20. Sicuteri, F. (1979): Headache as the most common disease of the antinociceptive system: Analogies with morphine abstinence. In: *Advances in Pain Research and Therapy, Vol. 3,* edited by J. J. Bonica, pp. 359–365. Raven Press, New York.
21. Sicuteri, F., Anselmi, B., and Del Bianco, P. L. (1978): Systemic non organic central pain: A new syndrome with decentralization supersensitivity. *Headache,* 18:133–136.
22. Sicuteri, F., Del Bianco, P. L., and Fanciullacci, M. (1966): Variazioni di sensibilità alla 5-HT e alle catecolamine durante l'attacco emicranico. Test delle venocostrizione. *Boll. Soc. It. Biol. Sper.,* 42:843–844.
23. Sneddon, J. M., and Turner, P. (1966): The effect of local guanethidine on the palpebral fissure and the pupil in thyrotoxicosis and its interaction with sympathomimetic amines. *Proc. Br. Physiol. Soc.,* 189:20–22.
24. Szabadi, E., Besson, J., and Bradshaw, L. W. (1975): Pupil responsiveness to tyramine in depressed patients treated with amitriptyline. *Br. J. Clin. Pharmacol.,* 2:362–363.
25. Turner, P. (1975): The human pupil as a model for clinical pharmacological investigations. *J. R. Coll. Physicians Lond.,* 9:165–172.

Advances in Neurology, Vol. 33, edited by
M. Critchley et al. Raven Press, New York © 1982

Iatrogenic Headache: The Hazard of Diagnostic Investigations

Brunon L. Imielinski

Department of Neurosurgery, Garyounis University, Benghazi, Libya

Diagnostic investigations in neurological sciences present the necessary evil, being, in many cases, indispensable but nevertheless encumbered by a risk of complications. One of the most common is headache, frequently of persistent character.

Cerebrospinal fluid (CSF) examination is a routine procedure in neurological, neurosurgical, and psychiatric units. In patients not harboring a space-occupying lesion it often causes headache, which is due to intracranial hypotension (10). The occurrence of this complication depends on individual susceptibility to irresolution of intracranial hydrodynamic conditions including intracranial pressure. Lumbar puncture is a simple manipulation, but if the entry is difficult, it becomes traumatic and results in the tear in the dura and arachnoid. This is responsible for a CSF leak in the days to follow, which causes or exacerbates the hypotensive syndrome. Even after an easy entry, the hole in the meninges produced by an ordinary LP needle may become a channel for a slow but steady CSF escape. It may be observed (1), and I have seen this many times, during lumbar disk surgery preceded by LP or myelography. This type of occult CSF leak is responsible for pressure coning in the case of space-occupying lesions despite very limited CSF tap during lumbar puncture itself (4).

Headache after cistern puncture is much less frequent, because in the erect position the pressure of CSF in the cistern is ordinarily zero or less (9).

The problem in question is much more far reaching in cases of the introduction of a contrast media into subarachnoid space. The most common positive contrast medium in present use is still ethyl iodophenylundecylate (Myodil, Pantopaque), which is often employed in quantities of 6 ml or more. It is supposed to be absorbtive at a rate of 1 ml/year but in my series of 150 lumbar myelographies it was still present intrathecally up to 5 years (in about 3% of cases). In consequence of belief in its absorbing capacity, the practice varies as to desirability of removing as much of the dye as possible after the examination. And indeed, pooling it in the lumbar curve and aspirating under TV monitor through the needle left in situ for that purpose is a time-consuming maneuver and not always successful. Unremoved Myodil or Pantopaque eventually sinks to the lower end of the theca and for a variable time remains mobile, which makes it possible to use it in rescreening. In due course the dye becomes immobilized and loculated by leptomeningeal adhesions. Some quantity slowly percolates into the nerve root sheaths and spreads along the proximal parts of the nerves. Removal of this type of dye should be attempted in order to avoid or minimize the meningeal reaction. In some cases this seems to be of idiosyncratic character. When severe, it creates the clinical picture of acute meningitis, with cloudy CSF containing many thousands of leukocytes and sterile (9). Escape of the dye into the intracranial subarachnoid spaces may lead to a leptomeningeal fibrosis sufficient to cause obstructive hydrocephalus (8). A high iodine content has been found in the basal aspect of the medulla in these patients (3). In my series of 150 myelographies with the use of this contrast media, the remnants of dye dispersed in the cisterna magna were encountered up to 5 years with the clinical picture of persistent headache in five cases (6). In the series of Davies (2), approximately one-half of 119 investigated patients who underwent myodil myelography experienced reactions immediately or within a few hours; in 14 (12%) symptoms were present 1 year or more after the examination. These investigations suggest an incidence of complications that prove that Myodil and Pantopaque are not always inert.

The next step toward evolving more safe contrast medium has been made by synthesizing Dimer-X (tocarmic acid). However absortive in the course of few hours, it has a serious drawback, for it must be introduced exclusively below the level of the medullary conus. The danger of exceeding this level lies in the possibility of spinal cord irritation, including spinal cord epilepsy. Headache during following days and even weeks is another common after effect.

The best contrast medium available today is, beyond question, Amipaque (metrizamide). The principles of this dye were elaborated by Ludwiczak et al. in 1969 (7), and it is produced by Nygaard, Oslo. It is an aqueous molecular solution that does not dissociate into anions and cations. In concentration of 170 mg of iodine/ml it is isotonic to CSF. Easily penetrating the fluid spaces and increasing the contrast degree of the brain, it proved to be useful in CT scanning also (5). The most unfavorable complication is epileptic seizure, reported in 0.05% of examined patients (7). In my experience with 80 Amipaque myelographies this has never occurred. The absorption of the dye is completed within 3 hr, and headache, if it occurs, is only transient. Unlike Dimer-X, it can be introduced at any level, which is the other great advantage of Amipaque.

In summary, it should be emphasized that the ideal contrast medium has not yet evolved and that the investigation should not continue without good reason (9). For example myelography is not necessary as a routine in cases of prolapsed lumbar disk. Some moderation is also advised in establishing indications to lumbar punctures.

REFERENCES

1. Brown, B. A., and Jones, O. W. (1962): *J. Neurosurg.,* 19:349.
2. Davies, F. L. (1956): *Lancet,* 2:747.
3. Erickson, T. C., and Van Baaren, H. J. (1953): J.A.M.A., 153:636.
4. Gillingham, F. J. *(personal communication).*
5. Hindmarsch, T. (1975): *Acta Radiol. Diagn.,* 16:146.
6. Imieliński, B. L. (1979): *(in press).*
7. Ludwiczak, R., Dobrzyńska, L., Czechlowski, B., et al. (1979): Myelography and ventriculography by the use of the contrast medium Amipaque. In: *Surgical Management of the Hypophysis and Pituitary Fossa. Spontaneous Intracerebral Haematomas,* edited by B. L. Imielinski. Gdansk.
8. Mason, M. S., and Raaf, J. (1962): *J. Neurosurg.,* 19:302.
9. Northfield, D. W. C. (1973): *The Surgery of the Central Nervous System.* Blackwell, Oxford.
10. Pickering, G. W. (1948): *Brain,* 71:274.

Advances in Neurology, Vol. 33, edited by
M. Critchley et al. Raven Press, New York © 1982

The Epidemiology of Disabling Headache

M. Goldstein and T. C. Chen

National Institute of Neurological and Communicative Disorders and Stroke, National Institutes of Health, Bethesda, Maryland 20014

It is neither appropriate nor productive to describe the importance of disabling headache to the readers of this volume. The fact of the importance of this problem, as measured by either incidence, prevalence, or morbidity, is sufficient. This chapter addresses the issues of disabling headache—both migrainous and nonmigrainous, from the perspective of population data. We have reviewed a number of published works relating to epidemiological aspects of disabling headache and summarize our impression of the strengths and inadequacies of the published information about prevalence, the characteristics of the afflicted population, and the identification of risk factors that may be associated with the occurrence of the headache syndrome or its acute exacerbations.

Epidemiologists and clinical observers often deal with different populations. The epidemiologist is concerned most with the disease in a general population, whereas the clinical observer is inclined to conduct his studies on the basis of patients in his practice; there are usually more serious cases in the patient population. Finally, we suggest research approaches that can provide improved data for approaching the clinical issues of etiology, prevention, and therapy.

DEMOGRAPHIC CHARACTERISTICS

Like the classic fable of the blind men each describing their individual perceptions of an elephant, clinicians and population scientists have usually described accurately what they looked for but only in terms of their own, rather specialized frame of reference. The criteria for descriptions of demographic characteristics—age, sex, social status, family history—have been relatively consistent among clinical and population studies; however, the bias in the selection of the population being studied and the limited definition of the class of headache under study raise serious questions about the extrapolation of findings to the general population. Thus too often two capable observers present data whose conclusions are in direct conflict with each other. If we avoid expecting of the data specific information that they were not designed to provide, provocative trends do become evident. During the past two decades, a number of population-based studies have been completed and provide us with useful insights about both the occurrence of and risk factors associated with disabling headache or migraine. A summary of these trends follows.

Incidence

There are no accurate or even useful data available about the number of new cases of disabling headache in general population groups, irrespective of whether headache is looked at from the viewpoint of degree of morbidity, supposed pathophysiological mechanism, or etiology. Two epidemiological reports in the published literature do provide us with some data that can be used to estimate the annual rate of new cases of disabling headache. Based on the data of age of onset of disabling/severe headache (65), the annual incidence rate of new cases in a nonclinical population can be estimated to be 1.32%; based on the data reported from a study following up a group of nonheadache children aged 7 to 15 from 1957 to 1971 (10), the annual rate of new cases of migraine and nonmigrainous headache can be estimated to be 1.19%. The validity of these figures remains to be explored; taken as they are, however, they indicate that approximately 1% of the general population each year may become new sufferers of disabling headache, including migraine.

Prevalence

There have been a number of recent studies on the prevalence of headache in general populations in Europe and the United States. If we plot these data presented in Table 1 and examine the ranges and the averaged values, we find, as seen in Fig. 1, a high prevalence of headache per se in both the general and patient populations; in other words, it is relatively rare to find someone who does not report having headaches. Also, women are somewhat more at risk than men. In the more severe class of headache, however, the disparity in prevalence rates between men and women increases, with women reporting a much higher prevalence of "severe" and "very severe" headaches than men. We are probably looking at more than a single syndrome, with severe and very severe headaches having different pathophysiological characteristics than the more general category. Also, the severity of the headache rather than the supposed mechanism may be a more useful index for differentiating among syndromes.

Migraine is a class of disabling headache that has captured the attention of clinicians and epidemiologists for several decades. Tables 2A and 2B provide us with a summary of the more recent result in the literature. Figure 2 shows the prevalence of migraine in these populations. In both children and adults, there are differences in prevalence between males and females, with females clearly more at risk than males as adults as compared to children. Despite the differences in classification of migrainous headache in these various studies, we still must recognize that adults have a substantially greater probability of experiencing migrainous headaches than do children or older children; also, the relatively small differences in prevalence by sex in children become sizable in adult life.

It has been noted in many population studies that the prevalence of both headache and migrane in adult populations decreases after middle age. Table 3 and Fig. 3 present the relationship of the prevalence of migraine with age in each sex. These figures are compiled from a number of series of prevalence-age data in migraine taken from the published literature. In plotting these figures, the level of average prevalence of each series of data was ignored; only the trend with age is presented. Examination of these trend plots indicates that during early ages, the prevalence of migraine increases rapidly

TABLE 1. *Prevalence of headache, severe headache and very severe headache*

Authors	Population and age range	Headache Male %	Headache Female %	Severe headache Male %	Severe headache Female %	Very severe headache Male %	Very severe headache Female %
Newland et al., 1978 England	General, city 18 yr. and over	73.1	81.4	13.0	20.8	6.5	11.3
Nikiforow et al., 1978 Finland	General, rural and urban 15 yr. and over	57.6	73.1	16.7	22.0	7.1	15.6
Philips, 1977 England	General practice, urban 16–60 yr.	74.3	88.6	—	—	—	—
Clark and Waters, 1974 England	General practice, city 15–64 yr.	83.6	90.4	14.7	26.6	7.1	11.2
Waters, 1974 Wales	General, urban and rural 21 yr. and over	63.5	78.4	12.4	22.5	6.6	11.6
Mills and Waters, 1974 England	General, isles 15–64 yr.	70.8	84.4	9.8	24.3	4.4	9.3
Markush, et al., 1975 U.S.	General, women only 15–44 yr.	—	76.4	—	—	—	15.5
Duebner, 1977 Wales	General, school 10–20 yrs.	74.4	81.5	—	—	—	—

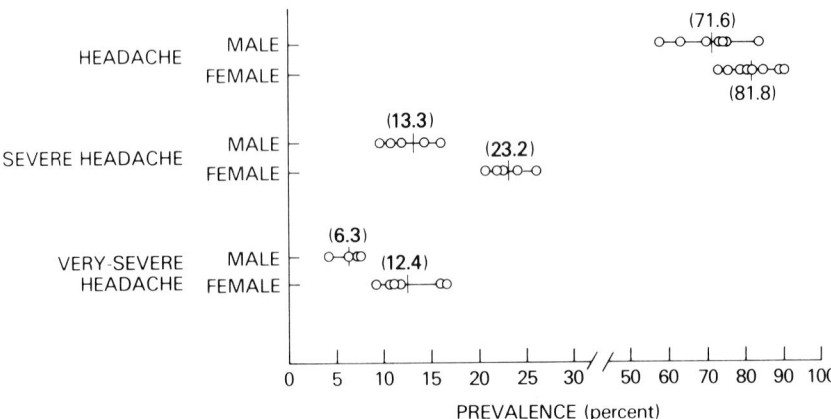

FIG. 1. Prevalence of headache, severe headache, and very severe headache. Numbers in parentheses indicate averaged values.

as age increases, reaches its peak at about ages 20 to 25, stays at the same level until about age 40, then declines steadily to a rather low prevalence in old age.

Disabling headache (exclusive of headache associated with brain tumors and stroke) and migraine become less prevalent at older ages. A number of hypotheses may explain this finding but remain to be tested. Sufferers of chronic disabling headache may die at an earlier age than do people who do not have headaches, thereby explaining the low prevalence with advanced age. This could be due to the morbid condition of the chronic headache sufferers, which may make them more vulnerable to attacks of other fatal diseases than the nonheadache population. Leviton et al. (31) reported that the risk for migraine sufferers dying before age 70 is 1.9 times higher than that of subjects without migraine. If this is generally true, we would expect that people in a general population who never had headache would be present more frequently in the older than in the younger age groups. The data of Ziegler et al. (65) support such a hypothesis.

In Table 4, the excess in percent of males or females aged 65 and over who never had a headache suggests that the lack of occurrence of headache may play a role in the probability of survival to older age. On the other hand, the low prevalence of migraine in the older ages can be interpreted partly by the hypothesis that some forms of migraine may be self-limiting, and certain groups of people become headache-free before reaching old age. In a study following up a small group of children and young adults with migraine during the period from 1957 to 1971, Bille (10) reported that 40% of the subjects became headache-free, and 32% showed improvement in the severity of headache; no such data are available from the adult population. If Bille's finding also applies to the adult population, then a certain portion of migrainous individuals in the general population could be expected to become headache-free with advancing age. In addition, since the onset of migraine is infrequent after middle age, fewer new cases would be added to the headache pool.

Finally, migrainous women tend to show striking decreases in migraine occurrence with menopause. It has been suggested that a hormonal factor may play a role in reducing the prevalence of migraine at older ages; however, factors other than hormonal changes occur concurrently with menopause in older age groups.

Again, headache is reported to be more prevalent in women than in men. The disparity

TABLE 2A. *Prevalence of migraine (adults)*

Authors	Population and age range	Definition (combination of symtptoms)	Migrainous headache Male %	Migrainous headache Female %
Newland et al., 1978 England	General, city 18 yr. and over	(1) + (2) + (3)	9.6	19.8
Clarke and Waters, 1974 England	General practice, city 15–65 yr.	(1) + (2) + (3)	7.1	15.3
Mills and Waters, 1974 England	General, islands 15–65 yr.	(1) + (2) + (3)	4.8	11.9
Green, 1977 England	General, working and school population	(1) + (6) + (2 or 3)	10.3	15.9
Markush et al., 1975 U.S.	General, women only 15–44 yr.	Any three or more of (1,2*,3,4)		9.0
Philips, 1977 England	General practice, urban 16–60 yr.	Any two or more of (1,2*,3)	9.2	17.1
Childs and Sweetham 1961, England	Factory employees Adults	(7) + (2) + (3)	4.9	13.2
Brewis et al., 1966 England	General, 15 yr. and over	(6) + (3) + absence from work or school	2.1	6.3
Dalsgaard-Nielsen, 1970 Denmark	General, school population 15–40 yr. and over	Doctors' interview and examination (prevalence values statistacally re-calculated)	8.4–11.2	9.5–18.8
Waters, 1974 Wales	General, urban and rural 21 yr. and over	Any combination of (1,2,3), prevalence values adjusted on clinical diagnosis	14.9	23.2
Dalsgaard-Nielsen, 1972 Denmark	Doctors 25–85 yr.	Doctors' own diagnosis	14.0	22.0
Waters, 1975 England	General practitioners 21–74 yr.	Doctors' diagnosis	13.3	25.4

(1) Unilateral pain; (2) preheadache warning; (2*) Major visual aura; (3) nausea/vomit; (4) throbbing pain; (5) positive family history; (6) repeated headache with pain-free intervals; (7) severe headache; (8) attack released by sleep.

TABLE 2B. *Prevalence of migrain (children)*

Authors	Population and age range	Definition (combination of symptoms)	Migranous headache Male %	Migranous headache Female %
Billie, 1962 Sweden	School children 7–15 yr.	(6) + any two or more of (1,2*,3,5)	3.4	4.5
Duebner, 1977 Wales	School children 10–15 yr.	(1) + (2) + (3)	3.3	5.2
Sillanpää, 1976	School children 7 yr.	(6) + any two or more of (1,2*,3,5)		3.2
Sparks, 1978	School children 10–18 yr.	(1) + (2*) + (3) + (5) + (8)	3.4	2.5
Brewis et al., 1966 England	General 5–15 yr.	(6) + (3) + absence from school or work	2.0	2.3
Dalsgaard-Nielsen 1972, Denmark	School children 7–15 yr.	Doctor's interview and examination (prevalence values statistically recalculated)	3.1–7.3	2.8–7.7
Ekbom et al., 1978 Sweden	Nonclinical, men only 18 yr.	(6) + any two or more of (1,2*,3,5)	1.7	

(1) Unilateral pain; (2) preheadache warning; (2*) major visual aura; (3) nausea/vomit; (4) throbbing pain; (5) positive family history; (6) repeated headache with pain-free intervals; (7) Severe headache; (8) Attack release by sleep.

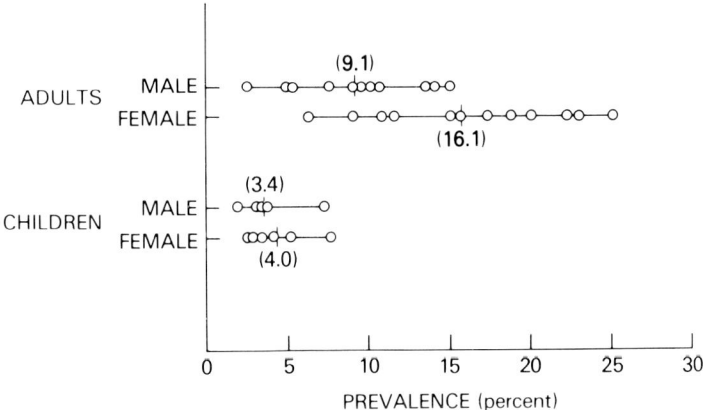

FIG. 2. Prevalence of migraine. Numbers in parentheses indicate averaged values.

in relative frequency of headache in the ratio female/male (F/M) increases as the severity class of the headache increases. Dalsgaard-Nielsen (18) and Bille (8) have indicated that the prevalence of migraine in boys and girls before puberty is about the same; as children approach adolescence and young adulthood, however, the prevalence in girls increases more rapidly than in boys. Figure 4 represents the trend of the sex ratio in prevalence of headache, in very severe headache, and in migraine with age, based on several series of prevalence data taken in the literature. Two phenomena deserve comment: (a) there is no apparent trend of a sex ratio for the prevalence of either headache in general or severe headache with age in the adult population; (b) the trend of the sex ratio for prevalence of migraine when it is relatively broadly defined (14,18,57) and represented in the lower curves appears to be less or not apparent with age. For some strictly defined migraine (12,46) represented in the two upper curves, the sex ratio demonstrates an increasing trend toward middle age and a decreasing trend after middle age. The interpretation of this phenomenon is unclear. It may be that, as compared with other age groups, middle-aged women seek a physician's advice or report their severe migrainous headache more often than do men of the same age. Whether this increased representation in women with age is valid or not is unknown.

A number of other demographic factors have been explored in relation to disabling headache. In general, there is no meaningful association between disabling headache and either educational background, intelligence, socioeconomic class, or marital status. Individual differences have been reported in these factors in limited studies, but the results are confounded by problems of definition and population selection. If these factors are important, more adequately designed protocols will need to be utilized to demonstrate any significance. One study of headache concerning a potential relationship with marital status (39) raises some interesting questions. In four marital status groups, undefined headache was most common in divorced men and married women and least common in both widows and widowers; conclusions remain to be drawn.

Many other factors have been investigated in limited retrospective studies of special segments of the population; the findings have generally been inconclusive. However, a few factors deserve consideration and comment.

TABLE 3. *Prevalence of migraine with age*

Authors		Prevalence (%)						
Waters, 1974 Wales	Age (yr)	21–34	35–54	55–64	65–75			
	Male	16.8	16.4	12.6	4.9			
	Female	30.1	26.0	16.6	10.3			
Clarke and Waters, 1974 England	Age (yr)	15–20	21–34	35–54	55–64			
Brewis et al., 1966 England	Age (yr.)	5–15	16–25	26–35	36–45	46–55	56–65	66+
	Male	2.0	2.2	2.9	1.9	1.9	2.0	0.6
	Female	2.3	6.0	7.0	8.1	6.0	5.4	4.0
Morbidity statistics[a], second national study, 1979 England and Wales	Age (yr.)	1–4	5–14	15–24	25–44	45–64	65–74	75+
	Male	0.3	4.7	7.0	6.8	4.3	2.6	1.0
	Female	—	4.7	13.0	18.9	13.8	4.5	1.3
Dalsgaard-Nielsen, 1970 Denmark	Age (yr.)	7–9	10–13	14–17	18–21	22–30	31–40	40+
	Male	3.1	4.5–6.0	7.3–8.4	9.4–10.0	10.6–11.0	11.2	
	Female	2.8	4.3–6.0	7.7–9.5	11.2–12.8	14.7–16.7	18.0–18.5	18.8

[a] Prevalence values are expressed by per thousand.

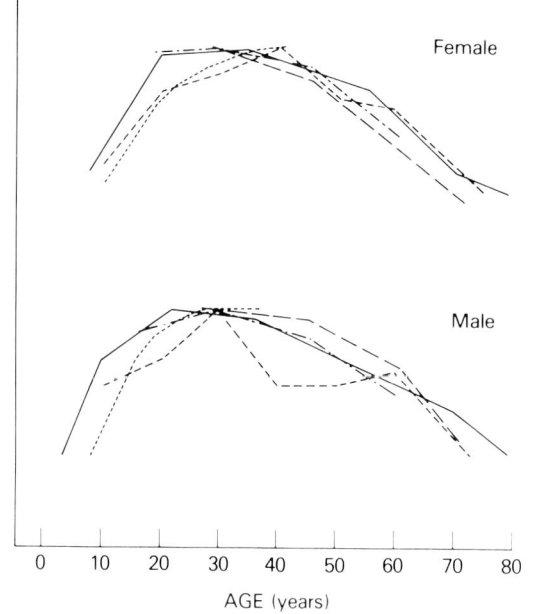

FIG. 3. Trend of prevalence of migraine with age.

FAMILY HISTORY

The issue of regarding migraine as a familial or genetic disorder continues to be controversial. A number of investigators, clinical and epidemiological, report findings of positive family history in migraine patients; other epidemiological studies, however, do not provide supportive evidence (33,56,64). A study by Ziegler et al. (64) involving a nonclinic twin population found the overall frequency of concordance of disabling or severe headache to be of no significant difference between monozygotic and dizygotic same sex twins. Lucas (33) reported similar findings in a study of migraine with a larger twin population, although the concordance rate for migraine in the monozygotic twins is significantly higher overall than that of dizygotic twins. The controversy about familial factors remains unsolved; but to put the present evidence in perspective, migraine might be considered a heterogeneous condition with some still-unidentified inherited predisposing factors that require interaction with the environment to produce a recognizable clinical syndrome (64,66).

TABLE 4. *Percent of people with life history of* absence of headaches

Age (yr)	Male		Female	
	Total No.	No headache %	Total No.	No headache %
15–24	46	8.7	94	4.2
25–39	145	8.3	404	3.0
40–54	153	9.8	320	7.5
55–64	80	15.0	190	19.5
65+	77	57.1	300	43.3

From ref. 65, with permission.

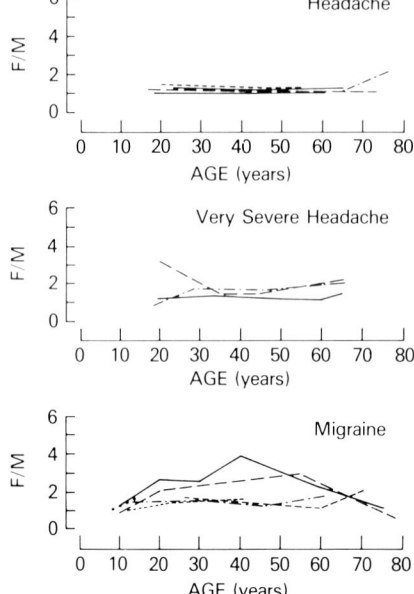

FIG. 4. Trend of sex ratio (F/M) in prevalence of headache, very severe headache, or migraine.

PSYCHOLOGICAL AND HORMONAL FACTORS

A number of studies indicate that persons with severe headache of any variety have histories of greater psychological stress, tension, and/or depression than those in non-headache populations. The interpretation of the association of headaches with stress, however, requires caution. Which is cause and which is effect? Are both related to a factor common to both headache and to psychological problems? Rees (44) reminds us that nothing specific in the life situation or environmental circumstances is directly associated with migraine. The important factor is the role of the patient's personality in dealing with life circumstances and his particular life situation.

A word about *menarche, menstruation,* and *contraception.* Although a number of studies suggest that severe headache and migraine are associated with hormonal factors in the female, well-designed, controlled studies are notable by their absence. The results from existing evaluations are not consistent. Failure to demonstrate a general relationship between headache or migraine with menarcheal status is particularly evident in recent studies in school children by Duebner (23), Moss and Waters (37), and Small and Waters (50). Also in adult women, menstrual disorders are not more evident in migraine subjects than in nonmigraine patients (17,34,39). Phillips (43), however, found that migraine was generally worse when the patient was on oral contraceptives and that the headache often assumed a cyclic pattern with occurrence most frequent between courses of medication. This provocative report should be evaluated in large-scaled studies.

OTHER RISK FACTORS

A number of reports claim that changes in weather conditions and that extremes of severity of weather can be precipitating factors for severe headaches of either the migrainous or nonmigrainous variety in a small portion of people with headache; temperature extremes, barometric changes, status of humidity, glare, and wind factor have all been implicated separately and in combination. Wilkinson and Woodrow (63) suggest that these factors may operate by means of a "stress response" rather than directly by themselves.

Any discussion of risk factors associated with severe headache would be incomplete without mentioning factors such as smoking, hypertension, and the common diseases generally considered to be related or contributory. The published literature on the association between smoking and severe headache is sparse and demands focused attention in well-designed studies. There are many excellent reasons to advise patients to stop smoking, but the data on smoking and headache clearly cannot be cited as one of them. The best that can be said at this time is that a few investigations indicate that there may be interesting connections between smoking and the onset of a severe headache, but the findings are not more than suggestive.

The data on the relationship between hypertension—diastolic or systolic, or both— and migraine headache depends on which authors are quoted. Some report that migrainous patients have a higher incidence of hypertension than does the general population; others report the contrary. Also, with the exception of situations in which there is a life-threatening rapid rise in diastolic pressure, there is little evidence that control of elevated blood pressure reduces the occurrence of severe headache. Perhaps recent national and international programs directed against hypertension will provide an opportunity to evaluate the results of hypertension control on the occurrence of severe headache; we point out that specific information about headache is rarely incorporated into protocols monitoring the results of these community programs.

In many clinical and pathophysiological classifications, the migraine syndrome is considered a cerebrovascular disorder and defined as a focal cerebral dysfunction commonly attributed to focal cerebral ischemia attributable to vasoconstriction. The relationship of either a history or the occurrence of migraine to subsequent cerebral infarction or hemorrhage remains to be demonstrated. Neither do we have reliable information about the effect on frequency of migraine headache of either having had a stroke or the removal of stroke risk factors. Headache per se is often reported as one of the presenting symptoms of stroke; since both stroke and migraine have many symptoms in common, a true relationship may exist. There is clearly a need to initiate carefully categorized, well-designed studies to explore these relationships.

A comment on *epilepsy.* No reliable evidence exists that there is any meaningful relationship between migraine and epilepsy. Also, a number of authors find that the often-stated relationship between migraine headache and allergy is considerably overrated.

Table 5 summarizes the factors associated with disabling headache; it is not specific to migraine headache.

CONCLUSION

This chapter emphasizes that severe headache, both migrainous and nonmigrainous, is an important health problem, yet we know little about it. In the past, a lack of definition and classification plagued comparisons of data and confused communications. However, because of the efforts of leaders in this area of medicine and research—many of whom are contributors to this volume—we should now be able to get on with the

TABLE 5. *Factors associated with headache*

Factor	Association with headache[a]
Demographic	
Age	+
Sex	+
Education	−
Intelligence	−
Social class	−
Marital status	−
Psychological	
Stress	+
Tension, anxiety, depression	+
Personality	(+)?
Familial and genetic	(+)?
Hormonal	
Menarche	(+)?
Menstruation	(+)?
Oral contraceptives	?
Seasonal and weather	(+)?
Smoking	−
Dietary	
Food	(+)?
Alcohol	(+)?
Tyramine	(+)?
Other diseases	
Hypertension	(+)?
Cerebrovascular diseases	(+)?
Epilepsy, multiple sclerosis	−
Asthma	−
Hayfever	−
Death at an earlier age	?

[a]+, significant association; − no apparent association; ?, association uncertain; (+)?, association in certain subgroup(s) of patients which needs to be identified.

job of defining and evaluating the several factors at play. In order to assist us, we urge the Neurosciences Program of the World Health Organization to establish an international classification of headache so that we can all use the same criteria in our studies and reports. Parallel to this, national or large-scale community surveys must be designed to collect a broad spectrum of data and needed information. This should include measuring the occurrence of both disabling and migraine headache in general populations and assessing the potential risk factors against appropriate controls in homogeneous subgroups. Also, several provocative leads about potential risk factors are associated with severe headache. Most have resulted from retrospective and case series evaluations. We now require prospective studies of both general populations and of suspected high risk groups in order to evaluate their respective roles in the occurrence of headache.

The prevalence of severe and disabling headache is high enough to make well-designed community studies of risk factors operationally and economically feasible. The issue is: Are the data to be obtained about disabling headache of enough significance to receive priority attention from scientists and research funding organizations?

REFERENCES

1. Andrasik, F., Holroyd, K. A., and Abell, T. (1979): Prevalence of headache within a college student population. A preliminary analysis. *Headache,* 19:384–387.
2. Appenzeller, O. (1972): Altitude headache. *Headache,* 12:126–129.
3. Bakal, D. A., and Kaganov, J. A. (1979): Symptom characteristics of chronic and non-chronic headache sufferers. *Headache,* 19:285–289.
4. Barlow, C. F. (1978): Migraine in childhood. *Res. Clin. Stud. Headache,* 5:34–36.
5. Barolin, G. S. (1966): Migraines and epilepsies—a relationship? *Epilepsia,* 7:53–66.
6. Barolin, G. S. (1970): Psychology and neuropsychology in migraine. *Res. Clin. Stud. Headache,* 3:126–153.
7. Basser, L. S. (1969): The relation of migraine and epilepsy. *Brain,* 92:285–300.
8. Bille, B. (1962): Migraine in school children. *Acta Pediatr. [Suppl. 136],* 51:1–151.
9. Bille, B. (1975): Epidemiology of migraine in children. *Dan. Med. Bull.,* 22:107–108.
10. Bille, B. (1975): The prognosis of migraine in childhood. *Dan. Med. Bull.,* 22:112.
11. Boisen, E. (1975): Stroke in migraine: Report on seven strokes associated with severe migraine attacks. *Dan. Med. Bull.,* 22:100–106.
12. Brewis, M., Poskanzer, D. C., Rolland, C., and Miller, H. (1966): Neurological disease in a English city. *Acta Neurol. Scand. [Suppl. 24],* 42:1–89.
13. Childs, A. J., and Sweetnam, M. T. (1961): A study of 104 cases in migraine. *Br. J. Indust. Med.,* 18:234–236.
14. Clarke, G. J. R., and Waters, W. E. (1974): Headache and migraine in a London general practice. In: *The Epidemiology of Migraine,* edited by W. E. Waters, pp. 23–34. Boehringer, Ingelheim, Bracknell-Berkshire.
15. Cohen, M. J. (1978): Psychophysiological studies of headache: Is there similarity between migraine and muscle contraction headache? *Headache,* 18:189–196.
16. Couch, J. R., Ziegler, D., and Hassanein, R. S. (1975): Evaluation of the relationship between migraine headache and depression. *Headache,* 15:41–50.
17. Crisp, A. H., Kalucy, R. S., McGuinness, B., Ralph, P. C., and Harris, G. (1977): Some clinical, social and psychological characteristics of migraine subjects in the general population. *Postgrad. Med. J.,* 53:691–697.
18. Dalsgaard-Nielsen, T. (1970): Some aspects of the epidemiology of migraine in Denmark. *Headache,* 10:14–23.
19. Dalsgaard-Nielsen, T., and Ulrich, J. (1972): Prevalence and heredity of migraine and migranoid headaches among 461 Danish doctors. *Headache,* 12:168–172.
20. Dalton, K. (1975): Food intake prior to a migraine attack—study of 2,313 spontaneous attacks. *Headache,* 15:188–193.
21. Daniels, L. E. (1965): Hypertension and vascular incidents during bouts of migraine. *Postgrad. Med.,* 38:381–391.
22. Douglas, R. M. (1964): Hypertension and headache. A survey of 231 treated hypertensive patients. *N.Z. Med. J.,* 63:70–76.
23. Duebner, D. C. (1977): An epidemiologic study of migraine and headache in 10–20 year olds. *Headache,* 17:173–180.
24. Edmeads, J. (1979): The headache of ischemic cerebrovascular disease. *Headache,* 19:345–349.
25. Ekbom, J., Ahlborg, B., and Schéle, R. (1978): Prevalence of migraine and cluster headache in Swedish men of 18. *Headache,* 18:9–19.
26. Friedman, A. P. (1976): The epidemiology of migraine. *Hemicrania,* 7:2–4.
27. Grant, E. C. (1979): Food allergies and migraine. *Lancet,* 1(8123):966–969.
28. Green, J. E. (1977): A survey of migraine in England, 1975–1976. *Headache,* 17:67–68.
29. Kugler, J., and Laub, M. (1978): Headache determination by meterotropic influences. *Res. Clin. Stud. Headache,* 6:117–122.
30. Lance, J. W., and Anthony, M. (1966): Some clinical aspects of migraine. A prospective survey of 500 patients. *Arch. Neurol.,* 15:356–361.
31. Leviton, A., Malvea, B., and Graham, J. R. (1974): Vascular diseases, mortality, and migraine in the parents of migraine patients. *Neurology,* 24:669–672.
32. Leviton, A. (1978): Epidemiology of headache. *Adv. Neurol.,* 19:341–351.
33. Lucas, R. N. (1977): Migraine in twins. *J. Psychosom. Res.,* 21:147–156.
34. Markush, R. E., Karp, H. R., Heyman, A., and O'Fallon, W. M. (1975): Epidemiological study of migraine symptoms in young women. *Neurology,* 25:430–435.
35. Monzoni, G. C., Terzano, M. G., and Mancia, D. (1979): Possible interference between migrainous and epileptic mechanisms in intercolated attacks, case report. *Eur. Neurol.,* 18(2):124–20.
36. Mills, C. H., and Waters, W. E. (1974): Headache and migraine on the isles of Scilly. In: *The Epidemiology of Migraine,* edited by W. E. Waters, pp. 23–34. Boehringer, Ingelheim, Bracknell-Berkshire.

37. Moss, G., and Waters, W. E. (1974): Headache and migraine in a girls' grammar school. In: *The Epidemiology of Migraine,* edited by W. E. Waters, pp. 49–58, Boehringer Ingelheim, Bracknell-Berkshire.

38. Newland, C. A., Illis, L. S., Robinson, P. K., Batchelor, B. G., and Waters, W. E. (1978): A survey of headache in an English city. *Res. Clin. Stud. Headache,* 5:1–20.

39. Nikiforow, R., and Hokkanen, E. (1978): An epidemiological study of headache in an urban and a rural population in Northern Finland. *Headache,* 8:137–145.

40. Nikiforow, R., and Hokkanen, E. (1979): Effect of headache on working ability: A survey of an urban and a rural population in Northern Finland. *Headache,* 19:214–218.

41. Ninch, B. (1970): Migraine and epilepsy. *Eur. Neurol.,* 3:168–178.

42. Philips, C. (1977): Headache in general practice. *Headache,* 16:322–329.

43. Phillips, B. M. (1971): Migraine and the pills. In: *Background to Migraine, 4th Migraine Symposium,* edited by J. N. Cumings, pp. 55–61. Springer-Verlag, New York.

44. Rees, W. L. (1971): Psychiatric and psychological aspects of migraine. In: *Background in Migraine, 4th Migraine Symposium,* edited by J. N. Cumings, pp. 45–53. Springer-Verlag, New York.

45. Rees, W. L. (1974): Personality and psychodynamic mechanism in migraine. *Psychother. Psychosom.,* 23:111–122.

46. Royal College of General Practitioners (1979): *Morbidity Statistics from General Practice 1971–1972, Second National Study.* Studies on Medical and Population Subjects No. 36. Her Majesty's Stationery Office, London.

47. Ruskin, N. (1978): Headache associated with organic diseases of the nervous system. *Med. Clin. North. Am.,* 62:459–466.

48. Schéle, R., Ahlborg, B., and Ekbom, K. (1978): Physical characteristics and allergic history in young men with migraine and other headaches. *Headache,* 18:80–86.

49. Sillanpää, M. (1976): Prevalence of migraine and other headache in Finnish children starting school. *Headache,* 15:288–290.

50. Small, P., and Waters, W. E. (1974): Headache and migraine in a comprehensive school. In: *The Epidemiology of Migraine,* edited by W. E. Waters, pp. 59–67. Boehringer Ingelheim, Bracknell-Bershire.

51. Somerville, B. M. (1972): A study of migraine in pregnancy. *Neurology (Minneap.),* 22:355–365.

52. Spark, J. P. (1978): The incidence of migraine in school children. A survey by the medical officers of school association. *Practitioner,* 221(1323):407–411.

53. Traub, Y. M., and Korczyn, A. D. (1978): Headache in patients with hypertension. *Headache,* 17:245–247.

54. Vijayan, N., Gould, S., and Watson, G. (1980): Exposure to sun and precipitation of migraine. *Headache,* 20:42–43.

55. Volans, G. N., and Castleden, C. M. (1976): The relationship between smoking and migraine. *Postgrad. Med. J.,* 52:80–82.

56. Waters, W. E. (1971): Migraine, intelligence, social class and familial prevalence. *Br. Med. J.,* ii:77–81.

57. Waters, W. E. (1974): The Pontypridd headache survey. *Headache,* 14:81–90.

58. Waters, W. E. (1975): Review of the epidemiology of migraine in adults. *Dan. Med. Bull.,* 22:86–88.

59. Waters, W. E. (1975): Epidemiological data relevant to prognosis in migraine in adults. *Dan. Med. Bull.,* 22:89–91.

60. Waters, W. E. (1975): Migraine in general practitioners. *Br. J. Prev. Soc. Med.,* 29:48–52.

61. Waters, W. E., and O'Connor, P. J. (1975): Prevalence of migraine. *J. Neurol. Neurosurg. Psychiatry,* 38:613–616.

62. Watkins, S. M., and Espir, M. (1969): Migraine and multiple sclerosis. *J. Neurol. Neurosurg. Psychiatry,* 32:35–37.

63. Wilkinson, M., and Woodrow, J. (1979): Migraine and weather. *Headache,* 19:375–378.

64. Ziegler, D. K., Hassanein, R. S., Harris, D., and Stewart, R. (1975): Headache in a non-clinic twin population. *Headache,* 14:213–218.

65. Ziegler, D. K., Hassanein, R. S., and Couch, J. R. (1977): Characteristics of life headache histories in a non-clinic population. *Neurology,* 27:265–269.

66. Ziegler, D. K. (1978): The epidemiology and genetics of migraine. *Res. Clin. Stud. Headache,* 5:21–33.

Advances in Neurology, Vol. 33, edited by
M. Critchley et al. Raven Press, New York © 1982

Monoamine Sensitivity of Smooth Muscle *In Vivo* in Nociception Disorders

P. L. Del Bianco, G. Franchi, B. Anselmi, and F. Sicuteri

Department of Clinical Pharmacology, University of Florence, Florence, Italy

The phenomena preceding or accompanying a migraine attack are considered to be of primary importance in the pathogenesis of the pain (2,11,14). Our group has been working on a new theory concerning the pathogenesis of headache, which hypothesizes a central neurochemical mechanism (21,22). The latest findings on the role of endorphins in the neuromodulation of certain central and peripheral functions support this hypothesis. The research that has demonstrated a close correlation between endorphins and the monoaminergic system is particularly stimulating. The isolated myenteric plexus/longitudinal muscle preparation from morphine-tolerant/dependent guinea pigs exhibits *in vitro* a normal sensitivity to serotonin (5-HT) and prostaglandin E, if kept in the presence of morphine; this sensitivity increases when morphine is removed or naloxone is added. Moreover, a strong jumping reaction is induced by intraventricular administration of monoamines in morphine-tolerant/dependent rats after naloxone but not in rats prewithdrawal (16,18).

These variations in sensitivity could be due to a receptor modification, or more likely, to changes in the effector cells (cyclic nucleotides), which are stimulated by receptor activation (13). These results demonstrate that morphine dependance/tolerance induces a neuronal supersensitivity revealed by morphine withdrawal. In animals, moreover, morphine inhibits norepinehprine (NE) release from the adrenergic terminal of the nictitating membrane and of the vas deferens (12,15). These findings support the hypothesis whereby normal endorphin activity is necessary for normal neuronal sensitivity to monoamine neurotransmitters (13).

Some years ago, an increased sensitivity to 5-HT and NE of the vein smooth muscle in migraine patients was demonstrated during the painful attack. This phenomenon was ascribed to a local deficiency of specific monoaminergic mediators (10,29). An increased sensitivity to phenylephrine and to aceclidine (cholinergic agonist) in migraineous patients was also observed at the level of the neuroirideal junction (5). In migraine patients, moreover, we detected (a) an increased sensitivity of certain brain areas to specific monoamines or correlated drugs, (b) an increased emetic effect of apomorphine, (c) an important orthostatic hypotension due to bromocriptine and ergotamine (dopaminergic agonists), (d) elementary or even structured hallucinations from nonhallucinogenic doses of LSD-25 or psylocibin, and (e) headache from fenfluramine (which induces a fall in the 5-HT and NE turnover). These findings reveal an enhanced reactivity of the peripheral and central monoamine receptors in migraine (6,8,9,26).

The therapeutic action of the ergot derivatives in migraine, if administered acutely (in the case of ergotamine) or chronically (methysergide, lisuride), is well known. This action depends on the capacity of these drugs to act, when given in low doses, as partial agonists to 5-HT, which is probably deficient during a migraine attack (3,19). Migraine, therefore, is a syndrome in which spontaneous phenomena of supersensitivity to monoamines and correlated drugs at central and peripheral levels are detectable. These considerations have suggested further investigation and experimental comparisons between the migraine attack and the morphine abstinence crisis. Both syndromes have phenomena and certain experimental findings in common (24,28).

The endorphin theory of headache suggests a failure of the endorphinergic system, due to a deficiency in brain enkephalin turnover, putatively associated to an opiate receptor dysfunction during the migraine attack (24).

COMPUTERIZED VENOTEST FINDINGS

Some functional aspects of the neurovascular junction in man can be investigated by using the computerized venotest (4,30). This technique quantifies the venospastic activity of some monoamines, such as 5-HT, NE, and dopamine (DA) and of their liberators, e.g., tyramine (TY). Increased monoamine venospastic activity during a migraine attack reaches its peak at the end of the crisis and reverts to normal in the pain-free period; 5-HT supersensitivity was more evident than that to NE and epinephrine (Fig. 1).

Spontaneous supersensitivity (in a few cases of impressive extent) to monoamines (5-HT, NE, DA, TY) was detected in central panalgesia, a syndrome characterized by systemic pains, psychic irritability, sensory hyperesthesia, and vegetative disorders (23). It occurs sometimes as a complication of serious and long-term headaches. In 50% of these patients, a chronic supersensitivity is notable; this is similar and sometimes even stronger than the supersensitivity detected at the end of a migraine attack (27).

An experimental situation, mimicking central panalgesia, can be induced in some headache sufferers (but not in normal subjects) by means of 5-HT deprivation. In fact parachlorophenylalanine (PCPA), a powerful and selective inhibitor of 5-HT synthesis, provokes a state of panalgesia reversible (after discontinuation of PCPA treatment) in 50% of the tested headache sufferers, which is indistinguishable from the spontaneous disorder. During the painful periods, these patients exhibit a vein supersensitivity to 5-HT only (20,25).

Using the computerized venotest, the effective pharmacological activity of ergot derivatives was definitely identified. These drugs are widely used in headache treatment with the conviction that they act only because of their antiserotonin and/or, in the case of ergotamine, vasospastic properties. These drugs are 5-HT antagonists when given in high doses; when given in low doses, they are partial agonists of the venospastic activity of 5-HT (7). It is interesting to note that the 5-HT agonist doses are roughly comparable with the levels of the drug circulating in the blood after the usual therapeutic administrations. Both ergotamine and lisuride, in minimal doses, act as partial 5-HT agonists (Figs. 2 and 3).

Exposure to opiates (see above) is accompanied by the development of increased latent neuronal monoamine supersensitivity, i.e., the kind of supersensitivity that is revealed by morphine withdrawal or by naloxone. Clinical analogies between a migraine attack and the morphine abstinence syndrome have suggested that the same kind of monoamine

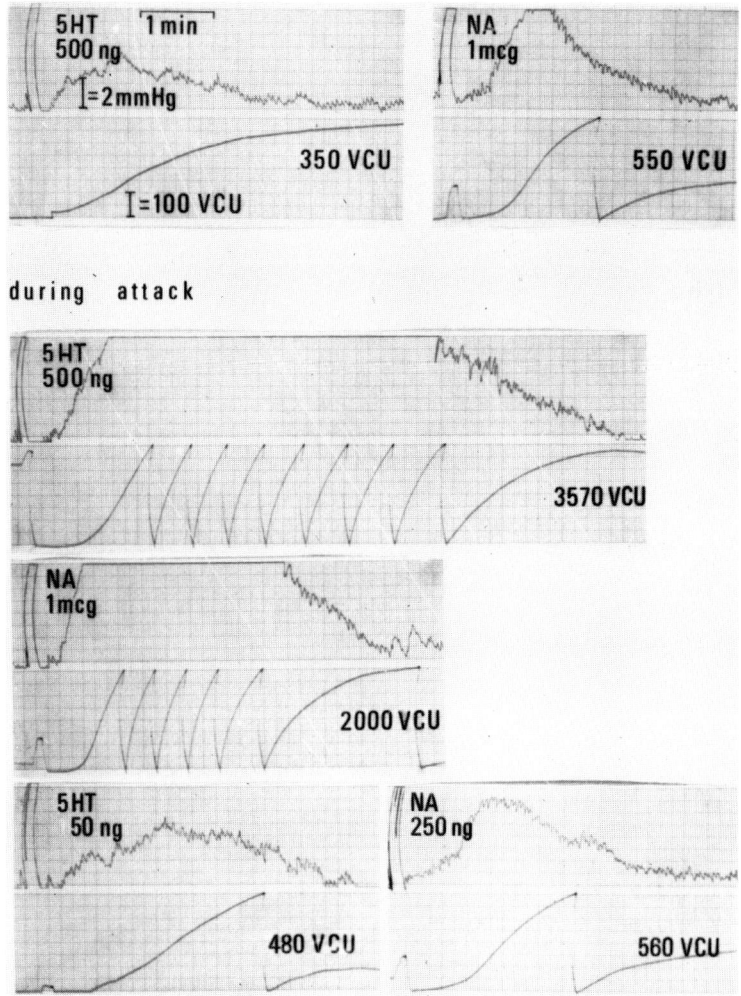

FIG. 1. In migraine patients during the pain-free period, 500 ng of 5-HT and 1 μg of NE (NA) are needed to achieve a threshold venospastic effect **(top)**. The same dose of 5-HT and NE during an attack provokes a high venospastic response, about 10 and 5 times higher, respectively, than those obtained in pain-free periods **(middle)**. During the attack, threshold effects are induced with doses 10 times lower in the case of 5-HT and 5 times lower in the case of NE **(bottom)**.

supersensitivity found in addicts during morphine abstinence might be encountered in headache patients during a migraine attack.

Volunteer headache patients were submitted to short and light morphine treatment (20 mg/day for 3 days); in all subjects, a venous supersensitivity to 5-HT and DA (but not to NE and TY) was observed in computerized venotests 12 hr after the last dose of morphine (in the absence of clinical symptoms of opiate abstinence). The computerized venotest was also carried out on six heroin addicts who had been hospitalized to undergo the naloxone test and the successive methadone treatment. These patients

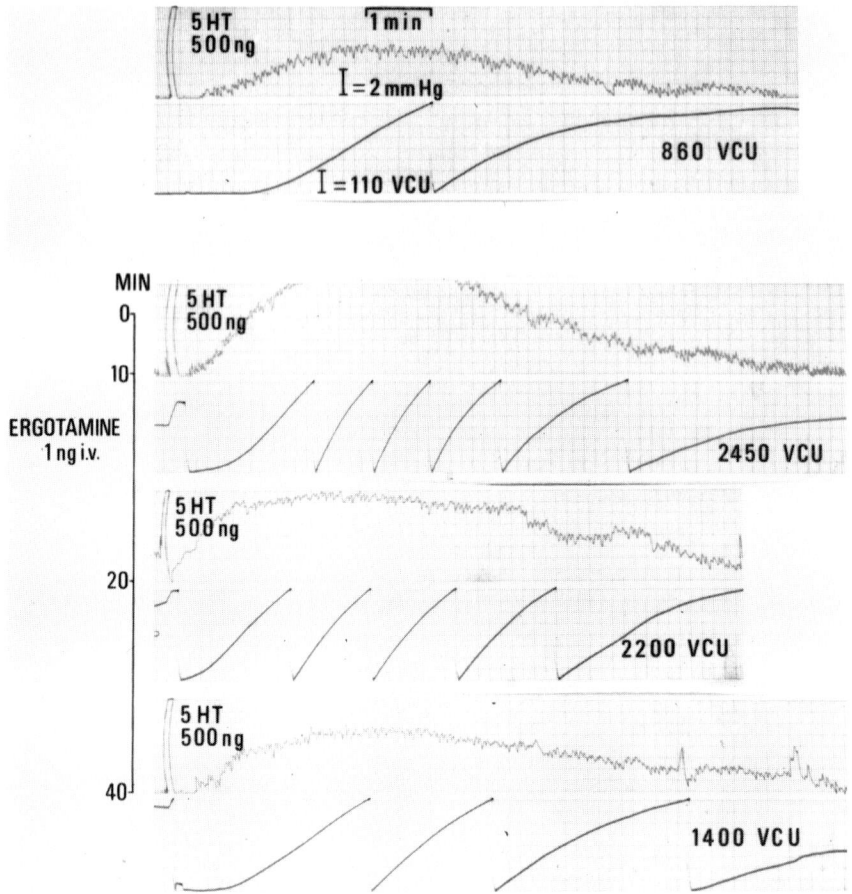

FIG. 2. Ergotamine tartrate in a very low dose (1 ng) induces an increase of 5-HT starting 10 min after administration and lasting about 20 to 30 min.

were tested 8 to 12 hr after their last dose of heroin, when the clinical signs of abstinence had not yet appeared or were very slight, and after naloxone administration (0.4 mg i.v.). During the same period, three central panalgesia, pentazocine-dependent patients (due to severity of the painful phenomena) were also under observation. In these patients, the computerized venotest was carried out 12 hr after the last dose of pentazocine and after naloxone (0.4 mg) locally administered into the same vein used for the test. In both heroin and pentazocine addicts, the computerized venotest revealed a supersensitivity (dramatic in a few cases: up to 1.000 times the normal rate) to 5-HT and DA even before naloxone administration and when the clinical signs of abstinence were still undetectable. The degree of supersensitivity varied from patient to patient, but the local administration of naloxone further enhanced the venous reactivity to 5-HT and DA. Normal venous sensitivity was observed in these patients to NE and TY. On the other hand, morphine (10 μg) injected into the same vein used for the test inhibited the venospastic activity of 5-HT and DA and the clinical signs of abstinence when present (Fig. 4).

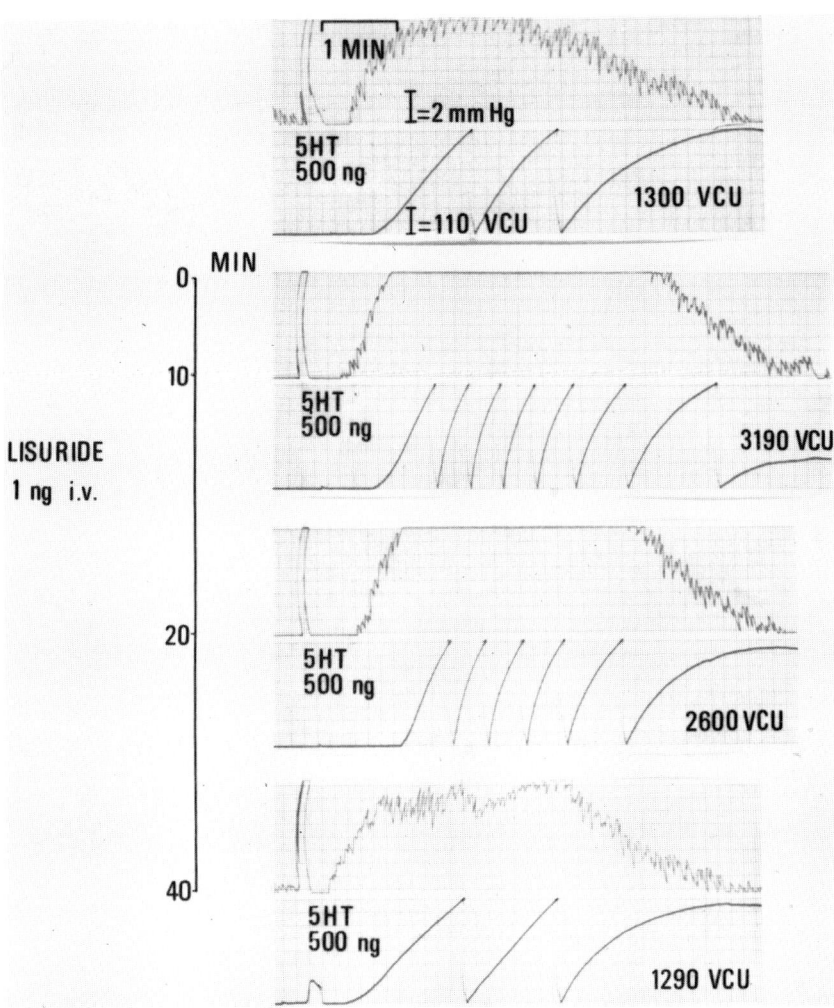

FIG. 3. Lisuride in low doses (1 ng) induces a potentiation of 5-HT venospasm starting 10 min after administration and lasting about 10 to 20 min.

COMMENT

The results can be summarized as follows: (a) At the end of a migraine attack, there is a supersensitivity in the neuromuscular junction of the human vein. (b) There are probably opiate receptors in the human vein capable of modifying the reactivity of the smooth muscle of the vessel to monoamines. (c) During chronic morphine or pentazocine treatment, supersensitivity of the smooth muscle of the human vein to monoamines (5-HT and DA) is detectable. This supersensitivity is revealed by naloxone and inhibited by morphine. (d) Vein supersensitivity precedes the clinical phenomena of abstinence and could be used as a diagnostic tool for the detection of drug addiction. (e) Supersensitivity to 5-HT and DA, as well as to NE, is present in migraine and in central spontaneous or pharmacologically induced panalgesia and might be related to a defect in the natural opiate mechanisms. (f) Ergot derivatives are confirmed as partial 5-HT

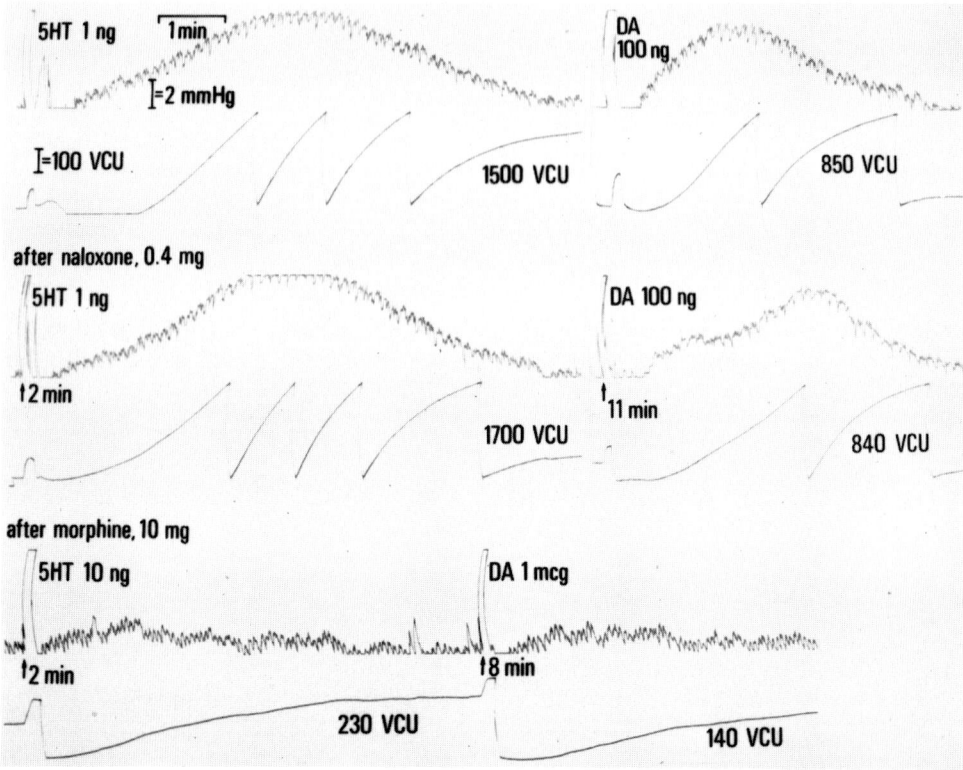

FIG. 4. Computerized venotest on a 21-year-old male morphine addict 8 hrs after the last morphine administration. A slight dose of 5-HT (1 ng) and DA (100 ng) induces a high increase of venous pressure **(top).** In this case, naloxone does not provoke any significant change **(middle).** After 10 μg morphine, a dose of 5-HT and DA 10 times higher is required to induce a mild venospastic response **(bottom).**

agonists. In very low doses, they significantly potentiate the venospastic activity of 5-HT. This result supports the hypothesis according to which these drugs also act at a central level on 5-HT-deficient neurons.

The most significant result of these studies is the confirmed existence of a monoamine supersensitivity in morphine addicts; this supersensitivity is closer to that of panalgesia patients than to that of migraine sufferers. It remains to be determined whether there are any correlations between the supersensitivity to monoamines observed in migraine subjects and addicts, as well as between the clinical picture of migraine and that of the abstinence syndrome. Migraine and addict supersensitivity phenomena differ in regard to degree of intensity, specificity, and time of appearance. NE supersensitivity is undetectable in addicts; 5-HT supersensitivity in migraineurs is lower than in addicts and appears only during the final stages of the painful attack.

A systemic cerebral and extracerebral fall in the endorphinergic activity at the beginning of the migraine attack promotes a prolonged leakage (because of incontinence due to poor opioid modulation) of the monoamines into the synaptic cleft and thus a depletion of the neuronal monoamines with consequent supersensitivity due to mediator deficiency. This could explain the delayed appearance of supersensitivity during a migraine attack, the venous monoamine sensitivity of migraine patients being normal during the pain-free periods.

This peripheral behavior is in accord with that of the endogenous opioids in the cerebrospinal fluid, which are at a normal level in the pain-free periods and fall during the migraine attack.

In addicts, the supersensitivity is constantly present but is unmasked by naloxone as well as by morphine withdrawal. In a situation of chronically reduced endorphin levels, as in the case of central panalgesia, venous supersensitivity to monoamines is constant and high. A monoamine supersensitivity, therefore, is revealed in the venous smooth muscle in man in two completely opposite conditions: in the chronic excess of exogenous opioids and in the chronic lack of endogenous opiates. The supersensitivity of the migraine attack putatively follows the fluctuating trend of the endorphinergic and monoaminergic systems that characterizes this syndrome.

SUMMARY

A significant degree of supersensitivity to 5-HT and DA was detected when carrying out the computerized venotest on migraine patients during an attack. A similar supersensitivity was observed during morphine abstinence and naloxone-precipitated withdrawal in addicts. Mild abstinence after slight and short morphine treatment provoked monoamine supersensitivity in volunteers. In these conditions, the administration of morphine inhibited the 5-HT and DA supersensitivity. In spontaneous central panalgesia, monoamine supersensitivity is detectable, as well as in panalgesia induced in headache sufferers by means of PCPA 5-HT deprivation. By means of the venotest, the ergot derivatives were confirmed as being partial 5-HT agonists. These drugs can also carry out their therapeutic activity by potentiating 5-HT at a central level in 5-HT-deficient neurons. The presence of opiate receptors in the human vein is stressed. The high supersensitivity of the venous smooth muscle to 5-HT and DA both in headache and systemic pain sufferers and during morphine withdrawal suggests a pathophysiological analogy between these conditions.

REFERENCES

1. Anselmi, B., Baldi, E., Casacci, F., and Salmon, S. (1980): Endogenous opioids in CSF and blood in idiopathic headache sufferers. *Headache*, 20:294–299.
2. Appenzeller, O. (1979): Headache: Clinical and pathogenetic aspect. *Advances in Pain Research and Therapy, Vol. 3*, edited by J. J. Donica et al, pp. 345–358. Raven Press, New York.
3. Curran, D. A., Hinterberger, H., and Lance, J. W. (1969): Methysergide. In: *Research and Clinical Studies in Headache*, edited by A. P. Friedman, pp. 74–122. Karger, Basel.
4. Del Bianco, P. L., and Sicuteri, F. (1978): Computerized venospasm: A method for exploring the neurovascular junction in man. *J. Pharmacol. Meth.*, 1:329–340.
5. Fanciullacci, M. (1978): Iris adrenergic impairment in idiopathic headache. *Headache*, 19:8–13.
6. Fanciullacci, M., Franchi, G., and Sicuteri, F. (1971): Amine biogene, cefalee essenziali ed allucinogeni (dietilamide dell'acido lisergico e psilocibina). *Atti 3° Congr. Naz. Soc. Ital. di Medicina Psicosomatica*, pp. 78–86.
7. Fanciullacci, M., Franchi, G., and Sicuteri, F. (1976): Ergotamine and methysergide as serotonin partial agonists in migraine. *Headache*, 16:226–231.
8. Fanciullacci, M., Michelacci, S., Curradi, C., and Sicuteri, F. (1980): Hyperresponsiveness of migraine patients to the hypotensive action of bromocriptine. *Headache*, 20:99–102.
9. Franchi, G. (1979): On the circulatory collapse from ergotamine during migraine attacks: A clinical pharmacological contribution. *Proceedings of the Fourth Meeting of the Italian Headache Society*, edited by F. Savoldi and G. Nappi, pp. 240–244, Fidia Research Laboratories, Abano Terme (Padova).

10. Franchi, G., Anselmi, B., and Michelacci, S. (1972): Change in serotonin and catecholamine vascular reactivity during migraine attack. In: *Research and Clinical Studies in Headache,* edited by A. P. Friedman, pp. 304–310. Karger, Basel.

11. Greppi, E., and Sicuteri, F. (1964): L'emicrania, motivi di fisiopatogenesi e terapia. In: *Relaz. 65° Congr. Soc. Ital. Medicina Internazionale,* edited by E. Greppi and F. Sicuteri, pp. 1–199. L. Pozzi, Rome.

12. Henderson, G. J., and Kosterlitz, H. W. (1975): The effect of morphine on the release of noradrenaline from the cat isolated nictitating membrane and the guinea-pig ileum myenteric plexus, longitudinal muscle preparation. *Br. J. Pharmacol.,* 53:505–509.

13. Herz, A., and Schulz, R. (1981): Neuronal supersensitivity during morphine withdrawal. *This volume.*

14. Heyck, H. (1969): Pathogenesis of migraine. *Research and Clinical Studies in Headache, Vol. 2,* edited by A. P. Friedman, pp. 1–28. Karger, Basel.

15. Hughes, J., Kosterlitz, H. W., and Leslie, F. M. (1975): Effect of morphine on adrenergic transmission in the mouse vas deferens. Assessment of agonist and antagonist potencies of narcotic analgesic. *Br. J. Pharmacol.,* 53:271–278.

16. Schultz, R., and Goldstein, A. (1973): Morphine tolerance and supersensitivity to 5-hydroxytryptamine in the myenteric plexus of the guinea-pig. *Nature,* 244:168–170.

17. Schultz, R., and Herz, A. (1976): Aspects of opiate dependence in the myenteric plexus of the guinea-pig. *Life Sci.,* 19:117–128.

18. Schulz, R., and Herz, A. (1977): Naloxone-precipitated withdrawal reveals sensitization neurotransmitters in morphine tolerant/dependent rats. *Naunyn Schmiederbergs Arch. Pharmacol.,* 299:95–99.

19. Sicuteri, F. (1959): Prophylactic and therapeutic properties of UML 491 in migraine. *Int. Arch. Allergy,* 15:300–307.

20. Sicuteri, F. (1971): Pain syndrome in man with p-chlorophenylalanine. *Pharmacol. Res. Commun.,* 3:401–407.

21. Sicuteri, F. (1976): Headache: Disruption of pain modulation. In: *Advances in Pain Research and Therapy, Vol. 1,* edited by J. J. Bonica and D. Albe-Fessard, pp. 881–885. Raven Press, New York.

22. Sicuteri, F. (1976): Headache as methonymy of non organic central pain. *Headache New Vistas,* edited by F. Sicuteri, pp. 19–67. Biochemical Press, Florence.

23. Sicuteri, F. (1978): Systemic non organic central pain (SNOCP): A new syndrome characterized by impressive 5-HT supersensitivity. *2nd World Congr. on Pain, Montreal,* August 27–September 1, p. 117 (abstr).

24. Sicuteri, F. (1979): Headache as the most common disease of the antinociceptive system: Analogies with morphine abstinence. In: *Advances in Pain Research and Therapy, Vol 3,* edited by J. J. Bonica and D. Albe-Fessard, pp. 359–365. Raven Press, New York.

25. Sicuteri, F., Anselmi, B., and Del Bianco, P. L. (1973): 5-Hydroxytryptamine, supersensitivity as a new theory of headache and central pain: A clinical pharmacological approach with p-chlorophenylalanine. *Psychopharmacology (Berlin),* 29:347–356.

26. Sicuteri, F., Anselmi, B., and Del Bianco, P. L. (1976): Fenfluramine headache. *Headache,* 16:185–188.

27. Sicuteri, F., Anselmi, B., and Del Bianco, P. L. (1978): Systemic non organic central pain: A new syndrome with decentralization supersensitivity. *Headache,* 18:133–136.

28. Sicuteri, F., Del Bianco, P. L., and Anselmi, B. (1979): Morphine abstinence and serotonin supersensitivity in man: Analogies with the mechanism of migraine? *Psychopharmacology (Berlin),* 65:205–209.

29. Sicuteri, F., Del Bianco, P. L., and Fanciullacci, M. (1966): Variazioni di sensibilità alla 5-HT ed alle catecolamine durante l'attacco emicranico: test della venocostrizione. *Boll. Soc. Ital. Biol. Sper.,* 42:843–844.

30. Sicuteri, F., Del Bianco, P. L., Fanciullacci, M., and Franchi, G. (1964): Il test della venocostrizione per la misura della sensibilità alla 5-idrossitriptamina e alle catecolamine nell'uomo. *Boll. Soc. Ital. Biol. Sper.,* 40:1,148.

Advances in Neurology, Vol. 33, edited by
M. Critchley et al. Raven Press, New York © 1982

Headache Induced by Freezing External Carotid Artery Branches

V. A. Fasano, G. Broggi, G. Lo Russo, and S. Zeme

Institute of Neurosurgery, University of Turin, Turin, Italy

In a previous work (1), we examined the effects of transitory cooling lasting 30 sec at a temperature varying from 0 to 10°C on the vessel walls of several branches of the external carotid artery (meedle superficial temporal and occipital arteries) and of cooling and freezing of the maxillary artery and its branches and of the mucosa surrounding the ganglion pterygopalatinum behind the inferior posterior wall of the sinus sphenoideus.

Temporary cooling of the meedle superficial temporal artery sometimes provokes pain in the temporal or frontal regions. In cases of cooling of the occipital artery, pain spread throughout the nucal region and along the free edge of the trapezium. More complete results were obtained by cooling the maxillary and sphenopalatina arteries.

Pain in these cases was evoked in the medial and posterior regions of the orbit, in the temporal and frontal regions, as was a homolateral nasal and lachrymal secretion accompanied by nausea. After a pain-free interval from 6 to 12 hr, the patient complained of a deep, intense pain, continuous in the same region. A temporary disappearance of pain was later seen.

These observations on cryosurgery for headache suggest some considerations for a physiopathological basis for the mechanism and distribution of pain: the external carotid artery and its branches (a) are mainly responsible for these types of headache; and (b) must be considered together and thus respond to stimuli.

REFERENCE

1. Fasano, V. A. (1976): Diagnostic researches and treatment with cryoprobe of non-migraine or trigeminal facial pain. *Min. Med.,* 67:1,845–1,849.

Advances in Neurology, Vol. 33, edited by
M. Critchley et al. Raven Press, New York © 1982

Hemicrania and Lateralized Cervicoscapular Muscular Hypertonicity

Jacques Boquet, Nicholas Moore, and Francis Boismare

Department of Pharmacology, Hôtel Dieu, Rouen, France

Systematic clinical examination of the cervical muscles in migraineurs led us to suspect a hypertonicity of these muscles, confirming the conclusions of Wolff (8) and Vaughan et al. (6). Since the hypertonicity was asymmetrical, we performed a bilateral electromyogram (EMG) recording to establish a possible correlation between the side of the muscular hypertonicity and the pain. Furthermore, an electrical examination in the second interosseous space of the hand was performed in order to demonstrate spasmophilia.

METHOD

Twenty male (3) or female (17) patients between 20 and 65 years of age were examined. Among these patients, 12 were suffering from common hemicrania; eight also presented with ophthalmic symptoms. In every patient, the side of the pain was noted and an EMG recording performed on the left and right trapezius muscles. This was always performed during a pain-free period, spontaneously after hyperventilation or during neck rotations, standing or in the recumbent position. Correlation between the side of the pain and the side of the muscular hypertonicity was analyzed by a chi square test on 17 subjects; three subjects suffering from bilateral muscular hypertonicity were excluded. An EMG was performed on the interosseous space of the hand to look for signs of spasmophilia.

RESULTS

Of the eight right-sided patients, five showed a cervical spine on the right side; of the nine left-sided patients, two cervical spines were seen. Clinical results showed eight right, nine left, and two either left or right sided hemicrania; in 17 of the 20 patients, we found a pain or a muscular tenderness of the trapezius muscles upon digital pressure on the same side as the headache. A spontaneous asymmetry (during the relaxed position) of the trapezius EMG recording was observed, with an increase of the activity on the same side as the pain in 50% of the patients.

During hyperventilation (Fig. 1) while standing or during rotational movements of the neck (Fig. 2) modifying the length of the cervical muscles, the correlation between the side of the pain and the hypertonic muscular side was 85% (Fig. 3) (Chi square, 16.99; $p < 0.001$). Finally, tetany symptoms were found in 80% of our subjects.

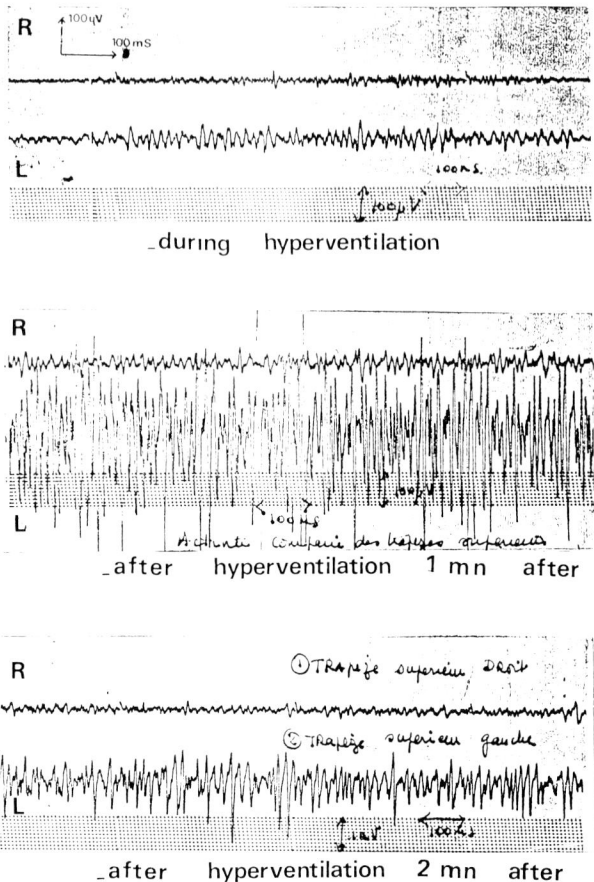

_during   hyperventilation

_after   hyperventilation   1 mn   after

_after   hyperventilation   2 mn   after

FIG. 1. Left hemicrania. Trapezius EMG recording shows an asymmetry increased by hyperventilation and remaining 2 min. after hyperventilation.

DISCUSSION

These data show the correlation between hemicrania and cervical muscular hypertonicity. A high degree of correlation exists between the side of the pain and the side of an increased tone of the cervical muscles, mainly in stimulating conditions (hyperventilation or active movements). Lateralized hypertonicity could be explained by an increased excitability in the cervical muscular proprioceptors and/or by a modification of the postural tonus of extrapyramidal origin, and/or by a modification of the fusorial system, perhaps mediated via the autonomic system (Fig. 4). The first two hypotheses are justified by the fact that stretching or tilting determines a lateralized (clinical and myographic) hyperactivity in the trapezius muscles on the painful side. The localization of the hypertonicity at the cervical level may be due to the high density of fusorial spindles in these muscles (1,5,7).

A modification of sympathetic activity in migraine sufferers has been established by Fanciulacci et al. (2), who have shown a postsynaptic hypersensitivity of the alpha-adrenergic receptors in the pupil. The same authors found, as did we, a correlation

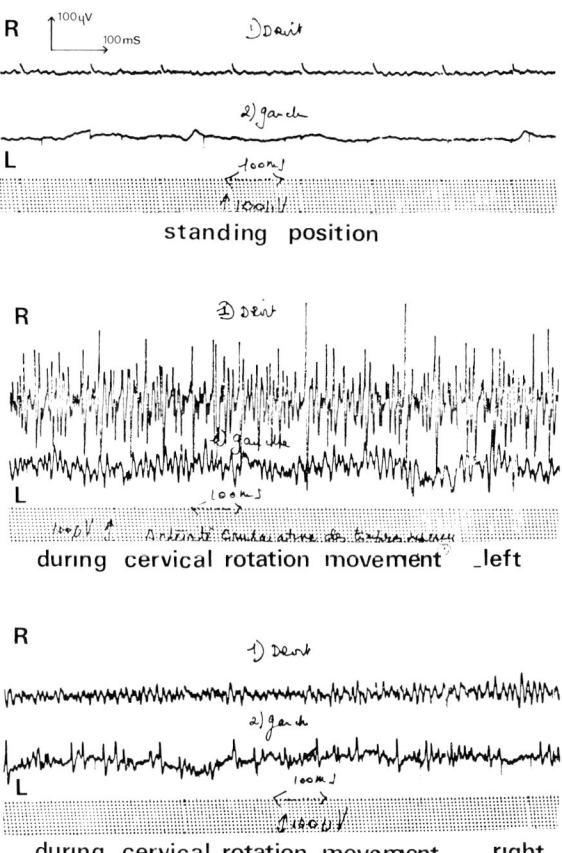

FIG. 2. Right hemicrania. Trapezius EMG recording is initially symmetrical (a) and becomes asymmetrical after cervical rotation to the left (b) but not the right (c).

n:19	MIGRAINE		
	side of the pain	L.side	R.side
CERVICAL HYPERTONICITY (EMG)	L.side	9	0
	R.side	0	8
	R + L side	1	1
	$\chi^2 = 16{,}99$	$P < 0{,}001$	

FIG. 3. Correlation between the side of the headache and the side of the trapezius muscle hypertonicity (n = number of patients).

HEMICRANIA

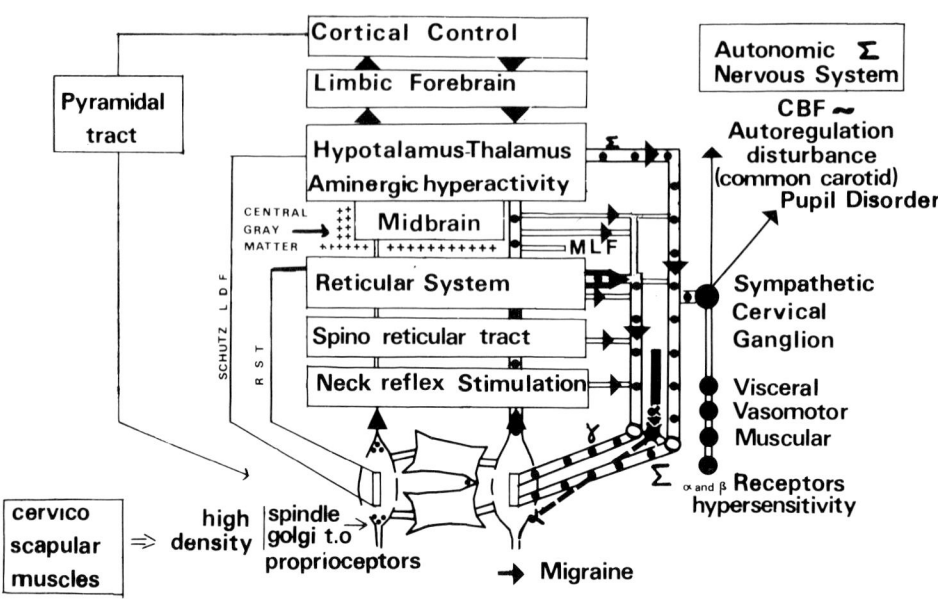

FIG. 4. Comparative pathophysiologic scheme showing the pathways conveying the nociceptive impulses during hemicrania and, on the left side, the increase of the sympathetic and gamma activity. SCHUTZ LDF, schutz fascicle (sympathetic pathway from the thalamohypothalamic system); RST, reticulospinal tract (descending gamma pathway from the reticular system); CBF, cerebral blood flow; ϵ; sympathetic system; γ; gamma system; golgi t.o., golgi tendon organ.

between the side of the iris muscle hypersensitivity and the side of the pain. It is known that the sympathetic system enhances the cervical muscular tone (3); thus it may be hypothesized that migraine sufferers are characterized by a lateralized adrenergic hypersensitivity capable of increasing the alpha mydriatic reaction (2), the muscular hypertonicity, and the reactivity of the brain vessels. It is not yet possible to establish whether the sympathetic and muscular disturbances have a common high origin (thalamolimbo hypothalamic) (4) or if there is an involvement phenomenon, since lower connections between the gamma system (reticulospinal tract) and the sympathetic system are possible (3). Furthermore, the facilitating role of the tetania, mainly during hyperventilation, should be explored.

SUMMARY

Clinical and EMG examination of the trapezius muscles in hemicrania showed a high degree of correlation (chi square, 16.99) between the side of the pain and the side of hemicrania. Muscular and/or sympathetic disturbances may be involved. This notion, which evokes the possibility of a lateralized disturbance of the sympathetic system, needs further study, mainly during pain periods, before it can be strictly established.

REFERENCES

1. Cooper, S., and Daniel, P. M. (1963): Muscle spindles in man, their morphology in the lumbricals and the deep muscles of the neck. *Brain,* 86:563–594.
2. Fanciulacci, M., Del Bianco, P. L., and Sicuteri, F. (1978): Iris and vein adrenoceptors in migraine and central panalgesia. In: *Recent Advances in the Pharmacology of Adrenoceptors,* edited by E. Szabadi, C. M. Bradshaw, and P. Bevan, pp. 295–303. Elsevier, New York.
3. Hinoki, M., and Niki, H. (1975): Neurotological studies on the role of the sympathetic nervous system in the formation of traumatic vertigo of cervical origin. *Acta Otolaryngol.,* 330:185–196.
4. Hinoki, M., Nakanishi, K., Ito, S., Ushio, N., and Ichibangase, T. (1978): "Neurotic vertigo" from the standpoint of neurotology. *Agressologie,* 19(4):269–286.
5. Richmond, F. J. R., and Abrahams, V. C. (1975): Morphology and distribution of muscle spindles in dorsal muscles of the cat neck. *J. Neurophysiol.,* 38:1,322–1,339.
6. Vaughan, R., Pall, M. L., and Haynes, S. N. (1977): Frontalis EMG response to stress in subjects with frequent muscle-contraction headaches. *Headache,* 16:313–318.
7. Voss, H. (1958): Zahl und Anordnung der Muskel spindeln in den unteren Zungenbeinmuskeln dem M. sternocleidomastoideus und den Bauch-und tiefen Nackenmuskeln. *Anat. Anz.,* 105:265–275.
8. Wolff, H. G. (1963): *Headache and Other Head Pain,* second edition. Oxford University Press, New York.

Subject Index